W9-CCI-612

7th edition

MEDICAL TERMINOLOGY

A WORD • BUILDING APPROACH

JANE RICE, RN, CMA-C

Medical Assisting Program Director, Retired
Georgia Northwestern Technical College
Rome, Georgia

Pearson

Boston   Columbus   Indianapolis   New York   San Francisco   Upper Saddle River
Amsterdam   Cape Town   Dubai   London   Madrid   Milan   Munich   Paris   Montreal   Toronto
Delhi   Mexico City   Sao Paulo   Sydney   Hong Kong   Seoul   Singapore   Taipei   Tokyo

Library of Congress Cataloging-in-Publication Data
Cataloging-in-Publication data on file with the Library of Congress.

Notice: The author and the publisher of this volume have taken care that the information and technical recommendations contained herein are based on research and expert consultation, and are accurate and compatible with the standards generally accepted at the time of publication. Nevertheless, as new information becomes available, changes in clinical and technical practices become necessary. The reader is advised to carefully consult manufacturers' instructions and information material for all supplies and equipment before use, and to consult with a healthcare professional as necessary. This advice is especially important when using new supplies or equipment for clinical purposes. The author and publisher disclaim all responsibility for any liability, loss, injury, or damage incurred as a consequence, directly or indirectly, of the use and application of any of the contents of this volume.

Publisher: Julie Levin Alexander
Publisher's Assistant: Regina Bruno
Editor-in-Chief: Mark Cohen
Development Editors: Lynda Hatch, Dynamic WordWorks
Associate Editor: Melissa Kerian
Assistant Editor: Nicole Ragonese
Editorial Assistant: Rosalie Hawley
Director of Marketing: David Gesell
Executive Marketing Manager: Katrin Beacom
Marketing Specialist: Michael Sirinides
Managing Production Editor: Patrick Walsh

Production Liaison: Christina Zingone
Production Editor: Patty Donovan, Laserwords Maine
Senior Media Editor: Amy Peltier
Media Project Manager: Lorena Cerisano/Julita Navarro
Manufacturing Manager: Alan Fischer
Art Director: Kristine Carney
Interior Designer: Lisa Delgado
Composition: Laserwords Maine
Printing and Binding: R.R. Donnelley/Roanoke
Cover Printer: Lehigh-Phoenix Color/Hagerstown

PEARSON

www.pearsonhighered.com

10 9 8 7 6 5 4 3 2 1
ISBN-13: 978-0-13-214802-3
ISBN-10: 0-13-214802-1

In special memory of
my parents,
Warren Galileo and
Elizabeth Styles Justice,
and my sister,
Betty Sue Nelson.

Contents in Brief

Preface

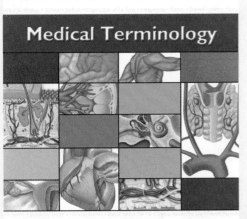

7th Edition

Medical Terminology

A Word-Building Approach

Jane Rice

This text has helped thousands of students over the years in successfully mastering the challenging yet exciting terminology of medicine. Its trademarks are twofold:

1. **A word-building approach.** A logical, simple system for learning medical vocabulary by building from word parts such as prefixes, suffixes, roots, and combining vowels.
2. **Accurate and complete coverage of human anatomy.** Concise coverage of all major body structures and functions, organized by system.

The 7th edition builds upon this framework and presents an exciting blend of fresh ideas merged with proven methods.

NEW TO THIS EDITION

Here is a summary of the key enhancements of the 7th edition:

- New tables of combining forms with meanings appear at the start of all body systems chapters. This makes it easier and faster for students to learn the foundations of key terms pertaining to each system.
- Visually updated "Building Your Medical Vocabulary" sections now include embedded photographs and color-coded word parts. This makes it easier for students to understand the meanings of terms and how they are assembled.
- Pink words in the "Building Your Medical Vocabulary" section of previous editions – denoting terms not built from word parts – have been changed to black for greater clarity.
- Consolidated, streamlined, and refined discussions of physiology throughout.
- An anatomy labeling activity has been added within each body system chapter. This reinforces the content and provides an opportunity for active learning.
- Coverage of obstetrics is now integrated within the Female Reproductive System chapter, rather than being set off as a separate chapter.
- "Life Span Considerations" features are now interspersed appropriately throughout each chapter wherever relevant, rather than being presented as a free-standing section.
- The "Pathology Checkpoint" section from previous editions has been eliminated.
- "FYI" features provide interesting medical tidbits to broaden knowledge and pique interest.
- The end-of-chapter "Practical Application" exercise has been expanded to include a variety of medical records, in addition to the SOAP feature from previous editions. These offer interaction with real-world medical terminology usage.

FEATURES AT A GLANCE

Here is a sneak peak at what makes *Medical Terminology: A Word Building Approach* so dynamic and trusted as a learning resource.

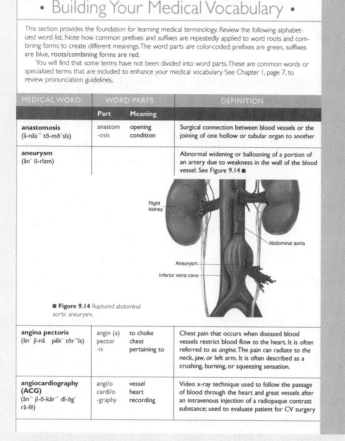

• Building Your Medical Vocabulary •

This section provides the foundation for learning medical terminology. Review the following alphabet-ized word list. Note how common prefixes and suffixes are repeatedly applied to word roots and com-bining forms to create different meanings. The word parts are color-coded: prefixes are green, suffixes are blue, roots/combining forms are red.

You will find that some terms have not been divided into word parts. These are common words or specialized terms that are included to enhance your medical vocabulary. See Chapter 1, page 7, to review pronunciation guidelines.

MEDICAL WORD	WORD PARTS		DEFINITION
	Part	Meaning	
anastomosis (ă-năs˝ tō-mō´sĭs)	anastom -osis	opening condition	Surgical connection between blood vessels or the joining of one hollow or tubular organ to another
aneurysm (ăn´ ū-rĭzm)			Abnormal widening or ballooning of a portion of an artery due to weakness in the wall of the blood vessel. See Figure 9.14 ■

Right kidney
Abdominal aorta
Aneurysm
Inferior vena cava

■ **Figure 9.14** Ruptured abdominal aortic aneurysm.

angina pectoris (ăn´ jĭ-nă pĕk´ tŏr˝ĭs)	angin (a) pector -is	to choke chest pertaining to	Chest pain that occurs when diseased blood vessels restrict blood flow to the heart. It is often referred to as *angina*. The pain can radiate to the neck, jaw, or left arm. It is often described as a crushing, burning, or squeezing sensation.
angiocardiography (ACG) (ăn˝ jĭ-ō-kăr´ dĭ-ŏg´ ră-fē)	angi/o cardi/o -graphy	vessel heart recording	Video x-ray technique used to follow the passage of blood through the heart and great vessels after an intravenous injection of a radiopaque contrast substance; used to evaluate patient for CV surgery

• **Building Your Medical Vocabulary** — This section is the heart of every chapter. It is an alphabet-ized word list that shows how word parts are built, pronounced, and defined.

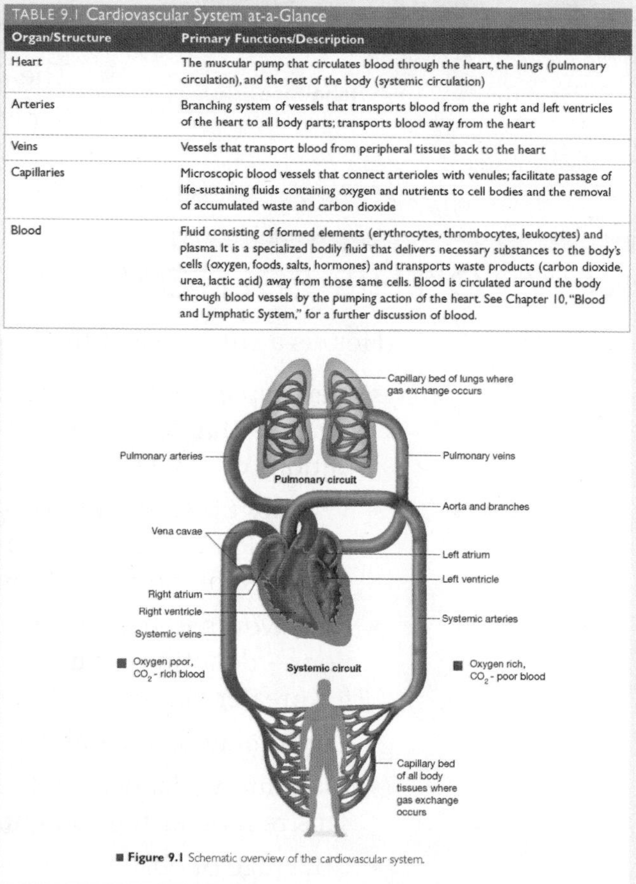

TABLE 9.1 Cardiovascular System at-a-Glance	
Organ/Structure	Primary Functions/Description
Heart	The muscular pump that circulates blood through the heart, the lungs (pulmonary circulation), and the rest of the body (systemic circulation)
Arteries	Branching system of vessels that transports blood from the right and left ventricles of the heart to all body parts; transports blood away from the heart
Veins	Vessels that transport blood from peripheral tissues back to the heart
Capillaries	Microscopic blood vessels that connect arterioles with venules; facilitate passage of life-sustaining fluids containing oxygen and nutrients to cell bodies and the removal of accumulated waste and carbon dioxide
Blood	Fluid consisting of formed elements (erythrocytes, thrombocytes, leukocytes) and plasma. It is a specialized bodily fluid that delivers necessary substances to the body's cells (oxygen, foods, salts, hormones) and transports waste products (carbon dioxide, urea, lactic acid) away from those same cells. Blood is circulated around the body through blood vessels by the pumping action of the heart. See Chapter 10, "Blood and Lymphatic System," for a further discussion of blood.

Capillary bed of lungs where gas exchange occurs
Pulmonary arteries
Pulmonary veins
Pulmonary circuit
Aorta and branches
Vena cavae
Left atrium
Right atrium
Left ventricle
Right ventricle
Systemic arteries
Systemic veins
■ Oxygen poor, CO_2 - rich blood
Systemic circuit
■ Oxygen rich, CO_2 - poor blood
Capillary bed of all body tissues where gas exchange occurs

■ **Figure 9.1** Schematic overview of the cardiovascular system.

• **Designed for Visual Learners** — Nearly every page is highlighted by a vibrant and instructive image. Examples include anatomi-cally precise diagrams, authentic medical pho-tographs, and engaging labeling activities.

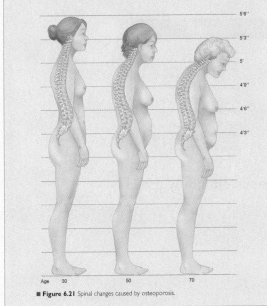

LIFE SPAN CONSIDERATIONS

With normal aging, individuals can lose 1.0–1.5 inches in height. Loss of more than 1.5 inches in height can be related to vertebral compression fractures and other issues due to osteoporosis. See Figure 6.21 ■

■ **Figure 6.21** Spinal changes caused by osteoporosis.

• **Lifespan Considerations** — These boxes provide interesting facts about the human body as it relates to the child and the older adult.

• Drug Highlights •

TYPE OF DRUG	DESCRIPTION AND EXAMPLES
anti-inflammatory agents	Relieves the swelling, tenderness, redness, and pain of inflammation. Such agents can be classified as steroidal (corticosteroids) and nonsteroidal.
corticosteroids (glucocorticoids)	Steroid substance with potent anti-inflammatory effects EXAMPLES: Depo-Medrol (methylprednisolone acetate), prednisone, and Delta-Cortef (prednisolone)
nonsteroidal (NSAIDs)	Agents used in the treatment of arthritis and related disorders EXAMPLES: Bayer aspirin (acetylsalicylic acid), MotrinIB (ibuprofen), Feldene (piroxicam), ketoprofen, and Naprosyn (naproxen)

• **Drug Highlights** — These sections present essential pharmacology information that relates to the subject of the chapter.

• Diagnostic and Lab Tests •

TEST	DESCRIPTION
angiography (ăn″ jē-ŏg′ ră-fē)	X-ray recording of a blood vessel after the injection of a radiopaque substance. Used to determine the patency of the blood vessels, organ, or tissue being studied. Types: aortic, cardiac, cerebral, coronary, digital subtraction (use of a computer technique), peripheral, pulmonary, selective, and vertebral.
cardiac catheterization (kăr′ dĭ-ăk kăth″ ĕ-tĕr-ĭ -z ā′ shŭn)	Medical procedure used to diagnose heart disorders. A tiny catheter is inserted into an artery in the arm or leg of the patient and is fed through this artery to the heart. Dye is then pumped through the catheter, enabling the physician to locate by x-ray any blockages in the arteries supplying the heart. See Figure 9.38 ■

• **Diagnostic and Lab Tests** — These sections present a snapshot of current tests and procedures that are used in the physical assessment and diagnosis of certain conditions/diseases.

• Abbreviations •

ABBREVIATION	MEANING	ABBREVIATION	MEANING
ACG	angiocardiography	IV	intravenous
AED	automated external defibrillator	LA	left atrium
AMI	acute myocardial infarction	LBBB	left bundle branch block
ASHD	arteriosclerotic heart disease	LD, LDH	lactic dehydrogenase
AST	aspartate aminotransferase	LDL	low-density lipoprotein
A-V, AV	atrioventricular; arteriovenous	LV	left ventricle
BBB	bundle branch block	MI	myocardial infarction
BP	blood pressure	MRI	magnetic resonance imaging
CABG	coronary artery bypass graft	MS	mitral stenosis
CAD	coronary artery disease	MV	mitral valve

• **Abbreviations** — These sections present commonly used abbreviations with their meanings.

• Study and Review • Study and Review • St

Anatomy and Physiology

Write your answers to the following questions.

1. List the organs of the urinary system.

a. _____   b. _____

c. _____   d. _____

2. State the vital function of the urinary system. _____

3. Define hilum. _____

4. Define renal pelvis. _____

5. The medulla is the _____ portion of the kidney.

6. Define nephron. _____

7. Each nephron consists of a _____ _____ and a _____

8. The malpighian corpuscle consists of _____ and _____

_____ .

9. Urine is formed by the process of _____ and _____ in the nephron.

10. An average of _____ to _____ mL of urine is voided daily.

11. Describe the ureters and state their function. _____

12. Describe the urinary bladder and state its function. _____

_____

13. The external urinary opening is the _____ .

14. Define urinalysis. _____

• **Study and Review** — A self-paced study guide section featuring a wide variety of study formats.

PRACTICAL APPLICATION
MEDICAL RECORD ANALYSIS

This exercise contains information, abbreviations, and medical terminology from an actual medical record or case study that has been adapted for this text. The names and any personal information have been created by the author. Read and study each form or case study and then answer the questions that follow. You may refer to Appendix III, Abbreviations and Symbols, on page A41 PRN.

OXFORD NEUROLOGICAL CENTER
7894 Hazelbrook Drive
Centreville, VA 30120
(123) 456-7890

Marcus James Madison, MD   Charles Robert Jones, MD   Nagoya T. Yung, MD

Summary Report

Patient: Brown, James E.   **Age:** 78   **Sex:** Male   **Date:** 05/19/xx

James E. Brown, age 78, has rather advanced Parkinson's disease, present for 7 years. It is affecting his activities of daily living (ADL). He has difficulty bathing, dressing, and has frequent falls. He has marked hesitancy on changing directions and unsteadiness with fatigue. He can brush his teeth and wash his face.

On neurological examination he did have mild to moderate impairment in cognition and short-term memory, although he is oriented to time, place, and person. He has a mild tremor, worse in the left arm than the right. He has rigidity in the upper extremities. He has marked difficulty in movement, with long delays in initiating movement and frequent freezing in place. He has postural instability. He has mild dysarthria (difficult articulation of speech) . His gait is characterized by shuffling strides. He can arise from a chair with difficulty only after multiple attempts. Deep tendon reflexes are symmetrical, and toes are downgoing. Cranial nerves are unremarkable.

He has been on Sinemet 25–100 mg tid for the last 6 years. I have asked him to increase his Sinemet dose to qid. Mr. Brown is to return to our office in 3 months.

Marcus James Madison, MD

• **Practical Application** — A case study section that challenges readers to apply their understanding of each chapter while interacting with medical records.

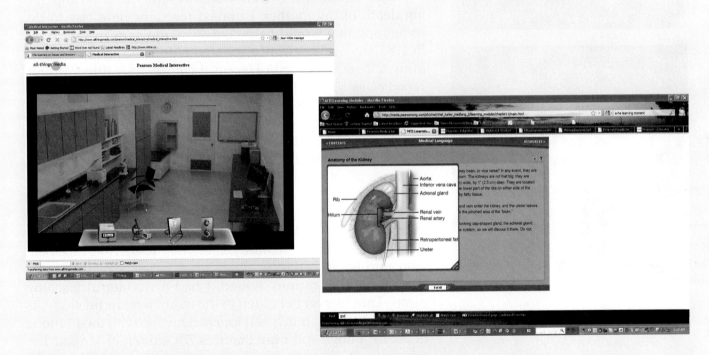

MYMEDICALTERMINOLOGYLAB

PEARSON
mymedicalterminologylab

The ultimate personalized learning tool is available at **www.mymedicalterminologylab.com**. This online course correlates with the text-book and is available for purchase separately or for a discount when packaged with the book. MyMedicalTerminologyLab is an immersive study experience that takes place within Pearson General Hospital—a virtual world of fun quizzes, word games, videos, and other self-study challenges. The system allows learners to track their own progress through the course and use a personalized study plan to achieve success.

MyMedicalTerminologyLab saves instructors time by providing quality feed-back, ongoing individualized assessments for students, and instructor resources all in one place. It offers instructors the flexibility to make technology an integral part of their course, or a supplementary resource for students.

Visit **www.mymedicalterminologylab.com** to log in to the course or purchase access. Instructors seeking more information about discount bundle options or for a demonstration, please contact your Pearson sales representative.

COMPREHENSIVE INSTRUCTIONAL PACKAGE

Perhaps the most gratifying part of an educator's work is the "aha" learning moment when the light bulb goes off and a student truly understands a concept—when a connection is made. Along these lines, Pearson is pleased to help instructors foster more of these educational connections by providing a complete battery of resources to support teaching and learning. Qualified adopters are eligible to receive a wealth of materials designed to help instructors prepare, present, and assess. For more information, please contact your Pearson sales representative or visit **www.pearsonhighered.com/educator**.

About the Author

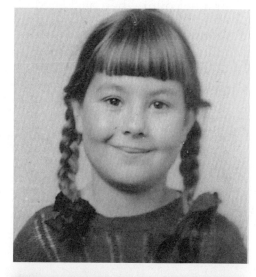

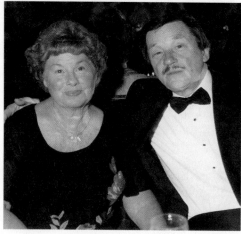

The year is 1947 and I am a little girl with brown hair that is braided into pigtails. I am very shy and afraid, for, you see, I am in the second grade and I cannot read. Not one little word. The teacher discovered this and made me sit on a tall metal stool in front of the classroom with a dunce cap on my head. Still to this day, I get very nervous when I have to get up in front of a crowd of people.

My mother taught me to read because back then, there were no special classes for children with learning disabilities. I did not learn "phonetics" but memorized everything. I still have trouble pronouncing words, but I can tell you all you want to know about a medical word.

After the death of two brothers, my father, and the impending death of my mother, I prayed for something else to do, something that would help take away the pain and the hurt. In 1982, my prayers were answered with a most precious gift: *Medical Terminology with Human Anatomy,* now titled *Medical Terminology: A Word-Building Approach,* which was first published in September 1985.

I owe so much to God and my best friend and husband, Charles Larry Rice. God continues to guide me in my writing. He provides me the knowledge and ability to organize, research, develop, and then to write. Larry, my husband of 45 years, is supportive and gives me the freedom to be an author. He is my love and hero. Also, I express my love to the flowers in my life: Melissa Rice-Noble, Doug Noble, and our grandchildren: Zachary, Benjamin, Jacob, Mary Katherine, Elizabeth Ann, and Emily Sarah.

Although I am now retired, I had a wonderful teaching career. I am forever beholden to the many wonderful students who taught me so much and touched my life with their unique qualities. I hope and pray that this 7th edition of *Medical Terminology: A Word-Building Approach* will enable you, the learner, to become the professional that you choose to be.

Jane Rice, RN, CMA-C

Acknowledgments

First, I would like to offer my warmest thanks to all of the individuals who have accepted *Medical Terminology: A Word-Building Approach* as their text. Over the past 26 years, I have been blessed with the gift of writing. It is my desire for this edition to make learning a wonderful experience for you, the learner and educator.

It has taken a "village" of people to create such a work of excellence. I want to express my gratitude to each person who worked so hard on this project and provided his or her unique talents to create and develop this edition. A sincere thank you to all the exceptional people at Pearson Health Science. To Lynda Hatch—You were with me all the way. Through your guidance and excellent work, this seventh edition of my "dream" has reached a new dimension. To Elena Mauceri—You have been with me through many a revision, and I cherish your assistance and friendship. To Mark Cohen—It is really you who made this edition what it is. Your continual support of my work has proven to be the driving force in making an excellent book the best it can be. To Melissa Kerian—Your supervision of the ancillary components exceeds all expectations. To Jason Smith, MD, Northwest Georgia Dermatology & Skin Surgery Center, Rome, Georgia —A special thank you for providing me with much of the art used for the integumentary system and oncology chapters.

Editorial Development Team

The content and format of *Medical Terminology: A Word Building Approach* are the result of an incredible collaboration of expert educators from all around. This book represents the collective insights, experience, and thousands of hours of work performed by members of this development team. Their influence will continue to have an impact for decades to come. Let us introduce the members of our team.

Adejoke Adenekan, MBBS (MD), MPH, MS
Bauder College
Atlanta, Georgia

Jana Allen, MT, BS
Volunteer State Community College
Gallatin, Tennessee

Michael Battaglia, Ms, Ed
Greenville Technical College
Greenville, South Carolina

Jeffery J. Betts, PhD
Central Michigan University
Mount Pleasant, Michigan

Mary Ellen Camire, PhD
University of Maine
Orono, Maine

Carol Charie, AA, CPC
The Salter School
Fall River, Massachusetts

Angela M. Corio, PT, MPT
Carolinas Rehabilitation
Charlotte, North Carolina

Lucinda A Drohn, RN, MSN
Liberty University
Lynchburg, Virginia

Jennifer Esch, BS, PA-C
Bryant and Stratton College
Milwaukee, Wisconsin

Pamela A. Eugene, BAS, RT (R)
Delgado Community College
New Orleans, Louisiana

Angie Hall, CPC, CMC, CMIS, CMOM, CHIT, CMA-A
Greenville Technical College
Greenville, South Carolina

Kelly Hannah, RN, MSN, MS
Western Iowa Tech Community College
Sioux City, Iowa

Glenda Hatcher, RN, BSN, CMA (AAMA)
Southwest Georgia Technical College
Thomasville, Georgia

Harold Horn, Professor
Lincoln Land Community College
Springfield, Illinois

Susan Horn, AAS, CMA
Indiana Business College
Lafayette, Indiana

Faraneh Javan, MD
West Valley College
Saratoga, California

Crystal Kitchens, MA, CMT
Richland Community College
Decatur, Illinois

Jean M. Krueger-Watson, PhD
Clark College
Vancouver, Washington

Jennifer Lamé, MPH, BS, RHIT
Southwest Wisconsin Technical
College
Fennimore, Wisconsin

Trisha LaPointe, PharmD,
BCPS
Massachusetts College of
Pharmacy and Health Sciences
Boston, Massachusetts

Lynette McCullough, MS
Griffin Technical College
Griffin, Georgia

Paulette Miller, RN, MS, RHIA
Illinois State University
Normal, Illinois

Katrina B. Myricks, MS
Holmes Community College
Ridgeland, Missouri

Cindy S. Neville, BS, RN, CPC
DuBois Business College
DuBois, Pennsylvania

Lawrence Newmann, DPM
Florida Atlantic University
Boca Raton, Florida

Karen Perryman, BA, RT
(R)(M), RDMS
Santa Rosa Junior College
Santa Rosa, California

Kathy Plitnick, RN, PhD,
CCRN
Byrdine F. Lewis School of
Nursing
Georgia State University
Atlanta, Georgia

Donna Jeanne Pugh,
BSN, RN
Florida Metropolitan
University
Jacksonville, Florida

Paula Silver, BS, PharmD
Medical Careers Institute
Newport News, Virginia

Abraham Solomon, MD
Florida Gulf Coast
University
Fort Myers, FL
Ave Maria University
Ave Maria, FL

Leeann Stahn, RHIT
Central Oregon Community
College
Bend, Oregon

Carolyn Stariha, RHIA
Houston Community College
Houston, Texas

Roland Tay, MD
Eastfield College
Mesquite, Texas

Joyce B. Thomas, CMA, AAS
Central Carolina Community
College
Pittsboro, North Carolina

Cynthia Thompson, BSRT, MA
Alamance Community College
Graham, North Carolina

Garnet Tomich, BA
San Diego, California

Richard Torres, PhD
Oregon Institute of Technology
Klamath Falls, Oregon

Carla Tyson-Howard, MHA,
RHIA
Houston Community College
Houston, Texas

Helen Weeks, MA, BAS, RMA
Henry Ford Community College
Dearborn, Michigan

Leesa Whicker, BA, CMA
Central Piedmont Community
College
Charlotte, North Carolina

Donna Williams, DNP, RN
Itawamba Community College
Fulton, Missouri

Kathy Zaiken, PharmD
Massachusetts College of
Pharmacy and Health Sciences
Boston, Massachusetts

A Commitment to Accuracy

As a learner embarking on a career in health care you probably already know how critically important it is to be precise in your work. Patients and co-workers will be counting on you to avoid errors on a daily basis. Likewise, we owe it to you—the reader—to ensure accuracy in this book. We have gone to great lengths to verify that the information provided in *Medical Terminology: A Word-Building Approach* is complete and correct. To this end, here are the steps we have taken:

1. **Editorial review** —We have assembled a large team of developmental consultants to critique every word and every image in this book. No fewer than 12 content experts have read each chapter for accuracy. In addition, some members of our developmental team were specifically assigned to focus on the precision of each illustration that appears in the book.

2. **Medical Illustrations** —A team of medically trained illustrators was hired to prepare each piece of art that graces the pages of this book. These illustrators have a higher level of scientific education than the artists for most textbooks, and they worked directly with the author and members of our development team to make sure that their work was clear, correct, and consistent with what is described in the text.

3. **Accurate Ancillaries** —The teaching and learning ancillaries are often as important to instruction as the textbook itself. Therefore we took steps to ensure accuracy and consistency of these components by reviewing every ancillary component.

While our intent and actions have been directed at creating an error-free text, we have established a process for correcting any mistakes that may have slipped past our editors. Pearson takes this issue seriously and therefore welcomes any and all feedback that you can provide along the lines of helping us enhance the accuracy of this text. If you identify any errors that need to be corrected in a subsequent printing, please send them to:

Pearson Health Science Editorial
Medical Terminology Corrections
One Lake Street
Upper Saddle River, NJ 07458

Thank you for helping Pearson reach its goal of providing the most accurate medical terminology textbooks available.

Detailed Contents

CHAPTER 9 CARDIOVASCULAR SYSTEM   259

CHAPTER 10 BLOOD AND LYMPHATIC SYSTEM   315

stem • Nervous System • Special Senses: The Ear • Sp
Senses: The Eye • Female Reproductive System with a
verview of Obstetrics • Male Reproductive System • C
ology • Radiology and Nuclear Medicine • Mental Hea

• Introduction to Medical Terminology • Suffixes

LEARNING OUTCOMES

On completion of this chapter, you will be able to:

1. Describe the fundamental elements that are used to build medical words.
2. List three guidelines that will assist you with the building and spelling of medical words.
3. Explain the use of abbreviations when writing and documenting data.
4. Analyze, build, spell, and pronounce medical words.
5. Identify and define selected abbreviations.
6. Describe selected medical and surgical specialties, giving the scope of practice and the physician's title.
7. Define HIPAA.
8. List and describe the general components of a patient's medical record.
9. List and describe the four parts of the SOAP chart note record.

plural suffix
combining form
abbreviation root
spelling pronunciation
prefix

Comprehension of Fundamental Word Structure

Medical terminology is the study of terms that are used in the art and science of medicine. It is a specialized language with its origin arising from the Greek influence on medicine. Hippocrates was a Greek physician who lived from 460 to 377 B.C. and whose vital role in medicine is still recognized today. He is called "the Father of Medicine" and is credited with establishing early ethical standards for physicians. Because of advances in scientific computerized technology, many new terms are coined daily; however, most of these terms are composed of word parts that have their origins in ancient Greek or Latin. Because of this foreign origin, it is necessary to learn the English translation of terms when learning the fundamentals of word structure.

FUNDAMENTALS OF WORD STRUCTURE

The fundamental elements in medical terminology are the component parts used to build medical words. The abbreviations used for component parts in this text are **P**, **prefix**; **R**, **root**; **CF**, **combining form**; and **S**, **suffix**. The key to learning medical terminology is through a word-building technique used in this text. Combining forms and word roots are integrated into each chapter of the text, according to body system or specialty area. Suffixes and prefixes are presented in Chapters 2 and 3 and then will continue to be repeated throughout the text. To build your medical vocabulary, all you have to do is recall the word parts that you have learned and then link them with the new component parts presented in each chapter.

Prefix

The term **prefix** means *to fix before* or *to fix to* the beginning of a word. A prefix can be a syllable or a group of syllables. Prefixes are united with or placed at the beginning of words to alter or modify their meanings or to create entirely new words. For example, the word **ex/cis/ion** means *the process of cutting out; surgical removal.* Note its component parts:

ex-	**P** or prefix meaning	out
cis	**R** or root meaning	to cut
-ion	**S** or suffix meaning	process

Word Root

A **root** is a word or word element from which other words are formed. It is the foundation of the word. The root conveys the central meaning of the word and forms the base to which prefixes and suffixes are attached for word modification.

For example, the word **mal/format/ion** means *the process of being badly shaped; deformed.* Note its component parts:

mal-	**P** or prefix meaning	bad
format	**R** or root meaning	a shaping
-ion	**S** or suffix meaning	process

Combining Form

A **combining form** is a word root to which a vowel has been added. A combining vowel (*a, e, i, o,* or *u*) links the root to the suffix or the word root to another root. The combining vowel does not have a meaning of its own. The vowel *o* is used more often than any other to make combining forms. Combining forms can be found at the beginning of a word or within the word.

For example, the word **chem/o/therapy** means *treatment of disease by using chemical agents.* Note the relationship of its component parts:

chem/o	**CF** or combining form meaning	chemical
-therapy	**S** or suffix meaning	treatment

Suffix

The term **suffix** means *to fasten on, beneath, or under.* A suffix can be a syllable or group of syllables united with or placed at the end of a word to alter or modify the meaning of the word or to create a new word. When you break down a word to understand it or when you give the meaning of the word or read its definition, you usually begin with the meaning of the suffix.

For example, the word **gastr/oma** means *a tumor of the stomach* and the word **gastr/itis** means *inflammation of the stomach:*

gastr	**R** or root meaning	stomach
-oma	**S** or suffix meaning	tumor
gastr	**R** or root meaning	stomach
-itis	**S** or suffix meaning	inflammation

Word roots and combining forms, together with their definitions, are included in each chapter according to the cell, tissue, organ, system, or element they describe. This arrangement makes it possible for you to form associations between medical terms and the various body systems. To reinforce the learning process, this text provides you a general anatomy and physiology overview for each of the body systems.

PRINCIPLES OF COMPONENT PARTS

As you learn definitions for prefixes, roots, combining forms, and suffixes, you will discover that some component parts have the same meanings as others. This occurs most often with words that relate to the organs of the body and the diseases that affect them. The existence of more than one component part for a particular meaning can be traced to differences in the Greek or Latin words from which they originated. Most of the terms for the body's organs originated from Latin words, whereas terms describing diseases that affect these organs have their origins in Greek. For example:

- **Uterus.** Latin word for one of the organs of the female reproductive system, the womb
- **Hyster.** Greek R (root) for womb
- **Hysterectomy.** Surgical excision of the womb from hyster R (root) meaning womb + -ectomy S (suffix) meaning surgical excision
- **Metr/i.** Greek CF (combining form) for uterus

- **Myometrium.** Muscular tissue of the uterus from my/o CF meaning muscle + metr/i CF meaning uterus + -um S meaning tissue

In this text, most definitions are worded in an attempt to establish a relationship with the meanings given for each word part. For example, the medical term **adhesion** is divided into two word parts: *adhes (R)*, which means stuck to, and *–ion (S)*, which means process. The definition given is "process of being stuck together." See page 8.

IDENTIFICATION OF MEDICAL WORDS

When identifying medical words, you will learn to distinguish among and select the appropriate component parts for the meaning of the word. For example, the word **microscope** means an instrument for examining small objects. Note the following: *micro- + -scope*; not *-scope + micro*. With the proper placement of component parts (P + S) the definition translates micro- = small and -scope = instrument for examining.

VOCABULARY WORDS

You will find that some terms have not been divided into word parts. These are common words or specialized terms that are included to enhance your medical vocabulary. These terms were selected because of their usage in medical records/reports, case studies, and in various medical and surgical specialty areas. For example, *abate*, which means to lessen, decrease, or cease. This term is used to note the lessening of pain or the decrease in severity of symptoms. *The patient's arthritic pain did not **abate**, even though she followed the prescribed treatment plan.* See page 8.

SPELLING

Medical words of Greek origin are often difficult to spell because many of them begin with a silent letter or have a silent letter within the word. The following are examples of words that begin with silent letters:

Silent Beginning	Pronounced	Medical Term	Pronunciation Guide
gn	n	**g**nathic	(năth′ ĭk)
kn	n	**k**nuckle	(nŭk′ ĕl)
mn	n	**m**nemonic	(nĭ-mŏn′ ĭk)
pn	n	**p**neumonia	(nū′ -mō′ nĭ-ă)
ps	s	**p**sychiatrist	(sĭ-kī′ ă-trĭst)
pt	t	**p**tosis	(tō′ sĭs)

The following are examples of medical terms that contain silent letters within the word:

Silent Letter	Medical Term	Pronunciation Guide
g	phle**g**m	(flĕm)
p	blepharo**p**tosis	(blĕf˝ ă-rō-tō´ sis)

Correct spelling is extremely important in medical terminology because the addition or omission of a single letter can change the meaning of a word to something entirely different. The following examples illustrate this point:

Term/Letter Change	Meaning of Term	Term/Letter Change	Meaning of Term
a**b**duct	To lead **away** from the middle	ar**t**eritis	Inflammation of an **artery**
a**d**duct	To lead **toward** the middle	ar**th**ritis	Inflammation of a **joint**

Prefixes and Suffixes That Are Frequently Misspelled

Following are some of the prefixes and suffixes that often contribute to spelling errors:

Prefix	Meaning	Suffix	Meaning
ante-	before, forward	**-poiesis**	formation
anti-	against	**-ptosis**	prolapse, drooping, sagging, falling down
ecto-	out, outside, outer	**-ptysis**	spitting
endo-	within, inner	**-rrhagia**	to burst forth, bursting forth
hyper-	above, beyond, excessive	**-rrhage**	to burst forth, bursting forth
hypo-	below, under, deficient	**-rrhaphy**	suture
inter-	between	**-rrhea**	flow, discharge
intra-	within	**-rrhexis**	rupture
para-	beside, alongside, abnormal	**-scope**	instrument for examining
peri-	around	**-scopy**	visual examination, to view, examine
per-	through	**-tome**	instrument to cut
pre-	before, in front of	**-tomy**	incision

Prefix	Meaning	Suffix	Meaning
pro-	before	**-tripsy**	crushing
super-	above, beyond	**-trophy**	nourishment, development
supra-	above, beyond		

Building and Spelling Medical Words

Follow these guidelines for building and spelling medical words.

1. If the suffix begins with a vowel, drop the combining vowel from the combining form and add the suffix. For example, gastr/*o* (stomach) + -*o*ma (tumor) becomes gastr*o*ma when we drop the *o* from gastr*o*.

2. If the suffix begins with a consonant, keep the combining vowel and add the suffix to the combining form. For example, lip/*o* (fat) + -lysis (destruction) becomes lip*o*lysis; we keep the *o* on the combining form lip*o*.

3. Keep the combining vowel between two or more roots in a term. For example, electr*o* (electricity) + cardi*o* (heart) + -gram (record) becomes electr*o*cardi*o*gram and we keep the two combining vowels.

FORMATION OF PLURAL ENDINGS

To change the following singular endings to plural endings, substitute the plural endings as illustrated:

Singular Ending	Plural Ending	Singular Ending	Plural Ending
a as in burs**a**	to **ae** as in burs**ae**	**ix** as in append**ix**	to **ices** as in append**ices**
ax as in thor**ax**	to **aces** as in thor**aces** or **es** as in thorax**es**	**nx** as in phala**nx**	to **ges** as in phalan**ges**
en as in foram**en**	to **ina** as in foram**ina**	**on** as in spermatozo**on**	to **a** as in spermatozo**a**
is as in cris**is**	to **es** as in cris**es**	**um** as in ov**um**	to **a** as in ov**a**
is as in ir**is**	to **ides** as in ir**ides**	**us** as in nucle**us**	to **i** as in nucle**i**
is as in femor**is**	to **a** as in femor**a**	**y** as in arter**y**	to **i** and add **es** as in arter**ies**

USE OF ABBREVIATIONS

An **abbreviation** is a process of shortening a word or phrase into appropriate letters. It is used as a form of communication in writing and documenting data. More than a thousand medical abbreviations are in use today and more will be created as new treatments and procedures are developed. When using abbreviations caution must be exercised. Many have more than one meaning, such as **ER,** which means *emergency room* and *endoplasmic reticulum,* and **PA,** which means *physician assistant, posteroanterior,* and *pernicious anemia.* It is essential that you use or translate the correct meaning for the abbreviation being used. If there is any question about which abbreviation to use, it is best to spell out the word or phrase and not use an abbreviation.

The Institute for Safe Medication Practice (ISMP) and the Joint Commission on Accreditation of Healthcare Organizations (JCAHO) developed a list of abbreviations considered to be dangerous because of the potential for misinterpretation. It is recommended that facilities using abbreviations for documentation keep a list of approved and unapproved abbreviations on hand and readily accessible. For more information on this list you can go to http://www.ismp.org or http://www.jointcommission.org.

In each chapter of this text, you will find selected abbreviations with their meanings. These abbreviations are in current use and are directly associated with the subject of the chapter. In the appendices, you will find an expanded alphabetical list of commonly used abbreviations and symbols. The abbreviations are presented using capital letters without periods except in those cases where lowercase letters and periods represent the norm or preferred method.

PRONUNCIATION

Pronunciation of medical words may seem difficult; however, it is very important to correctly pronounce medical words with the same or very similar sounds in order to convey their correct meanings. As in spelling, one mispronounced syllable can change the meaning of a medical word. The following guide will help you to pronounce each medical word in this text correctly.

PRONUNCIATION GUIDE	
This text uses a phonetically spelled pronunciation guide adapted from *Taber's Cyclopedic Medical Dictionary.* You should practice speaking each term aloud when working with the various lists of medical terms or vocabulary words.	
ACCENT MARKS	Marks used to indicate stress on certain syllables. *Example:* an″ tə -sep′ tik (antiseptic)
Single ′	Used to indicate stress on certain syllables; a single accent mark is called a *primary accent* and is used with the syllable that has the strongest stress (primary syllable).
Double ″	Used to indicate syllables that are stressed less than primary syllables; a double accent mark is called a *secondary accent.*
DIACRITICS	Marks placed over or under vowels to indicate the long or short sound of the vowel.
Macron ‾	Indicates the long sound of the vowel. *Example:* mī′ krō-skōp (microscope)
Breve ˘	Indicates the short sound of the vowel. *Example:* măks′ ĭ-măl (maximal)
Schwa ə	Indicates the uncolored, central vowel sound of most unstressed syllables. *Example:* bou′əl (bowel)

• Building Your Medical Vocabulary •

This section provides the foundation for learning medical terminology. Review the following alphabetized word list. Note how common prefixes and suffixes are repeatedly applied to word roots and combining forms to create different meanings. The word parts are color-coded: prefixes are green, suffixes are blue, roots/combining forms are red.

You will find that some terms have not been divided into word parts. These are common words or specialized terms that are included to enhance your medical vocabulary.

MEDICAL WORD	WORD PARTS		DEFINITION
	Part	Meaning	
abate (ă-bāt′)			To lessen, ease, decrease, or cease. Used to note the lessening of pain or the decrease in severity of symptoms. *The patient's arthritic pain did not **abate**, even though she followed the prescribed treatment plan.*
abnormal (AB) (ăb-nōr′ măl)	ab- norm -al	away from rule pertaining to	Pertaining to away from the norm or rule. A condition that is considered to be not normal.
abscess (ăb′ sĕs)			Localized collection of pus, which may occur in any part of the body
acute (ac) (ă-cūt′)			Sudden, sharp, severe; used to describe a disease that has a sudden onset, severe symptoms, and a short course
adhesion (ăd′ hē-zhŭn)	adhes -ion	stuck to process	Literally means *a process of being stuck together.* An abdominal adhesion usually involves the intestines and is caused by inflammation or trauma. This type of adhesion may cause an intestinal obstruction and require surgery.
afferent (ăf′ ĕrĕnt)			Carrying impulses toward a center
ambulatory (Amb) (ăm′ bŭ-lăh-tŏr″ ē)			Condition of being able to walk, not confined to bed
antidote (ăn′ tĭ-dōt)			Substance given to counteract poisons and their effects

MEDICAL WORD	WORD PARTS		DEFINITION
	Part	Meaning	
antipyretic (ăn″ tĭ-pī-rĕt´ ĭk)	anti- pyret -ic	against fever pertaining to	Pertaining to an agent that is used to lower an elevated body temperature (fever)
antiseptic (ăn″ tə-sĕp´ tĭk)	anti- sept -ic	against putrefaction pertaining to	Pertaining to an agent that works against sepsis (*putrefaction*); a technique or product used to prevent or limit infections
antitussive (ăn″ tĭ-tŭs´ ĭv)	anti- tuss -ive	against cough nature of, quality of	Pertaining to an agent that works against coughing
apathy (ăp´ ă-thē)			Condition in which one lacks feelings and emotions and is indifferent
asepsis (ā-sĕp´ sĭs)	a- -sepsis	without decay	Without decay; *sterile*, free from all living microorganisms
autoclave (ŏ´ tō-klāv)			An apparatus that sterilizes instruments and items using steam under pressure (15 pounds of pressure per square inch) to reach a heat of 250°F to 254°F for a specified time, such as 30 minutes for single wrapped items
autonomy (ăw-tŏ´ nōm-ē)	auto- nom -y	self law condition	Condition of being self-governed; to function independently
axillary (ax) (ăks´ ĭ-lār-ē)	axill -ary	armpit pertaining to	Pertaining to the armpit
biopsy (Bx) (bī´ ŏp-sē)	bi(o) -opsy	life to view	Surgical removal of a small piece of tissue for microscopic examination; used to determine a diagnosis of cancer or other disease processes in the body
cachexia (kă-kĕks´ ĭ-ă)	cac- -hexia	bad condition	Condition of ill health, malnutrition, and wasting. It may occur in chronic diseases such as cancer and pulmonary tuberculosis.

MEDICAL WORD	WORD PARTS		DEFINITION
	Part	Meaning	
centigrade (C) (sĕn´ tĭ-grād)	centi- -grade	one hundred, one hundredth a step	Literally means *having 100 steps* or *degrees;* unit of temperature measurement (Celsius scale) with a boiling point at 100° and a freezing point at 0°. Each degree of temperature change is 0.01 (1/100) of the scale.
centimeter (cm) (sĕn´ tĭ-mē-tĕr)	centi- -meter	one hundred, one hundredth measure	Unit of measurement in the metric system; one hundredth of a meter
centrifuge (sĕn´ trĭ-f ūj)	centr/i -fuge	center to flee	Device used in a laboratory to separate solids from liquids
chemotherapy (kē˝ mō-thĕr´ ă-pē)	chem/o -therapy	chemical treatment	The use of chemical agents in the treatment of disease, specifically drugs used in cancer therapy
chronic (krŏnik)			Pertaining to time; denotes a disease with little change or of slow progression; the opposite of acute
diagnosis (Dx) (dī˝ ăg-nō´ sĭs)	dia- -gnosis	through knowledge	Determination of the cause and nature of a disease
diaphoresis (dī˝ ă-f ō-rē´ sĭs)	dia- -phoresis	through to carry	To carry through sweat glands; *profuse sweating*
disease (dĭ-zēz´)			Literally means *lack of ease;* a pathological condition of the body that presents with a series of symptoms, signs, and laboratory findings peculiar to it and sets it apart from normal or other abnormal body states; a disruption of normal functioning of the body by a process that can be congenital, infectious, or the failure of normal activity to maintain and sustain health
disinfectant (dĭs˝ ĭn-fĕk´ tănt)	dis- infect -ant	apart to infect forming	Chemical substance that can be applied to objects to destroy pathogenic microorganisms, such as bacteria
efferent (ĕf´ ĕrĕnt)			Carrying impulses away from a center
empathy (ĕm´ pă-thē)			The ability to sense intellectually and emotionally the feelings of another person

MEDICAL WORD	WORD PARTS		DEFINITION
	Part	**Meaning**	
epidemic (ĕp″ i-dĕm′ ik)	epi- dem -ic	upon people pertaining to	Pertaining to among the people; the rapid, widespread occurrence of an infectious disease that can be spread by any pathological organism transmitted by and to humans, birds, insects, etc. In 2009 H1N1 (swine flu) reached an epidemic level, and in the same year the World Health Organization (WHO) declared a worldwide pandemic, with more than 207 countries and overseas territories or communities being affected.
etiology (ē″ tē-ŏl′ ō-jē)	eti/o -logy	cause study of	Study of the cause(s) of disease
excision (ĕk-sĭ′ zhŭn)	ex- cis -ion	out to cut process	Process of cutting out, surgical removal
febrile (fē′ brĭl)			Pertaining to fever, a sustained body temperature above 98.6°F
gram (g) (grăm)			Unit of weight in the metric system; a cubic centimeter or a milliliter of water is equal to the weight of a gram
heterogeneous (hĕt″ ĕr-ō-jē′ nĭ-ŭs)	hetero- gene -ous	different formation, produce pertaining to	Literally means *pertaining to a different formation;* composed of unlike substances; the opposite of homogeneous
illness (ĭl′ nĭs)			State of being sick
incision (ĭn-sĭzh′ ŭn)	in- cis -ion	in, into to cut process	Process of cutting into
kilogram (kg) (kĭl′ ō-grăm)	kil/o -gram	a thousand a weight	Unit of weight in the metric system; *1000 g;* a kilogram is equal to 2.2 lb
liter (L) (lē′ tĕr)			Unit of volume in the metric system; *1000 mL;* a liter is equal to 33.8 fl oz or 1.0567 qt

MEDICAL WORD	WORD PARTS		DEFINITION
	Part	**Meaning**	
macroscopic (măk″rō-skŏp´ĭk)	macr/o scop -ic	large to examine pertaining to	Pertaining to objects large enough to be examined by the naked eye
malaise (mă-lāz´)			A general feeling of discomfort, uneasiness; often felt by a patient who has a chronic disease
malformation (măl″fōr-mā´shŭn)	mal- format -ion	bad a shaping process	Literally means *a process of being badly shaped, deformed*; a structural defect that fails to form normal shape and therefore can affect the function; e.g., *cleft lip*
malignant (mă-lĭg´nănt)	malign -ant	bad kind forming	Literally means *formation of a bad kind*; growing worse, harmful, cancerous
maximal (măks´ĭ-măl)	maxim -al	greatest pertaining to	Pertaining to the greatest possible quantity, number, or degree
microgram (mcg) (mī´krō-grăm)	micro- -gram	small a weight	Unit of weight in the metric system; *0.001 mg*
microorganism (mī″krō-ōr´găn-ĭzm)	micro- organ -ism	small organ condition	Small living organisms that are not visible to the naked eye
microscope (mī´krō-skōp)	micro- -scope	small instrument for examining	Scientific instrument designed to view small objects
milligram (mg) (mĭl´ĭ-grăm)	milli- -gram	one-thousandth a weight	Unit of weight in the metric system; *0.001 g*
milliliter (mL) (mĭl´ĭ-lē″tĕr)	milli- -liter	one-thousandth liter	Unit of volume in the metric system; *0.001 L*
minimal (mĭn´ĭ-măl)	minim -al	least pertaining to	Pertaining to the least possible quantity, number, or degree
multiform (mŭl´tĭ-form)	multi- -form	many, much shape	Occurring in or having many shapes; an object that has more than one defined shape

TABLE 1.1 Selected Medical and Surgical Specialties (continued)

Specialty/Physician	Scope of Practice/Concentration	Word Parts of Specialty (-logy) and Physician (-ist)
Cardiology	Diseases of the heart, arteries, veins, and capillaries	cardi/o (heart), -logy (study of)
Cardiologist		-ist (one who specializes)
Dermatology (Derm)	Diseases of the skin	dermat/o (skin), -logy (study of)
Dermatologist		-ist (one who specializes)
Endocrinology	Diseases of the endocrine system (the glands and the hormones they secrete)	endo- (within), crin/o (to secrete), -logy (study of)
Endocrinologist		-ist (one who specializes)
Epidemiology	Epidemic diseases	epi- (upon), demi/o (people), -logy (study of)
Epidemiologist		-ist (one who specializes)
Family Practice (FP)	Care of members of the family regardless of age and/or sex	
Family Practitioner		
Gastroenterology	Diseases of the stomach and intestines	gastr/o (stomach), enter/o (intestine), -logy (study of)
Gastroenterologist		-ist (one who specializes)
Geriatrics	Study of aspects of aging	geront/o (old age), -logy (study of)
Gerontologist		-ist (one who specializes)
Gynecology (GYN)	Diseases of the female reproductive system	gynec/o (female), -logy (study of)
		-ist (one who specializes)
Gynecologist		
Hematology	Diseases of the blood and blood-forming tissues	hemat/o (blood), -logy (study of)
Hematologist		-ist (one who specializes)
Infectious Disease	Diseases caused by the growth of pathogenic microorganisms within the body	
Internal Medicine	Diseases of internal origin not usually treated surgically	intern (within), -al (pertaining to)
Internist		-ist (one who specializes)
Nephrology	Diseases of the kidney and urinary system	nephr/o (kidney), -logy (study of)
Nephrologist		-ist (one who specializes)

TABLE 1.1 Selected Medical and Surgical Specialties *(continued)*

Specialty/Physician	Scope of Practice/Concentration	Word Parts of Specialty (-logy) and Physician (-ist)
Neurology (Neuro)	Diseases of the nervous system	neur/o (nerve), -logy (study of)
Neurologist		-ist (one who specializes)
Obstetrics (OB)	Treatment of the female during pregnancy, childbirth, and postpartum	The Latin word element *obstetrix* means midwife.
Obstetrician		-ician (specialist, physician)
Oncology	Study of tumors	onc/o (tumor), -logy (study of)
Oncologist		-ist (one who specializes)
Ophthalmology	Diseases of the eye	ophthalm/o (eye), -logy (study of)
Ophthalmologist		-ist (one who specializes)
Orthopedic (Orth) Surgery (Orthopaedic)	Diseases and disorders involving locomotor structures of the body	orth/o (straight), ped (child), -ic (pertaining to)
Orthopedist		-ist (one who specializes)
(Orthopaedist)		-ist (one who specializes)
Otorhinolaryngology (ENT)	Diseases of the ear, nose, and larynx	ot/o (ear), rhin/o (nose), laryng/o (larynx) -logy (study of)
Otorhinolaryngologist		-ist (one who specializes)
Pathology (Path)	Study of structural and functional changes in tissues and organs caused by disease	path/o (disease), -logy (study of)
Pathologist		-ist (one who specializes)
Pediatrics (Peds)	Diseases of children	ped (child), iatr (treatment), -ic (pertaining to)
Pediatrician		-ician (specialist, physician)
Physical Medicine and Rehabilitation	Treatment of disease by physical agents	phys (nature), iatr (treatment)
Physiatrist		-ist (one who specializes)
Proctology	Diseases of the colon, rectum, and anus	proct/o (anus, rectum), -logy (study of)
Proctologist		-ist (one who specializes)
Psychiatry (Psych)	Diseases of the mind	psych/o (mind), iatr (treatment)
Psychiatrist		–ist (one who specializes)

TABLE 1.1 Selected Medical and Surgical Specialties *(continued)*

Specialty/Physician	Scope of Practice/Concentration	Word Parts of Specialty (-logy) and Physician (-ist)
Pulmonary Disease	Diseases of the lungs	pulmon/o (lung), -ary (pertaining to)
Pulmonologist		–ist (one who specializes)
Radiology	Study of radioactive substances and their relationship to prevention, diagnosis, and treatment of disease	radi/o (x-ray), -logy (study of)
Radiologist		–ist (one who specializes)
Rheumatology	Rheumatic diseases	rheumat/o (rheumatism), -logy (study of)
Rheumatologist		-ist (one who specializes)
Urology	Diseases of the urinary system	ur/o (urination), -logy (study of)
Urologist		-ist (one who specializes)

TABLE 1.2 Types of Surgical Specialties with Description of Practice

Surgical Specialty	Description of Practice
Surgery is defined as the branch of medicine dealing with manual and operative procedures for correction of deformities and defects, repair of injuries, and diagnosis and cure of certain diseases.	
Cardiovascular (CV)	Surgical repair and correction of cardiovascular dysfunctions
Colon and Rectum	Surgical repair and correction of colon and rectal dysfunctions
Cosmetic, Reconstructive, Plastic	Surgical repair, reconstruction, revision, or change of the texture, configuration, or relationship of contiguous structures of any part of the human body
General	Surgical repair and correction of various body parts and/or organs
Maxillofacial	Surgical treatment of diseases, injuries, and defects of the human mouth and dental structures
Neurologic	Surgical repair and correction of neurologic dysfunctions
Orthopedic (*Orthopaedic*)	Surgical prevention and repair of musculoskeletal dysfunctions
Thoracic	Surgical repair and correction of organs within the rib cage
Trauma	Surgical repair and correction of traumatic injuries
Vascular	Surgical repair and correction of vascular (vessels) dysfunctions

THE MEDICAL RECORD

The **medical record** is a written document of information describing a patient and his or her health care. This record contains the dates, observations, medical or surgical interventions, and treatment outcomes provided during hospitalization or a visit to a doctor's office. It includes information that the patient provides concerning his or her symptoms (Sx) and medical history, results of examinations, reports of x-rays and laboratory tests, diagnoses, and treatment plans.

This information is compiled and used by doctors, nurses, and other medical professionals to ensure that the patient receives quality health care. The physical medical record belongs to the health care provider, but the information in it belongs to the patient. The medical record serves as the following:

* Basis for planning care and treatment
* Means by which doctors, nurses, and others caring for the patient can communicate
* Legal document describing the care the patient received and can be used as evidence in court
* Means by which the patient or insurance company can verify that services billed were actually provided

In addition to information about physical health, these records may include private and confidential information about family relationships, sexual behavior, substance abuse, and even personal thoughts and feelings. This information is often keyed to a Social Security (SS) number and may be easily accessible to others because of a lack of consistent privacy protection in the use of Social Security numbers.

Information from medical records could influence one's credit, admission to educational institutions, and employment. It could also affect a person's ability to get health insurance or the rates paid for coverage. More important, having others know intimate details about a person's life can mean a loss of dignity and autonomy.

Health Insurance Portability and Accountability Act

Over a decade ago, Congress called on the Department of Health and Human Services (HHS) to issue patient privacy protections as part of the Health Insurance Portability and Accountability Act (HIPAA), which was passed in 1996. HIPAA is a set of rules that doctors, hospitals, and other health care providers must follow to help ensure that all medical records, medical billing, and patient accounts meet certain consistent standards with regard to documentation, handling, and privacy. In addition, HIPAA requires that all patients be able to access their own medical records, correct errors or omissions, and be informed about how personal information is shared or used and about privacy procedures.

HIPAA also includes provisions designed to encourage electronic transactions and requires safeguards to protect the security and confidentiality of health information. It covers health plans, health care clearinghouses, and those health care providers who conduct certain financial and administrative transactions (e.g., enrollment, billing, and eligibility verification) electronically.

Under the HIPAA Privacy Rule (45 CFR Parts 160 and 164), protected health information (PHI) is defined very broadly. PHI includes individually identifiable health information related to the past, present, or future physical or mental health or condition, the provision of health care to an individual, or the past, present, or future payment for the provision of health care to an individual. Even the fact that an individual received medical care is protected information under the regulation.

The Privacy Rule establishes a federal mandate for individual rights in health information, imposes restrictions on uses and disclosures of individually identifiable health information, and provides for civil and criminal penalties for violations. The complementary Security Rule includes standards for protection of health information in electronic form. For more information go to http://www.hhs.gov/ocr/hipaa.

Types and Components of a Medical Record

There are various types of medical records. They can be kept on paper, **microfilm** (photographs of records in a reduced size) or **microfiche** (sheets of microfilm), or in electronic form. Today, the electronic medical record (EMR) or electronic health record (EHR) is being utilized more by physicians and health care providers than in previous years. Sections contained within the medical record will vary according to the physician's preference, type of practice, cost, and regulatory requirements. Many of the EMR software programs have a prescription component that can be accessed by clicking on the prescription tab. This program can store thousands of drug names with their usual dosages. With just a few clicks, an entire prescription can be created.

A patient's medical record is often referred to as a *chart* or *file*. The general components of a patient's medical record include the following:

- **Patient Information Form.** Document that is filled out by the patient on the first visit to the physician's office and then updated as necessary, providing data that relates directly to the patient, including last name, first name, gender, date of birth (DOB), marital status, street address, city, state, zip code, telephone number, Social Security number, employment status, address and phone number of employer, name and contact information for the person who is responsible for the patient's bill, and vital information concerning who should be contacted in case of an emergency.
- **Medical History (Hx).** Document describing past and current history of all medical conditions experienced by the patient.
- **Physical Examination (PE).** Record that includes a current head-to-toe assessment of the patient's physical condition.
- **Consent Form.** Signed document by the patient or legal guardian giving permission for treatment.
- **Informed Consent Form.** Signed document by the patient or legal guardian that explains the purpose, risks, and benefits of a procedure and serves as proof that the patient was properly informed before undergoing a procedure.
- **Physician's Orders.** Record of the prescribed care, medications, tests, and treatments for a given patient.
- **Nurse's Notes.** Record of a patient's care that includes vital signs, particularly temperature (T), pulse (P), respiration (R) [TPR] and blood pressure (BP). The nurse's notes can also include treatments, procedures, and patient's responses to such care. See Figure 1.1 ■
- **Physician's Progress Notes.** Documentation given by the physician regarding the patient's condition, results of the physician's examination, summary of test results, plan of treatment, and updating of data as appropriate (assessment and diagnosis [Dx]).

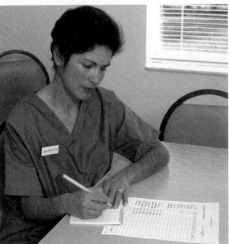

■ **Figure 1.1** Nurse's notes.

- **Consultation Reports.** Documentation given by specialists whom the physician has asked to evaluate the patient.
- **Ancillary/Miscellaneous Reports.** Documentation of procedures or therapies provided during a patient's care, such as physical therapy, respiratory therapy, or chemotherapy.
- **Diagnostic Tests/Laboratory Reports.** Documents providing the results of all diagnostic and laboratory tests performed on the patient.
- **Operative Report.** Documentation from the surgeon detailing the operation, including the preoperative and postoperative diagnosis, specific details of the surgical procedure, how well the patient tolerated the procedure, and any complications that occurred.
- **Anesthesiology Report.** Documentation from the attending anesthesiologist or anesthetist that includes a detailed account of anesthesia during surgery, which drugs were used, dose and time given, patient response, monitoring of vital signs, how well the patient tolerated the anesthesia, and any complications that occurred.
- **Pathology Report.** Documentation from the pathologist regarding the findings or results of samples taken from the patient, such as bone marrow, blood, or tissue.
- **Discharge Summary (also called Clinical Resumé, Clinical Summary, or Discharge Abstract).** Outline summary of the patient's hospital care, including date of admission, diagnosis, course of treatment and patient's response(s), results of tests, final diagnosis, follow-up plans, and date of discharge.

SOAP: Chart Note

The **SOAP—subjective, objective, assessment, plan—chart note** is a method of documentation employed by health care providers to write out notes in a patient's chart, along with other common formats, such as the admission note. Documenting patient encounters in the medical record is an integral part of medical/surgical practice workflow, starting with patient appointment scheduling, to writing out notes, to medical billing. The SOAP note is a method of displaying patient data in a concise, organized format and is written to improve communication among those caring for the patient. The length and focus of each component of a SOAP note varies depending on the specialty area. The four parts of a SOAP chart note follow.

1. **Subjective.** This describes the patient's current condition in narrative form and is information provided by the patient. It includes symptoms that the subject (patient) feels and describes to the health care professional. These symptoms arise within the individual and are not perceptible to an observer. Examples include pain, nausea, dizziness, tightness in the chest, lump in the throat, weakness of the legs, and "butterflies" in the stomach. The health care professional can see the physical reaction of the patient to the symptom but not the actual symptom. Subjective symptoms can be verbally expressed by a parent or a significant other. Also included in the subjective section is the patient's chief complaint (CC), presenting symptom, or presenting complaint stated by the patient and described in the patient's own words. This includes the concern that brings a patient to a doctor.

2. **Objective.** Symptoms that can be observed, such as those that are seen, felt, smelled, heard, or measured by the health care provider. Included in the objective analysis are the vital signs (TPR and BP) and data relating to the physical examination (PE) such as height (Ht), weight (Wt), general appearance,

condition of the lungs, heart, abdomen, musculoskeletal and nervous systems, and the skin. The results of laboratory and diagnostic tests may also be included. *Please note that it may be common practice for the nurse or other medical professional assisting the physician to record the patient's vital signs, allergies, and chief complaint at the top of the chart, instead of within the SOAP chart note.*

3. **Assessment.** Interpretation of the subjective and objective findings. Generally includes a diagnosis, including a differential diagnosis, possible diagnosis, or in some cases to rule out a disease/condition.

4. **Plan.** Includes the management and treatment regimen for the patient; may include laboratory tests, radiological tests, physical therapy, diet therapy, medications, medical and surgical interventions, patient referrals such as counseling and finding a support group, patient teaching, and follow-up directions.

A SOAP chart note should express current patient data, including the date of the visit, patient's name, date of birth, age, sex, and insurance carrier's name.

• Abbreviations •

ABBREVIATION	MEANING	ABBREVIATION	MEANING
AB	abnormal	HIPAA	Health Insurance Portability and Accountability Act of 1996
ABMS	American Board of Medical Specialties	Ht	height
ac	acute	Hx	history
Amb	ambulatory	kg	kilogram
ax	axillary	L	liter
BP	blood pressure	mcg	microgram
Bx	biopsy	mg	milligram
C	centigrade, Celsius	mL	milliliter
CC	chief complaint	Neuro	neurology
cm	centimeter	OB	obstetrics
CV	cardiovascular	Orth	orthopedics (orthopaedics)
Derm	dermatology	P	pulse
DOB	date of birth	Path	pathology
Dx	diagnosis	PE	physical examination
EHR	electronic health record	Peds	pediatrics
EMR	electronic medical record	PHI	protected health information
ENT	ear, nose, throat (larynx) (otorhinolaryngology)	Psych	psychiatry, psychology
FACP	Fellow of the American College of Physicians	R	respiration
		SOAP	subjective objective assessment plan
FACS	Fellow of the American College of Surgeons	SS	social security
		Sx	symptom
FP	family practice	T	temperature
g	gram	TPR	temperature, pulse, respiration
GI	gastrointestinal		
GYN	gynecology	Wt	weight
HHS	Health and Human Services	y/o	year(s) old

• Study and Review • Study and Review • Study and Review
Review • Study and Review • Study and Review • Stu
• Study and Review • Study and Review • Study a

Word Parts

PREFIXES

Give the definitions of the following prefixes.

1. a- _____
2. ab- _____
3. anti- _____
4. auto- _____
5. cac- _____
6. centi- _____
7. dia- _____
8. hetero- _____
9. mal- _____
10. micro- _____
11. milli- _____
12. multi- _____
13. neo- _____
14. para- _____
15. pro- _____
16. syn- _____
17. dis- _____
18. epi- _____
19. ex- _____
20. in- _____

ROOTS AND COMBINING FORMS

Give the definitions of the following roots and combining forms.

1. adhes _____
2. axill _____
3. centr/i _____
4. chem/o _____
5. format _____
6. gene _____
7. kil/o _____
8. macr/o _____
9. necr _____
10. nom _____
11. norm _____
12. onc/o _____
13. organ _____
14. pyret _____
15. pyr/o _____
16. radi/o _____

17. scop _____

18. sept _____

19. therm/o _____

20. top/o _____

21. tuss _____

22. infect _____

23. dem _____

24. eti/o _____

25. cis _____

26. malign _____

27. maxim _____

28. minim _____

29. palm _____

30. prophylact _____

SUFFIXES

Give the definitions of the following suffixes.

1. -al _____

2. -ary _____

3. -centesis _____

4. -drome _____

5. -form _____

6. -fuge _____

7. -genic _____

8. -gnosis _____

9. -grade _____

10. -gram _____

11. -graphy _____

12. -hexia _____

13. -ic _____

14. -ion _____

15. -ism _____

16. -ive _____

17. -liter _____

18. -logy _____

19. -meter _____

20. -osis _____

21. -ous _____

22. -pathy _____

23. -phoresis _____

24. -scope _____

25. -sepsis _____

26. -therapy _____

27. -ar _____

28. -y _____

Identifying Medical Terms

In the spaces provided, write the medical terms for the following meanings.

1. _____ Process of being stuck together

2. _____ Without decay

3. _____ Pertaining to the armpit

4. _____ Use of chemical agents in the treatment of disease

5. _____ Pertaining to a different formation

6. _____ Process of being badly shaped, deformed

7. _____ Scientific instrument designed to view small objects

8. _____ Occurring in or having many shapes

9. _____ New disease

10. _____ Study of tumors

Spelling

Circle the correct spelling of each medical term.

1. antseptic / antiseptic

2. autnomy / autonomy

3. centimeter / centmeter

4. diaphoresis / diphoresis

5. millgram / milligram

6. necrosis / necosis

7. parcentesis / paracentesis

8. radiology / radilogy

Matching

Select the appropriate lettered meaning for each of the following words.

_____ **1.** abate

_____ **2.** antipyretic

_____ **3.** cachexia

_____ **4.** diagnosis

_____ **5.** disease

_____ **6.** etiology

_____ **7.** illness

_____ **8.** prognosis

_____ **9.** prophylactic

_____ **10.** triage

a. Literally means *lack of ease*

b. State of being sick

c. Pertaining to protecting against disease or pregnancy

d. Pertaining to an agent that is used to lower an elevated body temperature (fever)

e. A system of prioritizing and classifying patient injuries to determine priority of need and treatment

f. To lessen, ease, decrease, or cease

g. Determination of the cause and nature of a disease

h. New disease

i. Literally means *a state of foreknowledge*

j. Condition of ill health, malnutrition, and wasting

k. Study of the cause(s) of disease

Abbreviations

Place the correct word, phrase, or abbreviation in the space provided.

1. AB _____

2. ax _____

3. biopsy _____

4. CV _____

5. Neuro _____

6. ear, nose, throat (otorhinolaryngology) _____

7. family practice _____

8. gram _____

9. GYN _____

10. Peds _____

Practical Application Exercise

Write your answers to the following questions about medical records.

1. Describe the *medical record*. _____

_____

2. Define *HIPAA*. _____

3. List 15 general components of a patient's medical record.

a. _____ b. _____

c. _____ d. _____

e. _____ f. _____

g. _____ h. _____

i. _____ j. _____

k. _____ l. _____

m. _____ n. _____

o. _____

4. List the four parts of the SOAP chart note record.

a. _____ b. _____

c. _____ d. _____

5. Assessment includes the _____ of the patient's condition.

6. The _____ includes the management and treatment regimen for the patient.

Special Senses: The Ear • Special Senses: The Eye • Fe
eproductive System with an Overview of Obstetrics •
e Reproductive System • Oncology • Radiology and N
ar Medicine • Mental Health • Introduction to Medical
ology • **Suffixes** • Prefixes • Organization of the Body

LEARNING OUTCOMES

On completion of this chapter, you will
be able to:

1. Recognize how suffixes are used when
   building medical words.
2. Identify adjective, noun, and diminutive
   suffixes.
3. Be aware of suffixes that have more than one
   meaning.
4. Recognize suffixes that pertain to
   pathological conditions.
5. Identify selected suffixes common to surgical
   and diagnostic procedures.
6. Analyze, build, spell, and pronounce medical
   words.

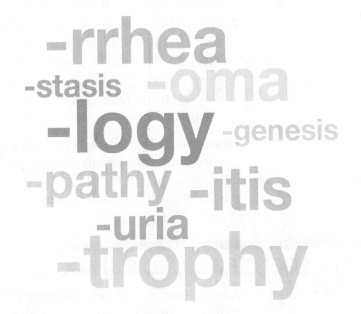

Overview of Suffixes

The term **suffix** means *to fasten on, beneath, or under.* A suffix can be a syllable or group of syllables united with or placed at the end of a word to alter or modify the meaning of the word or to create a new word. A suffix is connected to a root or to a combining form to make new words. For example, the suffix *-ic* (which means *pertaining to*) can be combined with the root *gastr* (which means *stomach*) to make the medical word *gastr/ic* (pertaining to the stomach) or the suffix *-itis* (which means *inflammation*) can be combined with the root *gastr* to make another medical word, *gastr/itis* (inflammation of the stomach).

A compound suffix is made up of more than one word component. It too is added to a root or a combining form to modify its meaning. For example, look at the suffix *-ectomy* (which means surgical excision). It is a combination of three word elements: *ec*, a prefix meaning out; *tom*, a root meaning to cut; and *-y,* a suffix meaning process. When the resulting suffix *-ectomy* is added to the root *gastr,* it forms the medical word *gastr/ectomy,* which means *surgical excision of the stomach* or literally *the process to cut out the stomach.*

Whenever you change the suffix, you alter the meaning of the word to which it is attached. For example, adding the suffix *-tomy* (incision) to the combining form *gastr/o* forms the medical word *gastr/o/tomy* (incision into the stomach). Notice that in the definition, the meaning associated with the suffix (incision) precedes the meaning associated with the combining form (stomach) to which it is attached. The term *gastr/o/tomy* means or can be read as *incision into* (the suffix) *the stomach* (the combining form).

Review the following guidelines, which were presented in Chapter 1. These will help you with the building and spelling of medical words.

1. If the suffix begins with a vowel, drop the combining vowel from the combining form and add the suffix. For example: gastr/*o* (stomach) + *-oma* (tumor) becomes gastr*o*ma when we drop the *o* from gastr*o*.

2. If the suffix begins with a consonant, keep the combining vowel and add the suffix to the combining form. For example, lip/*o* (fat) + *-lysis* (destruction) becomes lip*o*lysis, and we keep the *o* on the combining form lip*o*.

3. Keep the combining vowel between two or more roots in a term. For example, electr*o* (electricity) + cardi*o* (heart) + *-gram* (record) becomes electrocardi*o*gram, and we keep the combining vowels.

Here is a helpful tip: When giving the meaning of the word or reading its definition, you usually begin with the meaning of the suffix. Examples: gastr/**oma** is a **tumor** of the stomach; lip/o/**lysis** is the **destruction** of fat; electr/o/cardi/o/**gram** is a **record** of the electricity activity of the heart.

GENERAL USE SUFFIXES

A collection of suffixes common to medical terminology is listed in Table 2.1 ■ Note that all are preceded by a hyphen (-) to signify that they are to be linked to the end of a root or combining form. Example words are included for each suffix along with their definition. As you progress through this textbook, the understanding of word parts and the process of building medical words will become easier and easier for you. You do not need to learn all the word parts at one time or the definition of each example word. Start with 10 and then add 10 more and soon you will be surprised at how much you have learned.

TABLE 2.1 Selected Suffixes for General Use

Suffix	Meaning	Example Word	Definition
-algesia	condition of pain	an/*algesia*	Condition in which there is a lack of the sense of pain
-ant	forming	malign/*ant*	Refers to the spreading process of cancer from one area of the body to another
-ase	enzyme	amyl/*ase*	Enzyme that breaks down starch
-ate	use, action	exud/*ate*	Production of pus or serum
-blast	immature cell, germ cell	oste/o/*blast*	Bone-forming cell
-cide	to kill	sperm/i/*cide*	Agent that kills sperm
-crit	to separate	hemat/o/*crit*	Blood test that separates solids from plasma in the blood by centrifuging the blood sample
-cuspid	point	bi/*cuspid*	Having two points or cusps
-cyst	bladder, sac	blast/o/*cyst*	A structure formed in the early embryogenesis of mammals, after the formation of the morula, but before implantation
-cyte	cell	neur/o/*cyte*	Nerve cell, neuron
-dipsia	thirst	poly/*dipsia*	Excessive thirst
-drome	that which runs together	syn/*drome*	A group of signs and symptoms occurring together that characterize a specific disease or pathological condition
-er	relating to, one who	radi/o/graph/*er*	Person skilled in making x-ray records
-gen	formation, produce	muta/*gen*	Agent that causes a change in the genetic structure of an organism
-genesis	formation, produce	spermat/o/*genesis*	Formation of spermatozoa
-ide	having a particular quality	radi/o/nucl/*ide*	Radioactive species of an atomic nucleus identified by its atomic number, mass, and energy state
-ive	nature of, quality of	connect/*ive*	The nature of connecting or binding together

TABLE 2.1 Selected Suffixes for General Use *(continued)*

Suffix	Meaning	Example Word	Definition
-liter	liter	milli/*liter*	Unit of volume in the metric system; 0.001 L
-logy	study of	gynec/o/*logy*	Study of the female, especially the diseases of the female reproductive organs and the breasts
-lymph	clear fluid, serum, pale fluid	peri/*lymph*	Serum fluid of the inner ear
-or	one who, a doer	turg/*or*	Generally refers to the expected resiliency of the skin caused by the outward pressure of the cells and interstitial fluid. An evaluation of the skin turgor is an essential part of physical assessment.
-phil	attraction	bas/o/*phil*	White blood cell that has an attraction for a base dye
-stasis	control, stop, stand still	meta/*stasis*	Spreading process of cancer from a primary site to a secondary site
-therapy	treatment	hydro/*therapy*	Treatment using scientific application of water
-thermy	heat	dia/*thermy*	Treatment using high-frequency current to produce heat within a part of the body
-um	tissue, structure	epi/thel/i/*um*	Structure that covers the internal and external organs of the body and the lining of vessels, body cavities, glands, and organs
-uria	urination, condition of urine	hemat/*uria*	Presence of blood in the urine

GRAMMATICAL SUFFIXES

Grammatical suffixes are those that can be attached to a word root to form a part of speech, especially a noun or adjective, or to make a medical word singular or plural in its form. They are also used to indicate a diminutive form of a word that specifies a smaller version of the object indicated by the word root. You will find that many of these suffixes are the same as those used in the English language. See Tables 2.2–2.4 ∎

SUFFIXES THAT HAVE MORE THAN ONE MEANING

Some suffixes can have more than a single meaning, thereby making it a little more difficult when defining the medical terms to which they are attached. An alphabetical listing of some of these suffixes is included in Table 2.5 ∎

TABLE 2.2 Adjective Suffixes That Mean *Pertaining To*

Suffix	Word Analysis	Definition
-ac	card/i/*ac*	Pertaining to the heart
-ad	cephal/*ad*	Pertaining to the head
-al	con/genit/*al*	Pertaining to presence at birth
-ar	muscul/*ar*	Pertaining to the muscles
-ary	integument/*ary*	Pertaining to the skin (a covering)
-ic	norm/o/cephal/*ic*	Pertaining to a normal appearance of the head as used in the objective description during a physical examination
-ile	pen/*ile*	Pertaining to the penis
-ior	anter/*ior*	Pertaining to a surface or part situated toward the front of the body
-ose	grandi/*ose*	Pertaining to a feeling of greatness
-ous	edemat/*ous*	Pertaining to an abnormal condition in which the body tissues contain an accumulation of fluid
-tic	cyan/o/*tic*	Pertaining to an abnormal condition of the skin and mucous membranes caused by oxygen deficiency in the blood
-us	de/cubit/*us*	Pertaining to a bedsore
-y	cardi/o/pulmonar/*y*	Pertaining to the heart and lungs

TABLE 2.3 Noun Suffixes That Mean *Condition, Treatment,* or *Specialist*

Suffix	Word Analysis	Definition
-esis	enur/*esis*	Condition of involuntary emission of urine; bedwetting
-ia	a/lopec/*ia*	Condition of loss of hair; baldness
-iatry	pod/*iatry*	Treatment of diseases and disorders of the foot
-ician	obstetr/*ician*	Physician who specializes in treating the female during pregnancy, childbirth, and the postpartum
-ism	embol/*ism*	Condition in which a blood clot obstructs a blood vessel
-ist	cardi/o/log/*ist*	Physician who specializes in the study of the heart
-osis	hyper/hidr/*osis*	Condition of excessive sweating
-y	an/encephal/*y*	Congenital condition in which there is a lack of development of the brain

TABLE 2.4 Diminutive Suffixes That Mean *Small* or *Minute*

Suffix	Word Analysis	Definition
-cle	aur/i/*cle*	Literally means *small ear*
-icle	ventr/*icle*	Literally means *little belly;* a small cavity or chamber within a body or organ
-ole	bronchi/*ole*	One of the smaller subdivisions of the bronchial tubes
-ula	mac/*ula*	Small spot or discolored area of the skin
-ule	pust/*ule*	Small, elevated, circumscribed lesion of the skin that is filled with pus

TABLE 2.5 Selected Suffixes That Have More Than One Meaning

Suffix	Meanings
-ate	use, action, having the form of, possessing
-blast	immature cell, germ cell, embryonic cell
-ectasis	dilatation, dilation, distention, stretching, expansion
-gen	formation, produce
-genesis	formation, produce
-genic	formation, produce
-gram	a weight, mark, record
-ive	nature of, quality of
-lymph	serum, clear fluid, pale fluid
-lysis	destruction, separation, breakdown, loosening, dissolution
-penia	lack of, deficiency, abnormal reduction
-plasm	a thing formed, plasma
-plegia	stroke, paralysis, palsy
-ptosis	prolapse, drooping, falling down, sagging
-rrhea	flow, discharge
-scopy	to view, examine, visual examination
-spasm	tension, spasm, contraction
-staxis	dripping, trickling
-trophy	nourishment, development
-y	process, condition, pertaining to

SUFFIXES THAT PERTAIN TO PATHOLOGICAL CONDITIONS

Suffixes that carry meanings such as pain, weakness, swelling, softening, inflammation, and tumor are often combined with roots or combining forms to describe pathological conditions. Table 2.6 ■ is an alphabetical listing of some of the more frequently used suffixes associated with disease conditions and disorders.

TABLE 2.6	Selected Suffixes That Pertain to Pathological Conditions		
Suffix	**Meaning**	**Pathological Condition**	**Definition**
-algia	pain, ache	dent/*algia*	Pain in a tooth; toothache
-asthenia	weakness	neur/*asthenia*	Abnormal condition characterized by nervous weakness, exhaustion, and prostration that often follows depression
-betes	to go	dia/*betes*	General term used to describe diseases characterized by excessive discharge of urine
-cele	hernia, tumor, swelling	cyst/o/*cele*	Hernia of the bladder that protrudes into the vagina
-cusis	hearing	presby/*cusis*	Impairment of hearing that occurs with aging
-derma	skin	xer/o/*derma*	Dry skin
-dynia	pain, ache	ot/o/*dynia*	Pain in the ear, earache
-ectasis	dilation, distention	bronch/i/*ectasis*	Chronic dilation of a bronchus or bronchi, with a secondary infection that usually involves the lower portion of a lung
-edema	swelling	papill/*edema*	Swelling of the optical disk, usually caused by increased intracranial pressure (ICP)
-emesis	vomiting	hyper/*emesis*	Excessive vomiting
-ion	process	in/fect/*ion*	Process whereby a pathogenic (*disease producing*) microorganism invades the body, reproduces, multiplies, and causes disease
-itis	inflammation	burs/*itis*	Inflammation of a bursa (*padlike sac between muscles, tendons, and bones*)
-kinesis	motion	hyper/*kinesis*	Excessive muscular movement and motion; inability to be still; also known as hyperactivity
-lepsy	seizure	narc/o/*lepsy*	Chronic condition with recurrent attacks of uncontrollable drowsiness and sleep

TABLE 2.6 Selected Suffixes That Pertain to Pathological Conditions *(continued)*

Suffix	Meaning	Pathological Condition	Definition
-lexia	diction, word, phrase	dys/*lexia*	Condition in which an individual has difficulty in reading and comprehending written language
-malacia	softening	oste/o/*malacia*	Softening of the bones
-mania	madness	pyro/*mania*	Impulsive disorder consisting of a compulsion to set fires or to watch fires
-megaly	enlargement, large	acr/o/*megaly*	Characterized (in the adult) by marked enlargement and elongation of the bones of the face, jaw, and extremities
-mnesia	memory	a/*mnesia*	Condition in which there is a loss or lack of memory
-noia	mind	para/*noia*	Mental disorder characterized by highly exaggerated or unwarranted mistrust or suspiciousness
-oid	resemble	ster/*oid*	Literally means *resembling a solid substance*
-oma	tumor	carcin/*oma*	Malignant tumor arising in epithelial tissue
-opia	sight, vision	presby/*opia*	Vision defect in which parallel rays come to a focus beyond the retina; occurs normally with aging; farsightedness
-oxia	oxygen	hyp/*oxia*	Deficient amount of oxygen in the blood cells and tissues
-pathy	disease, emotion	retin/o/*pathy*	Any disease of the retina
-penia	deficiency	oste/o/*penia*	Deficiency of bone tissue, regardless of the cause
-pepsia	to digest	dys/*pepsia*	Difficulty in digestion; indigestion
-phagia	to eat, to swallow	a/*phagia*	Loss or lack of the ability to eat or swallow
-phasia	to speak, speech	dys/*phasia*	Impairment of speech caused by a brain lesion
-phobia	fear	acr/o/*phobia*	Fear of heights
-plasia	formation, produce	hyper/*plasia*	Excessive formation and growth of normal cells
-plasm	a thing formed, plasma	neo/*plasm*	New thing formed, such as an abnormal growth or tumor
-plegia	paralysis, stroke	hemi/*plegia*	Slight paralysis that affects one side of the body

TABLE 2.6 Selected Suffixes That Pertain to Pathological Conditions *(continued)*

Suffix	Meaning	Pathological Condition	Definition
-pnea	breathing	sleep a/*pnea*	Temporary cessation of breathing during sleep
-ptosis	drooping, prolapse, sagging	blephar/o/*ptosis*	Drooping of the upper eyelid(s)
-ptysis	spitting	hem/o/*ptysis*	Spitting up blood
-rrhage	bursting forth	hem/o/*rrhage*	Excessive bleeding; bursting forth of blood
-rrhea	flow, discharge	rhin/o/*rrhea*	Discharge from the nose
-rrhexis	rupture	my/o/*rrhexis*	Rupture of a muscle
-spasm	tension, spasm, contraction	my/o/*spasm*	Spasmodic contraction of a muscle
-trophy	nourishment, development	hyper/*trophy*	Literally means *excessive nourishment*

SUFFIXES ASSOCIATED WITH SURGICAL AND DIAGNOSTIC PROCEDURES

Suffixes with meanings such as puncture, surgical excision, instrument to measure, and new opening are often combined with roots or combining forms to describe surgical and/or diagnostic procedures. See Table 2.7 ■ for an alphabetical listing of some of the more frequently used suffixes associated with surgery and diagnosis.

TABLE 2.7 Selected Suffixes Used in Surgical and Diagnostic Procedures

Suffix	Meaning	Example Word	Definition
-centesis	surgical puncture	amni/o/*centesis*	Surgical puncture of the amniotic sac to obtain a sample of amniotic fluid containing fetal cells that are examined
-clasis	a break	oste/o/*clasis*	The intentional surgical fracture of a bone to correct a deformity
-desis	binding	arthr/o/*desis*	Surgical binding of a joint
-ectomy	surgical excision, surgical removal, resection	vas/*ectomy*	Surgical procedure in which the vas deferens are tied off and cut apart providing permanent sterility by preventing transport of sperm out of the testes
-gram	a weight, mark, record	dactyl/o/*gram*	Fingerprint

TABLE 2.7 Selected Suffixes Used in Surgical and Diagnostic Procedures (continued)

Suffix	Meaning	Example Word	Definition
-graph	instrument for recording	electr/o/cardi/o/graph	Medical diagnostic device used for recording the electrical impulses of the heart muscle
-graphy	recording	mamm/o/graphy	Process of obtaining x-ray pictures of the breast using a low-dose x-ray system
-ize	to make, to treat or combine with	an/esthet/ize	To induce a loss of feeling or sensation with the administration of an anesthetic
-lysis	destruction, separation, breakdown, loosening	lip/o/lysis	Destruction of fat
-meter	instrument to measure, measure	audi/o/meter	Medical instrument used to measure hearing
-metry	measurement	pelvi/metry	Measurement of the expectant mother's pelvic dimensions to determine whether it will be possible to deliver a fetus through the normal vaginal route
-opsy	to view	bi/opsy	Surgical removal of a small piece of tissue for microscopic examination
-pexy	surgical fixation	gastr/o/pexy	Surgical fixation of the stomach to the abdominal wall for correction of displacement
-pheresis	remove	plasma/pheresis	Removal of blood from the body and centrifuging it to separate the plasma from the blood and reinfusing the cellular elements back into the patient
-plasty	surgical repair	rhin/o/plasty	Surgical repair of the nose
-rrhaphy	suture	my/o/rrhaphy	Suture of a muscle wound
-scope	instrument for examining	ophthalm/o/scope	Medical instrument used to examine the interior of the eye
-scopy	visual examination, to view, examine	lapar/o/scopy	Visual examination of the abdominal cavity
-stomy	new opening	ile/o/stomy	Creation of a new opening through the abdominal wall into the ileum
-tome	instrument to cut	derma/tome	Instrument used to cut the skin for grafting
-tomy	incision	myring/o/tomy	Surgical incision of the tympanic membrane to remove unwanted fluids from the ear
-tripsy	crushing	lith/o/tripsy	Crushing of a kidney stone

• Building Your Medical Vocabulary •

This section provides the foundation for learning medical terminology. Review the following alphabetized word list. Note how common prefixes and suffixes are repeatedly applied to word roots and combining forms to create different meanings. The word parts are color-coded: prefixes are green, suffixes are blue, and **roots/combining forms are red**.

You will find that some terms have not been divided into word parts. These are common words or specialized terms that are included to enhance your medical vocabulary. See Chapter 1, page 7, to review pronunciation guidelines.

MEDICAL WORD	WORD PARTS		DEFINITION
	Part	**Meaning**	
abrasion (ă-brā´ zhŭn)	ab- ras -ion	away from to scrape off process	Process of scraping away from a surface, such as skin or teeth, by friction. An abrasion may be the result of trauma, such as a "skinned knee" or from a therapy, such as dermabrasion of the skin for removal of scar tissue. It can also occur from the wearing-down of a tooth from mastication (*chewing*).
anesthetize (ă-něs´ thĕ-tīz)	an- esthet -ize	without, lack of feeling, sensation to make	To induce a loss of feeling or sensation with the administration of an anesthetic
arousal (a-rou´ zel)	arous -al	alertness, to rise pertaining to	Pertaining to a state of alertness or consciousness
asymmetrical (ā-sĭ-mě´ -trĭ-kăl)	a- symmetric -al	lack of, without symmetry pertaining to	Unequal in size or shape. Without proportion of the body or parts of the body; different in placement or arrangement about an axis.
asystole (ă-sĭs´ tō-lē)	a- systole	without contraction	Literally means *without contraction* of the heart; a life-threatening cardiac condition characterized by the absence of electrical and mechanical activity in the heart.
comatose (kō´ mă-tōs)	comat -ose	a deep sleep pertaining to	Literally means *pertaining to a state of deep sleep* (coma); total lack of consciousness

MEDICAL WORD	WORD PARTS		DEFINITION
	Part	Meaning	
epithelium (ĕp″ ĭ-thē′ lē-ŭm)	epi- thel/i -um	upon, above nipple tissue, structure	Structure that covers the internal and external organs of the body and the lining of vessels, body cavities, glands, and organs. It is the layer of cells forming the outermost layer of the skin and the surface layer of mucous and serous membranes.
exogenous (ĕks-ŏj′ ĕ-nŭs)	ex (o)- gen -ous	out formation, produce pertaining to	Pertaining to originating outside the body or an organ of the body or produced from external causes, such as a disease caused by a bacterial or viral agent foreign to the body
grandiose (grăn′ dē-ōs)	grand/i -ose	great pertaining to	Pertaining to a feeling of *greatness*. In psychiatry, it refers to a person's unrealistic and exaggerated concept of self-worth, importance, wealth, and ability.
gynecoid (jĭn′ ĕ-koyd)	gynec -oid	female resemble	Literally means *to resemble a female*; gynecoid pelvis is the normal shape of the birth canal that allows for the exit of the average fetus
hypertrophy (hī-pĕr′ trŏ-f ē)	hyper- -trophy	excessive nourishment	Literally means *excessive nourishment*; the increase in the size of an organ, structure, or the body caused by an increase in the size of the cells rather than the number of cells; also called *overgrowth*
infection (ĭn-fĕk′ shŭn)	infect -ion	to infect process	Process whereby a pathogenic (*disease producing*) microorganism invades the body, reproduces, multiplies, and causes disease
irregular (ir-rĕg′ ū-lăr)	ir- regul -ar	not rule pertaining to	Pertaining to not being regular
nasolabial (nā″ zō-lā′ bĭ-ăl)	nas/o labi -al	nose lip pertaining to	Pertaining to the nose and lip
palpate (păl′ pāt)	palp -ate	touch use, action	To use the hands or fingers to examine by touch; to feel

MEDICAL WORD	WORD PARTS		DEFINITION
	Part	Meaning	
steroid (stĕr´oyd)	ster -oid	solid resemble	Literally means *resembling a solid substance;* applies to any one of a large group of substances chemically related to sterols; natural steroid hormones include the androgens, estrogens, and adrenal cortex secretions
trauma (traw´mă)			Physical injury or wound caused by external force, violence, or a toxic substance; also refers to psychological injury resulting from a severe emotional shock, which can cause disordered feelings and/or behavior
turgor (tur´jor)	turg -or	swelling one who	Generally refers to the expected resiliency of the skin caused by the outward pressure of the cells and interstitial fluid. An evaluation of the skin turgor is an essential part of physical assessment.

Identifying Suffixes

Underline the suffixes in the following medical words.

1. cardiac
2. cephalad
3. enuresis
4. obstetrician
5. bronchiole

6. pustule
7. dentalgia
8. diabetes
9. hyperemesis
10. hemoptysis

Defining Suffixes

Give the meaning of the following suffixes.

1. -asthenia _____
2. -ion _____
3. -itis _____
4. -malacia _____
5. -megaly _____
6. -pathy _____
7. -penia _____
8. -pepsia _____
9. -phobia _____
10. -rrhexis _____
11. -al _____
12. -ar _____
13. -ate _____
14. -ia _____
15. -ize _____
16. -oid _____
17. -or _____
18. -ose _____
19. -ous _____
20. -trophy _____
21. -um _____

Spelling

Circle the correct spelling of each medical term.

1. auricle / aurcle
2. bronchile / bronchiole
3. cardiologist / cardiolgist
4. cephalad / cephlad
5. cyanotic / cynoatic
6. embolsm / embolism
7. podiatry / podatry
8. pustle / pustule

Using Suffixes to Build Medical Words

Using a suffix from the following list, build the appropriate medical word.

-al   -ior   -ar   -ile
-ary   -osis   -ia   -ula
-icle   -us

1. Condition of excessive sweating   hyper/hidr/_____

2. Pertaining to muscles   muscul/_____

3. Small spot or discolored area of the skin   mac/_____

4. Condition of loss of hair   a/lopec/_____

5. Literally means *little belly*   ventr/_____

6. Pertaining to a bedsore   de/cubit/_____

7. Pertaining to the skin   integument/_____

8. Pertaining to the penis   pen/_____

9. Pertaining to present at birth   con/genit/_____

10. Pertaining to toward the front of the body   anter/_____

Identifying Medical Terms

In the spaces provided, write the medical terms for the following meanings.

1. _____ Process of scraping away from a surface

2. _____ To induce a loss of feeling or sensation

3. _____ Pertaining to a state of alertness or consciousness

4. _____ Unequal in size or shape

5. _____ Literally means *without contraction*

6. _____ Pertaining to a state of deep sleep

7. _____ Difficult articulation of speech

8. _____ Pertaining to a feeling of greatness

9. _____ To resemble a female

10. _____ To use the hands or fingers to examine by touch

PEARSON
mymedicalterminologylab™

MyMedicalTerminologyLab is a premium online homework management system that includes a host of features to help you study. Registered users will find:

- Fun games and activities built within a virtual hospital

- Powerful tools that track and analyze your results—allowing you to create a personalized learning experience

- Videos, flashcards, and audio pronunciations to help enrich your progress

- Streaming lesson presentations and self-paced learning modules

- A space where you and your instructors can view and manage your assignments

enses: The Ear • Special Senses: The Eye • Female Repro
ctive System with an Overview of Obstetrics • Male Re
ductive System • Oncology • Radiology and Nuclear M
cine • Mental Health • Introduction to Medical Termino
Suffixes • **Prefixes** • Organization of the Body • Integu

3

LEARNING OUTCOMES

On completion of this chapter, you will be able to:

1. Recognize how prefixes are used when building medical words.
2. Identify prefixes that are commonly used in medical terminology.
3. Recall prefixes that have more than one meaning.
4. Recognize prefixes that pertain to position or placement.
5. Identify selected prefixes that pertain to numbers and amounts.
6. Analyze, build, spell, and pronounce medical words.

sub- intra-
hydro- bi- mono-
anti- poly-
dys- endo- ex-
hyper-

Overview of Prefixes

The term **prefix** means *to fix before* or *to fix to the beginning* of a word. A prefix can be a syllable or a group of syllables. Prefixes are united with or placed at the beginning of words to alter or modify their meanings or to create entirely new words. For example, by adding the prefix *ab-* to the word *normal* the word **ab/norm/al** is created. As you know, there is a big difference between normal and abnormal. Ab/norm/al means *pertaining to away from the norm.* Remember that when giving the meaning of the word or reading its definition, you usually begin with the meaning of the suffix. Note the component parts of the word abnormal:

ab-	P or prefix meaning	away from
norm	R or root meaning	norm
-al	S or suffix meaning	pertaining to

Not all medical words have a prefix, but when they do, the prefix will alter or modify the meaning of the word. For example, see the following list of medical words that were formed by uniting various prefixes with a single suffix (*-pnea*).

Prefix	Suffix	Medical Word	Definition
a- (lack of)	-pnea (breathing)	*a*pnea	Temporary absence of (lack of) breathing
brady- (slow)	-pnea (breathing)	*brady*pnea	Slow breathing
dys- (difficult)	-pnea (breathing)	*dys*pnea	Difficult breathing
eu- (good, normal)	-pnea (breathing)	*eu*pnea	Good, normal breathing
hyper- (excessive)	-pnea (breathing)	*hyper*pnea	Excessive breathing
hypo- (deficient)	-pnea (breathing)	*hypo*pnea	Deficient breathing
tachy- (rapid)	-pnea (breathing)	*tachy*pnea	Rapid breathing

GENERAL USE PREFIXES

See Table 3.1 ■ for a collection of prefixes that are commonly used in medical terminology. These prefixes can be linked with a word root or a suffix.

TABLE 3.1 Selected Prefixes for General Use

Prefix	Meanings	Example Words	Definitions
a, an-	no, without, lack of, apart	*a*/mnes/ia	Condition in which there is a loss or lack of memory
		an/emia	Literally *a lack of red blood cells*
anti-, contra-	against	*anti*/gen	Invading foreign substance that induces the formation of antibodies
		contra/cept/ion	Process of preventing conception
auto-	self	*auto*/trans/fus/ion	Process of reinfusing a patient's own blood
brachy-	short	*brachy*/therapy	Radiation therapy in which the radioactive substance is inserted into a body cavity or organ. The source of radiation is located a short distance from the body area being treated.
brady-	slow	*brady*/card/ia	Abnormally slow heartbeat defined as less than 60 beats per minute
cac-, mal-	bad	*cac*/hexia	Condition of ill health, malnutrition, and wasting. It may occur in chronic diseases such as cancer and pulmonary tuberculosis.
		mal/format/ion	The process of being badly shaped, deformed
dia-	through, between	*dia*/gnosis	Determination of the cause and nature of a disease
dys-	bad, difficult, painful, abnormal	*dys*/meno/rrhea	Difficulty or painful monthly flow (menses or menstruation)
eu-	good, normal	*eu*/pnea	Good or normal breathing
ex-, exo-	out, away from	*ex*/cis/ion	Process of cutting out, surgical removal
		exo/crine	Pertains to a type of gland that secretes into ducts (duct glands); examples include sweat glands, salivary glands, mammary glands, stomach, liver, and pancreas

TABLE 3.1 Selected Prefixes for General Use *(continued)*

Prefix	Meanings	Example Words	Definitions
hetero-	different	*hetero*/sexu/al	Pertaining to the opposite sex; refers to an individual who has a sexual preference and relationship with the opposite sex
homeo-	similar, same, likeness, constant	*homeo*/stasis	State of equilibrium maintained in the body's internal environment; an important fundamental principle of physiology that permits a body to maintain a constant internal environment despite changes in the external environment
hydro-	water	*hydro*/cele	Accumulation of fluid in a saclike cavity
micro-	small	*micro*/cephal/us	Abnormally small head
oligo-	scanty, little	*oligo*/meno/rrhea	Scanty monthly flow (menses, menstruation)
pan-	all	*pan*/cyto/penia	Lack of the cellular elements of the blood
pseudo-	false	*pseudo*/cyesis	False pregnancy
sym-, syn-	together, with	*sym*/physis	State of growing together
		syn/cope	Temporary loss of consciousness caused by a lack of blood supply to the brain; also called *fainting*

PREFIXES THAT HAVE MORE THAN ONE MEANING

Just like suffixes, many prefixes have more than one meaning. See Table 3.2 ■ To be able to identify the correct meaning of the prefix, you will need to analyze the definition of the medical word. For example, in the medical word **dyspnea** (difficult breathing), *dys-* means difficult. Note that *dys-* also means bad, painful, or abnormal, but in dyspnea these meanings do not apply. As you learn the various component parts that are used to build medical words, you will acquire the knowledge to select and use the correct meaning for each word.

TABLE 3.2 Selected Prefixes That Have More Than One Meaning

Prefix	Meanings	Prefix	Meanings
a-, an-	no, not, without, lack of, apart	extra-	outside, beyond
ad-	toward, near, to	hyper-	above, beyond, excessive
bi-	two, double	hypo-	below, under, deficient
de-	down, away from	in-	in, into, not
di-	two, double	mega-	large, great
dia-	through, between, complete	meta-	beyond, over, between, change
dif-, dis-	apart, free from, separate	para-	beside, alongside, abnormal
dys-	bad, difficult, painful, abnormal	poly-	many, much, excessive
ec-, ecto-	out, outside, outer	post-	after, behind
end-, endo-	within, inner	pre-	before, in front of
ep-, epi-	upon, over, above	pro-	before, in front of
eu-	good, normal	super-	upper, above
ex-, exo-	out, away from	supra-	above, beyond

PREFIXES THAT PERTAIN TO POSITION OR PLACEMENT

Prefixes that carry meanings such as *away from, toward, before, above,* and *below* are often combined with roots and suffixes to describe a position or placement. See Table 3.3 ■ for an alphabetical listing of some of the more frequently used prefixes associated with position or placements.

TABLE 3.3 Prefixes That Pertain to Position or Placement

Prefix	Meanings	Example Words	Definitions
ab-	away from	*ab*/norm/al	Pertaining to away from the normal or rule
ad-	toward, near, to	*ad*/duct/or	Muscle that draws a part toward the middle
ana-	up, apart, backward	*ana*/phylaxis	Unusual or exaggerated allergic reaction to foreign proteins or other substances

TABLE 3.3 Prefixes That Pertain to Position or Placement *(continued)*

Prefix	Meanings	Example Words	Definitions
ante-	before, forward	*ante*/partum	Time between conception and before the onset of labor
cata-	down	*cata*/bol/ism	Literally *a casting down;* a breaking of complex substances into more basic elements
circum-, peri-	around	*circum*/cis/ion *peri*/cardi/al	Surgical process of removing the foreskin of the penis Pertaining to the pericardium, the sac surrounding the heart
endo-	within, inner	*endo*/card/itis	Inflammation of the endocardium (inner lining of the heart)
epi-	upon, above, over	*epi*/gastr/ic	Pertaining to the region above the stomach
ex-	out, away from	*ex*/cis/ion	Process of cutting out; surgical removal
extra-	outside, beyond	*extra*/corpore/al (circulation)	Pertaining to the circulation of the blood outside the body via a heart-lung machine or hemodialyzer
hyper-	above, beyond, excessive	*hyper*/tens/ion	High blood pressure
hypo-	below, under, deficient	*hypo*/tens/ion	Low blood pressure
inter-	between	*inter*/cost/al	Pertaining to between the ribs
intra-	within, into	*intra*/uter/ine	Pertaining to within the uterus
meso-	middle	*meso*/theli/oma	Malignant tumor of mesothelium (serous membrane of the pleura) caused by the inhalation of asbestos
para-	beside, alongside	*para*/plegia	Paralysis of the lower part of the body and of both legs
retro-	backward	*retro*/vers/ion	Process of being turned backward, such as the displacement of the uterus with the cervix pointed forward

TABLE 3.3	Prefixes That Pertain to Position or Placement *(continued)*		
Prefix	**Meanings**	**Example Words**	**Definitions**
sub-	below, under, beneath	*sub*/lingu/al	Pertaining to below the tongue
supra-	above, beyond, superior	*supra*/ren/al	Two small glands located on top (above) of each kidney, also called adrenal glands

PREFIXES THAT PERTAIN TO NUMBERS AND AMOUNTS

Prefixes with meanings such as *both, ten, double, many, half,* and *none* are often combined with roots or suffixes to describe numbers or amounts. See Table 3.4 ■ for an alphabetical list of some of the more frequently used prefixes associated with numbers and amounts.

TABLE 3.4	Prefixes That Pertain to Numbers and Amounts		
Prefix	**Meanings**	**Example Words**	**Definitions**
ambi-	both	*ambi*/later/al	Pertaining to both sides
bi-	two, double	*bi*/later/al	Pertaining to two sides
bin-	twice, two	*bin*/aur/al	Pertaining to both ears
centi-	one hundredth	*centi*/meter	Unit of measurement in the metric system; one hundredth of a meter
deca-	ten	*deca*/gram	A weight of 10 grams
di(s)-	two, apart	*dis*/locat/ion	Displacement of a bone from a joint
milli-	one thousandth	*milli*/liter	Unit of volume in the metric system; 0.001 L
mono-	one	*mono*/nucle/osis	Condition of excessive amounts of mononuclear leukocytes in the blood
multi-	many, much	*multi*/para	Refers to a woman who has given birth to two or more children and is written as Para 2 (3, 4, 5, etc.)
nulli-	none	*nulli*/para	Refers to a woman who has not given birth after more than 20 weeks of gestation and is written as Para 0

Prefix	Meanings	Example Words	Definitions
poly-	many	*poly*/uria	Excessive urination
primi-	first	*primi*/para	Refers to a woman who has had one birth at more than 20 weeks gestation, regardless of whether the infant is born alive or dead and is written as Para 1.
quadri-	four	*quadri*/plegia	Paralysis of all four extremities and usually the trunk due to injury to the spinal cord in the cervical spine
semi-, hemi-	half	*semi*/lun/ar,	Valves of the aorta and pulmonary artery; shaped like a crescent (half-moon)
		hemi/plegia	Paralysis of one half of the body when it is divided along the median sagittal plane
tri-	three	*tri*/som/y	Genetic condition of having three chromosomes instead of two that causes birth defects, such as Down syndrome
uni-	one	*uni*/later/al	Pertaining to one side

TABLE 3.4 Prefixes That Pertain to Numbers and Amounts *(continued)*

• Building Your Medical Vocabulary •

This section provides the foundation for learning medical terminology. Review the following alphabetized word list. Note how common prefixes and suffixes are repeatedly applied to word roots and combining forms to create different meanings. The word parts are color-coded: prefixes are green, suffixes are blue, and **roots/combining forms are red**.

You will find that some terms have not been divided into word parts. These are common words or specialized terms that are included to enhance your medical vocabulary. See Chapter 1, page 7, to review pronunciation guidelines.

MEDICAL WORD	WORD PARTS		DEFINITION
	Part	**Meaning**	
afebrile (ă-fĕb′ rĭl)	a- febr -ile	without fever pertaining to	Literally means *pertaining to without fever;* the patient's temperature would be within a normal range of 98.6°F
anicteric (ăn″ ĭk-tĕr′ ĭk)	an- icter -ic	without jaundice pertaining to	Term used to describe a condition that is without signs of jaundice (yellowish discoloration of the skin, whites of the eyes, mucous membranes and body fluids), such as anicteric hepatitis (a mild form of hepatitis in which there is no jaundice)
arrest (ă-rĕst′)			To stop, inhibit, restrain. A condition of being stopped, such as occurs in cardiac arrest when cardiac output and effective circulation stop.
bifurcate (bī′ fŭr-kāt)	bi- furc -ate	two fork use, action	Having two forks or two branches or two divisions; forked
binary (bī′ nār-ē)	bin- -ary	twice, two pertaining to	Literally means *to separate into two branches or composed of two elements or two structures.* The binary numeral system, or base-2 number system, represents numeric values using two symbols, 0 and 1, and is used internally by all modern computers.
concentration (kŏn-sĕn-trā′ shŭn)	con- centrat -ion	with, together center process	In psychology, the process of being able to bring to the center one thought and focus on it, while excluding other thoughts

MEDICAL WORD	WORD PARTS		DEFINITION
	Part	Meaning	
decompensation (dē-kŏm-pen-sā′ shŭn)	de- compensat -ion	down, away from to make good again process	Failure of a system. In cardiology—failure of the heart to maintain adequate circulation; in psychology—failure of the defense mechanism system that may occur during a relapsing of a mental condition.
enucleate (ē-nū′ klē-āt)			Literally means *to remove the kernel of.* It is used to describe the removal of the eyeball surgically or to remove a cataract surgically. It also means to remove a part or a mass in its entirety.
extraocular (ĕks″ tră-ŏk′ ū-lăr)	extra- ocul -ar	outside eye pertaining to	Pertaining to outside the eye, as used in describing the extraocular eye muscles. These are the muscles that control eye movement and eye coordination.
hyperactive (hī″ pĕr-ăk′ tĭv)	hyper- act -ive	excessive act nature of, quality of	Nature or quality of excessive activity; this can refer to the entire organism or to a particular entity such as the thyroid, heart, or muscles. It may also describe an individual who exhibits constant overactivity.
hypoplasia (hī″ pō-plā′ zē-ă)	hypo- -plasia	under formation	Underdevelopment of a tissue, organ, or body
insomnia (ĭn-sŏm′ nē-ah)	in- somn -ia	not sleep condition	Condition of not being able to sleep. People with insomnia can have difficulty falling asleep, wake up often during the night and have trouble going back to sleep, wake up too early in the morning, or experience unrefreshing sleep.
intermediary (ĭn″ tər-mē′ dē-er-ē)	inter medi -ary	between toward the middle pertaining to	Pertaining to situated between two bodies or occurring between two periods of time
latent (lă′ tə-nt)			Lying hidden; quiet, not active; for example, tuberculosis (TB) may be latent for extended periods of time and become active under certain conditions
lumen (lū′ měn)			Space within an artery, vein, intestine, or tube. It is also the hollow core of a hypodermic needle, which forms an oval-shaped opening when exposed at the beveled (flat, slanted surface) point.

MEDICAL WORD	WORD PARTS		DEFINITION
	Part	**Meaning**	
multifocal (mŭl˝ tĭ-fō´ kăl)	multi- foc -al	many focus pertaining to	Pertaining to or arising from many locations
occlusion (ŏ-kloo´ zhŭn)			Process of closing or state of being closed such as of a passage or lumen
parasternal (păr-ă-stĕrn´ ăl)	para- stern -al	beside sternum, breastbone pertaining to	Pertaining to either side of the sternum (breastbone)
patent (pă´ tĕnt)			Wide open; freely open; for example, a lumen would be patent (opposite of occlusion)
pericardial (pĕr-ĭ-kăr´ dē-ăl)	peri- cardi -al	around heart pertaining to	Pertaining to the pericardium (a fibrous sac surrounding the heart)
polydactyly (pŏl˝ ē-dăk´ tĭ-lē)	poly- dactyl -y	many finger or toe pertaining to	Pertaining to having more than the normal number of fingers and toes; for example, a person having six fingers or toes
premenstrual (prē-mĕn´ stroo-ăl)	pre- menstru -al	before to discharge the menses pertaining to	Pertaining to the number of days before the discharge of the menses (the monthly flow of bloody fluid from the endometrium via the vagina)
react (rē-ăkt´)	re- -act	again to act	Literally means *to act again*; to respond to a stimulus; to participate in a chemical reaction
regurgitation (rē-gŭr˝ jĭ-tā´ shŭn)	re- gurgitat -ion	backward to flood process	Process of a backward flow of solids or foods from the stomach to the mouth or the backflow of blood through a defective heart valve
sign (sīn)			Any objective clinical evidence of an illness or disordered function of the body. A sign can be seen, heard, measured, or felt by the examiner.
subacute (sŭb˝ ă-kūt´)	sub- acute	below sharp	Literally means *below sharp*. It is used to describe the course of a disease process or the healing process following tissue injury; designated as the mid-ground between acute and chronic.

MEDICAL WORD	WORD PARTS		DEFINITION
	Part	Meaning	
superinfection (soo˝ pĕr-ĭn-fĕk´ shŭn)	super- infect -ion	upper, above infect process	An infection following a previous infection produced by an overgrowth of a resistant strain of bacteria, fungi, or yeast. It can occur as an adverse effect of antibiotic usage or overusage.
symptom (sĭm´ tŭm)			Any perceptible change in the function of the body that indicates disease; symptoms may be acute, chronic, relapsing, remitting, and can have a systemic effect or local effect; they can be classified as objective (can be observed and measured), or subjective (felt and described by the patient) and cardinal (the vital signs: T, P, R, and BP).
unconscious (ŭn-kŏn´ shŭs)	un consci -ous	not aware pertaining to	An abnormal state in which the person is not aware of his or her environment. In this state the person experiences no sensory impressions and is unresponsive neurologically.

and Review • Study and Review • Study and Revie
Review • Study and Review • Study and Review • St
ew • **Study and Review** • Study and Review • Study

Identifying Prefixes

Underline the prefixes in the following medical words.

1. apnea	**2.** bradypnea	**3.** dyspnea	**4.** eupnea	**5.** hyperpnea
6. hypopnea	**7.** tachypnea	**8.** binary	**9.** concentration	**10.** extraocular

Defining Prefixes

Give the meaning of the following prefixes.

1. anti- _____	**2.** brachy- _____
3. dia- _____	**4.** hetero- _____
5. homeo- _____	**6.** hydro- _____
7. micro- _____	**8.** oligo- _____
9. pan- _____	**10.** pseudo- _____
11. a- _____	**12.** an- _____
13. bi- _____	**14.** bin- _____
15. con- _____	**16.** de- _____
17. extra- _____	**18.** hyper- _____
19. hypo- _____	**20.** in- _____
21. inter- _____	**22.** multi- _____
23. para- _____	**24.** peri- _____
25. poly- _____	**26.** pre- _____
27. re- _____	**28.** sub- _____
29. super- _____	**30.** un- _____

Spelling

Circle the correct spelling of each medical term.

1. biary / binary

2. concenteration / concentration

3. occlusion / occluson

4. parsternal / parasternal

5. percardial / pericardial

6. latent / latnet

7. patnt / patent

8. unconscious / unconsious

Using Prefixes to Build Medical Words

Using a prefix from the following list, build the appropriate medical word.

| an- | de- | hyper- | multi- | sub- |
| bi- | hypo- | inter- | poly- | un- |

1. Pertaining to without jaundice   _____ icteric

2. Nature of excessive activity   _____ active

3. Pertaining to arising from many locations   _____ focal

4. Failure of a system   _____ compensation

5. Pertaining to situated between two bodies   _____ mediary

6. Having two forks   _____ furcate

7. Pertaining to having more than the normal
   number of fingers and toes   _____ dactyly

8. Underdevelopment of a tissue, organ, or body   _____ plasia

9. Below sharp   _____ acute

10. Pertaining to not being aware   _____ conscious

Identifying Medical Terms

In the spaces provided, write the medical terms for the following meanings.

1. _____ Pertaining to without fever

2. _____ Pertaining to outside the eye

3. _____ Condition of not being able to sleep

4. _____ To stop, inhibit, restrain

5. _____ To remove the kernel of

6. _____ Space within an artery, vein, intestine, or tube

7. _____ Wide open

8. _____ To act again

9. _____ Any objective evidence of an illness

10. _____ Any perceptible change in the function of the body that indicates disease

---

^{PEARSON} mymedicalterminologylab

MyMedicalTerminologyLab is a premium online homework management system that includes a host of features to help you study. Registered users will find:

- Fun games and activities built within a virtual hospital

- Powerful tools that track and analyze your results—allowing you to create a personalized learning experience

- Videos, flashcards, and audio pronunciations to help enrich your progress

- Streaming lesson presentations and self-paced learning modules

- A space where you and your instructors can view and manage your assignments

ar • Special Senses: The Eye • Female Reproductive Sy
with an Overview of Obstetrics • Male Reproductive
m • Oncology • Radiology and Nuclear Medicine • Me
l Health • Introduction to Medical Terminology • Suffixe
refixes • **Organization of the Body** •

4

LEARNING OUTCOMES

On completion of this chapter, you will be
able to:

1. Define terms that describe the body and its
   structural units.

2. List the systems of the body and the organs
   in each system.

3. Define terms that are used to describe
   direction, planes, and cavities of the body.

4. Understand word analysis as it relates to
   head-to-toe assessment.

5. Analyze, build, spell, and pronounce medical
   words.

6. Comprehend the drugs highlighted in this
   chapter.

7. Identify and define selected abbreviations.

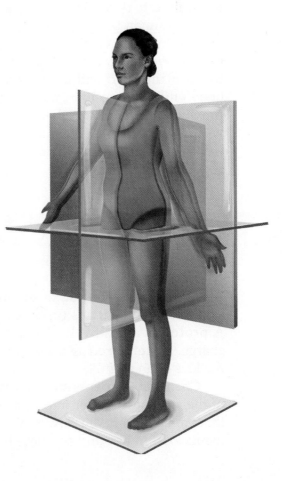

COMBINING FORMS OF THE ORGANIZATION OF THE BODY

adip/o	fat	**kary/o**	cell's nucleus
andr/o	man	**later/o**	side
anter/o	toward the front	**medi/o**	toward the middle
bi/o	life	**organ/o**	organ
caud/o	tail	**path/o**	disease
cran/i	cranium	**phen/o**	to show
cyt/o	cell	**physi/o**	nature
dist/o	away from the point of origin	**poster/o**	behind, toward the back, back
dors/o	backward	**proxim/o**	near the point of origin
hist/o	tissue	**somat/o**	body
hydr/o	water	**ventr/o**	near or on the belly side of the body
infer/o	below		
inguin/o	groin	**viscer/o**	body organs

Anatomy and Physiology

This chapter introduces you to terms describing the body and its structural units. To aid you, these terms have been grouped into two major sections: The first offers an overview of the units that make up the human body, and the second covers terms used to describe anatomical positions and locations.

The human body is made up of atoms, molecules, organelles, cells, tissues, organs, and systems. See Figure 4.1 ■ All of these parts normally function together in a unified and complex process known as **homeostasis** (a state of equilibrium that is maintained within the body's internal environment). This means that the body's fluid composition, its volume and characteristics, its temperature (T), blood pressure (BP), and the exchange of oxygen (O_2) and carbon dioxide (CO_2) remain within normal limits. By maintaining homeostasis, the cells of the body are in an environment that meets their needs and permits them to function optimally under changing conditions.

HUMAN BODY: LEVELS OF ORGANIZATION

Atoms

An **atom** is the smallest, most basic chemical unit of an element. It consists of a nucleus that contains protons and neutrons and is surrounded by electrons. A **proton** is a positively charged particle; a **neutron** is without any electrical charge. An **electron** is a negatively charged particle that revolves about the nucleus of an atom.

Chemical elements are made up of atoms, which can be classified on the basis of their atomic number into groups called elements. An **element** is a substance that cannot be broken down by chemical means into any other substance. Elements exist in free and combined states. More than 100 have been identified.

LEVEL

EXAMPLES

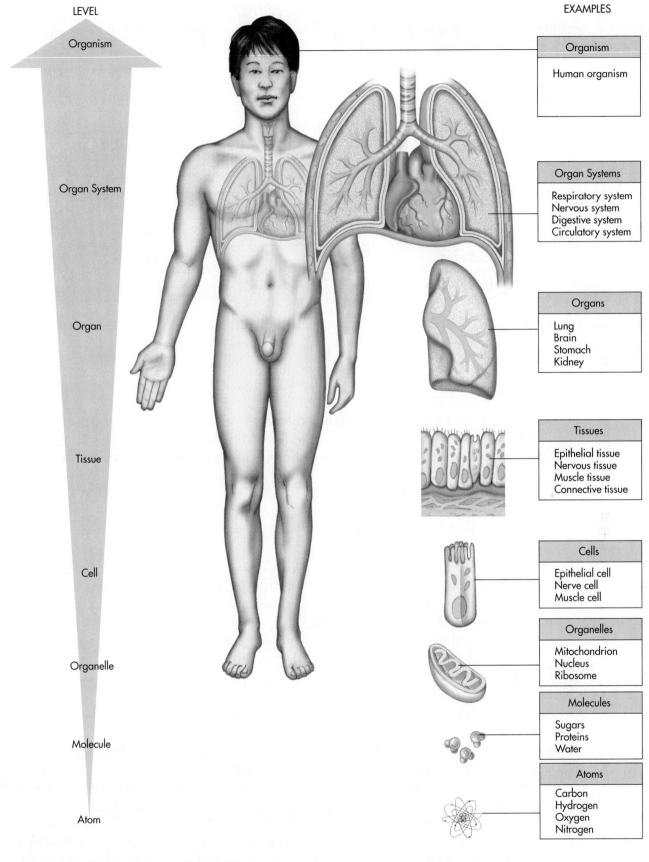

Organism
Human organism

Organ Systems
Respiratory system
Nervous system
Digestive system
Circulatory system

Organs
Lung
Brain
Stomach
Kidney

Tissues
Epithelial tissue
Nervous tissue
Muscle tissue
Connective tissue

Cells
Epithelial cell
Nerve cell
Muscle cell

Organelles
Mitochondrion
Nucleus
Ribosome

Molecules
Sugars
Proteins
Water

Atoms
Carbon
Hydrogen
Oxygen
Nitrogen

Organism

Organ System

Organ

Tissue

Cell

Organelle

Molecule

Atom

■ **Figure 4.1** Human body: levels of organization.

TABLE 4.1 Elements Found in the Human Body

Symbol	Element	Symbol	Element
Al	Aluminum	Mn	Manganese
C	Carbon	Mg	Magnesium
Ca	Calcium	N	Nitrogen
Cl	Chlorine	O or O_2	Oxygen
Co	Cobalt	P	Phosphorus
Cu	Copper	K	Potassium
F	Fluorine	Na	Sodium
H	Hydrogen	S	Sulfur
I	Iodine	Zn	Zinc
Fe	Iron		

Elements found in the human body include aluminum, carbon, calcium, chlorine, cobalt, copper, fluorine, hydrogen, iodine, iron, manganese, magnesium, nitrogen, oxygen, phosphorus, potassium, sodium, sulfur, and zinc. The mass of the human body is made up of just six elements: oxygen, carbon, hydrogen, nitrogen, calcium, and phosphorus. See Table 4.1 ■

Molecules

A **molecule** is a chemical combination of two or more atoms that form a specific chemical compound. In a water molecule (H_2O), oxygen forms polar covalent (sharing of electrons) bonds with two hydrogen atoms. **Water** is a tasteless, clear, odorless liquid that makes up 65% of a male's body weight and 55% of a female's body weight. Water is the most important constituent of all body fluids, secretions, and excretions. It is an ideal transportation medium for inorganic and organic compounds.

Cells

The body consists of millions of cells working individually and with each other to sustain life. For the purposes of this book, **cells** are considered the basic building blocks for the various structures that together make up a human being. There are several types of cells, each specialized to perform specific functions. The size and shape of a cell are generally related directly to its function. See Figure 4.2 ■

For example, cells forming the skin overlap each other to form a protective barrier, whereas nerve cells are usually elongated with branches connecting to other cells for the transmission of sensory impulses. Despite these differences, however, cells can generally be said to have a number of common components. The common parts of the cell are the cell membrane, cytoplasm, and nucleus. See Figure 4.3 ■ and Table 4.2 ■

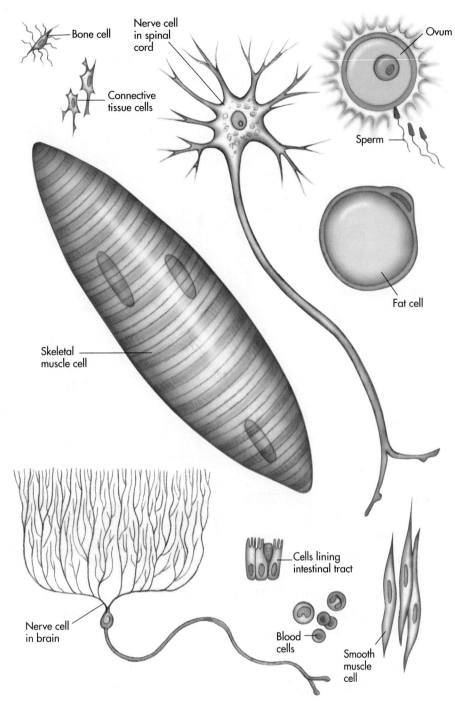

Bone cell

Connective
tissue cells

Nerve cell
in spinal
cord

Ovum

Sperm

Fat cell

Skeletal
muscle cell

Nerve cell
in brain

Cells lining
intestinal tract

Blood
cells

Smooth
muscle
cell

■ **Figure 4.2** Cells are the basic building blocks of the human body. They have many different shapes and vary in size and function. These examples show the range of forms and sizes with the dimensions they would have if magnified approximately 500 times.

Cell Membrane

The outer covering of the cell is called the **cell membrane.** Cell membranes have the capability of allowing some substances to pass into and out of the cell while denying passage to other substances. This selectivity allows cells to receive nutrition and dispose of waste just as a human being eats food and disposes of waste.

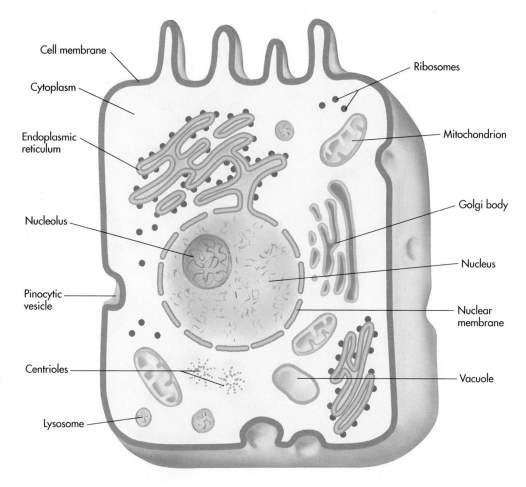

■ **Figure 4.3** Major parts of a cell.

Cytoplasm

Cytoplasm is the substance between the cell membrane and the nuclear membrane. It is a jellylike material that is mostly water. The cytoplasm provides storage and work areas for the cell. The work and storage elements of the cell, called *organelles* (little organs), are the endoplasmic reticulum (ER), ribosomes, Golgi apparatus, mitochondria, lysosomes, and centrioles.

Nucleus

The **nucleus** is responsible for the cell's metabolism, growth, and reproduction. It is the central portion of the cell that contains the **chromosomes** (microscopic bodies that carry the genes that determine hereditary characteristics). A single gene makes up each segment of deoxyribonucleic acid (DNA) and is located in a specific site on the chromosome. The human body has 23 pairs of chromosomes. A **genome** is the complete set of genes and chromosomes tucked inside each of the body's trillions of cells. Genes determine an individual's physical traits such as hair, skin, and eye color, body structure, and metabolic activity.

Stem Cells

Stem cells are the precursors of all body cells. Stem cells have three general properties: They are capable of dividing and renewing themselves for long periods, they are unspecialized, and they can give rise to specialized cell types. Some primary sources of stem cells include embryos, adult tissues, and umbilical cord blood. An embryonic

TABLE 4.2 Major Cell Structures and Primary Functions

Cell Structures	Primary Functions
Cell membrane	Protects the cell; provides for communication via receptor proteins; surface proteins serve as positive identification tags; allows some substances to pass into and out of the cell while denying passage to other substances; this selectivity allows cells to receive nutrition and dispose of waste
Cytoplasm	Provides storage and work areas for the cell; the work and storage elements of the cell, called *organelles,* are the ribosomes, endoplasmic reticulum, Golgi apparatus, mitochondria, lysosomes, and centrioles
Ribosomes	Make enzymes and other proteins; nicknamed "protein factories"
Endoplasmic reticulum (ER)	Carries proteins and other substances through the cytoplasm
Golgi apparatus	Chemically processes the molecules from the endoplasmic reticulum and then packages them into vesicles; nicknamed "chemical processing and packaging center"
Mitochondria	Involved in cellular metabolism and respiration; provides the principle source of cellular energy and is the place where complex, energy-releasing chemical reactions occur continuously; nicknamed "power plants"
Lysosomes	Contain enzymes that can digest food compounds; nicknamed "digestive bags"
Centrioles	Play an important role in cell reproduction
Cilia	Hairlike processes that project from epithelial cells; help propel mucus, dust particles, and other foreign substances from the respiratory tract
Flagellum	"Tail" of the sperm that enables the sperm to "swim" or move toward the ovum
Nucleus	Controls every *organelle* (little organ) in the cytoplasm; contains the genetic matter necessary for cell reproduction as well as control over activity within the cell's cytoplasm; responsible for the cell's metabolism, growth, and reproduction

cell is an unspecialized cell that can turn itself into any type of tissue. It is derived primarily from frozen **in vitro** (in glass, as in a test tube) fertilization embryos. An adult stem cell is a more specialized cell found in many kinds of tissue, such as bone marrow, skin, and the liver. An umbilical cord cell is a rich source of precursors of mature blood cells. It is obtained from cord blood at the time of birth.

Stem cells can now be grown and transformed into specialized cells with characteristics consistent with cells of various tissues such as muscles or nerves through cell culture. Highly plastic adult stem cells from a variety of sources, including umbilical cord blood and bone marrow, are used in medical therapies, which are often referred to as **regenerative** or **reparative medicine.**

Tissues

A **tissue** is a grouping of similar cells that together perform specialized functions. There are four basic types of tissue in the body: **epithelial, connective, muscle,** and **nerve.** Each of the four basic tissues has several subtypes named for their shape, appearance, arrangement, or function. The following sections describe the four basic types of tissue.

Epithelial Tissue

Epithelial tissue appears as sheetlike arrangements of cells, sometimes several layers thick, that form the outer surfaces of the body and line the body cavities and the principal tubes and passageways leading to the exterior. These cells form the secreting portions of glands and their ducts and are important parts of certain sense organs. There are six main functions of epithelial tissue:

1. **Protection.** Protect underlying tissue from mechanical injury, harmful chemicals and pathogens, and excessive water loss.
2. **Sensation.** Sensory stimuli are detected by specialized epithelial cells found in the skin, eyes, ears, and nose and on the tongue.
3. **Secretion.** In glands, epithelial tissue is specialized to secrete specific chemical substances such as enzymes, hormones, and lubricating fluids.
4. **Absorption.** Certain epithelial cells lining the small intestine absorb nutrients from the digestion of food.
5. **Excretion.** Epithelial tissues in the kidney excrete waste products from the body and reabsorb needed materials from the urine. Sweat is also excreted from the body by epithelial cells in the sweat glands.
6. **Diffusion.** Simple epithelium (found in the walls of capillaries and lungs) promotes the diffusion of gases, liquids, and nutrients.

Connective Tissue

The most widespread and abundant of the body tissues, **connective tissue** forms the supporting network for the organs of the body, sheaths the muscles, and connects muscles to bones and bones to joints. Bone is a dense form of connective tissue.

Muscle Tissue

There are three types of muscle tissue:

1. **Skeletal muscle** or *voluntary muscle* is striated in appearance and is anchored by tendons to bone. They are used to effect skeletal movement such as locomotion and in maintaining posture. An average adult male is made up of 42% skeletal muscle and an average adult female is made up of 36% (as a percentage of body mass).
2. **Smooth muscle** or *involuntary muscle* is found within the walls of organs and structures such as the esophagus, stomach, intestines, bronchi, uterus, urethra, bladder, blood vessels, and the arrector pili in the skin. Unlike skeletal muscle, smooth muscle is not under conscious control and is under the control of the autonomic nervous system.
3. **Cardiac muscle** is also an involuntary muscle and is a specialized form of striated tissue found only in the heart. Cardiac muscle is under the control of the autonomic nervous system.

Nerve Tissue

Nerve tissue consists of nerve cells (neurons) and supporting cells called *neuroglia*. It has the properties of excitability and conductivity and functions to control and coordinate the activities of the body.

Organs

Multiple different tissues serving a common purpose or function make up structures called **organs.** Examples are the brain, skin, or heart.

Systems

A group of different organs functioning together for a common purpose is called a **system.** The various body systems function in support of the body as a whole. Figure 4.4 ■ shows the organ systems of the body.

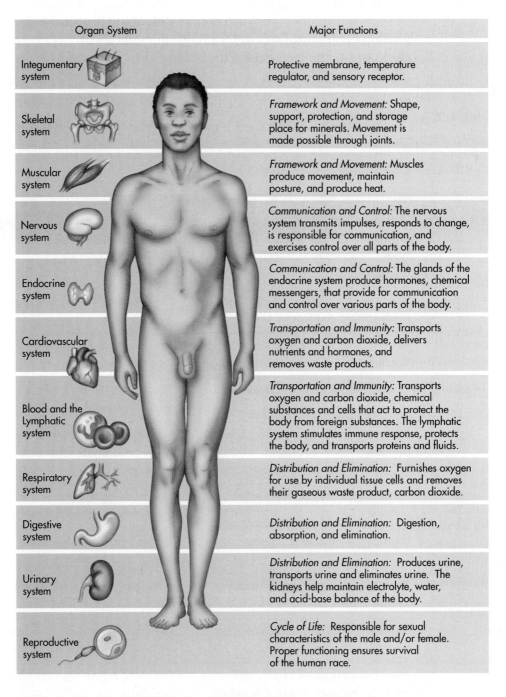

Organ System	Major Functions
Integumentary system	Protective membrane, temperature regulator, and sensory receptor.
Skeletal system	*Framework and Movement:* Shape, support, protection, and storage place for minerals. Movement is made possible through joints.
Muscular system	*Framework and Movement:* Muscles produce movement, maintain posture, and produce heat.
Nervous system	*Communication and Control:* The nervous system transmits impulses, responds to change, is responsible for communication, and exercises control over all parts of the body.
Endocrine system	*Communication and Control:* The glands of the endocrine system produce hormones, chemical messengers, that provide for communication and control over various parts of the body.
Cardiovascular system	*Transportation and Immunity:* Transports oxygen and carbon dioxide, delivers nutrients and hormones, and removes waste products.
Blood and the Lymphatic system	*Transportation and Immunity:* Transports oxygen and carbon dioxide, chemical substances and cells that act to protect the body from foreign substances. The lymphatic system stimulates immune response, protects the body, and transports proteins and fluids.
Respiratory system	*Distribution and Elimination:* Furnishes oxygen for use by individual tissue cells and removes their gaseous waste product, carbon dioxide.
Digestive system	*Distribution and Elimination:* Digestion, absorption, and elimination.
Urinary system	*Distribution and Elimination:* Produces urine, transports urine and eliminates urine. The kidneys help maintain electrolyte, water, and acid-base balance of the body.
Reproductive system	*Cycle of Life:* Responsible for sexual characteristics of the male and/or female. Proper functioning ensures survival of the human race.

■ **Figure 4.4** Organ systems of the body with major functions.

ANATOMICAL LOCATIONS AND POSITIONS

Four primary reference systems have been adopted to provide uniformity to the anatomical description of the body. These reference systems are **direction, planes, cavities,** and **structural unit.** The standard **anatomical position** for the body is erect, head facing forward, arms by the sides with palms to the front. Left and right are from the subject's point of view, not the examiner's.

Direction

Directional and positional terms describe the location of organs or body parts in relationship to one another. They are used in describing physical assessment of a patient's presenting complaints and in pinpointing the location of a given sign or symptom. Table 4.3 ■ lists the terms used to describe direction and position.

Planes

The terms defined on the next page are used to describe the imaginary planes that are depicted in Figure 4.5 ■ as passing through the body and dividing it into various sections.

TABLE 4.3 Directional and Positional Terms

Term	Description	Example
Superior	Above, in an upward direction, toward the head	The head is superior to the neck of the body.
Inferior	Below or in a downward direction; more toward the feet or tail	The feet are inferior to the head of the body.
Anterior (ventral)	In front of or before, the front side of the body	The breasts are located on the anterior side of the body.
Posterior (dorsal)	Toward the back, back side of the body	The nape is the back of the neck and is located on the posterior side of the body.
Cephalic	Pertaining to the head; superior in position	A cephalic presentation is one in which any part of the head of the fetus is presented during delivery.
Caudal	Pertaining to the tail; inferior in position	The cauda equina (horse's tail) is a bundle of spinal nerves below the end of the spinal cord
Medial	Nearest the midline or middle	The umbilicus is a depressed point in the medial area of the abdomen.
Lateral	To the side, away from the middle	In the anatomical position, the arm is located on the lateral side of the body.
Proximal	Nearest the point of attachment or near the beginning of a structure	The proximal end of the humerus (upper bone of the arm) joins with part of the shoulder bone.
Distal	Away from the point of attachment or far from the beginning of a structure	The distal end of the humerus joins with part of the elbow.

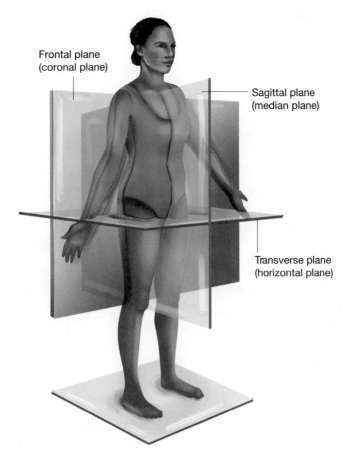

Frontal plane
(coronal plane)

Sagittal plane
(median plane)

Transverse plane
(horizontal plane)

■ **Figure 4.5** Planes of the body.

- **Midsagittal plane.** Vertically divides the body as it passes through the midline to form a **right half** and **left half.**
- **Transverse** or **horizontal plane.** Any plane that divides the body into **superior** and **inferior** portions.
- **Coronal** or **frontal plane.** Any plane that divides the body at right angles to the midsagittal plane. The coronal plane divides the body into **anterior** (ventral) and **posterior** (dorsal) portions.

Cavities

A **cavity** is a hollow space containing body organs. Body cavities are classified into two groups according to their location. On the front are the **ventral cavity** or **anterior cavity** and on the back are the **dorsal cavity** or **posterior cavity.** The various cavities found in the human body are depicted in Figure 4.6 ■

Ventral Cavity

The ventral cavity is the hollow portion of the human torso extending from the neck to the pelvis and containing the heart and the organs of respiration, digestion, reproduction, and elimination. The ventral cavity can be subdivided into three distinct areas: thoracic, abdominal, and pelvic.

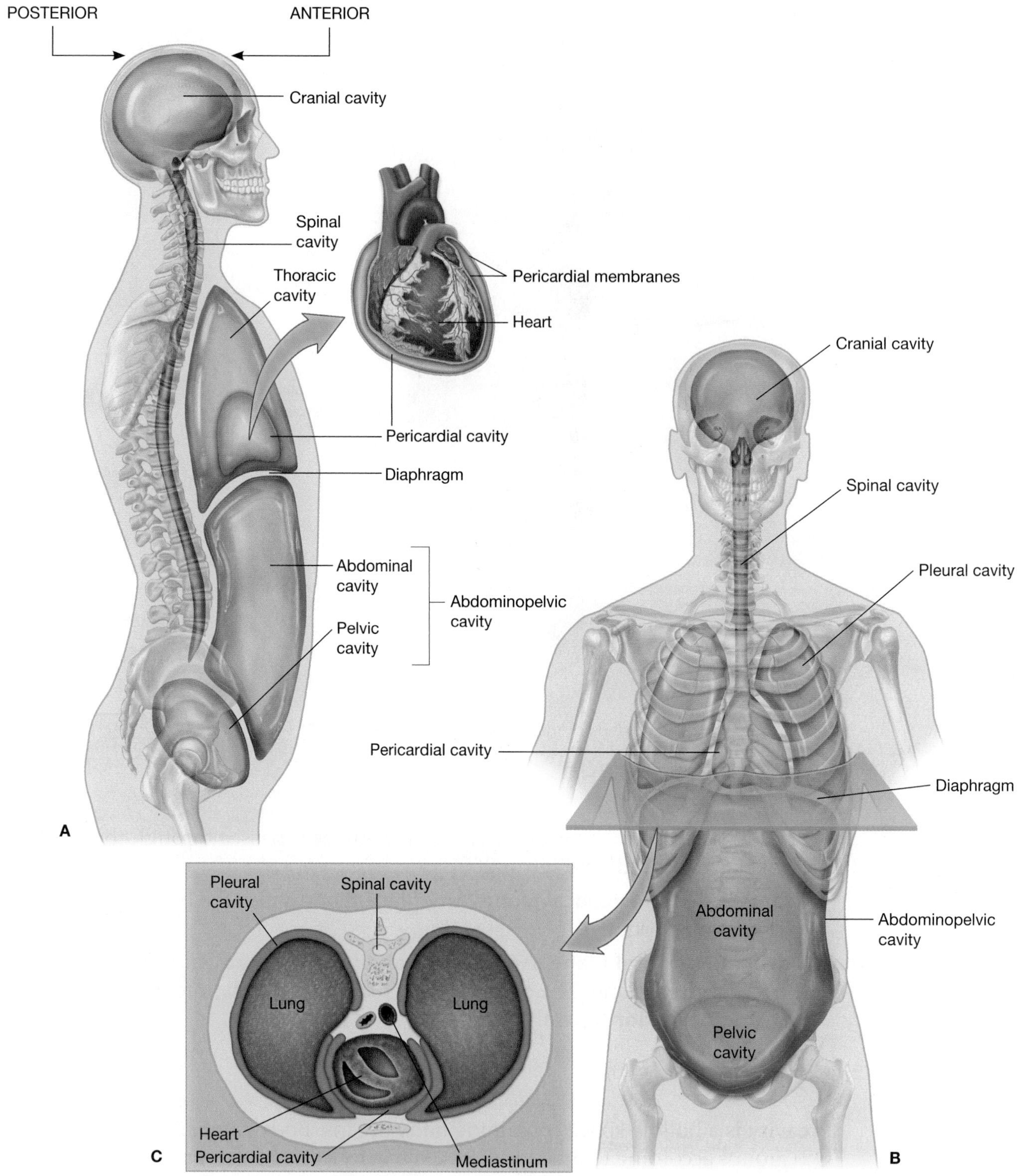

POSTERIOR ANTERIOR

Cranial cavity

Spinal cavity

Thoracic cavity

Pericardial membranes

Heart

Pericardial cavity

Diaphragm

Abdominal cavity

Abdominopelvic cavity

Pelvic cavity

A

Cranial cavity

Spinal cavity

Pleural cavity

Pericardial cavity

Diaphragm

Abdominal cavity

Abdominopelvic cavity

Pelvic cavity

B

Pleural cavity | Spinal cavity

Lung | Lung

Heart
Pericardial cavity

Mediastinum

C

■ **Figure 4.6** Body cavities. (A) Lateral view of a sagittal section through the body. (B) Anterior view of a frontal section through the body. (C) A transverse section through the lower thoracic cavity.

- **Thoracic cavity.** The area of the chest containing the heart and the lungs. Within this cavity, the space containing the **heart** is called the **pericardial** cavity and the spaces surrounding each **lung** are known as the **pleural** cavities. Other organs located in the thoracic cavity are the esophagus, trachea, thymus, and certain large blood and lymph vessels.

- **Abdominal cavity.** The space below the diaphragm, commonly referred to as the *belly*; contains the stomach, intestines, and other organs of digestion.
- **Pelvic cavity.** The space formed by the bones of the pelvic area; contains the organs of reproduction and elimination.

Dorsal Cavity

Containing the structures of the nervous system, the dorsal cavity is subdivided into the cranial cavity and the spinal cavity.

- **Cranial cavity.** The space in the skull containing the brain.
- **Spinal cavity.** The space within the bony spinal column that contains the spinal cord and spinal fluid.

Abdominopelvic Cavity

The **abdominopelvic cavity** is the combination of the abdominal and pelvic cavities. It is divided into nine regions.

Nine Regions of the Abdominopelvic Cavity

As a ready reference for locating visceral organs, anatomists divided the abdominopelvic cavity into nine regions (see Figure 4.7A ■). A tic-tac-toe pattern drawn across the abdominopelvic cavity delineates these regions:

- **Right hypochondriac.** Upper right region at the level of the ninth rib cartilage
- **Left hypochondriac.** Upper left region at the level of the ninth rib cartilage
- **Epigastric.** Region over the stomach
- **Right lumbar.** Right middle lateral region
- **Left lumbar.** Left middle lateral region
- **Umbilical.** In the center, between the right and left lumbar region; at the navel
- **Right iliac (inguinal).** Right lower lateral region
- **Left iliac (inguinal).** Left lower lateral region
- **Hypogastric.** Lower middle region below the navel

Abdomen Divided into Quadrants

The **abdomen** is divided into four corresponding regions that are used for descriptive and diagnostic purposes. By using these regions, one may describe the exact location of pain, a skin lesion, surgical incision, and/or abdominal tumor. See Figure 4.7B ■

- **Right upper quadrant (RUQ).** Contains the right lobe of the liver, gallbladder, part of the pancreas, and part of the small and large intestines
- **Left upper quadrant (LUQ).** Contains the left lobe of the liver, stomach, spleen, part of the pancreas, and part of the small and large intestines
- **Right lower quadrant (RLQ).** Contains part of the small and large intestines, appendix, right ovary, right fallopian tube, right ureter
- **Left lower quadrant (LLQ).** Contains part of the small and large intestines, left ovary, left fallopian tube, left ureter

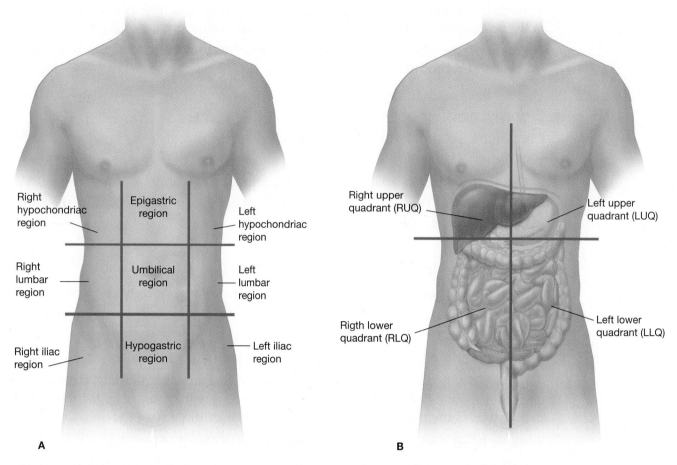

■ **Figure 4.7** (A) The nine regions of the abdominopelvic cavity. (B) The four regions of the abdomen, which are referred to as *quadrants.*

Note: Some organs, such as the urinary bladder and uterus, are located half in the right quadrant and half in the left quadrant. These organs are generally referred to as being in the *midline* of the body.

HEAD-TO-TOE ASSESSMENT

The terminology associated with head-to-toe assessment can be useful when studying the organization of the body and in understanding information contained in a patient's medical record. Body areas, along with their word parts and/or related terminology, are provided to enhance your learning process. See Table 4.4 ■

TABLE 4.4 Body Area Terminology

Body Area	Word Part(s)	Body Area	Word Part(s)
abdomen (belly)	abdomin/o	back	poster/o
ankle (tarsus)	tars/o	bones	oste/o
arm	brach/i	breast	mast/o; mamm/o

TABLE 4.4 Body Area Terminology (continued)

Body Area	Word Part(s)	Body Area	Word Part(s)
cheek	bucc/o	navel	umbilic/o; omphal/o
chest	thorac/o	neck	cervic/o
ear	ot/o	nerves	neur/o
elbow	cubital; olecran/o	nose	rhin/o; nas/o
eye	ophthalm/o; ocul/o; opt/o	ribs	cost/o
finger	dactyl/o	side	later/o
foot	pod/o	skin	derm/a; dermat/o; derm/o; cutane/o
gums	gingiv/o	skull	crani/o
hand	manus; chir/o	stomach	gastr/o
head	cephal/o	teeth	dent/i
heart	cardi/o	temples	tempor/o
hip or hip joint	coxa	thigh bone	femor/o
leg	crur/o	throat	pharyng/o
liver	hepat/o	thumb	pollex
lungs	pulm/o; pulmon/o; pneum/o; pneumon/o	tongue	lingu/o; gloss/o
mouth	or/o	wrist	carp/o
muscles	muscul/o		

Anatomy and Physiology Labeling

Identify the structures shown below by filling in the blanks.

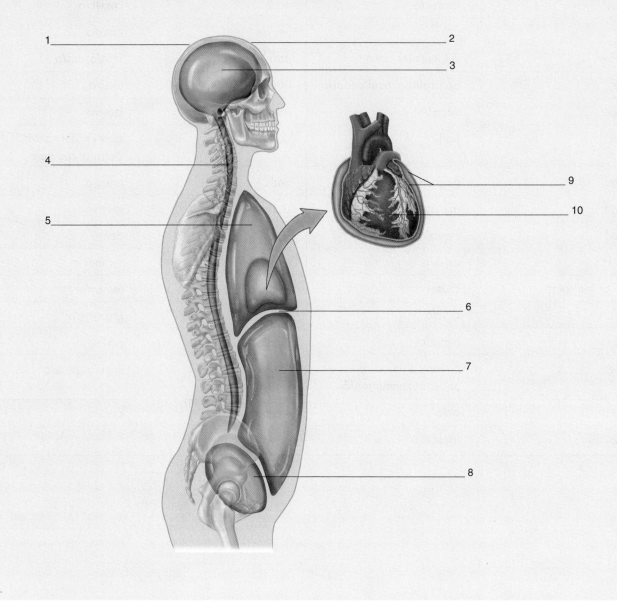

1_____ 2

3

4_____

5_____

9

10

6

7

8

• Building Your Medical Vocabulary •

This section provides the foundation for learning medical terminology. Review the following alphabetized word list. Note how common prefixes and suffixes are repeatedly applied to word roots and combining forms to create different meanings. The word parts are color-coded: prefixes are green, suffixes are blue, roots/combining forms are red.

You will find that some terms have not been divided into word parts. These are common words or specialized terms that are included to enhance your medical vocabulary. See Chapter 1, page 7, to review pronunciation guidelines.

MEDICAL WORD	WORD PARTS		DEFINITION
	Part	Meaning	
adipose (ăd˝ ĭ-pōs)	adip -ose	fat pertaining to	Pertaining to fatty tissue throughout the body
ambilateral (ăm˝ bĭ-lăt´ ĕr-ăl)	ambi- later -al	both side pertaining to	Pertaining to both sides
anatomy (ăn-ăt´ ō-mē)	ana- -tomy	up; apart incision	Literally means *to cut up* or *to cut apart*; the study of the structure of an organism such as humans. A specialist in the field of anatomy can learn about the structure of the human body by cutting it apart. This process is called **dissection.**
android (ăn´ droyd)	andr -oid	man resemble	To resemble man
anterior (an-tĕr´ ē-ōr)	anter -ior	toward the front pertaining to	Pertaining to a surface or part situated toward the front of the body
apex (ā´ pĕks)			Pointed end of a cone-shaped structure
base (bās)			Lower part or foundation of a structure
bilateral (bĭ-lăt´ ĕr-ăl)	bi- later -al	two side pertaining to	Pertaining to two sides
biology (bī-ŏl´ ō-jē)	bi/o -logy	life study of	Study of life

MEDICAL WORD	WORD PARTS		DEFINITION
	Part	**Meaning**	
caudal (kŏd´ ăl)	caud -al	tail pertaining to	Pertaining to the tail
center (sĕn´ tĕr)			Midpoint of a body or activity
chromosome (krō-mō-sōm)	chromo- -some	color body	Microscopic bodies in the nucleus that carry the genes that determine hereditary characteristics
cilia (sĭl´ ē-ă)			Hairlike processes that project from epithelial cells; they help propel mucus, dust particles, and other foreign substances from the respiratory tract
cranial (krā-nē-ăl)	cran/i -al	cranium pertaining to	Pertaining to the cranium (the portion of the skull that contains the brain)
cytology (sĭ-tŏl´ ō-jē)	cyt/o -logy	cell study of	Study of cells
deep			Far down from the surface
dehydrate (dē-hī´ drāt)	de- hydr -ate	down, away from water use, action	To remove water; to lose or be deprived of water from the body; to become dry
diffusion (di-fū´ zhŭn)	dif- fus -ion	apart to pour process	The process whereby particles in a fluid move from an area of high concentration to an area of lower concentration, resulting in an even distribution of the particles in the fluid
distal (dĭs´ tăl)	dist -al	away from the point of origin pertaining to	Farthest from the center or point of origin
dorsal (dōr´ săl)	dors -al	backward pertaining to	Pertaining to the back side of the body
ectomorph (ĕk´ tō-morf)	ecto- -morph	outside form, shape	Slender physical body form; linear physique
endomorph (ĕn˝ dō-morf)	endo- -morph	within form, shape	Round and soft physical body form
filtration (fĭl-trā´ shŭn)	filtrat -ion	to strain through process	Process of filtering or straining particles from a solution

MEDICAL WORD	WORD PARTS		DEFINITION
	Part	**Meaning**	
gene (jēn)			Hereditary unit that transmits and determines one's characteristics or hereditary traits
histology (hĭs-tŏl´ ō-jē)	hist/o -logy	tissue study of	Study of tissue
homeostasis (hō˝ mē-ō-stā´ sĭs)	homeo- -stasis	similar, same control, stop, stand still	State of equilibrium maintained in the body's internal environment; an important fundamental principle of physiology that permits a body to maintain a constant internal environment despite changes in the external environment
horizontal (hŏr´ ă-zŏn´ tăl)	horizont -al	horizon pertaining to	Pertaining to the horizon, of or near the horizon, lying flat, even, level
human genome (hŭ´ măn jē´ nōm)			Complete set of genes and chromosomes tucked inside each of the body's trillions of cells
inferior (ĭn-fē´ rē-or)	infer -ior	below pertaining to	Pertaining to below or in a downward direction
inguinal (ĭng´ gwĭ-năl)	inguin -al	groin pertaining to	Pertaining to the groin, of or near the groin
internal (ĭntĕr´ nal)	intern -al	within pertaining to	Pertaining to within or the inside
karyogenesis (kăr˝ i-ō-jĕn´ ĕ-sĭs)	kary/o -genesis	cell's nucleus formation, produce	Formation of a cell's nucleus
lateral (Lat, lat) (lăt´ ĕr-ăl)	later -al	side pertaining to	Pertaining to the side
medial (mē´ dēal)	medi -al	toward the middle pertaining to	Pertaining to the middle or midline
mesomorph (mĕs´ ō-morf)	meso- -morph	middle form, shape	Well-proportioned body form marked by predominance of tissue derived from the mesoderm (the middle layer of cells in the developing embryo)
organic (or-găn´ ĭk)	organ -ic	organ pertaining to	Pertaining to an organ or organs; pertaining to or derived from vegetable or animal forms of life

MEDICAL WORD	WORD PARTS		DEFINITION
	Part	**Meaning**	
pathology (pă-thŏl´ ō-jē)	path/o -logy	disease study of	Study of disease
perfusion (pur-fū´ zhŭn)	per- fus -ion	through to pour process	Literally means *a process of pouring through;* as passing of a fluid through spaces; to supply the body with nutritive fluid via the bloodstream
phenotype (fē´ nō-tīp)	phen/o -type	to show type	Physical appearance or type of makeup of an individual
physiology (fiz˝ i-ŏl´ ō-jē)	physi/o -logy	nature study of	Study of the function (nature) of living organisms; anatomy and physiology (A&P) is the combination of the study of the anatomy and physiology of the human body
posterior (pŏs-tē´ rĭ-ōr)	poster -ior	behind, toward the back pertaining to	Pertaining to the back part of a structure; toward the back
protoplasm (prō-tō-plăzm)	proto- -plasm	first a thing formed, plasma	Essential matter inside of a living cell
proximal (prŏk´ sĭm-ăl)	proxim -al	near the point of origin pertaining to	Nearest the center or point of origin; nearest the point of attachment
somatotrophic (sō˝ mă-tō-trŏf´ ĭk)	somat/o troph -ic	body a turning pertaining to	Pertaining to stimulation of body growth
superficial (sŭ˝ pĕr-fĭsh´ ăl)			Pertaining to the surface, on or near the surface
superior (sŭ-pēr´ rĭ-ōr)	super- -ior	upper, above pertaining to	Pertaining to above or in an upward direction
systemic (sis-tĕm´ ĭk)	system -ic	composite whole pertaining to	Pertaining to the body as a whole
topical (tŏp´ ĭ-kăl)	topic -al	place pertaining to	Pertaining to a place, definite locale

MEDICAL WORD	WORD PARTS		DEFINITION
	Part	Meaning	
unilateral (ŭ″ nĭ-lăt′ ĕr-ăl)	uni- later -al	one side pertaining to	Pertaining to one side
ventral (věn′ trăl)	ventr -al	near the belly side pertaining to	Pertaining to the front side of the body, abdomen, belly surface
vertex (věr′ těks)			Top or highest point; top or crown of the head
visceral (vĭs′ ĕr-ăl)	viscer -al	body organs pertaining to	Pertaining to body organs enclosed within a cavity, especially abdominal organs

• Drug Highlights •

A **drug** is a chemical substance that can alter or modify the functions of a living organism.

There are thousands of drugs that are available as over-the-counter (OTC) medicines and do not require a prescription. A prescription is a written legal document that gives directions for compounding, dispensing, and administering a medication to a patient.

In general, there are five medical uses for drugs. These are therapeutic, diagnostic, curative, replacement, and preventive or prophylactic.

Therapeutic use. Used in the treatment of a disease or condition, such as an allergy, to relieve the symptoms or to sustain the patient until other measures are instituted.

Diagnostic use. Certain drugs are used in conjunction with radiology to allow the physician to pinpoint the location of a disease process.

Curative use. Certain drugs, such as antibiotics, kill or remove the causative agent of a disease.

Replacement use. Certain drugs, such as hormones and vitamins, are used to replace or supplement substances normally found in the body.

Preventive or **prophylactic use.** Certain drugs, such as immunizing agents, are used to ward off or lessen the severity of a disease.

drug names   Most drugs may be cited by their chemical, generic, and trade or brand (proprietary) name. The *chemical name* is usually the formula that denotes the composition of the drug. It is made up of letters and numbers that represent the drug's molecular structure. The *generic name* is the drug's official name and is descriptive of its chemical structure and is written in lowercase letters. A generic drug can be manufactured by more than one pharmaceutical company. When this is the case, each company markets the drug under its own unique trade or brand name. A *trade* or *brand name* (*proprietary*) is registered by the U.S. Patent Office as well as approved by the U.S. Food and Drug Administration (FDA). A trade or brand name is capitalized.

Example: Chemical name: 4-hydroxyl-2-methyl-N-2-pyridinyl-2H-1, 2-benzothiazine3-carboxamide 1, 1-dioxide

Generic name: piroxicam

Trade or Brand name: Feldene (nonsterioidal anti-inflammatory drug)

undesirable actions of drugs

Most drugs have the potential for causing an action other than their intended action. For example, antibiotics that are administered orally may disrupt the normal bacterial flora of the gastrointestinal (GI) tract and cause gastric discomfort. This type of reaction is known as a *side effect*. An *adverse reaction* is an unfavorable or harmful unintended action of a drug. For example, the adverse reaction of Demerol may be light-headedness, dizziness, sedation, nausea, and sweating. A *drug interaction* can occur when one drug potentiates (increases the action) or diminishes the action of another drug. Drugs can also interact with foods, alcohol, tobacco, and other substances.

medication order and dosage

The *medication order* is given for a specific patient and denotes the name of the drug, the dosage, the form of the drug, the time for or frequency of administration, and the route by which the drug is to be given.

The *dosage* is the amount of medicine that is prescribed for administration. The form of the drug can be liquid, solid, semisolid, tablet, capsule, transdermal therapeutic patch, etc.

The *route of administration* can be by mouth, by injection, into the eye(s), ear(s), nostril(s), rectum, vagina, etc. It is important for the patient to know when and how to take a medication.

• Abbreviations •

ABBREVIATION	MEANING	ABBREVIATION	MEANING
abd	abdomen	GI	gastrointestinal
A&P	anatomy and physiology	H$_2$O	water
CO$_2$	carbon dioxide	LAT, lat	lateral
DNA	deoxyribonucleic acid	LLQ	left lower quadrant
ENT	ear, nose, throat (otorhinolaryngology)	LUQ	left upper quadrant
		O or O$_2$	oxygen
ER	endoplasmic reticulum (as used in this chapter); also means emergency room	OTC	over-the-counter (drugs)
		RLQ	right lower quadrant
		RUQ	right upper quadrant

Anatomy and Physiology

Write your answers to the following questions.

1. The _____ consist of millions of _____ working individually and with each other to _____ life.

2. The outer covering of the cell is known as the _____ , which has the capability of allowing some substances to pass into and out of the cell.

3. The common parts of the cell are the _____ , _____ , and _____ .

4. Three functions of the cell's nucleus are _____ , _____ , and _____ .

5. An _____ is an unspecialized cell that can turn itself into any type of tissue.

6. List the six functions of epithelial tissue.

   a. _____   b. _____

   c. _____   d. _____

   e. _____   f. _____

7. _____ tissue is the most widespread and abundant of the four body tissues.

8. Name the three types of muscle tissue.

   a. _____   b. _____

   c. _____

9. Two properties of nerve tissue are _____ and _____ .

10. Define *organ*. _____ .

11. Define *body system*. _____ .

12. Name the organ systems listed in this text.

   a. _____   b. _____

   c. _____   d. _____

   e. _____   f. _____

g. _____   h. _____

i. _____   j. _____

k. _____

13. Define the following directional terms.

   a. superior _____   **b.** anterior _____

   c. posterior _____   **d.** cephalic _____

   e. medial _____   **f.** lateral _____

   g. proximal _____   **h.** distal _____

14. The _____ vertically divides the body. It passes through
    the midline to form a right and left half.

15. The _____ plane is any plane that divides the body into superior and inferior portions.

16. The _____ plane is any plane that divides the body at right angles to the plane
    described in Question 14.

17. List the three distinct cavities that are located in the ventral cavity.

   a. _____   **b.** _____

   c. _____

18. Name the two distinct cavities located in the dorsal cavity.

   a. _____   **b.** _____

Word Parts

PREFIXES

Give the definitions of the following prefixes.

1. ambi- _____   **2.** ana- _____

3. bi- _____   **4.** chromo- _____

5. de- _____   **6.** dif- _____

7. ecto- _____   **8.** endo- _____

9. homeo- _____   **10.** meso- _____

11. per- _____   **12.** proto- _____

13. uni- _____   **14.** super- _____

ROOTS AND COMBINING FORMS

Give the definitions of the following roots and combining forms.

1. adip _____
2. andr _____
3. bi/o _____
4. caud _____
5. cyt _____
6. cyt/o _____
7. fus _____
8. hist/o _____
9. hydr _____
10. kary/o _____
11. later _____
12. path/o _____
13. physi/o _____
14. pin/o _____
15. somat/o _____
16. topic _____
17. troph _____
18. viscer _____
19. anter _____
20. cran/i _____
21. dist _____
22. dors _____
23. filtrat _____
24. horizont _____
25. infer _____
26. inguin _____
27. intern _____
28. later _____
29. medi _____
30. organ _____
31. phen/o _____
32. poster _____
33. proxim _____
34. system _____
35. ventr _____

SUFFIXES

Give the definitions for the following suffixes.

1. -al _____
2. -ate _____
3. -genesis _____
4. -ic _____
5. -ion _____
6. -logy _____
7. -morph _____
8. -oid _____
9. -ose _____
10. -plasm _____
11. -some _____
12. -stasis _____

13. -tomy _____ **14.** -ior _____

15. -ad _____ **16.** -type _____

Identifying Medical Terms

In the spaces provided, write the medical terms for the following meanings.

1. _____ To resemble man

2. _____ Pertaining to two sides

3. _____ Study of cells

4. _____ Slender physical body form

5. _____ Formation of a cell's nucleus

6. _____ Pertaining to the stimulation of body growth

7. _____ Pertaining to one side

Spelling

Circle the correct spelling of each medical term.

1. adipose / adpose

2. caual / caudal

3. cytology / cytlogy

4. diffusion / difusion

5. histology / histlogy

6. mesmorph / mesomorph

7. perfusion / prefusion

8. proximal / proxmal

9. somattrophic / somatotrophic

10. unilateral / unlateral

Matching

Select the appropriate lettered meaning for each of the following words.

_____ 1. ambilateral

_____ 2. anatomy

_____ 3. atom

_____ 4. chromosome

_____ 5. cilia

_____ 6. homeostasis

_____ 7. human genome

_____ 8. phenotype

_____ 9. physiology

_____ 10. vertex

a. Hairlike processes that project from epithelial cells

b. Top or highest point

c. Pertaining to both sides

d. Study of the structure of an organism such as a human

e. Smallest, most basic chemical unit of an element

f. Microscopic bodies that carry the genes that determine hereditary characteristics

g. Complete set of genes and chromosomes

h. Physical appearance or type of makeup of an individual

i. State of equilibrium maintained in the body's internal environment

j. Study of the nature of a living organism

k. Study of disease

Abbreviations

Place the correct word, phrase, or abbreviation in the space provided.

1. abd _____

2. A & P _____

3. DNA _____

4. ear, nose, throat _____

5. gastrointestinal _____

6. H_2O _____

7. LLQ _____

8. oxygen _____

9. over-the-counter (drugs) _____

10. RUQ _____

PEARSON mymedicalterminologylab

MyMedicalTerminologyLab is a premium online homework management system that includes a host of features to help you study. Registered users will find:

- Fun games and activities built within a virtual hospital
- Powerful tools that track and analyze your results—allowing you to create a personalized learning experience
- Videos, flashcards, and audio pronunciations to help enrich your progress
- Streaming lesson presentations and self-paced learning modules
- A space where you and your instructors can view and manage your assignments

emale Reproductive System with an Overview of Obste
s • Male Reproductive System • Oncology • adiology
d Nuclear Medicine • Mental Health • Introduc on to
cal Terminology • Suffixes • Prefixes • Organizati n of
Body • **Integumentary System** • Skeletal System •

5

LEARNING OUTCOMES

On completion of this chapter, you will
be able to:

1. Describe the integumentary system
   and its accessory structures.

2. List the functions of the skin.

3. Analyze, build, spell, and pronounce
   medical words.

4. Comprehend the drugs highlighted
   in this chapter.

5. Describe diagnostic and laboratory tests
   related to the integumentary system.

6. Identify and define selected abbreviations.

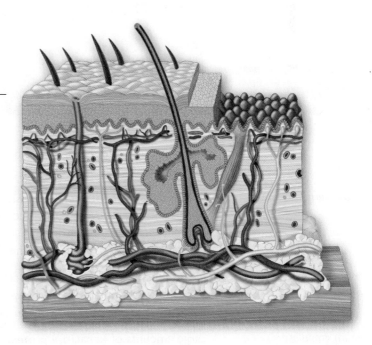

COMBINING FORMS OF THE INTEGUMENTARY SYSTEM

acr/o	extremity	**kerat/o**	horn
aden/o	gland	**leuk/o**	white
albin/o	white	**melan/o**	black
ang/i	vessel	**myc/o**	fungus
carcin/o	cancer	**onych/o**	nail
caus/o	heat	**pachy/o**	thick
cellul/o	little cell	**pedicul/o**	a louse
cutane/o	skin	**plak/o**	plate
derm/a	skin	**prurit/o**	itching
derm/o	skin	**rhytid/o**	wrinkle
dermat/o	skin	**scler/o**	hard, hardening
erythr/o	red	**seb/o**	oil
follicul/o	little bag	**therm/o**	hot, heat
hidr/o	sweat	**trich/o**	hair
icter/o	jaundice	**vuls/o**	to pull
integument/o	a covering	**xanth/o**	yellow
kel/o	tumor	**xer/o**	dry

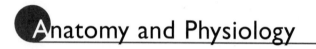

Anatomy and Physiology

The integumentary system is composed of the skin, the largest organ of the body, and its accessory structures, the hair, nails, sebaceous glands, and sweat glands. Table 5.1 ■ provides an at-a-glance look at the integumentary system.

TABLE 5.1 Integumentary System at-a-Glance

Organ/Structure	Primary Functions/Description
Skin	Protection, regulation, sensation, and secretion
Epidermis	Outer protective covering of the body that can be divided into five strata (*in order as the layers evolve and mature*)
Stratum germinativum	Innermost epidermal layer responsible for regeneration of the epidermis. Damage to this layer, as in severe burns, necessitates the use of skin grafts (SG). **Melanin**, the pigment that gives color to the skin, is formed in this layer. The more abundant the melanin, the darker the color of the skin.
Stratum spinosum	Means "spiny layer." Each time a stem cell divides, one of the daughter cells is pushed into this layer. Contains Langerhans cells, which are responsible for stimulating a defense against invading microorganisms and superficial skin cancers.
Stratum granulosum	Large amounts of **keratin**, a protein substance, is made. In humans, keratin is the basic structural component of hair and nails.
Stratum lucidum	Present in thick skin of the palms and soles. Cells are flattened, densely packed, and filled with keratin.

Organ/Structure	Primary Functions/Description
TABLE 5.1 Integumentary System at-a-Glance (*continued*)	
Stratum corneum	Outermost, horny layer, consisting of dead cells. Cells active in the **keratinization** process, during which the cells lose their nuclei and become hard or horny. Forms protective covering for the body
Dermis	Nourishes the epidermis, provides strength, and supports blood vessels
Papillae	Produce ridges that are one's fingerprints
Subcutaneous tissue	Supports, nourishes, insulates, and cushions the skin
Hair	Provides sensation and some protection for the head. Hair around the eyes, in the nose, and in the ears filters out foreign particles.
Nails	Protects ends of fingers and toes
Sebaceous (oil) glands	Lubricates the hair and skin
Sudoriferous (sweat) glands	Secretes sweat or perspiration, which helps to cool the body by evaporation. Sweat also rids the body of waste.

FUNCTIONS OF THE SKIN

The **skin** is the external covering of the body. In an average adult, it covers more than 3,000 square inches of surface area, weighs more than 6 pounds, and is the largest organ of the body. The skin is well supplied with blood vessels and nerves and has four main functions: protection, regulation, sensation, and secretion.

Protection

The skin serves as a protective membrane against invasion by bacteria and other potentially harmful agents that could try to penetrate into deeper tissues. It protects against mechanical injury of delicate cells located beneath its epidermis or outer covering. The skin also serves to inhibit excessive loss of water and electrolytes and provides a reservoir for storing food and water. The skin guards the body against excessive exposure to the sun's ultraviolet rays by producing a protective pigmentation, and it helps to produce the body's supply of vitamin D.

Regulation

The skin serves to raise or lower body temperature as necessary. When the body needs to lose heat, the blood vessels in the skin dilate, bringing more blood to the surface for cooling by **radiation**. At the same time, the sweat glands are secreting more sweat for cooling by means of **evaporation**. Conversely, when the body needs to conserve heat, the reflex actions of the nervous system cause the skin's blood vessels to constrict, thereby allowing more heat-carrying blood to circulate to the muscles and vital organs.

Sensation

The skin contains millions of microscopic nerve endings that act as **sensory receptors** for pain, touch, heat, cold, and pressure. When stimulation occurs, nerve impulses are sent to the cerebral cortex of the brain. The nerve endings in the skin are specialized according to the type of sensory information transmitted and, once this information reaches the brain, it triggers any necessary response. For example, touching a hot surface with the hand causes the brain to recognize the senses of **touch**, **heat**, and **pain** and results in the immediate removal of the hand from the hot surface.

Secretion

The skin contains millions of sweat glands, which secrete **perspiration** or **sweat**, and **sebaceous glands**, which secrete **oil** (sebum) for lubrication. Perspiration is largely water with a small amount of salt and other chemical compounds. This secretion, when left to accumulate, causes body odor, especially where it is trapped among hairs in the axillary region. **Sebum** is an oily secretion that acts to protect the body from dehydration and possible absorption of harmful substances.

LIFE SPAN CONSIDERATIONS

Before birth, **vernix caseosa**, a cheeselike substance, covers the fetus. At first, the fetal skin is transparent and blood vessels are clearly visible. In about 13–16 weeks, downy lanugo hair begins to develop, especially on the head. At 21–24 weeks, the skin is reddish and wrinkled and has little subcutaneous fat. At birth, the subcutaneous glands are developed, and the skin is smooth and pink. Newborns have less subcutaneous fat than adults; therefore, they are more sensitive to heat and cold.

LAYERS OF THE SKIN

The skin is essentially composed of two layers, the epidermis and the dermis. See Figure 5.1 ■

Epidermis

The **epidermis** is the outer layer of skin. The thickness of the epidermis varies in different types of skin. It is the thinnest on the eyelids at 0.05 mm and the thickest on the palms and soles at 1.5 mm.

The **epidermis** can be divided into five strata: the stratum germinativum, the stratum spinosum, the stratum granulosum, the stratum lucidum, and the stratum corneum. See Table 5.1 for the functions, descriptions, and locations of these strata within the epidermis.

Dermis

Sometimes called the **corium** or **true skin**, the **dermis** is composed of connective tissue containing lymphatics, nerves and nerve endings, blood vessels, sebaceous and sweat glands, elastic fibers, and hair follicles. It is divided into two layers: the

LIFE SPAN CONSIDERATIONS

As a person ages, the skin becomes looser as the dermal papilla becomes thinner. Collagen and elastic fibers of the upper dermis decrease and skin loses its elastic tone and wrinkles more easily.

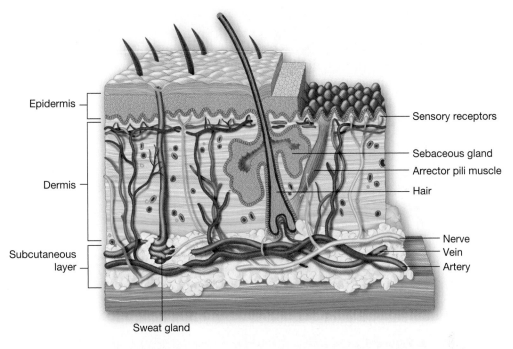

■ **Figure 5.1** The integument: the epidermis, dermis, subcutaneous tissue, and its appendages.

upper layer or **papillary layer** and the **lower layer** or **reticular layer**. The papillary layer is arranged into parallel rows of microscopic structures called **papillae**, which produce the ridges of the skin that are one's fingerprints or footprints. The reticular layer is composed of white fibrous tissue that supports the blood vessels. The dermis is attached to underlying structures by the **subcutaneous tissue** (see Figure 5.1). This tissue supports, nourishes, insulates, and cushions the skin.

ACCESSORY STRUCTURES OF THE SKIN

The hair, nails, sebaceous glands, and sweat glands are the accessory structures of the skin.

Hair

A **hair** is a thin, threadlike structure formed by a group of cells that develop within a hair **follicle** or **socket**. See Figure 5.2 ■ Each hair is composed of a **shaft**, which is the visible portion, and a **root**, which is embedded within the follicle. At the base of each follicle is a loop of capillaries enclosed within connective tissue called the **hair papilla**. The **pilomotor muscle** attaches to the side of each follicle. When the skin is cooled or the individual has an emotional reaction, the skin often forms

LIFE SPAN CONSIDERATIONS

By age 50, approximately half of all people have some gray hair. Scalp hair thins in women and men. The hair becomes dry and often brittle. Some older women may have an increase in facial hair due to hormonal changes. Some men may have an increase in hair of the nares (nostrils), eyebrows, or helix of the ear. In addition to the changes in the skin and hair, nails can flatten and become discolored, dry, and brittle.

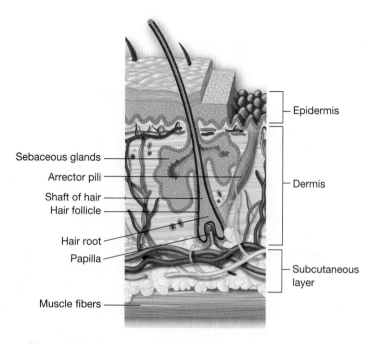

■ **Figure 5.2** Cross-section of skin and a hair follicle. Note the shaft of the hair, the root, and papilla.

"gooseflesh" as a result of contraction by these muscles. Hair is distributed over the whole body with the exception of the palms of the hands, soles of the feet, and the penis. It is thicker on the scalp and thinner on the other parts of the body. Hair around the eyes, in the nose, and in the ears serves to filter out foreign particles. Hair grows at approximately 0.5 inch a month, and its growth is not affected by cutting.

Nails

Fingernails and **toenails** are horny cell structures of the epidermis and are composed of hard keratin. A nail consists of a **body**, a **root**, and a **matrix** or **nailbed** (Figure 5.3 ■). The white, crescent-shaped area of the nail is the **lunula** (little moon). Nail growth may vary with age, disease, and hormone deficiency. Average growth is 1 mm per week, and a lost fingernail usually regenerates in $3\frac{1}{2}$ to $5\frac{1}{2}$ months. A lost toenail may require 6–8 months for regeneration.

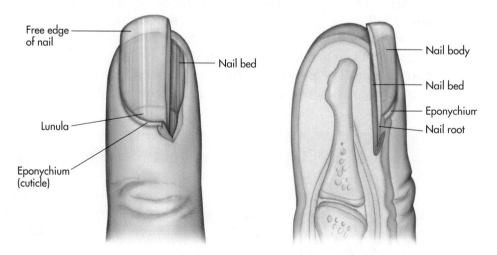

■ **Figure 5.3** The fingernail, an appendage of the integument.

Sebaceous (Oil) Glands

The oil-secreting glands of the skin are called **sebaceous glands**. They have tiny ducts that open into the hair follicles, and their secretion, **sebum**, lubricates the hair as well as the skin. The amount of secretion is controlled by the endocrine system and varies with age, puberty, and pregnancy.

Sudoriferous (Sweat) Glands

Sweat glands (coiled, tubular glands) are distributed over the entire surface of the body with the exception of the margin of the lips, glans penis, and the inner surface of the prepuce. The skin contains two types of sweat glands, apocrine and merocrine. These names refer to the mechanism of secretion. Apocrine sweat glands are located in the armpits (axillae), around the nipples, and in the groin. They secrete their products into hair follicles. Apocrine sweat glands begin secreting at puberty. Merocrine sweat glands are coiled tubular glands that discharge their secretions directly onto the surface of the skin. The adult integument contains 2 to 5 million merocrine sweat glands, with the most numerous being in the palms of the hands and soles of the feet. Sweat glands secrete sweat or perspiration, which helps to cool the body by evaporation. Sweat also rids the body of waste through the pores of the skin. Left to accumulate, sweat becomes odorous by the action of bacteria. Under ordinary circumstances the body can lose about 0.5 L or more of fluid per day through sweat.

Anatomy and Physiology Labeling

Identify the structures shown below by filling in the blanks.

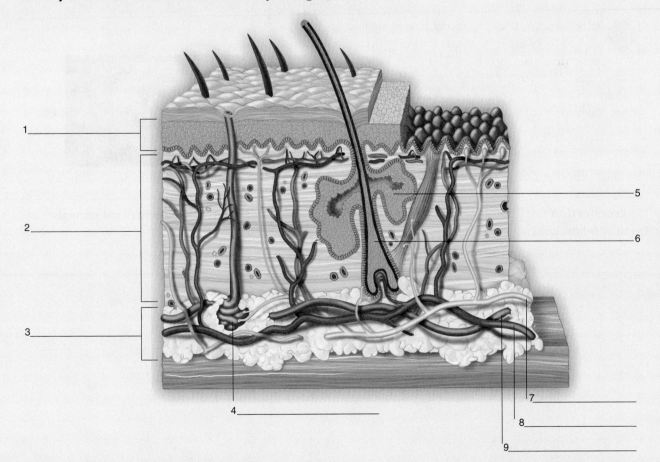

1 _____

2 _____

3 _____

4 _____

5 _____

6 _____

7 _____

8 _____

9 _____

• Building Your Medical Vocabulary •

This section provides the foundation for learning medical terminology. Review the following alphabetized word list. Note how common prefixes and suffixes are repeatedly applied to word roots and combining forms to create different meanings. The word parts are color-coded: prefixes are green, suffixes are blue, roots/combining forms are red.

You will find that some terms have not been divided into word parts. These are common words or specialized terms that are included to enhance your medical vocabulary. See Chapter 1, page 7, to review pronunciation guidelines.

MEDICAL WORD	WORD PARTS		DEFINITION
	Part	**Meaning**	
acne (ăk′ nē)			Inflammatory condition of the sebaceous glands and the hair follicles; *pimples*. See Figure 5.4 ■ ■ **Figure 5.4** Acne. (Courtesy of Jason L. Smith, MD)

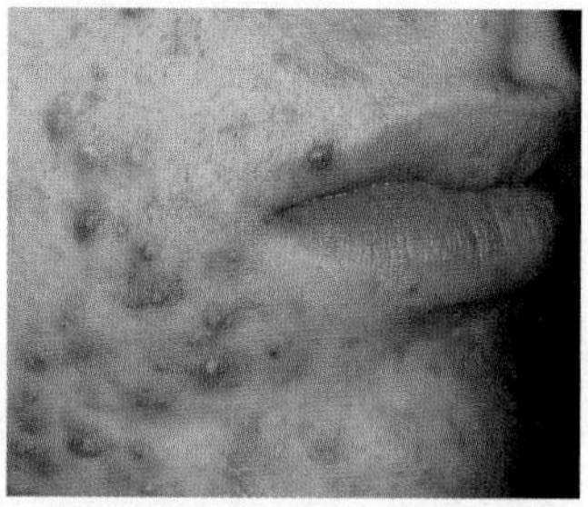

fyi Acne fulminans is a rare type of acne in teenage boys, marked by inflamed, tender, ulcerative, and crusting lesions of the upper trunk and face. It has a sudden onset and is characterized by fever, leukocytosis (elevated white blood cells), and an elevated sedimentation rate. About 50% of the cases have inflammation of several joints. See Figure 5.5 ■

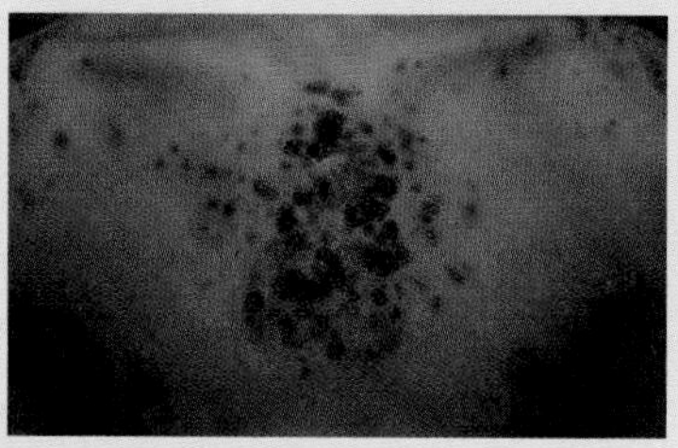

■ **Figure 5.5** Acne fulminans. (Courtesy of Jason L. Smith, MD)

MEDICAL WORD	WORD PARTS		DEFINITION
acrochordon (ăk″ rō-kor′ dŏn)	acr/o chord -on	extremity cord pertaining to	Small outgrowth of epidermal and dermal tissue; *skin tags*

MEDICAL WORD	WORD PARTS		DEFINITION
	Part	**Meaning**	
actinic dermatitis (ăk-tĭn´ ĭk dĕr˝ mă-tī´ tĭs)	actin -ic dermat -itis	ray pertaining to skin inflammation	Inflammation of the skin caused by exposure to radiant energy, such as x-rays, ultraviolet light, and sunlight. See Figure 5.6 ■

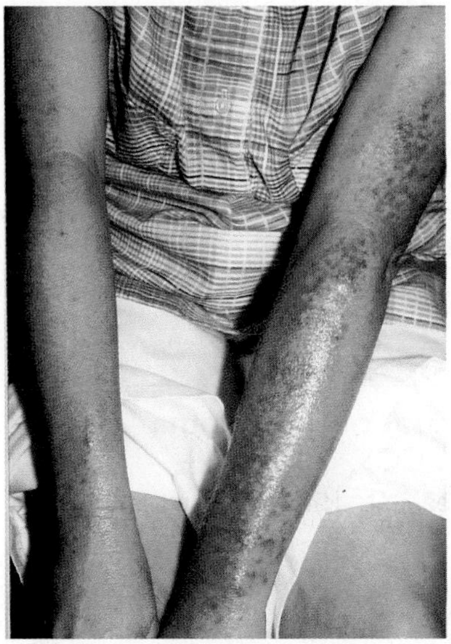

■ **Figure 5.6** Photodermatitis.

(Courtesy of Jason L. Smith, MD)

albinism (ăl´ bĭn-ĭsm)	albin -ism	white condition	Genetic condition in which there is partial or total absence of pigment in skin, hair, and eyes
alopecia (al˝ ō-pē´ shĭ-ă)	a- lopec -ia	without, lack of fox mange condition	Absence or loss of hair, especially of the head; baldness; *alopecia areata* is loss of hair in defined patches usually involving the scalp. See Figure 5.7 ■ Male pattern alopecia begins in the frontal area and proceeds until only a horseshoe area of the hair remains in the back and temples. See Figure 5.8 ■

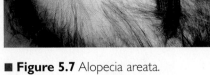

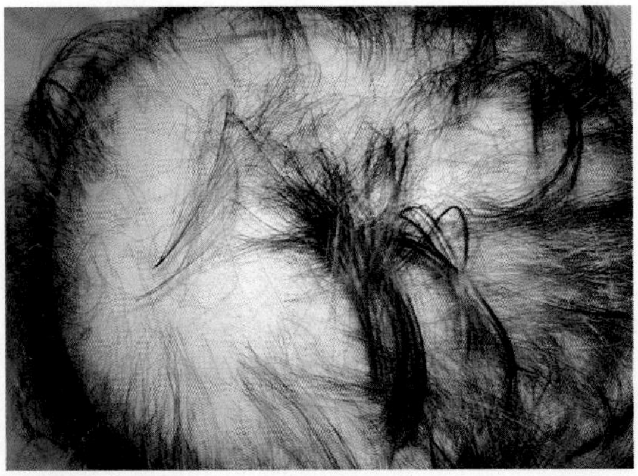

■ **Figure 5.7** Alopecia areata.

(Courtesy of Jason L. Smith, MD)

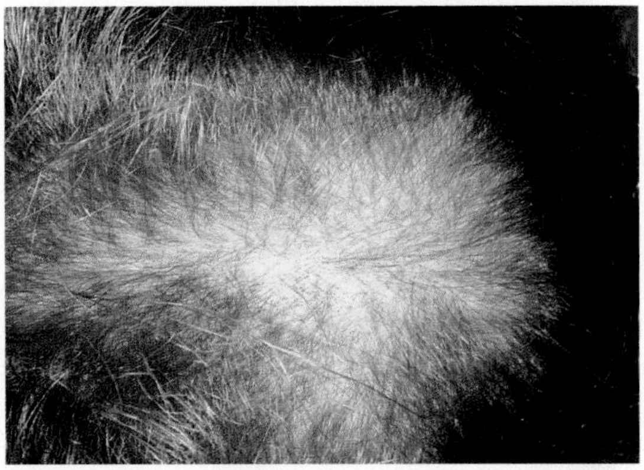

■ **Figure 5.8** Male pattern alopecia. (Courtesy of Jason L. Smith, MD)

MEDICAL WORD	WORD PARTS		DEFINITION
	Part	**Meaning**	
anhidrosis (ăn″ hĭ-drō′ sĭs)	an- hidr -osis	without, lack of sweat condition	Abnormal condition in which there is a lack of or complete absence of sweating. May be congenital or disease related, generalized or localized, temporary or permanent.
autograft (ŏ-tō-grăft)	auto- -graft	self pencil, grafting knife	Graft taken from one part of the patient's body and transferred to another part of that same patient
avulsion (ă-vŭlshŭn)	a- vuls -ion	away from to pull process	Process of forcibly tearing off a part or structure of the body, such as a finger or toe
basal cell carcinoma (BCC) (bā′ săl kăr″ sĭ-nō″ mă)			Epithelial malignant tumor of the skin that rarely metastasizes. It usually begins as a small, shiny papule and enlarges to form a whitish border around a central depression. See Figure 5.9 ■

LIFE SPAN CONSIDERATIONS

Premalignant and malignant skin lesions increase with aging and with overexposure to the sun. Carcinomas appear frequently on the nose, eyelid, or cheek. Basal cell carcinomas (BCC) account for 80% of the skin cancers seen in the older adult. These cancers are generally slow growing but should be surgically removed as soon as possible.

■ **Figure 5.9** Basal cell carcinoma. (Courtesy of Jason L. Smith, MD)

bite

Injury in which a part of the skin is torn by an insect, animal, or human, resulting in a combination of an abrasion, puncture, or laceration. See Figures 5.10 ■, 5.11 ■, and 5.12 ■

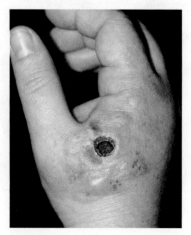

■ **Figure 5.10** Brown recluse spider bites.
(Courtesy of Jason L. Smith, MD)

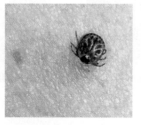

■ **Figure 5.11** Tick bite.
(Courtesy of Jason L. Smith, MD)

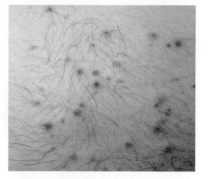

■ **Figure 5.12** Flea bites.
(Courtesy of Jason L. Smith, MD)

MEDICAL WORD	WORD PARTS		DEFINITION
	Part	Meaning	
boil			Acute, infected, painful nodule formed in the subcutaneous layers of the skin, gland, or hair follicle; most often caused by the invasion of staphylococci; *furuncle*
bulla (bŭl′ lă)			Larger blister; *a bleb.* See Figure 5.13 ■

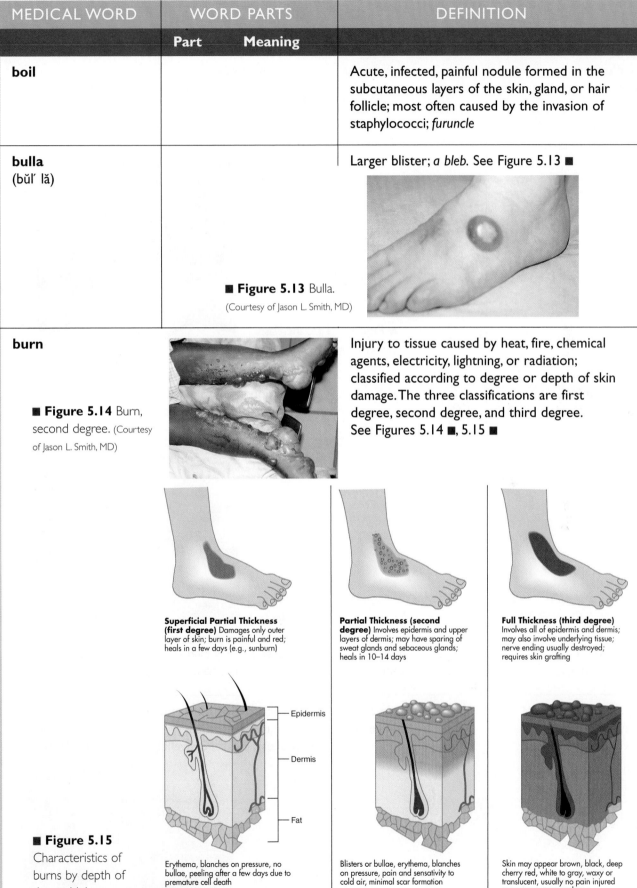

■ **Figure 5.13** Bulla.
(Courtesy of Jason L. Smith, MD)

burn

■ **Figure 5.14** Burn, second degree. (Courtesy of Jason L. Smith, MD)

Injury to tissue caused by heat, fire, chemical agents, electricity, lightning, or radiation; classified according to degree or depth of skin damage. The three classifications are first degree, second degree, and third degree. See Figures 5.14 ■, 5.15 ■

■ **Figure 5.15** Characteristics of burns by depth of thermal injury.

Superficial Partial Thickness (first degree) Damages only outer layer of skin; burn is painful and red; heals in a few days (e.g., sunburn)

Partial Thickness (second degree) Involves epidermis and upper layers of dermis; may have sparing of sweat glands and sebaceous glands; heals in 10–14 days

Full Thickness (third degree) Involves all of epidermis and dermis; may also involve underlying tissue; nerve ending usually destroyed; requires skin grafting

Epidermis

Dermis

Fat

Erythema, blanches on pressure, no bullae, peeling after a few days due to premature cell death

Blisters or bullae, erythema, blanches on pressure, pain and sensativity to cold air, minimal scar formation

Skin may appear brown, black, deep cherry red, white to gray, waxy or translucent, usually no pain injured area may appear sunken

MEDICAL WORD	WORD PARTS		DEFINITION
	Part	**Meaning**	
callus (kăl′ ŭs)			Hardened skin
candidiasis (kăn″ dĭ-dī′ ă-sĭs)			Infection of the skin or mucous membranes with any species of *Candida* but chiefly *Candida albicans*. *Candida* is a genus of yeasts and was formerly called *Monilia*. See Figure 5.16 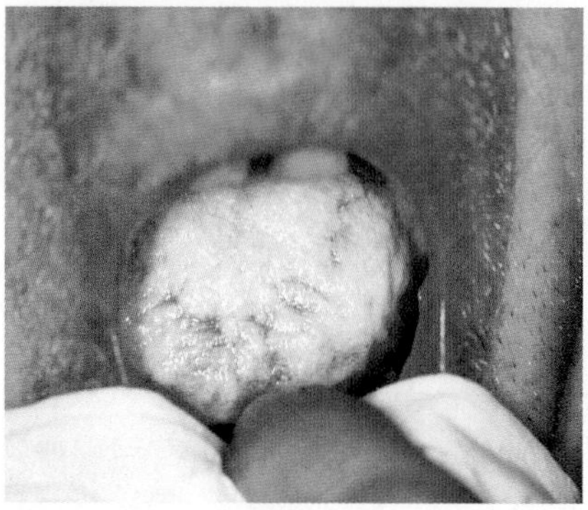 ■ ■ **Figure 5.16** Candidiasis. (Courtesy of Jason L. Smith, MD)
carbuncle (kăr′ bŭng″ kl)			Infection of the subcutaneous tissue, usually composed of a cluster of boils. See Figure 5.17 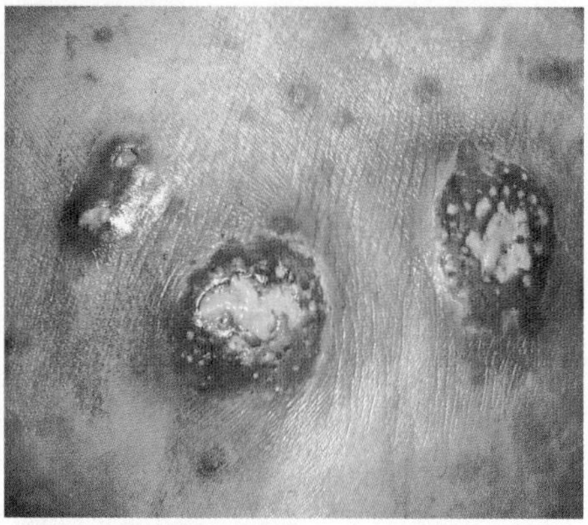 ■ ■ **Figure 5.17** Carbuncles. (Courtesy of Jason L. Smith, MD)
causalgia (kŏ-săl′ jĭ-ă)	caus -algia	heat pain	Intense burning pain associated with trophic skin changes in the hand or foot after trauma to the part
cellulitis (sĕl-ū-lī′ tĭs)	cellul -itis	little cell inflammation	An acute, diffuse inflammation of the skin and subcutaneous tissue characterized by local heat, redness, pain, and swelling. See Figure 5.18 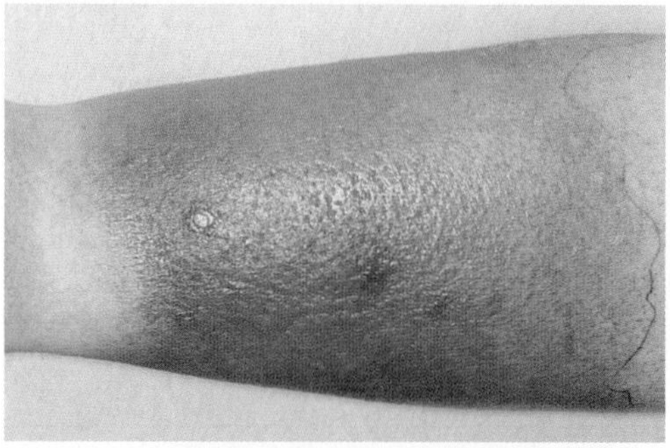 ■ ■ **Figure 5.18** Cellulitis. (Courtesy of Jason L. Smith, MD)

MEDICAL WORD	WORD PARTS		DEFINITION
	Part	Meaning	
cicatrix (sĭk´ ă-trĭks)			Scar left after the healing of a wound
comedo (kŏm´ ē-dō)			Blackhead
corn (korn)			Condition of horny induration and thickening of the skin that may be soft or hard depending on location. Caused by pressure, friction, or both from ill-fitting shoes.
cryosurgery (krī˝ ō-sĕr´ jĕr-ē)			Technique of using subfreezing temperature (usually with liquid nitrogen) to produce well-demarcated areas of cell injury and destruction
cutaneous (kū-tā´ nē-ŭs)	cutane -ous	skin pertaining to	Pertaining to the skin
cyst (sĭst)			Closed sac that contains fluid, semifluid, or solid material
debridement (da-brē-mōn)			Removal of foreign material or damaged or dead tissue, especially in a wound. It is used to promote healing and to prevent infection.
decubitus (decub) ulcer (dē-kū´ bĭ-tŭs ŭl´ sĕr)	de- cubit -us	down to lie pertaining to	An area of skin and tissue that becomes injured or broken down. Also known as a bedsore or pressure ulcer. The literal meaning of the word *decubitus* is a *lying down*. See Figure 5.19 ■ Also see types of skin signs in Figure 5.40 ■

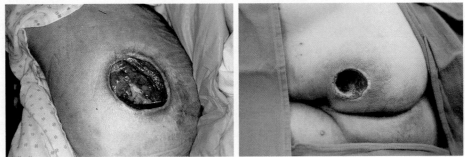

■ **Figure 5.19** Decubitus ulcer staging. (Courtesy of Sandra Quigley, Children's Hospital, Boston, MA)

MEDICAL WORD	WORD PARTS		DEFINITION
	Part	Meaning	
dehiscence (dē-hĭs´ ĕns)			Surgical complication where there is separation or bursting open of a surgical wound. See Figure 5.20 ■
dermabrasion (dĕrm´ ă-brā˝ zhŭn)			Surgical procedure to remove acne scars, nevi, tattoos, or fine wrinkles on the skin by using sandpaper, wire brushes, or other abrasive materials on an anesthetized epidermis
dermatitis (dĕr˝ mă-tī´ tĭs)	dermat -itis	skin inflammation	Inflammation of the skin. See Figure 5.21 ■

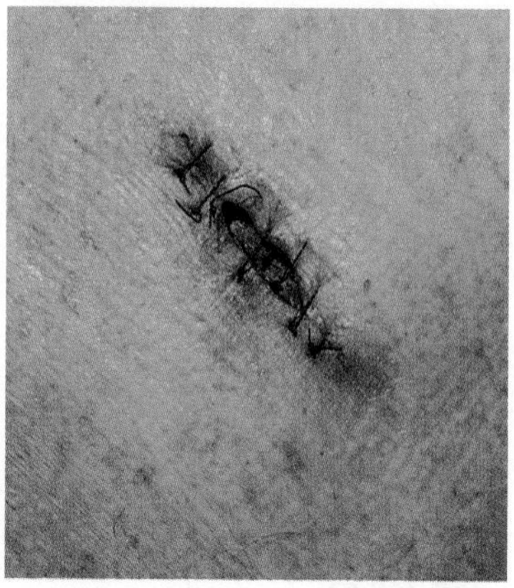

■ **Figure 5.20** Wound dehiscence, back. (Courtesy of Jason L. Smith, MD)

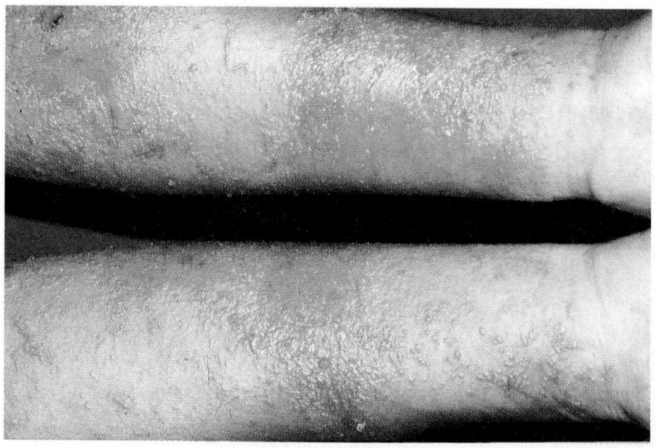

■ **Figure 5.21** Dermatitis; poison ivy. (Courtesy of Jason L. Smith, MD)

fyi To help prevent contact dermatitis with poison ivy, learn to recognize and avoid poison ivy. One form of poison ivy is a low plant usually found in groups of many plants and looks like weeds growing from 6 to 30 inches high. The other form is a "hairy" vine that grows up a tree. Each form has stems with three leaves. See Figure 5.22 ■ There is an old saying people should remember: "Leaflets three, let it be." If in contact with poison ivy, oak, or sumac, wash skin immediately with soap and water to remove oleoresin within 15 minutes of exposure. Also, wash all clothing including gloves, jackets, shoes, and shoelaces as soon as possible. Oleoresin, the extract of the plant, can be active for 6 months on surfaces such as clothing.

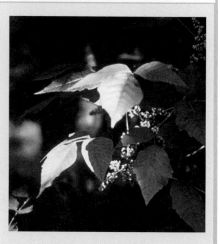

■ **Figure 5.22** Poison ivy plant.

MEDICAL WORD	WORD PARTS		DEFINITION
	Part	**Meaning**	
dermatologist (dĕr´ mah-tol´ ŏ -jĭst)	dermat/o log -ist	skin study of one who specializes	Physician who specializes in the study of the skin
dermatology (Derm) (dĕr˝ mah-tol´ ŏ -jē)	dermat/o -logy	skin study of	Study of the skin
dermatome (dĕr˝ mah-tōm)	derm/a -tome	skin instrument to cut	Surgical instrument used to cut the skin for grafting
dermomycosis (dĕr´ mō-mĭ-kō´ sĭs)	derm/o myc -osis	skin fungus condition	Skin condition caused by a fungus
ecchymosis (ĕk-ĭ-mō´ sĭs)	ec- chym -osis	out juice condition	Abnormal condition in which the blood seeps into the skin causing discolorations ranging from blue-black to greenish yellow
eczema (ĕk´ zĕ-mă)			An acute or chronic inflammatory skin disorder characterized by erythema, papules, vesicles, pustules, scales, crusts, or scabs alone or in combination. The most promising treatment involves nonsteroidal skin medications classified as topical immunomodulators (TIMS) or topical calcineurin (a protein phosphatase) inhibitor.
erythema (ĕr˝ ĭ-thē´ mă)			Redness of the skin; may be caused by capillary congestion, inflammation, heat, sunlight, or cold temperature. *Erythema infectiosum* is known as Fifth disease, a mild, moderately contagious disease caused by the human parvovirus B-19. It is most commonly seen in school-age children and is thought to be spread via respiratory secretions from infected persons. See Figure 5.23 ■

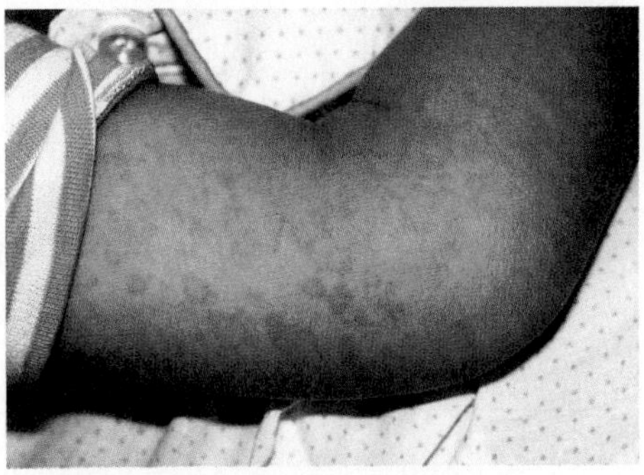

■ **Figure 5.23** Erythema infectiosum, Fifth disease.
(Courtesy of Jason L. Smith, MD)

MEDICAL WORD	WORD PARTS		DEFINITION
	Part	**Meaning**	
erythroderma (ĕ-rĭth″ rō-dĕr′ -mă)	erythr/o -derma	red skin	Abnormal redness of the skin occurring over widespread areas of the body
eschar (ĕs′ kăr)			Slough, scab
excoriation (ĕks-kō″ rē-ā′ shŭm)	ex- coriat -ion	out corium process	Abrasion of the epidermis by scratching, trauma, chemicals, or burns
exudate (ĕks′ ū-dāt)			Production of pus or serum
folliculitis (fō-lĭk″ ū-lī′ tĭs)	follicul -itis	little bag inflammation	Inflammation of a follicle or follicles. See Figure 5.24 ■

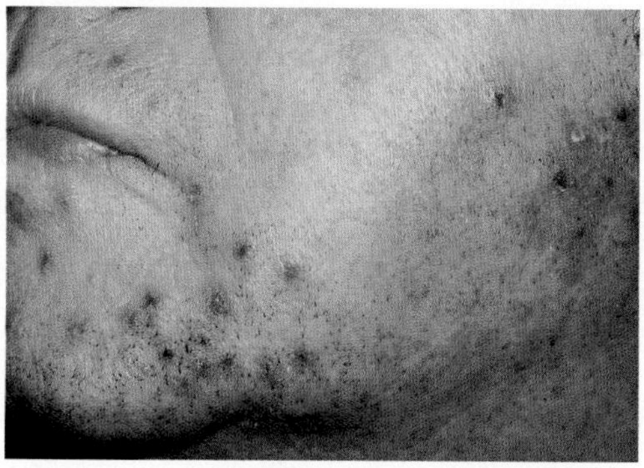

■ **Figure 5.24** Staphylococcal folliculitis. (Courtesy of Jason L. Smith, MD)

gangrene (găng′ grēn)			Literally means *an eating sore*. It is a necrosis, or death, of tissue or bone that usually results from a deficient or absent blood supply to the area.
herpes simplex (hĕr′ pēz sĭm′ plĕks)			An inflammatory skin disease caused by a herpes virus (Type I); *cold sore or fever blister.* See Figure 5.25 ■

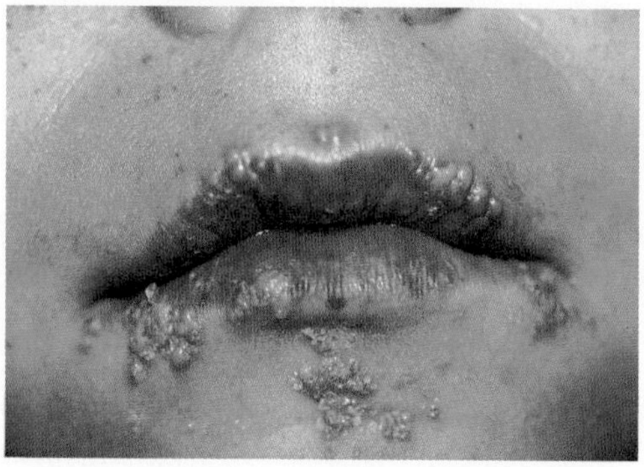

■ **Figure 5.25** Herpes labialis. (Courtesy of Jason L. Smith, MD)

hidradenitis (hī-drăd-ĕnī′ tĭs)	hidr aden -itis	sweat gland inflammation	Inflammation of the sweat glands

MEDICAL WORD	WORD PARTS		DEFINITION
	Part	**Meaning**	
hives (hīvz)			Eruption of itching and burning swellings on the skin; *urticaria*. See Figure 5.26 ■

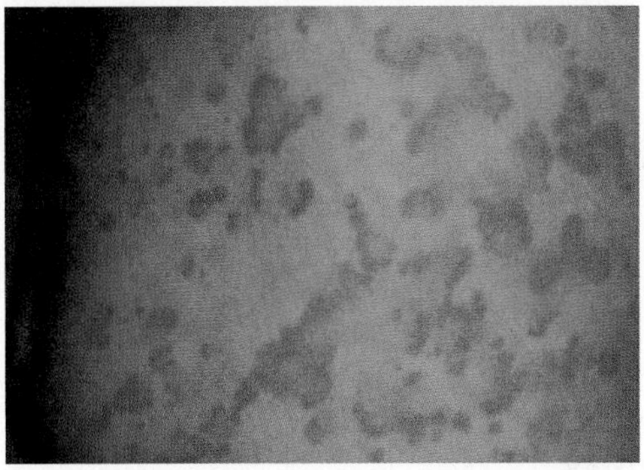

■ **Figure 5.26** Urticaria hives.
(Courtesy of Jason L. Smith, MD)

MEDICAL WORD	WORD PARTS		DEFINITION
hyperhidrosis (hī″ pĕr-hī-drō′ sĭs)	hyper- hidr -osis	excessive sweat condition	Abnormal condition of excessive sweating
hypodermic (hī″ pō-dĕr′mĭk)	hypo- derm -ic	under skin pertaining to	Pertaining to under the skin or inserted under the skin, as a hypodermic injection
icteric (ik-tĕr′ ik)	icter -ic	jaundice pertaining to	Pertaining to jaundice
impetigo (ĭm″ pĕ-tī′ gō)			Skin infection marked by vesicles or bullae; usually caused by streptococci (strep) or staphylococci (staph). See Figure 5.27 ■

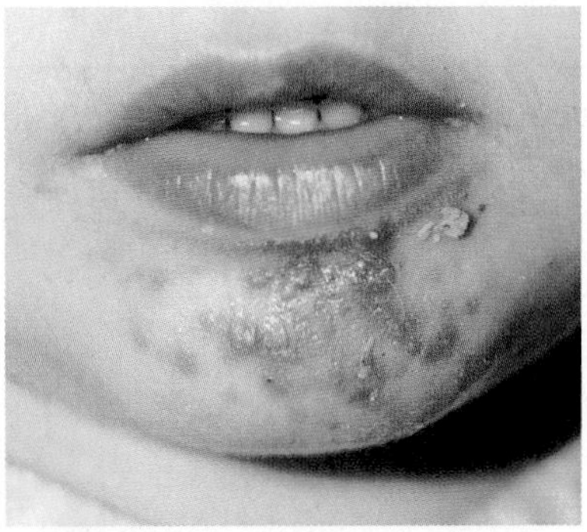

■ **Figure 5.27** Impetigo.
(Courtesy of Jason L. Smith, MD)

MEDICAL WORD	WORD PARTS		DEFINITION
integumentary (ĭn-tĕg″ ū-mĕn′ tă-rē)	integument -ary	a covering pertaining to	Covering; the skin, consisting of the dermis and the epidermis
intradermal (ID) (in″trăh-dĕr′ măl)	intra- derm -al	within skin pertaining to	Pertaining to within the skin, as an intradermal injection
jaundice (jawn′ dĭs)	jaund -ic(e)	yellow pertaining to	Yellow; a symptom of a disease in which there is excessive bile in the blood; the skin, whites of the eyes, and mucous membranes are yellow; *icterus*

MEDICAL WORD	WORD PARTS		DEFINITION
	Part	**Meaning**	
keloid (kē′ lŏ yd)	kel -oid	tumor resemble	Overgrowth of scar tissue caused by excessive collagen formation. See Figure 5.28 ■ ■ **Figure 5.28** Keloid. (Courtesy of Jason L. Smith, MD)
lentigo (lĕn-tī′ gō)			A flat, brownish spot on the skin sometimes caused by exposure to the sun and weather; *freckle*
leukoderma (lū″ kō-dĕr′ mă)	leuk/o -derma	white skin	Localized loss of pigmentation of the skin
leukoplakia (lū″ kō-plā′ kē-ă)	leuk/o plak -ia	white plate condition	White spots or patches formed on the mucous membrane of the tongue or cheek; the spots are smooth, hard, and irregular in shape and can become malignant
lupus (lū′ pŭs)			Originally used to describe a destructive type of skin lesion; current usage of the word is usually in combination with the words *vulgaris* or *erythematosus*, (e.g., *lupus vulgaris* or *lupus erythematosus*)
melanocarcinoma (mĕl″ ă-nō-kar″ sĭn-ō′ mă)	melan/o carcin -oma	black cancer tumor	Cancerous tumor that has black pigmentation
melanoma (mĕl″ ă-nō′ mă)	melan -oma	black tumor	Cancer that develops in the pigment cells of the skin; malignant black mole or tumor. See Figure 5.29 ■ Often the first sign of melanoma is change in the size, shape, or color of a mole. The **ABCDs** of melanoma describe the changes that can occur in a mole using the letters: **A**—asymmetry; the shape of one half does not match the other. **B**—border; the edges are ragged, notched, or blurred. **C**—color; is uneven. Shades of black, brown, or tan are present. Areas of white, red, or blue may be seen. **D**—diameter; there is a change in size.

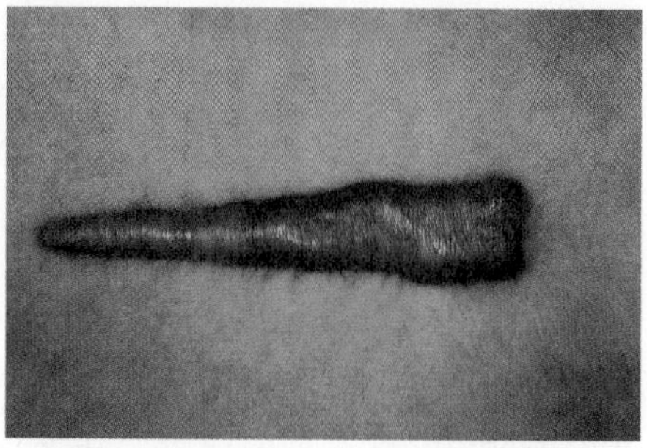

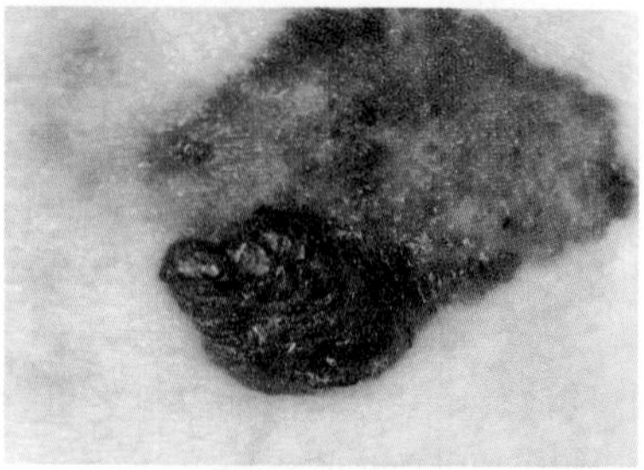

■ **Figure 5.29** Melanoma, forearm.
(Courtesy of Jason L. Smith, MD)

MEDICAL WORD	WORD PARTS		DEFINITION
	Part	Meaning	
miliaria (mĭl-ē-ā´ rē-ă)	miliar -ia	millet (tiny) condition	Called *prickly heat*; commonly seen in newborns and/or infants. It is caused by excessive body warmth. There is retention of sweat in the sweat glands, which have become blocked or inflamed, and then rupture or leak into the skin. Miliaria appears as a rash with tiny pinhead-sized papules, vesicles, and/or pustules. See Figure 5.30 ■

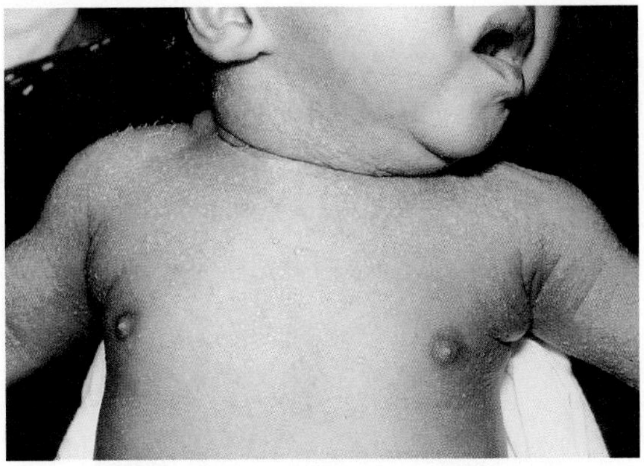

■ **Figure 5.30** Miliaria. (Courtesy of Jason L. Smith, MD)

mole (mōl)			Pigmented, elevated spot above the surface of the skin; a *nevus*. See Figure 5.31 ■

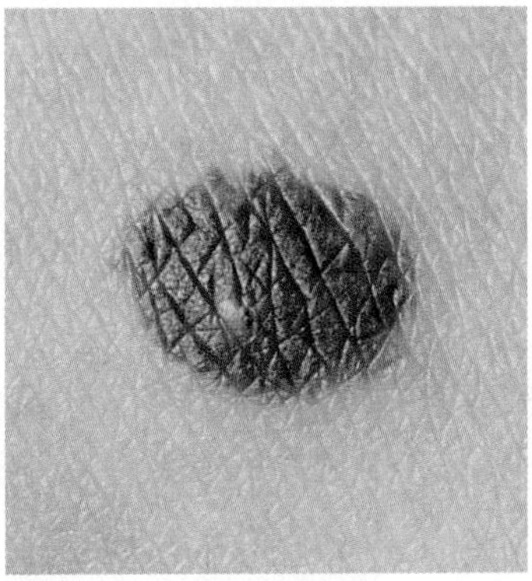

■ **Figure 5.31** Nevus mole.
(Courtesy of Jason L. Smith, MD)

onychitis (ŏn˝ ĭ-kī´ tĭs)	onych -itis	nail inflammation	Inflammation of the nail
onychomycosis (ŏn˝ ĭ-kō-mī-kō´ sĭs)	onych/o myc -osis	nail fungus condition	A fungal infection of the nails. See Figure 5.32 ■

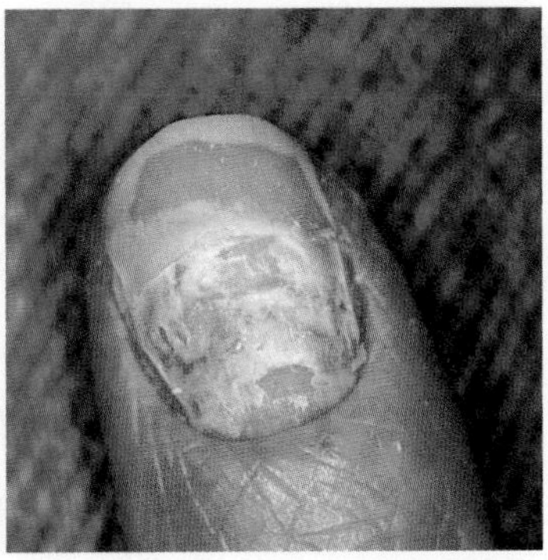

■ **Figure 5.32** Onychomycosis.
(Courtesy of Jason L. Smith, MD)

pachyderma (păk-ē-der´ mă)	pachy -derma	thick skin	Thick skin

MEDICAL WORD	WORD PARTS		DEFINITION
	Part	Meaning	
paronychia (păr″ ō-nĭk´ ĭ-ă)	par- onych -ia	around nail condition	Infectious condition of the marginal structures around the nail
pediculosis (pĕ-dĭk″ ū-lō´ sĭs)	pedicul -osis	a louse condition	Condition of infestation with lice. See Figure 5.33 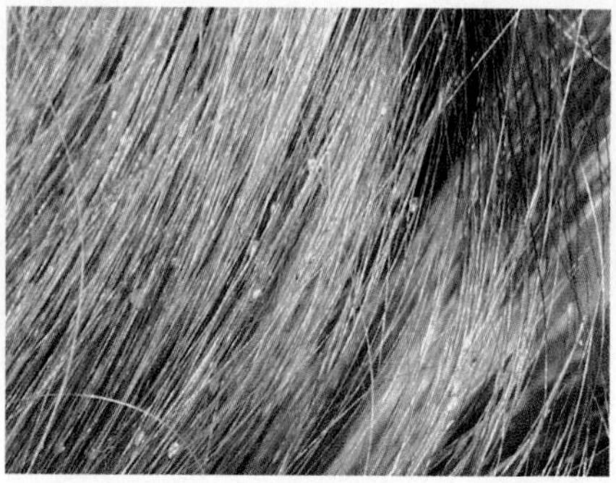 ∎ ∎ **Figure 5.33** Pediculosis capitis. (Courtesy of Jason L. Smith, MD)
petechiae (pē-tē´ kĭ-ē)			Small, pinpoint, purplish hemorrhagic spots on the skin
pruritus (proo-rī´ tŭs)	prurit -us	itching ˘ pertaining to	Severe itching
psoriasis (sō-rī´ ă-sĭs)	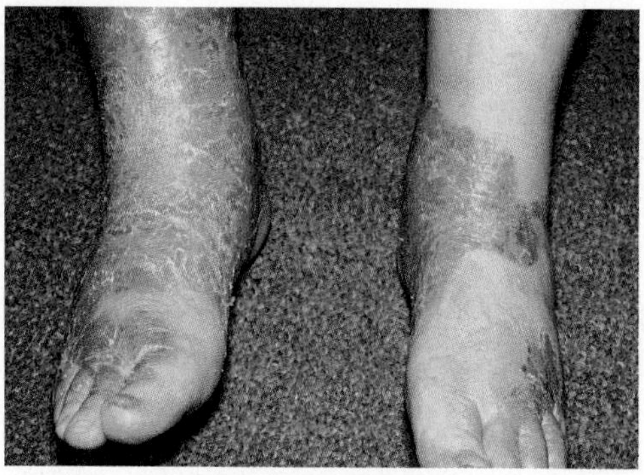 ∎ **Figure 5.34** Psoriasis, lower extremities. (Courtesy of Jason L. Smith, MD)		Chronic skin condition characterized by frequent episodes of redness, itching, and thick, dry scales on the skin. See Figure 5.34 ∎
purpura (pur´ pū-ra)	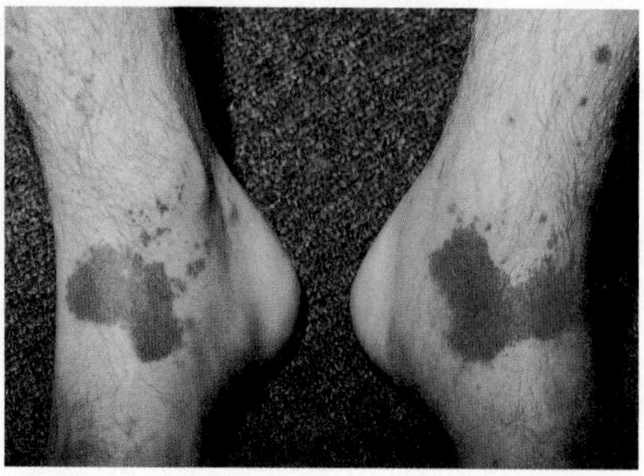 ∎ **Figure 5.35** Purpura. (Courtesy of Jason L. Smith, MD)		Purplish discoloration of the skin caused by extravasation of blood into the tissues. See Figure 5.35 ∎

MEDICAL WORD	WORD PARTS		DEFINITION
	Part	**Meaning**	
rhytidoplasty (rĭt´ ĭ-dō-plăs˝ tē)	rhytid/o -plasty	wrinkle surgical repair	Plastic surgery for the removal of wrinkles
rosacea (rō-zā´ sē-ă)			A chronic disease of the skin of the face marked by varying degrees of papules, pustules, erythema, telangectasia, and hyperplasia of the soft tissues of the nose; usually occurs in middle-aged and older people. See Figure 5.36 ■ ■ **Figure 5.36** Rosacea. (Courtesy of Jason L. Smith, MD)
roseola (rō-zē´ ō-lă)			Any rose-colored rash marked by *maculae* or red spots on the skin. See Figure 5.37 ■ ■ **Figure 5.37** Roseola. (Courtesy of Jason L. Smith, MD)
rubella (roo-bĕl´ lă)			Systemic disease caused by a virus and characterized by a rash and fever; also called *German measles* and *three-day measles*
rubeola (roo-bē´ ō-lă)			Contagious disease characterized by fever, inflammation of the mucous membranes, and rose-colored spots on the skin; also called *measles*

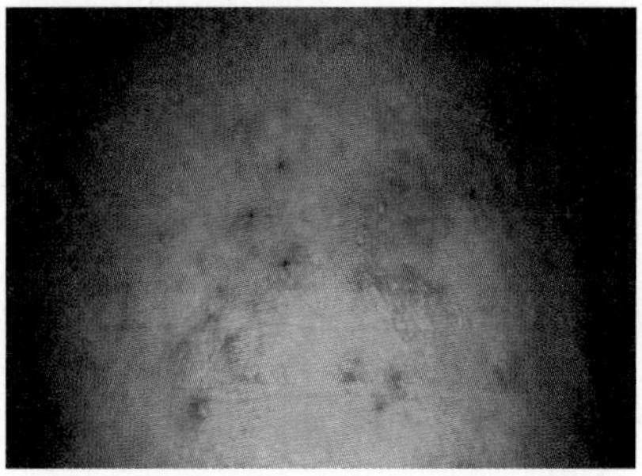

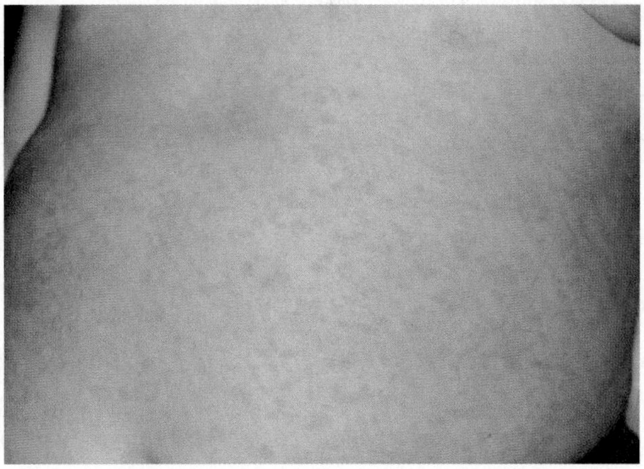

MEDICAL WORD	WORD PARTS		DEFINITION
	Part	Meaning	
scabies (skā′ bēz) or (skā′ bĭ-ēz)			Contagious skin disease characterized by papules, vesicles, pustules, burrows, and intense itching; it is caused by an arachnid, *Sarcoptes scabiei, variety hominis,* the itch mite, and is also called *the itch.* See Figure 5.38 ■

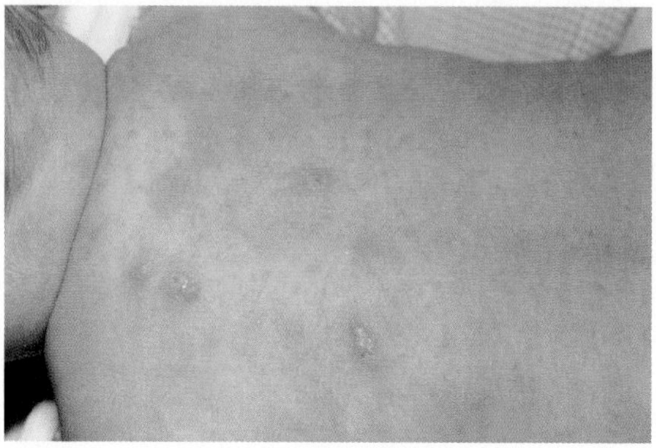

■ **Figure 5.38** Scabies.
(Courtesy of Jason L. Smith, MD)

scar			Mark left by the healing process of a wound, sore, or injury
scleroderma (skli rō-děr′ mă)	scler/o -derma	hard, hardening skin	Chronic condition with hardening of the skin and other connective tissues of the body
seborrhea (sĕb″ or-ē′ ă)	seb/o -rrhea	oil flow	Excessive flow (secretion) of oil from the sebaceous glands
sebum (sē′ bŭm)			Fatty or oily secretion produced by the sebaceous glands
senile keratosis (sĕn′ ĭ′ l kĕr″ ă-tō′ sĭs)	senile kerat -osis	old horn condition	Condition occurring in older people wherein there is dry skin and localized scaling caused by excessive exposure to the sun. See Figure 5.39 ■

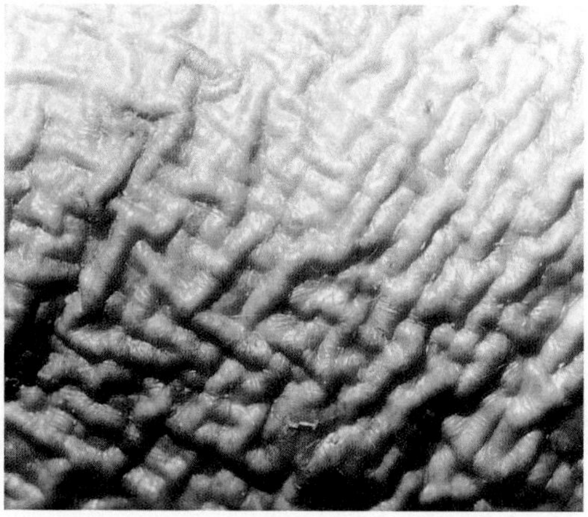

■ **Figure 5.39** Photoaging solar elastosis; senile keratosis.
(Courtesy of Jason L. Smith, MD)

MEDICAL WORD	WORD PARTS		DEFINITION
	Part	**Meaning**	
skin signs (skĭn sīgns)			Objective evidence of an illness or disorder. They can be seen, measured, or felt. Types of skin signs are shown and described in Figure 5.40 ■

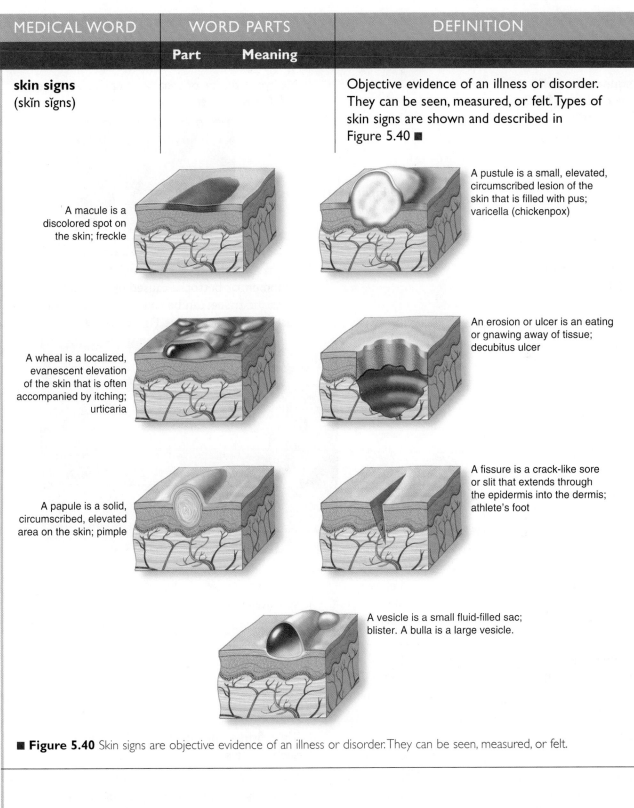

■ **Figure 5.40** Skin signs are objective evidence of an illness or disorder. They can be seen, measured, or felt.

MEDICAL WORD	WORD PARTS		DEFINITION
	Part	**Meaning**	
squamous cell carcinoma (SCC) (skwā′mŭs sel kărsĭ-nō′mă)			Malignant tumor of squamous epithelial tissue. See Figure 5.41 ■ ■ **Figure 5.41** Squamous cell carcinoma. (Courtesy of Jason L. Smith, MD)
striae *(plural)* (strī′ē)			Streaks or lines on the breasts, thighs, abdomen, or buttocks caused by weakening of elastic tissue; can be caused by obesity or result of pregnancy. See Figure 5.42 ■ ■ **Figure 5.42** Striae. (Courtesy of Jason L. Smith, MD)
subcutaneous (Sub-Q, sub Q) (sŭb kū-tā′ nē-ŭs)	sub- cutane -ous	below skin pertaining to	Pertaining to below the skin, as a subcutaneous injection
subungual (sŭb-ŭng′ gwăl)	sub- ungu -al	below nail pertaining to	Pertaining to below the nail
taut (tŏt)			Tight, firm; to pull or draw tight a surface, such as the skin
telangiectasia (tĕl-ăn″ jē-ĕk-tā′ zē-ă)	tel ang/i -ectasia	end, distant vessel dilatation	A vascular lesion formed by dilatation of a group of small blood vessels that may appear as a *birthmark*
thermanesthesia (thĕrm″ ăn-ĕs-thē′ zē-ă)	therm an- -esthesia	hot, heat without, lack of sensation	Inability to distinguish between the sensations of heat and cold

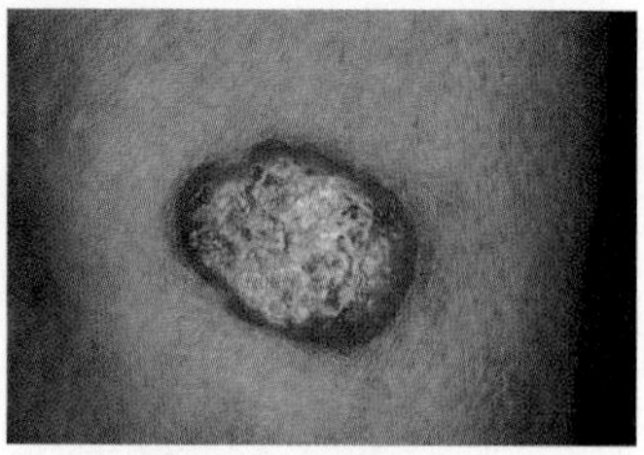

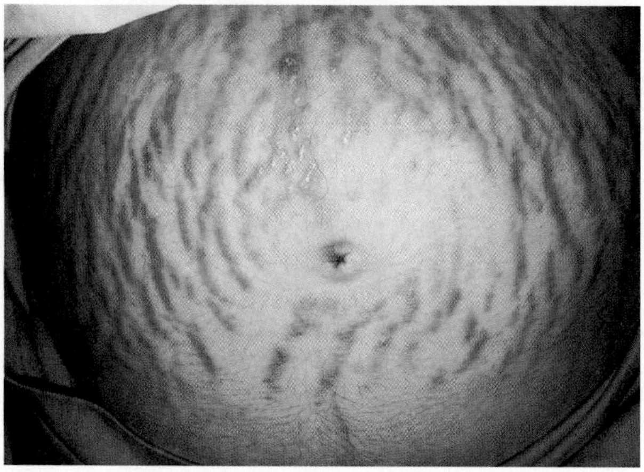

MEDICAL WORD	WORD PARTS		DEFINITION
	Part	Meaning	
tinea (tĭn′ ē-ă) 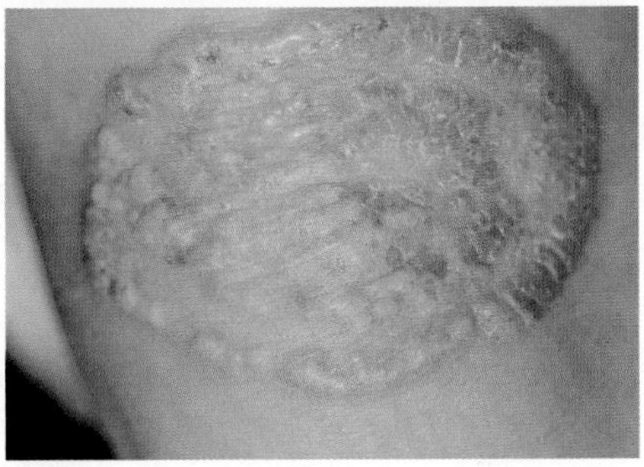			Contagious skin diseases affecting both humans and domestic animals, caused by certain fungi and marked by the localized appearance of discolored, scaly patches on the skin; also called *ringworm*. See Figure 5.43 ■
trichomycosis (trĭk″ ō-mi-kō′ sĭs)	trich/o myc -osis	hair fungus condition	Fungal condition of the hair
ulcer (ŭl′ sĕr) 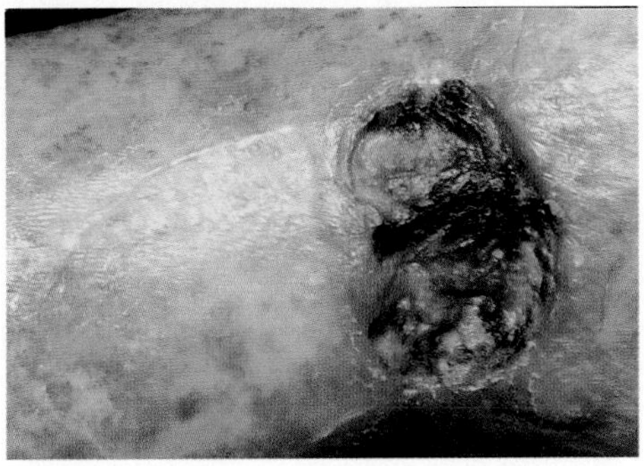			Open lesion or sore of the epidermis or mucous membrane. See Figure 5.44 ■
varicella (văr″ i-sĕl′ ă)			Contagious viral disease characterized by fever, headache, and a crop of red spots that become macules, papules, vesicles, and crusts; also called *chickenpox*. See Figure 5.45 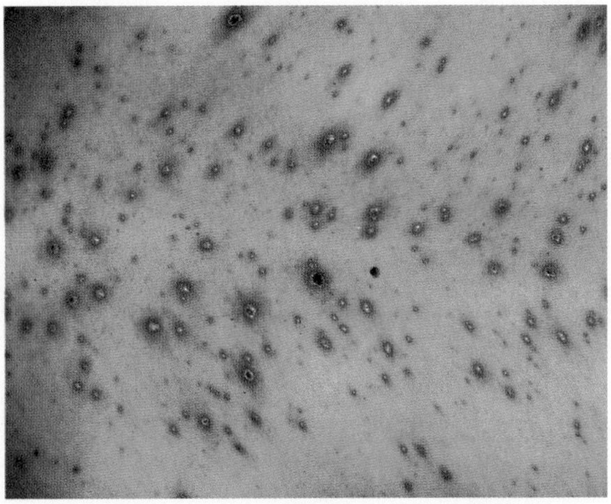 ■

■ **Figure 5.43** Tinea corporis.
(Courtesy of Jason L. Smith, MD)

■ **Figure 5.44** Leg ulcer radiation site. (Courtesy of Jason L. Smith, MD)

■ **Figure 5.45** Varicella chickenpox.
(Courtesy of Jason L. Smith, MD)

MEDICAL WORD	WORD PARTS		DEFINITION
	Part	**Meaning**	
vitiligo (vĭt″ ĭl-ĭ′ gō)			Skin condition characterized by milk-white patches surrounded by areas of normal pigmentation
wart			A skin lesion with a rough papillomatous surface (of viral origin) on the epidermis; *verruca*. A plantar wart, known as *verruca plantaris*, occurs on a pressure-bearing area, especially the sole of the foot. See Figure 5.46 ■

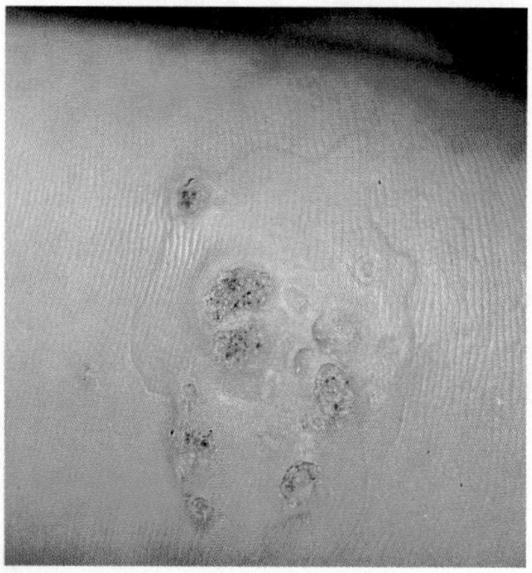

■ **Figure 5.46** Plantar wart. (Courtesy of Jason L. Smith, MD)

MEDICAL WORD	WORD PARTS		DEFINITION
wound (woond)			Injury to soft tissue caused by trauma; generally classified as open or closed
xanthoderma (zăn″ thō-děr′ mă)	xanth/o -derma	yellow skin	Yellowness of the skin
xanthoma (zăn thō′ mă)	xanth -oma	yellow tumor	Literally means *yellow tumor;* a soft, rounded plaque or nodule, usually on the eyelids, especially near the inner canthus
xeroderma (zē″ rō-děr′ mă)	xer/o -derma	dry skin	Dry skin
xerosis (zē″ rō′ sĭs)	xer -osis	dry condition	Abnormal dryness of skin, mucous membranes, or the conjunctiva

LIFE SPAN CONSIDERATIONS

Skin conditions can be acute or chronic, local or systemic. Dryness (**xerosis**) and itching (**pruritus**) are common in older adults. Certain children's skin conditions are associated with age, such as **miliaria** in babies and **acne** in adolescents.

• Drug Highlights •

TYPE OF DRUG	DESCRIPTION AND EXAMPLES
emollients	Substances that are generally oily in nature. These substances are used for dry skin caused by aging, excessive bathing, and psoriasis. EXAMPLE: Desitin
keratolytics	Agents that cause or promote loosening of horny (keratin) layers of the skin. These agents may be used for acne, warts, psoriasis, corns, calluses, and fungal infections. EXAMPLES: Duofilm, Keralyt, and Compound W
local anesthetic agents	Agents that inhibit the conduction of nerve impulses from sensory nerves and thereby reduce pain and discomfort. These agents may be used topically to reduce discomfort associated with insect bites, burns, and poison ivy. EXAMPLES: Solarcaine and Xylocaine
antihistamine agents	Agents that act to prevent the action of histamine. Used to help relieve symptoms, such as itching, in allergic responses and contact dermatitis. EXAMPLE: diphenhydramine (Benadryl)
antipruritic agents	Agents that prevent or relieve itching EXAMPLES: Topical—PBZ (tripelennamine HCl); Oral—Benadryl (diphenhydramine HCl) and Atarax (hydroxyzine HCl)
antibiotic agents	Agents that destroy or stop the growth of microorganisms. These agents are used to prevent infection associated with minor skin abrasions and to treat superficial skin infections and acne. Several antibiotic agents are combined in a single product to take advantage of the different antimicrobial spectrum of each drug. EXAMPLES: Neosporin, Polysporin, and Mycitracin
antifungal agents	Agents that destroy or inhibit the growth of fungi and yeast. These agents are used to treat fungus and/or yeast infection of the skin, nails, and scalp. EXAMPLES: Equate antifungal cream (clotrimazole) and Lamisil (terbinafine)
antiviral agents	Agents that combat specific viral diseases. EXAMPLES: Zovirax (acyclovir) is used in the treatment of herpes simplex virus types 1 and 2, varicella-zoster, Epstein–Barr, and cytomegalovirus. *Relenza* (zanamivir) has antiviral activity against influenza A and B viruses. Tamiflu (oseltamivir phosphate) has antiviral activity against the H1N1 virus (swine flu).

TYPE OF DRUG	DESCRIPTION AND EXAMPLES
anti-inflammatory agents	Agents used to relieve the swelling, tenderness, redness, and pain of inflammation. Topically applied corticosteroids are used in the treatment of dermatitis and psoriasis. EXAMPLES: Carmol HC (hydrocortisone acetate; urea) and Temovate (clobetasol propionate) Oral corticosteroids are used in the treatment of contact dermatitis, such as in poison ivy, when the symptoms are severe. EXAMPLE: Sterapred (prednisone) 12-day unipak
antiseptic agents	Agents that prevent or inhibit the growth of pathogens. Antiseptics are generally applied to the surface of living tissue to reduce the possibility of infection, sepsis, or putrefaction. EXAMPLES: Isopropyl alcohol and Zephrian (benzalkonium chloride)
other drugs	Retin-A (tretinoin) is available as a cream, gel, or liquid. It is used in the treatment of acne vulgaris. Rogaine (minoxidil) is available as a topical solution to stimulate hair growth. It was first approved as a treatment of male pattern baldness. Botulinum Toxin Type A (Botox Cosmetic) is approved by the FDA to temporarily improve the appearance of moderate to severe frown lines between the eyebrows (glabellar lines). Small doses of a sterile, purified botulinum toxin are injected into the affected muscles and block the release of the chemical acetylcholine that would otherwise signal the muscle to contract. The toxin thus temporarily paralyzes or weakens the injected muscle.

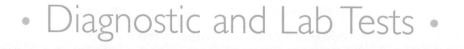

• Diagnostic and Lab Tests •

TEST	DESCRIPTION
tuberculosis skin tests (tū-bĕr″ kū-lō′ sĭs)	Performed to identify the presence of the *Tubercle bacilli*. The tine, Heaf, or Mantoux test are used. The tine and Heaf tests are intradermal tests performed using a sterile, disposable, multiple-puncture lancet. The tuberculin is on metal tines that are pressed into the skin. A hardened raised area at the test site 48–72 hours later indicates the presence of the pathogens in the body. In the Mantoux test 0.1 mL of purified protein derivative (PPD) tuberculin is intradermally injected. Test results are read 48–72 hours after administration.

TEST	DESCRIPTION
scratch (epicutaneous) or prick test (skrăch)	Involves the placement of a suspected allergen in the uppermost layers of the epidermis. One technique used is to place a drop of the allergen on the skin of the forearm or back. Pass a sterile lancet or needle through the drop, and prick the skin no deeper than the uppermost layers of the epidermis. Redness or swelling at the scratch site within 10 minutes indicates allergy to the substance. This indicates that the test result is positive. If no reaction occurs, the test result is negative.
sweat test (chloride) (swĕt)	Performed on sweat to determine the level of chloride concentration on the skin. In **cystic fibrosis (CF)**, which is an inherited disease that affects the pancreas, respiratory system, and sweat glands, there is an increase in skin chloride.
Tzanck test (tsănk)	Microscopic examination of a small piece of tissue that has been surgically scraped from a pustule. The specimen is placed on a slide and stained, and the type of viral infection can be identified.
wound culture (woond)	Performed on wound exudate to determine the presence of microorganisms and to identify the specific type. An effective antibiotic can be prescribed for identified microbes.
biopsy (Bx) (bī´ŏp-sē)	The obtaining of a small piece of living tissue for microscopic examination. May be obtained surgically, through a needle and syringe, hollow punch, brush, or stereotactically. Used to establish a diagnosis, especially to distinguish between benign and malignancy conditions.
sedimentation rate (ESR) (sĕd˝-ĭmĕn-tā´shŭn-rāt)	Blood test to determine the rate at which red blood cells settle in a long, narrow tube. The distance the RBCs settle in 1 hour is the rate. Higher or lower rate can indicate certain disease conditions.

• Abbreviations •

ABBREVIATION	MEANING	ABBREVIATION	MEANING
BCC	basal cell carcinoma	**MD**	medical doctor
Bx	biopsy	**mm**	millimeter
CF	cystic fibrosis	**PC**	professional corporation
Cm	centimeter	**PPD**	purified protein derivative
decub	decubitus	**SCC**	squamous cell carcinoma
Derm	dermatology	**SG**	skin graft
DOB	date of birth	**SSN**	Social Security number
Dx	diagnosis	**staph**	staphylococcus
HCl	hydrochloric acid	**strep**	streptococcus
Hx	history	**Sub-Q, sub Q**	subcutaneous
ID	intradermal	**TIMs**	topical immunomodulators
I&D	incision and drainage	**UV**	ultraviolet

and Review • Study and Review • Study and Review
Review • Study and Review • Study and Review • Stu
w • Study and Review • Study and Review • Study a

Study and Review •

Study and Review • Study a

Anatomy and Physiology

Write your answers to the following questions.

1. Name the primary organ of the integumentary system. _____

2. Name the four accessory structures of the integumentary system.

   a. _____   **b.** _____

   c. _____   **d.** _____

3. State the four main functions of the skin.

   a. _____   **b.** _____

   c. _____   **d.** _____

4. The skin is essentially composed of two layers, the _____ and the
_____ .

5. Name the five strata of the epidermis.

   a. _____   **b.** _____

   c. _____   **d.** _____

   e. _____

6. _____ is a protein substance that is the basic structural component of hair and nails.

7. _____ is a pigment that gives color to the skin.

8. The _____ is known as the *corium* or *true skin*.

9. Name the two layers of the part of the skin described in question 8.

   a. _____   **b.** _____

10. The crescent-shaped white area of the nail is the _____.

Word Parts

PREFIXES

Give the definitions of the following prefixes.

1. a-, an- _____
2. auto- _____
3. ec- _____
4. de- _____
5. ex- _____
6. hyper- _____
7. hypo- _____
8. intra- _____
9. par- _____
10. sub- _____

ROOTS AND COMBINING FORMS

Give the definitions of the following roots and combining forms.

1. acr/o _____
2. actin _____
3. aden _____
4. albin _____
5. carcin _____
6. caus _____
7. chym _____
8. coriat _____
9. cutane _____
10. derm _____
11. derm/a _____
12. dermat _____
13. dermat/o _____
14. derm/o _____
15. lopec _____
16. erythr/o _____
17. hidr _____
18. icter _____
19. kel _____
20. kerat _____
21. leuk/o _____
22. log _____
23. melan _____
24. melan/o _____
25. myc _____
26. onych _____
27. cellul _____
28. onych/o _____
29. pachy _____
30. pedicul _____
31. chord _____
32. rhytid/o _____

33. scler/o _____

34. seb/o _____

35. senile _____

36. therm _____

37. vuls _____

38. trich/o _____

39. ungu _____

40. xanth/o _____

41. xer/o _____

42. cubit _____

43. follicul _____

44. integument _____

45. jaund _____

46. plak _____

47. miliar _____

48. prurit _____

49. tel _____

50. ang/i _____

SUFFIXES

Give the definitions of the following suffixes.

1. -al _____

2. -algia _____

3. -on _____

4. -us _____

5. -derma _____

6. -ary _____

7. -esthesia _____

8. -graft _____

9. -ia _____

10. -ic _____

11. -ion _____

12. -ism _____

13. -ist _____

14. -itis _____

15. -logy _____

16. -ectasia _____

17. -oid _____

18. -oma _____

19. -osis _____

20. -ous _____

21. -plasty _____

22. -rrhea _____

23. -tome _____

Identifying Medical Terms

In the spaces provided, write the medical terms for the following meanings.

1. _____ Inflammation of the skin caused by exposure to actinic rays

2. _____ Pertaining to the skin

3. _____ Inflammation of the skin

4. _____ Study of the skin

5. _____ Severe itching

6. _____ Condition of excessive sweating

7. _____ Pertaining to under the skin

8. _____ Pertaining to jaundice

9. _____ Inflammation of the nail

10. _____ Thick skin

11. _____ Inability to distinguish between the sensations of heat and cold

12. _____ Yellowness of the skin

Spelling

Circle the correct spelling of each medical term.

1. caualgia / causalgia

2. dermomcosis / dermomycosis

3. ecchymosis / echymosis

4. exoriation / excoriaton

5. hyperhidrosis / hyprhidrosis

6. melnoma / melanoma

7. oncyhomyosis / onychomycosis

8. rhytdoplasty / rhytidoplasty

9. sleroderma / scleroderma

10. sebrrhea / seborrhea

Matching

Select the appropriate lettered meaning for each of the following words.

_____ 1. acne

_____ 2. alopecia

_____ 3. cicatrix

_____ 4. comedo

_____ 5. decubitus

_____ 6. dehiscence

_____ 7. exudate

_____ 8. leukoplakia

_____ 9. petechiae

_____ 10. pruritus

a. Small, pinpoint, purplish hemorrhagic spots on the skin

b. Production of pus or serum

c. Severe itching

d. Inflammatory condition of the sebaceous gland and the hair follicles

e. Scar left after the healing of a wound

f. Loss of hair, baldness

g. White spots or patches formed on the mucous membrane of the tongue or cheek

h. Blackhead

i. Separation or bursting open of a surgical wound

j. Bedsore

k. Slough, scab

Abbreviations

Place the correct word, phrase, or abbreviation in the space provided.

1. basal cell carcinoma _____

2. Bx _____

3. decub _____

4. ID _____

5. incision and drainage _____

6. PPD _____

7. skin graft _____

8. staph _____

9. strep _____

10. topical immunomodulators _____

Diagnostic and Laboratory Tests

Select the best answer to each multiple-choice question. Circle the letter of your choice.

1. An intradermal test performed using a sterile, disposable, multiple puncture lancet is:
   a. sweat test
   b. Mantoux test
   c. tine test
   d. Tzanck test

2. A test done on wound exudate to determine the presence of microorganisms is:
   a. sweat test
   b. biopsy
   c. Tzanck test
   d. wound culture

3. A microscopic examination of a small piece of tissue that has been surgically scraped from a pustule is:
   a. Tzanck test
   b. sweat test
   c. biopsy
   d. wound culture

4. Tests performed to identify the presence of the *Tubercle bacilli* include the:
   a. tine, Heaf, and sweat
   b. tine, Heaf, and Mantoux
   c. tine, Tzanck, and Mantoux
   d. tine, Mantoux, and sweat

5. The _____ test used to determine the level of chloride concentration on the skin is:
   a. sweat
   b. Tzanck
   c. tine
   d. Mantoux

PRACTICAL APPLICATION

MEDICAL RECORD ANALYSIS

This exercise contains information, abbreviations, and medical terminology from an actual medical record or case study that has been adapted for this text. The names and any personal information have been created by the author. Read and study each form or case study and then answers the questions that follow. You may refer to Appendix III, Abbreviations and Symbols, on page A41.

SOUTH SIDE PATHOLOGY, PC
315 West Eighth Street, Rome, GA 30165
Phone: 123-456-7890
Frank Jones Smith, MD, Laboratory Director

Surgical Pathology Report

Patient: Frances Marie Melton   **Case Number:** 104589
SSN: 000-00-0000   **Collected:** 02/11/xx
DOB: 1/31/39   **Sex:** Female   **Received:** 02/12/xx
Age: 72
Signed: Scott Parker, MD
Northside Dermatology
103 John Maddox Drive
Rome, GA 30165

Clinical Information:

---

1. Hemorrhagic papule   Dx: BCC
2. Translucent papule with telangiectasia   Dx: BCC

Diagnosis:

1. Skin of left nasal dorsum, shave biopsy-actinic keratosis.
2. Skin of right mid back, shave biopsy-basal cell carcinoma.

Gross Description:

1. Two containers, the first labeled "left nasal dorsum," have within a brown and white 4 × 5 mm superficial skin shave. With margins inked, this is bisected and entirely submitted.
2. The second labeled "right mid back" has within a 0.5 × 0.7 cm superficial skin shave. With margins inked, this is trisected and entirely submitted.

Microscopic Description:

1. Sections show keratinocyte atypical involving the lower layers of the epidermis as well as solar elastosis (breakdown of elastic tissue due to apparent excessive sun exposure) and parakeratosis (incomplete keratinization due to apparent excessive sun exposure). The actinic keratosis has proliferative features.
2. Sections show a mixed superficial and micronodular form of basal cell carcinoma featuring focal pigmentation. The lesion extends to the base of the shave.

Frank Jones Smith, MD
Pathologist
(Case signed 02/14/20xx)

Medical Record Questions

Place the correct answer in the space provided.

1. What is the abbreviation for diagnosis? _____

2. What does the abbreviation BCC mean? _____

3. Define papule. _____

4. What is the medical term that means dilatation of small blood vessels that may appear as a birthmark?

_____

5. What is the medical term that means breakdown of elastic tissue due to apparent excessive sun exposure?

_____

LEARNING OUTCOMES

On completion of this chapter, you will be able to:

1. List the primary functions of bones.

2. Explain various types of body movements that occur at the diarthrotic joints.

3. Contrast the male pelvis to that of the female pelvis.

4. Define fracture and state the various types.

5. Analyze, build, spell, and pronounce medical words.

6. Comprehend the drugs highlighted in this chapter.

7. Describe diagnostic and laboratory tests related to the skeletal system.

8. Identify and define selected abbreviations.

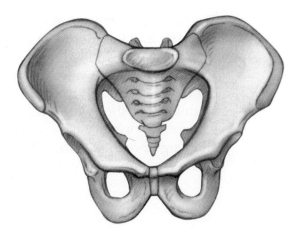

COMBINING FORMS OF THE SKELETAL SYSTEM

acetabul/o	acetabulum	lumb/o	loin, lower back
acr/o	extremity	mandibul/o	lower jawbone
ankyl/o	stiffening, crooked	maxill/o	jawbone
arthr/o	joint	menisc/i	crescent
burs/o	a pouch	myel/o	bone marrow
calcan/e	heel bone	oste/o	bone
carcin/o	cancer	patell/o	kneecap
carp/o	wrist	ped/o	foot
cartilagin/o	cartilage	phalang/e	phalanges (finger/toe bones)
chondr/o	cartilage	rach/i	spine
clavicul/o	clavicle, collarbone	rad/i	radius
coccyg/e	coccyx, tailbone	radi/o	x-ray
coccyg/o	coccyx, tailbone	rheumat/o	discharge
coll/a	glue	sacr/o	sacrum
cost/o	rib	sarc/o	flesh
crani/o	skull	scapul/o	shoulder blade
dactyl/o	finger or toe	scoli/o	curvature
femor/o	femur	spin/o	spine
fibul/o	fibula	spondyl/o	vertebra
fixat/o	fastened	stern/o	sternum, breastbone
humer/o	humerus	tendon/o	tendon
ili/o	ilium	tibi/o	tibia
isch/i	ischium, hip	tract/o	to draw
kyph/o	a hump	uln/o	ulna, elbow
lamin/o	lamina (thin plate)	vertebr/o	vertebra
lord/o	bending, curve, swayback	xiph/o	sword

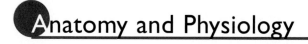

Anatomy and Physiology

The human adult skeletal system is composed of 206 bones that, with **cartilage**, **tendons**, and **ligaments**, make up the **framework** or skeleton of the body. The skeleton can be divided into two main groups of bones: the **axial skeleton** consisting of 80 bones and the **appendicular skeleton** with the remaining 126 bones. The principal bones of the axial skeleton are the skull, spine, ribs, and sternum. The shoulder girdle, arms, and hands and the pelvic girdle, legs, and feet are the primary bones of the appendicular skeleton. Table 6.1 ■ provides an at-a-glance look at the skeletal system. See Figure 6.1 ■ for an anterior view of the skeleton.

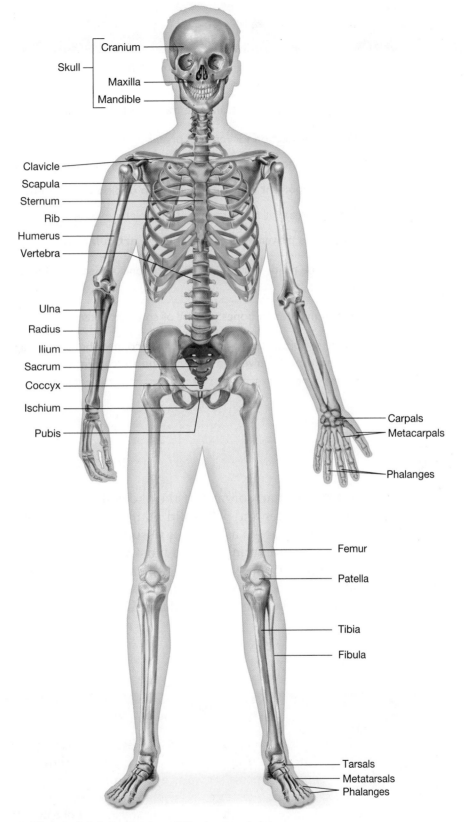

■ **Figure 6.1** Anterior view of the human skeleton.

TABLE 6.1 Skeletal System at-a-Glance	
Organ/Structure	**Primary Functions/Description**
Bones	• Primary organs of the skeletal system, which are composed of approximately 50% water and 50% solid matter • Provide shape, support, and the framework of the body • Provide protection for internal organs • Serve as a storage place for mineral salts, calcium, and phosphorus • Play an important role in the formation of blood cells (**hematopoiesis**) • Provide areas for the attachment of skeletal muscles • Help make movement possible through **articulation**
Cartilage	• Forms the major portion of the embryonic skeleton and part of the skeleton in adults
Tendons	• Attach muscles to bones; consist of connective tissue
Ligaments (lig)	• Bands of fibrous connective tissue that connect bones, cartilages, and other structures; also serve as a place for the attachment of fascia

BONES

The **bones** are the primary organs of the skeletal system; they are composed of approximately 50% water and 50% solid matter. The solid matter in bone is a calcified, rigid substance known as **osseous tissue**. This tissue is a relatively hard and lightweight composite material, formed mostly of calcium phosphate. While bone is essentially brittle, it does have a significant degree of elasticity, contributed chiefly by collagen. All bones consist of living and dead cells embedded in the mineralized organic **matrix** (the intercellular substance of bone) that makes up the osseous tissue.

LIFE SPAN CONSIDERATIONS

Bone begins to develop during the second month of fetal life as cartilage cells enlarge, break down, disappear, and are replaced by bone-forming cells called **osteoblasts**. Most bones of the body are formed by this process, known as **endochondral ossification**. In this process, the bone cells deposit organic substances in the spaces vacated by cartilage to form bone matrix. As this process proceeds, blood vessels form within the bone and deposit salts such as calcium phosphate and phosphorus that serve to harden the developing bone. After age 35, both men and women will normally lose 0.3–0.5% of their bone density per year as part of the aging process.

Classification of Bones

Bones are classified according to their shapes. See Figure 6.2 ■ Table 6.2 ■ classifies the bones and gives an example of each type.

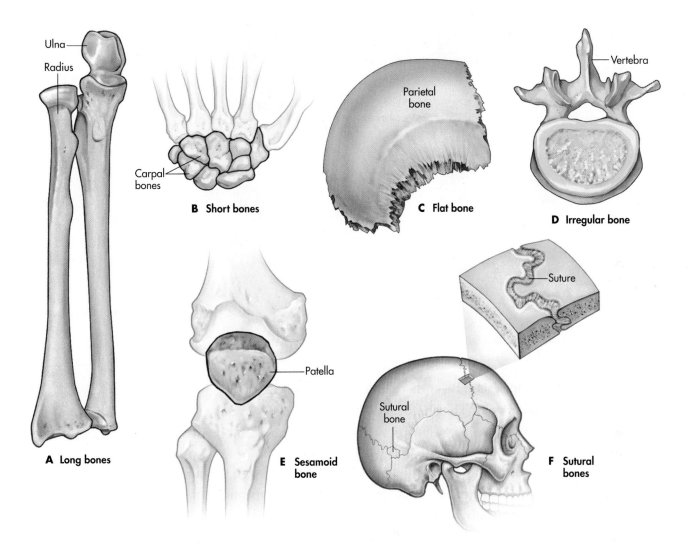

■ **Figure 6.2** Classification of bones by shape.

TABLE 6.2 Classifications of Bone	
Bone	**Example**
Flat	Ribs, scapula (shoulder blade), parts of the pelvic girdle, bones of the skull
Long	Tibia (shin bone), femur (thigh bone), humerus, radius
Short	Carpals, tarsals
Irregular	Vertebrae, ossicles of the ear
Sesamoid	Patella (kneecap)
Sutural or Wormian	Between the flat bones of the skull

Structure of a Long Bone

Long bones, such as the tibia, femur, humerus, or radius, have most of the features found in all bones. These features are listed here and shown in Figure 6.3 ■

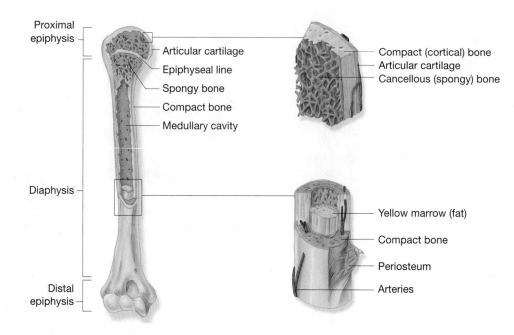

■ **Figure 6.3** Features found in a long bone.

- **Epiphysis**. The ends of a developing bone.
- **Diaphysis**. The shaft of a long bone.
- **Periosteum**. A fibrous vascular membrane that forms the covering of bones except at their articular (joint) surfaces.
- **Compact bone**. The dense, hard layer of bone tissue.
- **Medullary canal**. A narrow space or cavity throughout the length of the diaphysis.
- **Endosteum**. A tough, connective tissue membrane lining the medullary canal and containing the bone marrow.
- **Cancellous or spongy bone.** The reticular network that makes up most of the volume of bone.

LIFE SPAN CONSIDERATIONS

The **epiphyseal plate**, also known as the growth plate or physis, is a thin disc of hyaline cartilage (the type that makes up the embryonic skeleton) positioned between the epiphysis and diaphysis. In children, this is the center of longitudinal bone growth. It is possible to determine the biological age of a child from the development of epiphyseal ossification centers as shown radiographically. See Figure 6.4 ■ About 3 years after the onset of puberty, the ends of the long bones (**epiphyses**) knit securely to their shafts (**diaphysis**). Once growth is completed and an individual reaches full maturity and stature, the epiphyseal plate becomes the epiphyseal line.

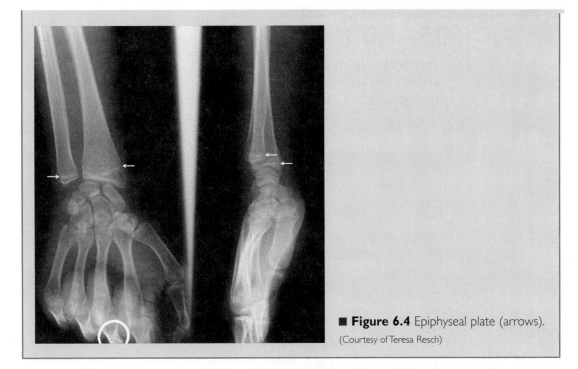

■ **Figure 6.4** Epiphyseal plate (arrows).
(Courtesy of Teresa Resch)

Bone Markings

Certain commonly used terms describe the **markings of bones**. These markings are listed and described in Table 6.3 ■ so you can better understand their roles in joining bones together, providing areas for muscle attachments, and serving as a passageway for blood vessels, ligaments, and nerves.

TABLE 6.3 Bone Markings	
Marking	**Description of the Bone Structure**
Condyle	Rounded projection that enters into the formation of a joint, articulation
Crest	Ridge on a bone
Fissure	Slitlike opening between two bones
Foramen	Opening in the bone for blood vessels, ligaments, and nerves
Fossa	Shallow depression in or on a bone
Head	Rounded end of a bone
Meatus	Tubelike passage or canal
Process	Enlargement or protrusion of a bone
Sinus	Air cavity within certain bones
Spine	Pointed, sharp, slender process
Sulcus	Groove, furrow, depression, or fissure
Trochanter	Either of the two bony projections below the neck of the femur
Tubercle	Small, rounded process
Tuberosity	Large, rounded process

JOINTS AND MOVEMENT

A **joint (jt)** is an articulation, a place where two or more bones connect. Figure 6.5 ■ shows the knee joint. The manner in which bones connect determines the type of movement possible at the joint.

LIFE SPAN CONSIDERATIONS

Various age-related joint changes that occur in the older person are due to diminished viscosity of the synovial fluid, degeneration of collagen and elastin cells, outgrowth of cartilaginous clusters in response to continuous wear and tear, and formation of scar tissues and calcification in the joint capsules. **Osteoarthritis** often results from years of accumulated wear and tear on joints and tends to occur more frequently in the hips, knees, and finger joints.

Classification of Joints

Joints are classified as follows:

- **Synarthrosis (Fibrous).** Does not permit movement. The bones are in close contact with each other, but there is no joint cavity. An example is a *cranial suture.*

- **Amphiarthrosis (Cartilaginous).** Permits very slight movement. An example of this type of joint is a *vertebra.*

- **Diarthrosis (Synovial).** Allows free movement in a variety of directions. A synovial membrane lines the joint and produces synovial fluid, which lubricates the joint. Examples of this type of joint are the *knee, hip, elbow, wrist,* and *foot.*

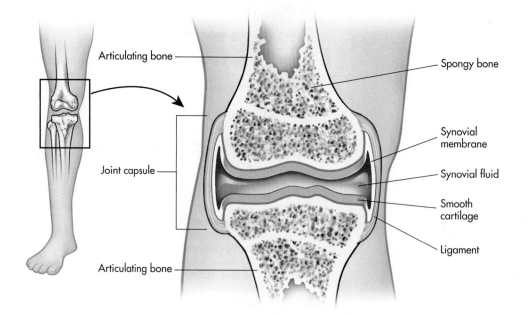

Articulating bone

Joint capsule

Articulating bone

Spongy bone

Synovial membrane

Synovial fluid

Smooth cartilage

Ligament

■ **Figure 6.5** Knee joint.

Joint Movements

The following terms describe types of body movement that occur at the **diarthrotic joints** (see Figure 6.6 ■):

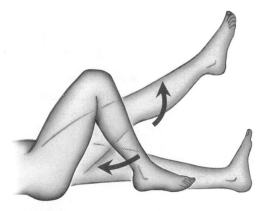

■ **Figure 6.6 A** Flexion and Extension
Flexion–Bending a limb.
Extension–Straightening a flexed limb.

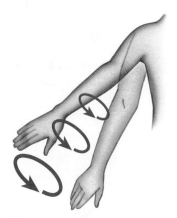

■ **Figure 6.6 B** Circumduction
Circumduction–Moving a body part in a circular motion.

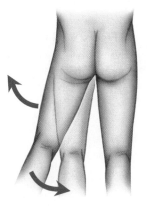

■ **Figure 6.6 C** Abduction and Adduction
Abduction–Moving a body part away from the middle.
Adduction–Moving a body part toward the middle.

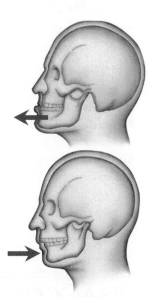

■ **Figure 6.6 D** Protraction and Retraction
Protraction–Moving a body part forward.
Retraction–Moving a body part backward.

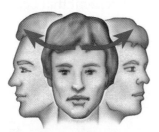

■ **Figure 6.6 E** Rotation
Rotation–Moving a body part around
a central axis.

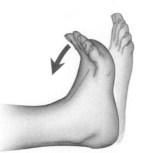

■ **Figure 6.6 F** Dorsiflexion
Dorsiflexion–Bending a body part backward.

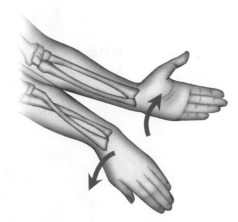

■ **Figure 6.6 G** Pronation and Supination
Pronation–Lying prone (face downward);
also turning the palm downward.
Supination–Lying supine (face upward);
also turning the palm or foot upward.

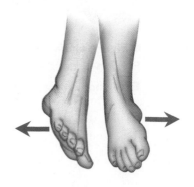

■ **Figure 6.6 H** Eversion and Inversion
Eversion–Turning outward.
Inversion–Turning inward.

VERTEBRAL COLUMN

The **vertebral column** is composed of a series of separate bones (**vertebrae**) connected in such a way as to form four spinal curves. These curves have been identified as the cervical, thoracic, lumbar, and sacral. The *cervical curve* consists of the first seven vertebrae, the *thoracic curve* consists of the next 12 vertebrae, the *lumbar curve* consists of the next five vertebrae, and the *sacral curve* consists of the sacrum and coccyx (tailbone) (see Figure 6.7 ■).

It is known that a curved structure has more strength than a straight structure. The spinal curves of the human body are most important because they help support the weight of the body and provide the balance that is necessary to walk on two feet.

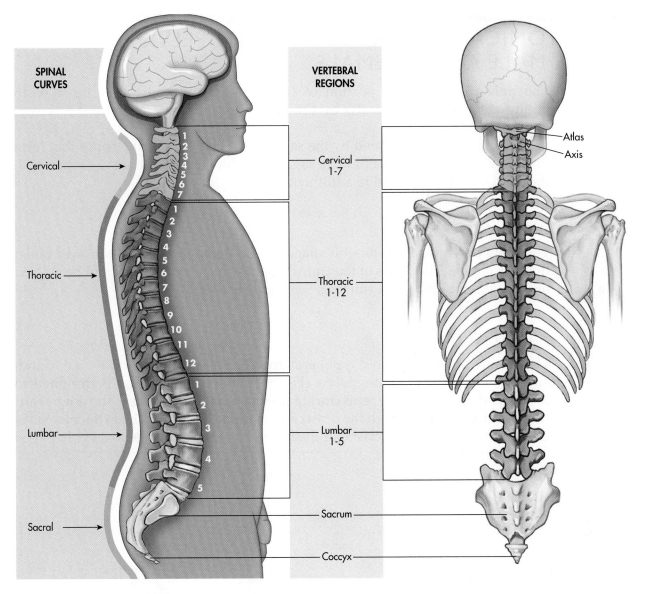

SPINAL CURVES

Cervical

Thoracic

Lumbar

Sacral

VERTEBRAL REGIONS

Cervical 1-7

Thoracic 1-12

Lumbar 1-5

Sacrum

Coccyx

Atlas
Axis

1 2 3 4 5 6 7
1 2 3 4 5 6 7 8 9 10 11 12
1 2 3 4 5

■ **Figure 6.7** Vertebral (spinal) column.

LIFE SPAN CONSIDERATIONS

Young children who are beginning to walk often have a pot-bellied stance because of a lumbar lordosis. This posture usually disappears around 5 years of age. After 6 years of age, the spine has normal thoracic convex (arched; curved evenly) and lumbar concave (rounded; hollowed out) curves. See Figure 6.8 ■

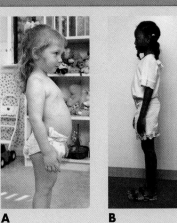

■ **Figure 6.8** Normal development of posture and spinal curves. (A) Toddler: Protruding abdomen; lumbar lordosis. (B) School-age child: Height of shoulders and hips is level; balanced thoracic convex and lumbar concave curves.

A   B

ANATOMICAL DIFFERENCES IN THE PELVIS OF A MALE AND A FEMALE

The **pelvis** is the lower portion of the trunk of the body. It forms a basin bound anteriorly and laterally by the hip bones and posteriorly by the sacrum and coccyx.

The bony pelvis is formed by the sacrum, the coccyx, and the bones that form the hip and pubic arch, the ilium, pubis, and ischium. These bones are separate in the child but become fused in adulthood.

Male Pelvis

The **male pelvis** (android type) is shaped like a *funnel*, forming a narrower outlet than the female. The bones of the android pelvis are generally thick and heavy and more suited for lifting and running. See Figure 6.9A ■

Female Pelvis

The **female pelvis** (gynecoid type) is shaped like a *basin*. It can be oval to round, and is wider than the male pelvis (Figure 6.9B ■). Its structure is designed to accommodate the average fetus during pregnancy and to facilitate the downward passage of the fetus through the birth canal during childbirth. The **gynecoid** pelvis is a type of pelvis characteristic of the normal female and is the ideal pelvic type for childbirth.

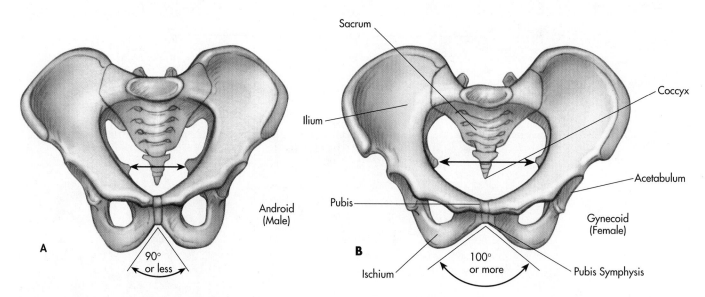

■ **Figure 6.9** (A) The male pelvis (android) is shaped like a funnel, forming a narrower outlet than the female. (B) The female pelvis (gynecoid) is shaped like a basin.

FRACTURES

A crack or break in the bone is called a **fracture (Fx).** A fracture is classified according to its external appearance, the site of the fracture, and the nature of the crack or break in the bone. Important fracture types are shown in Figure 6.10 ■

Many fractures fall into more than one category. For example, Colles' fracture is a transverse fracture, but depending on the injury, it can also be a comminuted fracture that can be either open or closed. The following provides a summary of the types of fractures:

Type of Fracture	Description	Figure 6.10A–6.10L
Closed, or simple	A completely internal break that does not involve a break in the skin (x-ray of the tibia and fibula). Note the break in the fibula (smaller bone).	
Open, or compound	The fracture projects through the skin and there is a possibility of infection or hemorrhage; more dangerous than a closed fracture	
Transverse	Breaks the shaft of a bone across its longitudinal axis; the break is in the fibula, the smaller bone (note that images A and C are the same)	
Comminuted	Shatters the affected part into a multitude of bony fragments (x-ray of the femur bone)	
Greenstick	Only one side of the shaft is broken, and the other is bent (like a greenstick); usually occurs in children whose long bones have not fully ossified	
Spiral	Produced by twisting stresses that are spread along the length of a bone (note the break in the humerus)	

Type of Fracture	Description	Figure 6.10A–6.10L
Colles'	A break in the distal portion of the radius; often the result of reaching out to cushion a fall	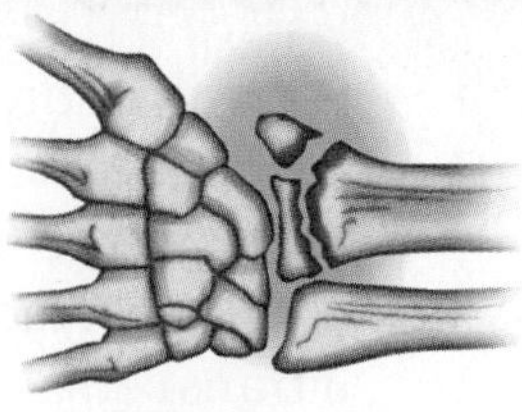 G
Pott's	Occurs at the ankle and affects both bones of the lower leg (fibula and tibia)	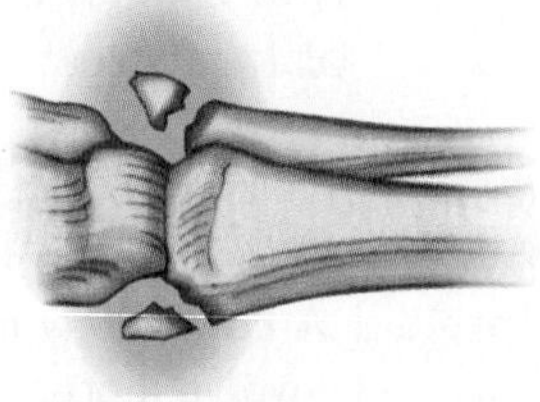 H
Compression	Occurs in vertebrae subjected to extreme stresses, as when one falls and lands on his or her bottom	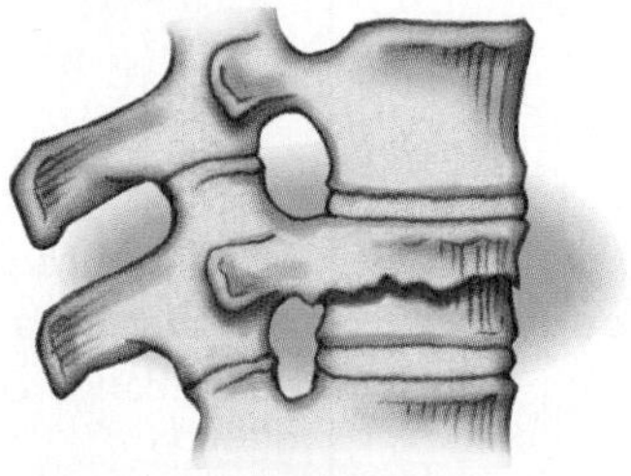 I
Vertebral compression	Fractures of the spine (vertebra) can cause severe "band-like" pain that radiates from the back to the sides of the body; often occur in patients with osteoporosis. Over the years, repeated spinal fractures can lead to chronic lower back pain as well as loss of height or curving of the spine due to collapse of the vertebrae. The collapse gives individuals a hunched-back appearance of the upper back, often called a "dowager's hump" because it commonly is seen in elderly women.	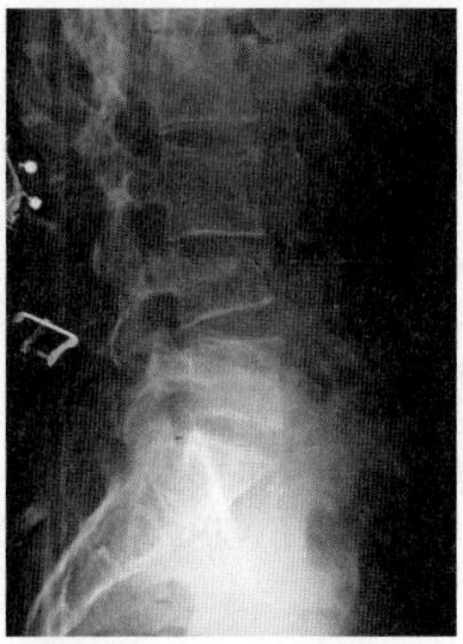 J
Epiphyseal	Usually occurs through the growth plate where the matrix is undergoing calcification and chondrocytes (cartilage cells) are dying; this type of fracture is seen in children	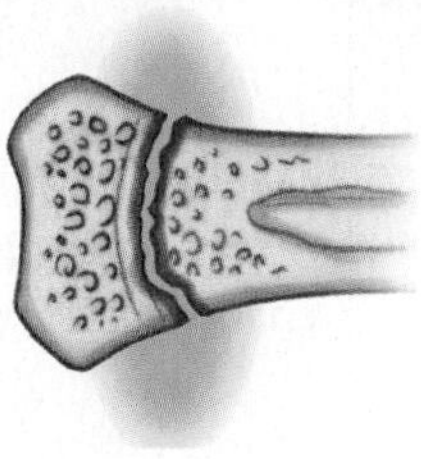 K
Stress	Usually occurs during the course of normal activity; some patients with osteoporosis develop stress fractures of the feet while walking or stepping off a curb	
Hip	Typically occurs as a result of a fall; with osteoporosis, hip fractures can occur as a result of trivial accidents	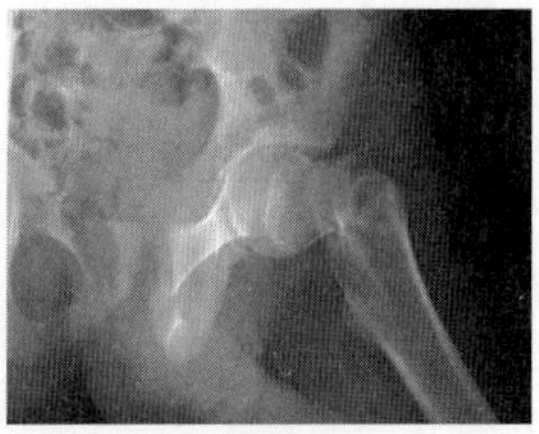 L

Anatomy and Physiology Labeling

Identify the structures shown below by filling in the blanks.

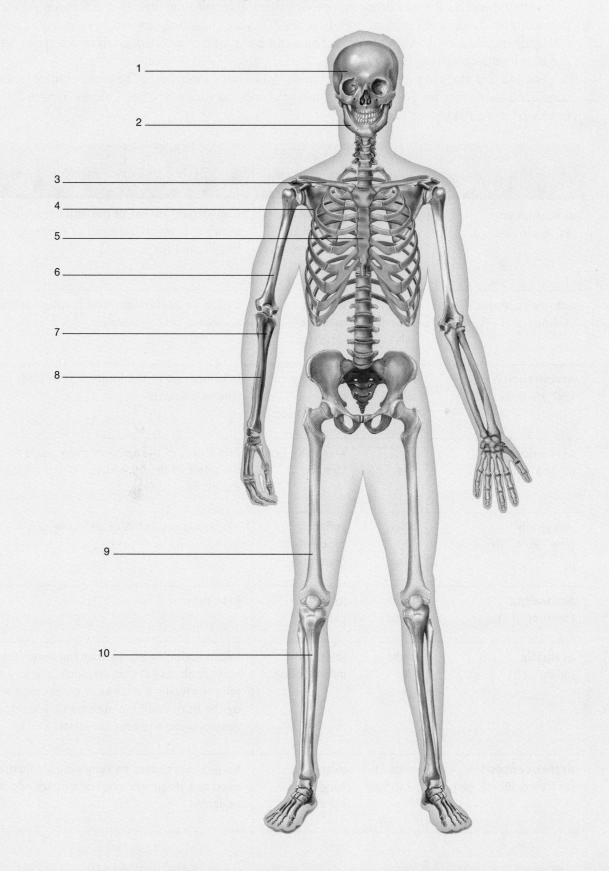

1 _____

2 _____

3 _____

4 _____

5 _____

6 _____

7 _____

8 _____

9 _____

10 _____

• Building Your Medical Vocabulary •

This section provides the foundation for learning medical terminology. Review the following alphabetized word list. Note how common prefixes and suffixes are repeatedly applied to word roots and combining forms to create different meanings. The word parts are color-coded: prefixes are green, suffixes are blue, roots/combining forms are red.

You will find that some terms have not been divided into word parts. These are common words or specialized terms that are included to enhance your medical vocabulary. See Chapter 1, page 7, to review pronunciation guidelines.

MEDICAL WORD	WORD PARTS		DEFINITION
	Part	**Meaning**	
acetabulum (ăs″ ĕ-tăb′ ū-lŭm)	acetabul -um	acetabulum, hip socket structure, tissue	Cup-shaped socket of the innominate bone (hip bone) into which the head of the femur (thighbone) fits
achondroplasia (ă -kŏn″ drō-plā′ sĭ-ă)	a- chondr/o -plasia	without cartilage formation	Defect in the formation of cartilage at the epiphyses of long bones
acroarthritis (ăk″ rō-ăr-thrī′ tĭs)	acr/o arthr -itis	extremity joint inflammation	Inflammation of the joints of the hands or feet (the extremities)
acromion (ă -krō′ mĭ-ŏn)	acr -omion	extremity, point shoulder	Projection of the spine of the scapula that forms the point of the shoulder and articulates with the clavicle
ankylosis (ăng″ kĭ-lō′ sĭs)	ankyl -osis	stiffening, crooked condition	Abnormal condition of stiffening of a joint
arthralgia (ăr-thrăl′ jĭ-ă)	arthr -algia	joint pain	Joint pain
arthritis (ăr-thrī′ tĭs)	arthr -itis	joint inflammation	Inflammation of a joint that can result from various disease processes, such as injury to a joint (including fracture), an attack on the joints by the body itself (an autoimmune disease), or general wear and tear on joints
arthrocentesis (ăr″ thrō-sĕn-tē′ sĭs)	arthr/o -centesis	joint surgical puncture	Surgical procedure to remove joint fluid; may be used as a diagnostic tool or as part of a treatment regimen

MEDICAL WORD	WORD PARTS		DEFINITION
	Part	**Meaning**	
arthroplasty (ăr″ thrō-plăs′ tē)	arthr/o -plasty	joint surgical repair	Surgical procedure used to repair a joint
arthroscope (ăr-thrŏs′ kōp)	arthr/o -scope	joint instrument for examining	Surgical instrument used to examine the interior of a joint
bone marrow transplant			Surgical procedure used to transfer bone marrow from a donor to a patient
bursa (bŭr′ sah)			Padlike sac between muscles, tendons, and bones that is lined with synovial membrane and contains a fluid, *synovia*
bursitis (bŭr-sī′ tĭs)	burs -itis	a pouch inflammation	Inflammation of a bursa
calcaneal (kăl-kā′ nē-ăl)	calcan/e -al	heel bone pertaining to	Pertaining to the heel bone
calcium (Ca) (kăl′ sĭ-ŭm)			Mineral that is essential for bone growth, teeth development, blood coagulation, and many other functions. The daily recommendations of calcium by age group are: 1–3 years 500 mg 4–8 years 800 mg 9–18 years 1300 mg 19–50 years 1000 mg 50+ years 1200 mg
carpal (kăr′ pəl)	carp -al	wrist pertaining to	Pertaining to the wrist bones. There are two rows of four bones in the wrist for a total of eight wrist bones.

MEDICAL WORD	WORD PARTS		DEFINITION
	Part	Meaning	
carpal tunnel syndrome			Abnormal condition caused by compression of the median nerve by the carpal ligament due to injury or trauma to the area, including repetitive movement of the wrists; symptoms: soreness, tenderness, weakness, pain, tingling, and numbness at the wrist. See Figure 6.11 ■

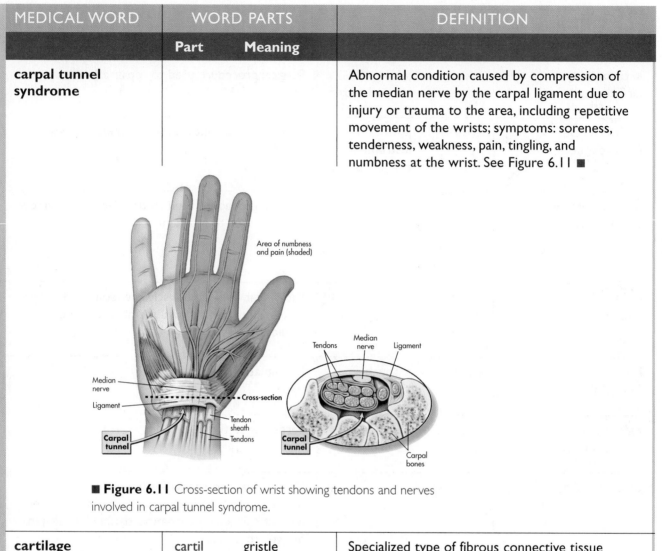

■ **Figure 6.11** Cross-section of wrist showing tendons and nerves involved in carpal tunnel syndrome.

cartilage (kär´ tǐ-lǐj)	cartil	gristle	Specialized type of fibrous connective tissue found at the ends of bone; forms the major portions of the embryonic skeleton before birth
	-age	related to	
cast			Type of material made of plaster of paris, fiberglass, sodium silicate, starch, or dextrin used to immobilize a fractured bone, a dislocation, or a sprain. See Figure 6.12 ■

■ **Figure 6.12** This girl has a long leg cast, which was applied after surgery to correct her clubfoot.

MEDICAL WORD	WORD PARTS		DEFINITION
	Part	**Meaning**	
chondral (kŏn´ drăl)	chondr -al	cartilage pertaining to	Pertaining to cartilage
chondrocostal (kŏn″ drō-kŏs´ tăl)	chondr/o cost -al	cartilage rib pertaining to	Pertaining to the rib cartilage
clavicular (klă-vĭk´ ū-lăr)	clavicul -ar	clavicle, collar bone pertaining to	Pertaining to the clavicle (*collar bone*)
coccygeal (kŏk-sĭj´ ĭ-ăl)	coccyg/e -al	coccyx, tailbone pertaining to	Pertaining to the coccyx (*tailbone*)
coccygodynia (kŏk-sĭ-gō-dĭn´ ĭ-ă)	coccyg/o -dynia	coccyx, tailbone pain	Pain in the coccyx (*tailbone*)
collagen (kŏl´ ă-jĕn)	coll/a -gen	glue formation, produce	Fibrous insoluble protein found in the connective tissue, skin, ligaments, and cartilage
connective	connect -ive	to bind together nature of	Literally means *the nature of connecting or binding together*
costal (kăst´ əl)	cost -al	rib pertaining to	Pertaining to the rib
costosternal (kăs″ tō-stĕr´ năl)	cost/o stern -al	rib sternum pertaining to	Pertaining to a rib and the sternum
craniectomy (krā″ nĭ-ĕk´ tŏ-mē)	crani -ectomy	skull surgical excision	Surgical excision of a portion of the skull. *Note that the suffix begins with a vowel: drop the (o) from the combining form and add –ectomy to form craniectomy.*
craniotomy (krā″ nĭ-ŏt´ ō-mē)	crani/o -tomy	skull incision	Surgical incision made into the skull
dactylic (dăk´ tĭl´ ĭk)	dactyl -ic	finger or toe pertaining to	Pertaining to the finger or toe

MEDICAL WORD	WORD PARTS		DEFINITION
	Part	**Meaning**	
dactylogram (dăk-til′ə grăm)	dactyl/o -gram	finger or toe mark, record	Medical term for fingerprint
dislocation (dĭs″ lō-kā′ shŭn)	dis- locat -ion	apart to place process	Displacement of a bone from a joint
femoral (fĕm′ ŏr-ăl)	femor -al	femur pertaining to	Pertaining to the femur; the *thigh bone,* the longest bone in the body
fibular (fĭb′ ū-lăr)	fibul -ar	fibula pertaining to	Pertaining to the fibula; the *smaller of the two lower leg bones*
fixation (fĭks-ā′ shŭn)	fixat -ion	fastened process	Process of holding or fastening in a fixed position; making rigid, immobilizing
flatfoot			Abnormal flatness of the sole and arch of the foot; also known as *pes planus*
genu valgum (jē′ nū văl gŭm)			Medical term for knock-knee. See Figure 6.13A ■
genu varum (jē′ nū vā′ rŭm)			Medical term for bowleg. See Figure 6.13B ■

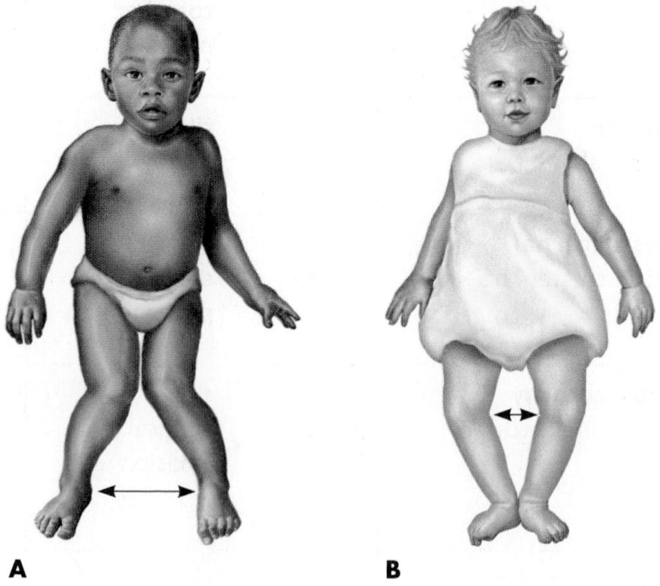

■ **Figure 6.13** (A) Genu valgum, or knock-knee. Note that the ankles are far apart when the knees are together. (B) Genu varum, or bowleg. The legs are bowed so that the knees are far apart as the child stands.

A   B

MEDICAL WORD	WORD PARTS		DEFINITION
	Part	**Meaning**	
gout (gowt) 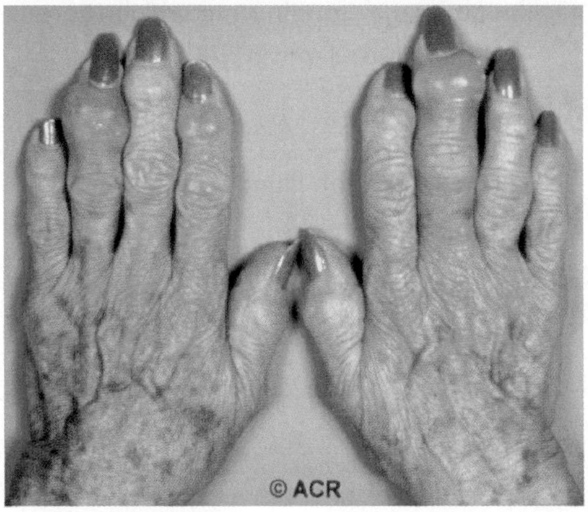	 ■ **Figure 6.14** Gout of the finger joint. (Source: Reprinted from the Clinical Slide Collection on the Rheumatic Diseases, © 1991, 1995. Used by permission of the American College of Rheumatology.)		Hereditary metabolic disease that is a form of acute arthritis, which is marked by joint inflammation. It is caused by hyperuricemia, excessive amounts of uric acid in the blood, and deposits of urates of sodium (uric acid crystals) in and around the joints. It usually affects the great toe first, but can be seen in the finger, knee, or foot joints. See Figure 6.14 ■
hallux (hăl″ ŭks)			Medical term for the big or great toe
hammertoe (hăm′ er-tō)	 ■ **Figure 6.15** Hammertoe.		An acquired flexion deformity of the interphalangeal joint. See Figure 6.15 ■
humeral (hū′ měr-ăl)	humer -al	humerus pertaining to	Pertaining to the humerus (*upper arm bone*)

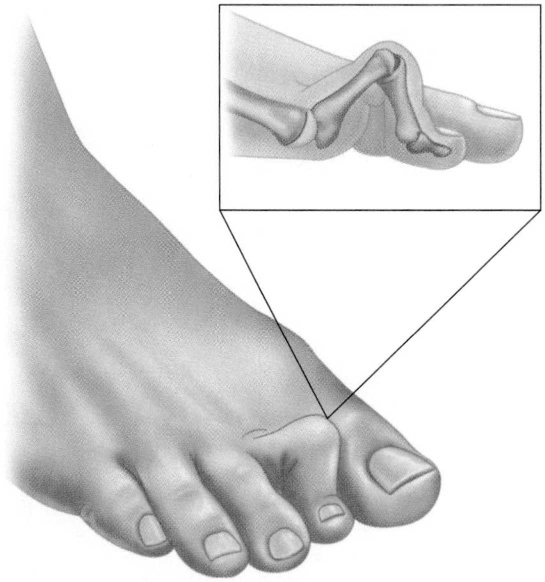

MEDICAL WORD	WORD PARTS		DEFINITION
	Part	Meaning	
hydrarthrosis (hi″ drăr-thrō′ sĭs)	hydr- arthr -osis	water joint condition	An abnormal condition in which there is an accumulation of watery fluid in the cavity of a joint
iliac (ĭl′ ē-ăk)	ili -ac	ilium pertaining to	Pertaining to the ilium
iliosacral (ĭl″ ĭ-ō-sā′ krăl)	ili/o sacr -al	ilium sacrum pertaining to	Pertaining to the ilium and the sacrum
intercostals (ĭn″ tēr-käs′ tăl)	inter cost -al	between rib pertaining to	Pertaining to the space between two ribs
ischial (ĭs′ kĭ-al)	isch/i -al	ischium, hip pertaining to	Pertaining to the ischium, hip
ischialgia (ĭs″ kĭ-ăl′ jĭ-ă)	isch/i -algia	ischium, hip pain	Pain in the ischium, hip
kyphosis (kĭ-fō′ sĭs)	kyph -osis	a hump condition	Condition in which the normal thoracic curvature becomes exaggerated, producing a "humpback" appearance. It can be caused by a congenital defect, a disease process such as tuberculosis and/or syphilis, malignancy, compression fracture, faulty posture, osteoarthritis, rheumatoid arthritis, rickets, osteoporosis, or other conditions. See Figure 6.16A ■

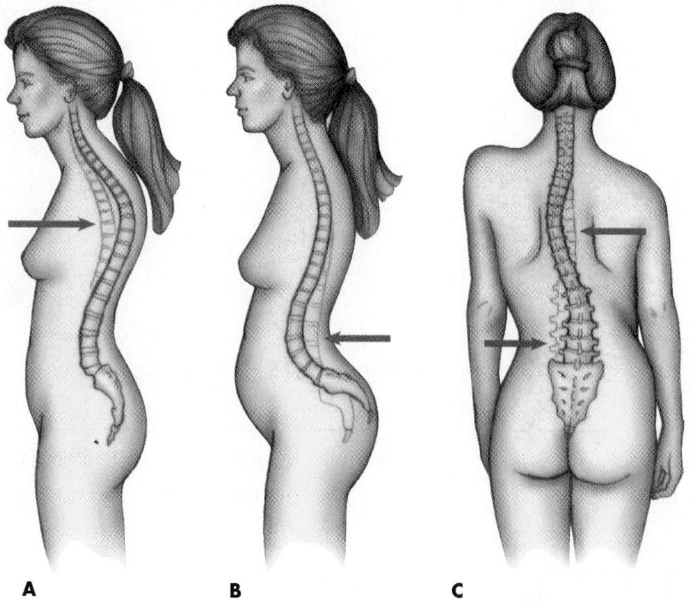

■ **Figure 6.16** Abnormal curvatures of the spine: (A) kyphosis; (B) lordosis; and (C) scoliosis.

A   B   C

MEDICAL WORD	WORD PARTS		DEFINITION
	Part	Meaning	
laminectomy (lăm″ ĭ-něk′ tō-mē)	lamin -ectomy	lamina (thin plate) surgical excision	Surgical excision of a vertebral posterior arch
ligament (lig) (lĭg′ ă-měnt)			Band of fibrous connective tissue that connects bones, cartilages, and other structures; also serves as a place for the attachment of fascia
lordosis (lŏr-dō′ sĭs)	lord -osis	bending, curve, swayback condition	An abnormal anterior curvature of the lumbar spine. This condition can be referred to as *swayback* because the abdomen and buttocks protrude due to an exaggerated lumbar curvature. See Figure 6.16B ■
lumbar (lŭm′ băr)	lumb -ar	loin, lower back pertaining to	Pertaining to the loins (*lower back*)
lumbodynia (lŭm″ bō-dĭn′ ĭ-ă)	lumb/o -dynia	loin, lower back pain	Pain in the loins (*lower back*)
mandibular (măn-dĭb′ ū-lăr)	mandibul -ar	lower jawbone pertaining to	Pertaining to the lower jawbone
maxillary (măk′ sĭ-lěr″ē)	maxill -ary	jawbone pertaining to	Pertaining to the upper jawbone
meniscus (měn-ĭs′ kŭs)	menisc -us	crescent structure	Crescent-shaped interarticular fibrocartilage structure found in certain joints, especially the lateral and medial *menisci* (semilunar cartilages) of the knee joint
metacarpals (mět″ ă-kär′ pəl)	meta- carp -al	beyond wrist pertaining to	Pertaining to the bones of the hand. There are five radiating bones in the fingers.
metacarpectomy (mět″ ă-kär-pěk′ tō-mē)	meta- carp -ectomy	beyond wrist surgical excision	Surgical excision of one or more bones of the hand

MEDICAL WORD	WORD PARTS		DEFINITION
	Part	**Meaning**	
myelitis (mī-ĕ-lī′ tĭs)	myel -itis	bone marrow inflammation	Inflammation of the bone marrow
myeloma (mī-ē-lō′ mă)	myel -oma	bone marrow tumor	Tumor of the bone marrow
myelopoiesis (mī′ ĕl-ō-poy-ē′ sĭs)	myel/o -poiesis	bone marrow formation	Formation of bone marrow
olecranal (ō-lĕk′ răn-ăl)	olecran -al	elbow pertaining to	Pertaining to the elbow
osteoarthritis (OA) (ŏs″ tē-ō-ăr-thrī′ tĭs)	oste/o arthr -itis	bone joint inflammation	Inflammation of the bone and joint; the most common type of arthritis in the United States and in people over 55 years of age. Women are more likely to suffer from this condition. See Figure 6.17 ■

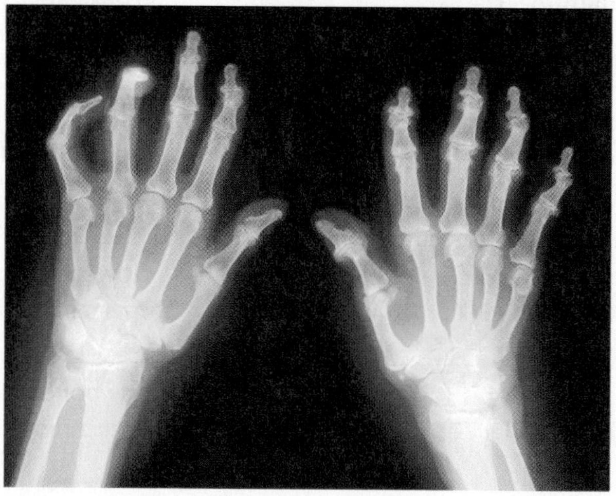

■ **Figure 6.17** X-ray showing typical joint changes associated with osteoarthritis.
(Source: Getty Images/Stone Allstock.)

MEDICAL WORD	WORD PARTS		DEFINITION
osteoblast (ŏs′ tē-ō-blăst″)	oste/o -blast	bone immature cell, germ cell	Bone-forming cell
osteocarcinoma (ŏs″ tē-ō-kăr″ sĭn-ō mă)	oste/o carcin -oma	bone cancer tumor	Cancerous tumor of a bone
osteochondritis (ŏs″ tē-ō-kŏn-drī′ tĭs)	oste/o chondr -itis	bone cartilage inflammation	Inflammation of bone and cartilage
osteogenesis (ŏs″ tē-ō-jĕn′ ĕ-sĭs)	oste/o -genesis	bone formation	Formation of bone

MEDICAL WORD	WORD PARTS		DEFINITION
	Part	**Meaning**	
osteomalacia (ŏs″ tē-ō-măl-ā′ shĭ-ă)	oste/o -malacia	bone softening	Softening of bones
osteomyelitis (ŏs″ tē-ō-mī″ ĕl-ī′ tĭs)	oste/o myel -itis	bone bone marrow inflammation	Inflammation of the bone marrow. See Figure 6.18 ■

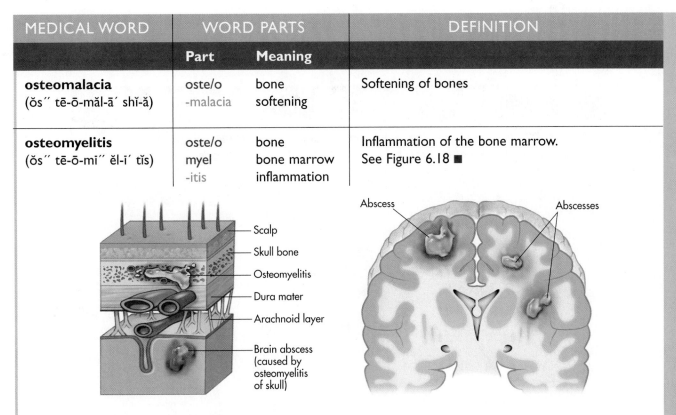

■ **Figure 6.18** Abscess of the brain due to osteomyelitis.

osteopenia (ŏs″ tē-ō-pē′ nĭ-ă)	oste/o -penia	bone deficiency	Deficiency of bone tissue, regardless of the cause
osteoporosis (ŏs″ tē-ō-por-ō′ sĭs)	oste/o por -osis	bone a passage condition	Abnormal condition characterized by a decrease in the density of bones, decreasing their strength and causing fragile bones, which can result in fractures. Estrogen is important in maintaining bone density in women. When estrogen levels drop after menopause, loss of bone density accelerates. Accelerated bone loss after menopause is a major cause of osteoporosis in women. It is most common in women after menopause, when it is called postmenopausal osteoporosis, but may also develop in men. See Figure 6.19 ■

■ **Figure 6.19** (A) Normal spongy bone. (B) Spongy bone with osteoporosis, which is characterized by a loss of bone material.

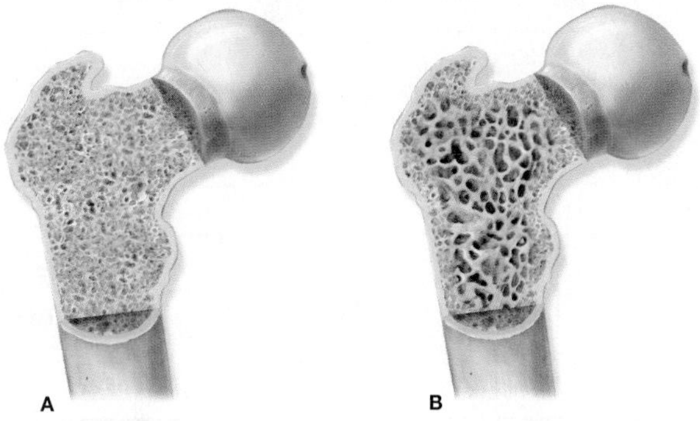

MEDICAL WORD	WORD PARTS		DEFINITION
	Part	**Meaning**	

LIFE SPAN CONSIDERATIONS

With normal aging, individuals can lose 1.0–1.5 inches in height. Loss of more than 1.5 inches in height can be related to vertebral compression fractures and other issues due to osteoporosis. See Figure 6.20 ■

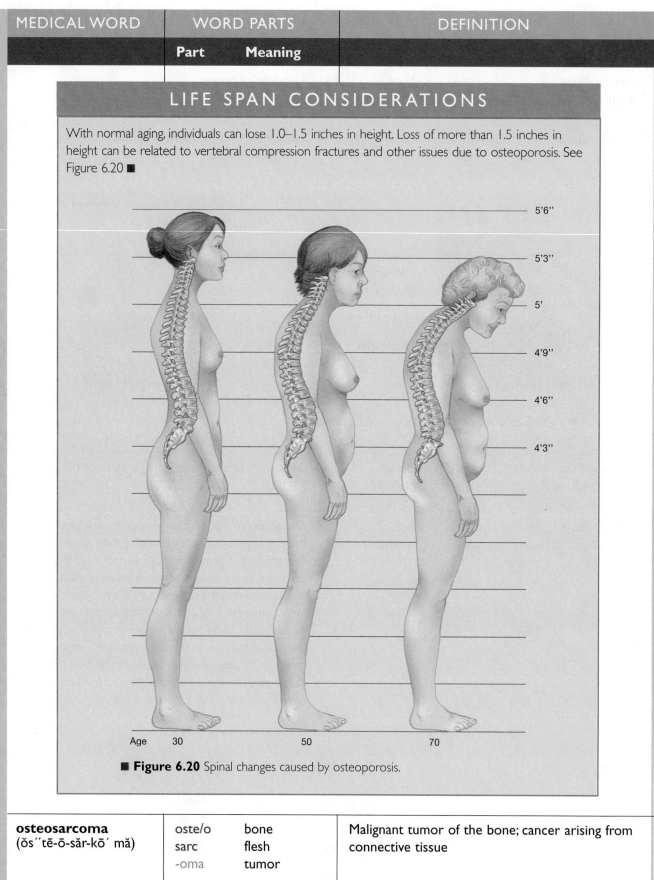

■ **Figure 6.20** Spinal changes caused by osteoporosis.

| osteosarcoma (ŏs″tē-ō-săr-kō′ mă) | oste/o
sarc
-oma | bone
flesh
tumor | Malignant tumor of the bone; cancer arising from connective tissue |

MEDICAL WORD	WORD PARTS		DEFINITION
	Part	Meaning	
osteotome (ŏs´ tē-ō-tōm´´)	oste/o -tome	bone instrument to cut	Surgical instrument used for cutting bone
patellar (pă-těl´ ăr)	patell -ar	kneecap pertaining to	Pertaining to the patella; the *kneecap*
pedal (pěd´ l)	ped -al	foot pertaining to	Pertaining to the foot
periosteoedema (pěr´´ ĭ-ŏs´´ tē-ō-ĕ-dē´ mă)	peri- oste/o -edema	around bone swelling	Swelling around a bone
phalangeal (fā-lăn´ jē-ăl)	phalang/e -al	phalanges (finger/toe bones) pertaining to	Pertaining to the bones of the fingers and the toes
phosphorus (P) (fŏs´ fō-rŭs)	phos phor -us	light carrying pertaining to	Mineral that is essential in bone formation, muscle contraction, and many other functions
polyarthritis (pŏl´´ ē-ăr-thrī´ tĭs)	poly- arthr -itis	many, much joint inflammation	Inflammation of more than one joint
rachigraph (rā´ kĭ-grăf)	rach/i -graph	spine instrument for recording	Instrument used to measure the curvature of the spine
radial (rā´ dĭ-ăl)	rad/i -al	radius pertaining to	Pertaining to the radius (lateral lower arm bone in line with the thumb). *A radial pulse can be found on the thumb side of the arm.*
radiograph (rā´ dĭ-ō-grăf)	radi/o -graph	x-ray record, instrument for recording	Film or record on which an x-ray image is produced
reduction (rē-dŭk´ shŭn)	re- duct -ion	back to lead process	Manipulative or surgical procedure used to correct a fracture or hernia

MEDICAL WORD	WORD PARTS		DEFINITION
	Part	**Meaning**	
rheumatoid arthritis (RA) (roo´ mă-toyd ăr-thrĭ´ tĭs)	rheumat -oid arthr -itis	discharge resemble joint inflammation	Chronic autoimmune disease characterized by inflammation of the joints, stiffness, pain, and swelling, which results in crippling deformities. See Figures 6.21 ■ and 6.22 ■

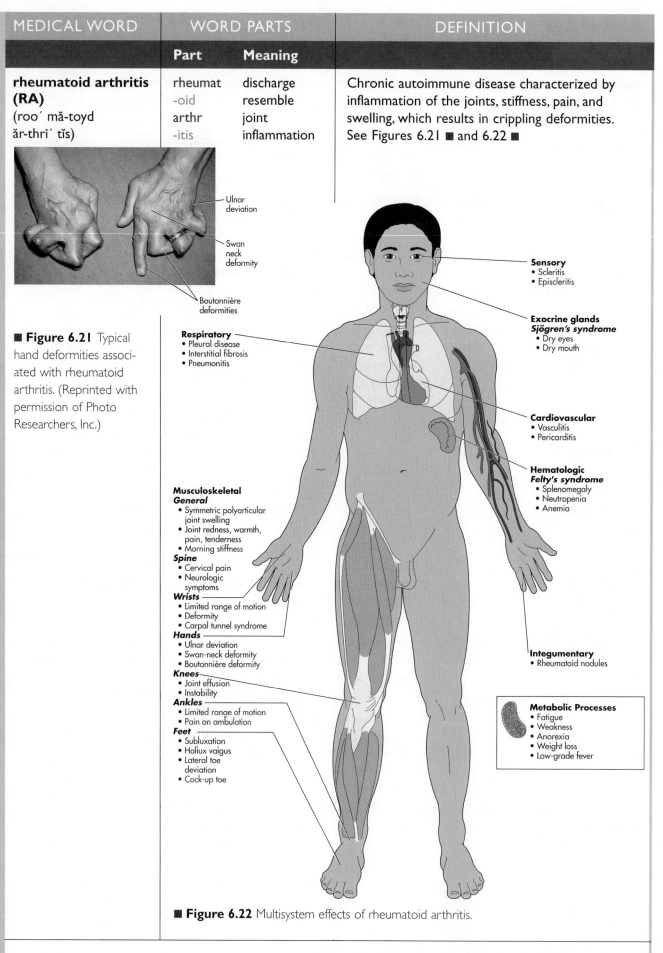

Ulnar deviation

Swan neck deformity

Boutonnière deformities

■ **Figure 6.21** Typical hand deformities associated with rheumatoid arthritis. (Reprinted with permission of Photo Researchers, Inc.)

Sensory
• Scleritis
• Episcleritis

Exocrine glands
Sjögren's syndrome
• Dry eyes
• Dry mouth

Cardiovascular
• Vasculitis
• Pericarditis

Hematologic
Felty's syndrome
• Splenomegaly
• Neutropenia
• Anemia

Integumentary
• Rheumatoid nodules

Respiratory
• Pleural disease
• Interstitial fibrosis
• Pneumonitis

Musculoskeletal
General
• Symmetric polyarticular joint swelling
• Joint redness, warmth, pain, tenderness
• Morning stiffness
Spine
• Cervical pain
• Neurologic symptoms
Wrists
• Limited range of motion
• Deformity
• Carpal tunnel syndrome
Hands
• Ulnar deviation
• Swan-neck deformity
• Boutonnière deformity
Knees
• Joint effusion
• Instability
Ankles
• Limited range of motion
• Pain on ambulation
Feet
• Subluxation
• Haliux valgus
• Lateral toe deviation
• Cock-up toe

Metabolic Processes
• Fatigue
• Weakness
• Anorexia
• Weight loss
• Low-grade fever

■ **Figure 6.22** Multisystem effects of rheumatoid arthritis.

MEDICAL WORD	WORD PARTS		DEFINITION
	Part	Meaning	
rickets (rĭk´ ĕts)			Abnormal condition that can occur in children and is caused by a lack of vitamin D
scapular (skăp´ ū-lăr)	scapul -ar	shoulder blade pertaining to	Pertaining to the shoulder blade
scoliosis (skō″ lĭ-ō´ sĭs)	scoli -osis	curvature condition	An abnormal lateral curvature of the spine. The characteristic signs include asymmetry of the trunk, uneven shoulders and hips, a one-sided rib hump, and a prominent scapula. See Figure 6.23 ■ and Figure 6.16C ■

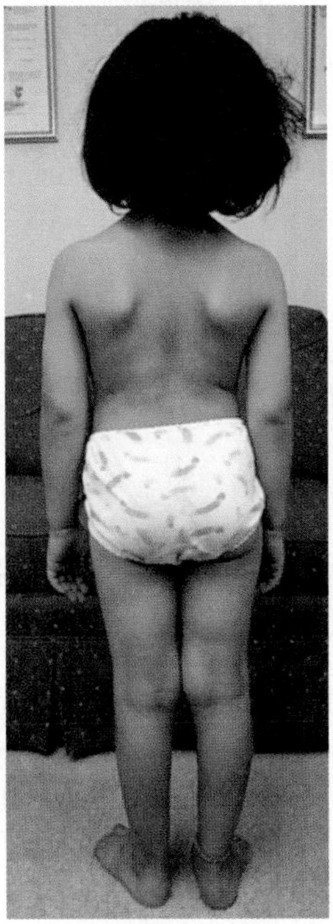

■ **Figure 6.23** Does this child have legs of different lengths or scoliosis? Look at the level of the iliac crests and shoulders to see if they are level. See the more prominent crease at the waist on the right side? This child could have scoliosis.

MEDICAL WORD	WORD PARTS		DEFINITION
spinal (spī´ năl)	spin -al	spine pertaining to	Pertaining to the spine
splint			Appliance used for fixation, support, and rest of an injured body part
spondylitis (spŏn-dĭl-ī´ tĭs)	spondyl -itis	vertebra inflammation	Inflammation of one or more vertebrae
sprain			A traumatic injury to the tendons, muscles, or ligaments around a joint characterized by pain, swelling, and discoloration

MEDICAL WORD	WORD PARTS		DEFINITION
	Part	**Meaning**	
spur			Sharp or pointed projection, as on a bone
sternal (stĕr´ năl)	stern -al	sternum, breastbone pertaining to	Pertaining to the sternum (*breastbone*)
sternotomy (stĕr-nŏt´ ō-mē)	stern/o -tomy	sternum, breastbone incision	Surgical incision of the sternum (*breastbone*)
subclavicular (sŭb˝ klă-vĭk´ ū-lăr)	sub- clavicul -ar	under, beneath clavicle, collar bone pertaining to	Pertaining to beneath the clavicle (*collar bone*)
subcostal (sŭb-kŏs´ tăl)	sub- cost -al	under, beneath rib pertaining to	Pertaining to beneath the ribs
submaxilla (sŭb˝măk-sĭl´ă)	sub- maxilla	under, beneath jaw	Below the jaw or mandible
symphysis (sĭm´ fĭ-sĭs)	sym- -physis	together growth	Literally means *growing together;* a joint in which adjacent bony surfaces are firmly united by fibrocartilage. An example is the *symphysis pubis,* where the bones of the pelvis have grown together.
tendonitis (tĕn´ dŭ-nī tĭs)	tendon -itis	tendon inflammation	Inflammation of a tendon
tennis elbow			Chronic condition characterized by elbow pain caused by excessive pronation and supination activities of the forearm; usually caused by strain, as in playing tennis
tibial (tĭb´ ĭ-ăl)	tibi -al	tibia pertaining to	Pertaining to the tibia; the *shin bone.* Larger of the two bones of the lower leg.

MEDICAL WORD	WORD PARTS		DEFINITION
	Part	Meaning	
traction (Tx) (trăk´ shŭn)	tract -ion	to draw process	Process of drawing or pulling on bones or muscles to relieve displacement and facilitate healing. See Figure 6.24 ■

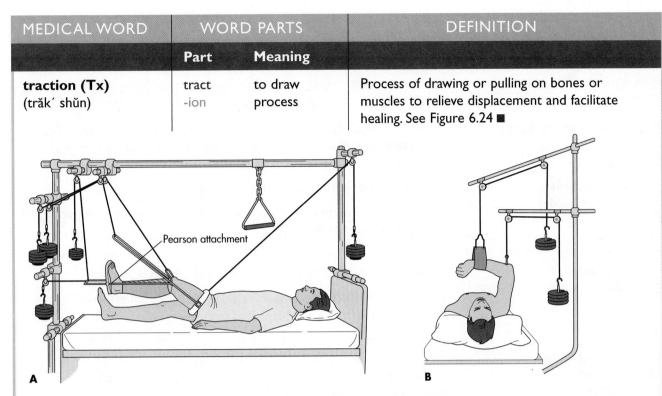

Pearson attachment

A

B

■ **Figure 6.24** Traction is the application of a pulling force to maintain bone alignment during fracture healing. Different fractures require different types of traction. (A) Balanced suspension traction is commonly used for fractures of the femur. (B) Skeletal traction, in which the pulling force is applied directly to the bone, may be used to treat fractures of the humerus.

MEDICAL WORD	WORD PARTS		DEFINITION
ulnar (ŭl´ năr)	uln -ar	ulna, elbow pertaining to	Pertaining to the ulna (medial lower arm bone), or to the nerve or artery named from it. *The ulna is located on the little finger side of the arm.*
ulnocarpal (ŭl˝ nō-kăr´ păl)	uln/o carp -al	ulna, elbow wrist pertaining to	Pertaining to the ulna side of the wrist
vertebral (věr´ tě-brăl)	vertebr -al	vertebra pertaining to	Pertaining to a vertebra
vertebrosternal (věr˝ tě-brō-ster´ năl)	vertebr/o stern -al	vertebra sternum pertaining to	Pertaining to a vertebra and the sternum
xiphoid (zĭf´ oyd)	xiph -oid	sword resemble	Literally means *resembling a sword*. The xiphoid process is the lowest portion of the sternum; a sword-shaped cartilaginous process supported by bone.

• Drug Highlights •

TYPE OF DRUG	DESCRIPTION AND EXAMPLES
anti-inflammatory agents	Relieves the swelling, tenderness, redness, and pain of inflammation. Such agents can be classified as steroidal (corticosteroids) and nonsteroidal.
corticosteroids (glucocorticoids)	Steroid substance with potent anti-inflammatory effects EXAMPLES: Depo-Medrol (methylprednisolone acetate), prednisone, and Delta-Cortef (prednisolone)
nonsteroidal (NSAIDs)	Agents used in the treatment of arthritis and related disorders EXAMPLES: Bayer aspirin (acetylsalicylic acid), MotrinIB (ibuprofen), Feldene (piroxicam), ketoprofen, and Naprosyn (naproxen)
disease-modifying antirheumatic drugs (DMARDs)	Can influence the course of the disease progression; therefore, their introduction in early rheumatoid arthritis is recommended to limit irreversible joint damage. EXAMPLES: gold preparation Ridaura (auranofin); antimalarial Plaquenil Sulfate (hydroxychloroquine sulfate); a chelating agent Cuprimine (penicillamine) and the immunosuppressants Trexall (methotrexate sodium), Imuran (azathioprine), and Cytoxan (cyclophosphamide)
COX-2 inhibitors	Cyclooxygenase (COX) is an enzyme involved in many aspects of normal cellular function and in the inflammatory response. COX-2 is found in joints and other areas affected by inflammation as occurs with osteoarthritis and rheumatoid arthritis. Inhibition of COX-2 reduces the production of compounds associated with inflammation and pain. EXAMPLES: Celebrex (celecoxib) and Mobic (meloxicam)
antitumor necrosis factor (anti-TNF) drugs	These drugs have evolved out of the biotechnology industry and seem to slow, if not halt altogether, the destruction of the joints by disrupting the activity of tumor necrosis factor (TNF), a substance involved in the body's immune response. EXAMPLE: Enbrel (etanercept)
agents used to treat gout	Acute attacks of gout are treated with colchicine. Once the acute attack of gout has been controlled, drug therapy to control hyperuricemia can be initiated. EXAMPLES: Benemid (probenecid) and Zyloprim (allopurinol)

TYPE OF DRUG	DESCRIPTION AND EXAMPLES
agents used to treat or prevent postmenopausal osteoporosis	
antiresorptive agents	Antiresorptive agents decrease the removal of calcium from bones. *Fosamax* reduces the activity of the cells that cause bone loss and increases the amount of bone in most patients. *Actonel* inhibits osteoclast-mediated bone resorption and modulates bone metabolism. To receive the clinical benefits of either of these drugs the patient must be informed and follow the prescribed drug regimen. EXAMPLES: Fosamax (alendronate), Actonel (risedronate), Evista (raloxifene), Boniva (ibandronate), Calcimar (calcitonin), and Reclast (zoledronate)
estrogen hormone therapy (EHT)	After menopause, EHT has been shown to prevent bone loss, increase bone density, and prevent bone fractures. It is useful in preventing osteoporosis in postmenopausal women. EXAMPLES: Premarin, Estrace, Estratest (oral estrogen), Estraderm, Vivelle (transdermal estrogen via skin patch) Estrogen also is available in combination with progesterone as pills and patches.
analgesics	Agents that relieve pain. They are classified as narcotic or non-narcotic.
narcotic	EXAMPLES: Demerol (meperidine HCl) and morphine sulfate
non-narcotic	EXAMPLES: Tylenol (acetaminophen), aspirin, ibuprofen (Advil, Motrin, Nuprin), and Naprosyn (naproxen)

• Diagnostic and Lab Tests •

TEST	DESCRIPTION
arthrography (ăr-thrŏg´ ră-fē)	Diagnostic examination of a joint (usually the knee) in which air and then a radiopaque contrast medium are injected into the joint space, x-rays are taken, and internal injuries of the meniscus, cartilage, and ligaments can be seen if present.
arthroscopy (ăr-thrŏs´ kō-pē)	Process of examining internal structures of a joint via an arthroscope; usually done after an arthrography and before joint surgery. See Figure 6.25 ■

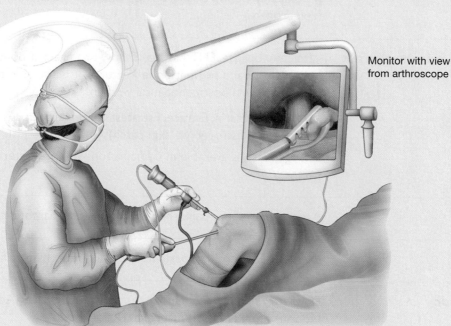

Monitor with view
from arthroscope

■ **Figure 6.25** Arthroscopic surgery involves the surgery of a joint with the use of a flexible arthroscope and other surgical tools. In this example, the surgeon inserts the arthroscope to evaluate the damage to the knee joint and then uses instruments to perform the necessary procedure.

TEST	DESCRIPTION
dual-energy x-ray absorptiometry scan (DXA) (ăb-sorp´ shē-ŏm´ ĕt-rĕ)	Test used to measure bone mass or bone mineral density; used for diagnosing osteoporosis, formerly known as DEXA. The bone density of the patient is compared to the average peak bone density of young adults of the same sex and race. This score is called the *T score,* and it expresses the bone density in terms of the number of standard deviations (SD) below peak young adult bone mass. Osteoporosis is defined as a bone density T score of −2.5 or below. Osteopenia (between normal and osteoporosis) is defined as a bone density T score between −1 and −2.5.

TEST	DESCRIPTION

LIFE SPAN CONSIDERATIONS

In women, osteoporosis is defined by the World Health Organization (WHO) as a bone mineral density −2.5 standard deviations (SDs) below peak bone mass (compared to an average 25- to 35-year-old healthy female of the same ethnicity) as measured by a dual energy x-ray absorptiometry (DXA) scan. The standard deviation is the difference between the BMD and that of the healthy young adult. This result is the T score. Positive T scores indicate the bone is stronger than normal; negative T scores indicate the bone is weaker than normal. The risk for bone fracture doubles with every SD below normal. Thus, a person with a BMD of 1 SD below normal (T score of −1) has twice the risk for bone fracture as a person with a normal BMD. A person with a T score of −2 has four times the risk for bone fracture as a person with a normal BMD. People with a high risk for bone fracture can be treated with the goal of preventing future fractures. A DXA scan is recommended every 2 years after osteoporosis is diagnosed to evaluate effectiveness of treatment.

TEST	DESCRIPTION
goniometry (gō″ nē-ŏm′ ĕt-rē)	Measurement of joint movements, especially range of motion (ROM) and angles via a goniometer. See Figure 6.26 ∎ 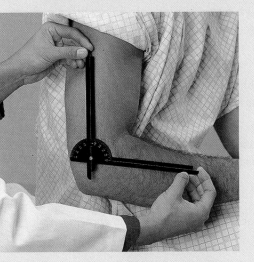 ∎ **Figure 6.26** Using a goniometer to measure joint ROM.
photon absorptiometry (fō′ tŏn ăb-sorp′ shē-ŏm′ ĕt-rĕ)	Bone scan that uses a low beam of radiation to measure bone mineral density and bone loss in the lumbar vertebrae; useful in monitoring osteoporosis.
thermography (thĕr-mŏg′ ră-fē)	Process of recording heat patterns of the body's surface; can be used to investigate the pathophysiology of rheumatoid arthritis.
x-ray	Examination of bones using an electromagnetic wave of high energy produced by the collision of a beam of electrons with a target in a vacuum tube; used to identify fractures and pathological conditions of the bones and joints such as rheumatoid arthritis, spondylitis, and tumors. See Figures 20.6 on page 727, 20.9 on page 730, and 20.15 on page 734.

TEST	DESCRIPTION
alkaline phosphatase blood test (ăl´ kă-lĭn fŏs´ fă-tās)	Blood test to determine the level of alkaline phosphatase; increased level in osteoblastic bone tumors, rickets, osteomalacia, and during fracture healing.
antinuclear antibodies (ANA) (ăn˝ tĭ-nū´ klē-ăr ăn´ tĭ-bŏd˝ ēs)	Present in a variety of immunological diseases; positive result can indicate rheumatoid arthritis, lupus, and other autoimmune diseases.
bone mineral density test (BMD)	Test used to measure bone mass or bone mineral density. Several different machines measure bone density. Peripheral machines measure density in the finger, wrist, kneecap, shin bone, and heel. Central machines measure density in the hip, spine, and total body.
calcium (Ca) blood test	Calcium level of the blood can be increased in metastatic bone cancer, acute osteoporosis, prolonged immobilization, and during fracture healing; can be decreased in osteomalacia and rickets.
C-reactive protein blood test (CRP) (sē-rē-ăk˝ tĭv prō´ tē-in)	Positive result can indicate rheumatoid arthritis, acute inflammatory change, and widespread metastasis.
phosphorus (P) blood test (fŏs´ fō-rŭs)	Phosphorus level of the blood can be increased in osteoporosis and fracture healing.
serum rheumatoid factor (RF) (sē´ rŭm roo´ mă-toyd)	Immunoglobulin present in the serum of 50–95% of adults with rheumatoid arthritis.
uric acid blood test (ū´ rĭk ăs´ ĭd)	Uric acid is increased in gout, arthritis, multiple myeloma, and rheumatism.

• Abbreviations •

ABBREVIATION	MEANING	ABBREVIATION	MEANING
ACL	anterior cruciate ligament	LLC	long leg cast
ANA	antinuclear antibodies	LLCC	long leg cylinder cast
AP	anteroposterior	NSAIDs	nonsteroidal anti-
BMD	bone mineral density (test)		inflammatory drugs
C1	cervical vertebra, first	OA	osteoarthritis
C2	cervical vertebra, second	ORTHO	orthopedics, orthopaedics
C3	cervical vertebra, third	P	phosphorus
Ca	calcium	PCL	posterior cruciate ligament
CDH	congenital dislocation of hip	PEMFs	pulsing electromagnetic
CRP	C-reactive protein blood test		fields
DJD	degenerative joint disease	PWB	partial weight bearing
DMARDs	disease-modifying	RA	rheumatoid arthritis
	antirheumatic drugs	RF	rheumatoid factor
DXA	dual-energy x-ray	ROM	range of motion
(formerly DEXA)	absorptiometry scan	SAC	short arm cast
EHT	estrogen hormone therapy	SD	standard deviation
Fx	fracture	SLC	short leg cast
JRA	juvenile rheumatoid arthritis	SPECT	single photon emission
jt	joint		computed tomography
KJ	knee jerk	T1	thoracic vertebra, first
L1	lumbar vertebra, first	T2	thoracic vertebra, second
L2	lumbar vertebra, second	T3	thoracic vertebra, third
L3	lumbar vertebra, third	TMJ	temporomandibular joint
LAC	long arm cast	TNF	tumor necrosis factor
lig	ligament	Tx	Traction

Anatomy and Physiology

Write your answers to the following questions.

1. The skeletal system is composed of _____ bones.

2. Name the two main divisions of the skeletal system.

   a. _____   b. _____

3. Name five classifications of bone and give an example of each.

   a. _____ Example: _____

   b. _____ Example: _____

   c. _____ Example: _____

   d. _____ Example: _____

   e. _____ Example: _____

4. State the six main functions of bones.

   a. _____   b. _____

   c. _____   d. _____

   e. _____   f. _____

5. Define the following features of a long bone.

   a. Epiphysis _____

   b. Diaphysis _____

   c. Periosteum _____

   d. Compact bone _____

   e. Medullary canal _____

   f. Endosteum _____

   g. Cancellous or spongy bone _____

162

6. Match the term in the left column with its definition from the right. Place the correct number from the right column in the space provided in the left column.

_____ **1.** Meatus   **a.** Air cavity within certain bones

_____ **2.** Head   **b.** Shallow depression in or on a bone

_____ **3.** Tuberosity   **c.** Pointed, sharp, slender process

_____ **4.** Process   **d.** Large, rounded process

_____ **5.** Condyle   **e.** Groove, furrow, depression, or fissure

_____ **6.** Tubercle   **f.** Tubelike passage or canal

_____ **7.** Crest   **g.** Opening in the bone for blood vessels, ligaments, and nerves

_____ **8.** Trochanter   **h.** Rounded projection that enters into the formation of a joint, articulation

_____ **9.** Sinus   **i.** Ridge on a bone

_____ **10.** Fissure   **j.** Small, rounded process

_____ **11.** Fossa   **k.** Rounded end of a bone

_____ **12.** Spine   **l.** Slitlike opening between two bones

_____ **13.** Foramen   **m.** Enlargement or protrusion of a bone

_____ **14.** Sulcus   **n.** Either of the two bony projections below the neck of the femur

7. Name the three classifications of joints.

a. _____   **b.** _____

c. _____

8. _____ is moving a body part away from the middle.

9. Adduction is _____ .

10. _____ is moving a body part in a circular motion.

11. Dorsiflexion is _____ .

12. _____ is turning outward.

13. Extension is _____ .

14. _____ is bending a limb.

15. Inversion is _____ .

16. _____ is lying face downward.

17. Protraction is _____.

18. _____ is moving a body part backward.

19. Rotation is _____.

20. _____ is lying face upward.

Word Parts

PREFIXES

Give the definitions of the following prefixes.

1. a- _____
2. dis- _____
3. hydr- _____
4. inter- _____
5. meta- _____
6. peri- _____
7. poly- _____
8. sub- _____
9. sym- _____
10. re- _____

ROOTS AND COMBINING FORMS

Give the definitions of the following roots and combining forms.

1. acetabul _____
2. cartil _____
3. acr _____
4. acr/o _____
5. ankyl _____
6. arthr _____
7. arthr/o _____
8. burs _____
9. calcan/e _____
10. locat _____
11. carcin _____
12. carp _____
13. carp/o _____
14. chondr _____
15. chondr/o _____
16. clavicul _____
17. fixat _____
18. coccyg/e _____
19. coccyg/o _____
20. coll/a _____
21. duct _____
22. connect _____
23. cost _____
24. cost/o _____

25. menisci _____

26. phos _____

27. crani _____

28. crani/o _____

29. dactyl _____

30. dactyl/o _____

31. femor _____

32. phor _____

33. fibul _____

34. radi/o _____

35. humer _____

36. ili _____

37. ili/o _____

38. isch/i _____

39. kyph _____

40. lamin _____

41. lord _____

42. lumb _____

43. lumb/o _____

44. mandibul _____

45. maxill _____

46. maxilla _____

47. myel _____

48. myel/o _____

49. rheumat _____

50. olecran _____

51. oste/o _____

52. patell _____

53. tract _____

54. ped _____

55. phalang/e _____

56. por _____

57. rachi _____

58. radi _____

59. sacr _____

60. sarc _____

61. scapul _____

62. scoli _____

63. scoli/o _____

64. spin _____

65. spondyl _____

66. stern _____

67. stern/o _____

68. tenon _____

69. tibi _____

70. uln _____

71. uln/o _____

72. vertebr _____

73. vertebr/o _____

74. xiph _____

SUFFIXES

Give the definitions of the following suffixes.

1. -ac _____ **2.** -al _____

3. -algia _____ **4.** -ar _____

5. -ary _____ **6.** -blast _____

7. -centesis _____ **8.** -age _____

9. -ion _____ **10.** -dynia _____

11. -ectomy _____ **12.** -edema _____

13. -gen _____ **14.** -genesis _____

15. -gram _____ **16.** -graph _____

17. -ic _____ **18.** -itis _____

19. -ive _____ **20.** -scope _____

21. -malacia _____ **22.** -us _____

23. -oid _____ **24.** -oma _____

25. -omion _____ **26.** -osis _____

27. -penia _____ **28.** -physis _____

29. -plasia _____ **30.** -plasty _____

31. -poiesis _____ **32.** -tome _____

33. -tomy _____ **34.** -um _____

Identifying Medical Terms

In the spaces provided, write the medical terms for the following meanings.

1. _____ Inflammation of the joints of the hands or feet

2. _____ Abnormal condition of stiffening of a joint

3. _____ Inflammation of a joint

4. _____ Pertaining to the heel bone

5. _____ Pertaining to cartilage

6. _____ Pain in the coccyx

7. _____ Pertaining to the rib

8. _____ Surgical excision of a portion of the skull

9. _____ Pertaining to the finger or toe

10. _____ Surgical instrument used for cutting bone

11. _____ Pertaining to the space between two ribs

12. _____ Pain in the hip

13. _____ Pertaining to the loins

14. _____ Tumor of the bone marrow

15. _____ Inflammation of the bone and joint

16. _____ Inflammation of the bone marrow

17. _____ Deficiency of bone tissue

18. _____ Pertaining to the foot

19. _____ Literally means resembling a sword

Spelling

Circle the correct spelling of each medical term

1. acrmoin / acromion

2. arthroscope / arthrscope

3. bursitis / buritis

4. chondrocostal / chondrcostal

5. conective / connective

6. cranotomy / craniotomy

7. dislocation / dislocaton

8. ischial / ischal

9. melyitis / myelitis

10. osteoporosis / osteoprosis

11. phosphous / phosphorus

12. patellar / patelar

13. phalangeal / phalangal

14. rachgraph / rachigraph

15. scolosis / scoliosis

16. spondylitis / spondlitis

17. symphysis / symphsis

18. tendnits / tendonitis

19. ulncarpal / ulnocarpal

20. vertebral / vertbral

Matching

Select the appropriate lettered meaning for each of the following words.

_____ **1.** arthroscope

_____ **2.** carpal tunnel syndrome

_____ **3.** fixation

_____ **4.** gout

_____ **5.** hammertoe

_____ **6.** kyphosis

_____ **7.** metacarpal

_____ **8.** rickets

_____ **9.** tennis elbow

_____ **10.** ulnar

a. Abnormal condition that can occur in children and is caused by a lack of vitamin D

b. An acquired flexion deformity of the interphalangeal joint

c. Hereditary metabolic disease that is a form of acute arthritis

d. Chronic condition characterized by elbow pain that is caused by excessive pronation and supination activities of the forearm

e. Making rigid, immobilizing

f. Pertaining to the elbow

g. Pertaining to the bones of the hand

h. In this condition, the normal thoracic curvature becomes exaggerated, producing a "humpback" appearance

i. Surgical instrument used to examine the interior of a joint

j. Abnormal condition caused by compression of the median nerve by the carpal ligament

k. Pertaining to the knee

Abbreviations

Place the correct word, phrase, or abbreviation in the space provided.

1. congenital dislocation of hip _____

2. degenerative joint disease _____

3. LLC _____

4. OA _____

5. pulsing electromagnetic fields _____

6. RA _____

7. single photon emission computed tomography _____

8. T 1 _____

9. TMJ _____

10. traction _____

Diagnostic and Laboratory Test

Select the best answer to each multiple-choice question. Circle the letter of your choice.

1. _____ is a diagnostic examination of a joint in which air and then a radiopaque contrast medium are injected into the joint space, x-rays are taken, and internal injuries of the meniscus, cartilage, and ligaments may be seen, if present.
   a. Arthroscopy   **c.** Arthrography
   b. Goniometry   **d.** Thermography

2. The process of recording heat patterns of the body's surface is:
   a. arthrography   **c.** goniometry
   b. arthroscopy   **d.** thermography

3. _____ is increased in gout, arthritis, multiple myeloma, and rheumatism.
   a. Calcium   **c.** Uric acid
   b. Phosphorus   **d.** Alkaline phosphatase

4. _____ level of the blood can be increased in osteoporosis and fracture healing.
   a. Antinuclear antibodies   **c.** Uric acid
   b. Phosphorus   **d.** Alkaline phosphatase

5. _____ is/are present in a variety of immunological diseases.
   a. Alkaline phosphatase   **c.** C-reactive protein
   b. Antinuclear antibodies   **d.** Uric acid

PRACTICAL APPLICATION

MEDICAL RECORD ANALYSIS

This exercise contains information, abbreviations, and medical terminology from an actual medical record or case study that has been adapted for this text. The names and any personal information have been created by the author. Read and study each form or case study and then answer the questions that follow. You may refer to Appendix III, Abbreviations and Symbols, on page A41.

Clear Shot Imaging Services
Phone (123) 456-7890

NAME: BELL, CRYSTAL JANE   ORD: 07DX00145

DATE OF BIRTH: 5/26/37

CLINICAL DATA: v49.81   POST MENO

REQUESTING PHYSICIAN: Kyle Preston, MD

EXAM CODE: XRDXA/76075   ORDER DATE: 03/19/xx

LOCATION: SHORTER MEDICAL

EXAM: XR DXA, BONE DENSITY SCAN 03/19/xx

BONE DENSITOMETRY, 3/19/xx

Routine bone densitometry of the lumbar spine and both hips was performed. The results of the examination expressed as standard deviations (SD) from the mean bone mineral density (BMD) are as follows:

Spine (L1-L4) T-score	0.6	Z-score	1.7
Femoral neck T-score	−2.3	Z-score	−0.8

Impression:

There is a discrepancy between the lumbar spine and hips due to what I believe is spondylosis. The hips are of a more accurate reading and is considered with osteopenia. Follow-up in 18–24 months is recommended.

DICTATED: Lions, Daniel

TECHNOLOGIST: 303768

transcribed: rs 03/19/xx

24599

VERIFIED: Daniel Lions, MD

Medical Record Questions

Place the correct answer in the space provided.

1. What is the meaning of DXA? _____

2. What does the abbreviation BMD mean? _____

3. What does the abbreviation L1 mean? _____

4. What is the medical term that means deficiency of bone tissue? _____

5. What is the exam code for this bone density scan? _____

PEARSON
mymedicalterminologylab

MyMedicalTerminologyLab is a premium online homework management system that includes a host of features to help you study. Registered users will find:

- Fun games and activities built within a virtual hospital
- Powerful tools that track and analyze your results—allowing you to create a personalized learning experience
- Videos, flashcards, and audio pronunciations to help enrich your progress
- Streaming lesson presentations and self-paced learning modules
- A space where you and your instructors can view and manage your assignments

verview of Obstetrics • Male Reproductive System •
ology • Radiology and Nuclear Medicine • Mental Health
troduction to Medical Terminology • Suffixes • Prefixes
rganization of the Body • Integumentary System • Skel
l System • **Muscular System**

Muscular System

LEARNING OUTCOMES

On completion of this chapter, you will
be able to:

1. Describe the muscular system.

2. Describe the three basic types of muscle
   tissue.

3. Explain the primary functions of muscles.

4. Analyze, build, spell, and pronounce medical
   words.

5. Comprehend the drugs highlighted in this
   chapter.

6. Describe diagnostic and laboratory tests
   related to the muscular system.

7. Identify and define selected abbreviations.

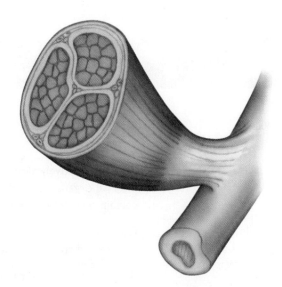

COMBINING FORMS OF THE MUSCULAR SYSTEM

agon/o	agony, a contest	**path/o**	disease
amputat/o	to cut through	**prosth/e**	an addition
brach/i	arm	**rhabd/o**	rod
cleid/o	clavicle	**rotat/o**	to turn
clon/o	turmoil	**sarc/o**	flesh
duct/o	to lead	**scler/o**	hardening
dactyl/o	finger or toe	**stern/o**	sternum
dermat/o	skin	**synov/o**	synovial
fasci/o	a band	**ten/o**	tendon
fibr/o	fiber	**therm/o**	hot, heat
is/o	equal	**ton/o**	tone, tension
metr/o	to measure	**tors/o**	twisted
muscul/o	muscle	**tort/i**	twisted
my/o(s)	muscle	**troph/o**	a turning
neur/o	nerve	**volunt/o**	will

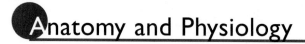

Anatomy and Physiology

The muscular system is composed of all the **muscles** in the body and works in coordination with the skeletal and nervous systems. Muscles provide the mechanism for movement of the body and locomotion from one place to another. In addition to causing movement, muscles produce heat and help the body maintain posture and stability. There are three basic types of muscles: skeletal, smooth, and cardiac. Table 7.1 ■ provides an at-a-glance look at the muscular system.

The muscles are the primary tissues of the system. They make up approximately 42% of a person's body weight and are composed of long, slender cells known as **fibers**. Muscle fibers are of different lengths and shapes and vary in color from white to deep red. Each muscle consists of a group of fibers held

TABLE 7.1 Muscular System at-a-Glance

Organ/Structure	Primary Functions/Description
Muscles	Cause movement, help to maintain posture, and produce heat
Skeletal muscles	Produces various types of body movement through contractility, extensibility, and elasticity
Smooth muscles	Produce relatively slow contraction with greater degree of extensibility in the internal organs, especially organs of the digestive, respiratory, and urinary tract, plus certain muscles of the eye and skin, and walls of blood vessels
Cardiac muscle	Contraction of the myocardium, which is controlled by the autonomic nervous system and specialized neuromuscular tissue located within the right atrium
Tendons	Bands of connective tissue that attach muscles to bones

together by connective tissue and enclosed in a fibrous sheath or **fascia**. See Figure 7.1 ∎

Each fiber within a muscle receives its own nerve impulses and has its own stored supply of glycogen, which it uses as fuel for energy. Muscle must be supplied with proper nutrition and oxygen to perform properly; therefore, blood and lymphatic vessels permeate its tissues.

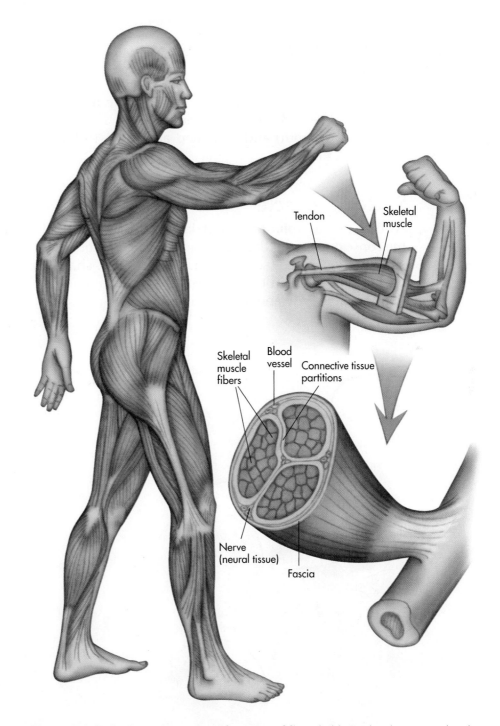

∎ **Figure 7.1** Skeletal muscle consists of a group of fibers held together by connective tissue. It is enclosed in a fibrous sheath (fascia).

TYPES OF MUSCLES

Skeletal muscle, smooth muscle, and cardiac muscle are the three basic types of muscles in the body. They are composed of different types of muscle tissue (e.g., striated or smooth) and classified according to their functions and appearance (Figure 7.2 ■).

Skeletal Muscle

Also known as **voluntary** or **striated** muscles, **skeletal muscles** are controlled by the conscious part of the brain and attach to the bones. These muscles have a cross-striped appearance (striated) and vary in size, shape, arrangement of fibers, and means of attachment to bones. Selected skeletal muscles are listed with their functions in Table 7.2 ■ and shown in Figure 7.3 ■

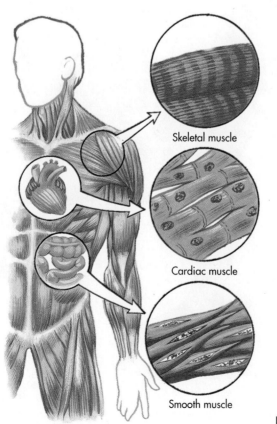

Skeletal muscle

Cardiac muscle

Smooth muscle

■ **Figure 7.2** Types of muscle tissue.

TABLE 7.2 Selected Skeletal Muscles

Muscle	Direction	Action
Sternocleidomastoid	Anterior	Rotates and laterally flexes neck
Trapezius	Anterior/posterior	Draws head back and to the side; rotates scapula
Deltoid	Anterior/posterior	Raises and rotates arm
Rectus femoris	Anterior	Extends leg and assists flexion of thigh
Sartorius	Anterior	Flexes and rotates the thigh and leg
Tibialis anterior	Anterior	Dorsiflexes foot and increases the arch in the beginning process of walking
Pectoralis major	Anterior	Flexes, adducts, and rotates arm
Biceps brachii	Anterior	Flexes arm and forearm and supinates forearm
External oblique	Anterior	Contracts abdomen and viscera (internal organs)
Rectus abdominis	Anterior	Compresses or flattens abdomen
Gastrocnemius	Anterior/posterior	Plantar flexes foot and flexes knee
Soleus	Anterior	Plantar flexes foot
Triceps	Posterior	Extends forearm
Latissimus dorsi	Posterior	Adducts, extends, and rotates arm; used during swimming
Gluteus medius	Posterior	Abducts and rotates thigh
Gluteus maximus	Posterior	Extends and rotates thigh
Biceps femoris	Posterior	Flexes knee and rotates it outward
Semitendinosus	Posterior	Flexes and rotates leg; extends thigh
Semimembranosus	Posterior	Flexes and rotates leg; extends thigh
Achilles tendon	Posterior	Plantar (sole of the foot) flexion and extension of ankle

There are over 600 skeletal muscles in the body that, through contractility, extensibility, excitability, and elasticity, are responsible for the movement of the body. **Contractility** allows muscles to change shape to become shorter and thicker. With **extensibility**, living muscle cells can be stretched and extended. They become longer and thinner. In **excitability**, muscles receive and respond to stimulation. With **elasticity**, once the stretching force is removed, a living muscle cell returns to its original shape.

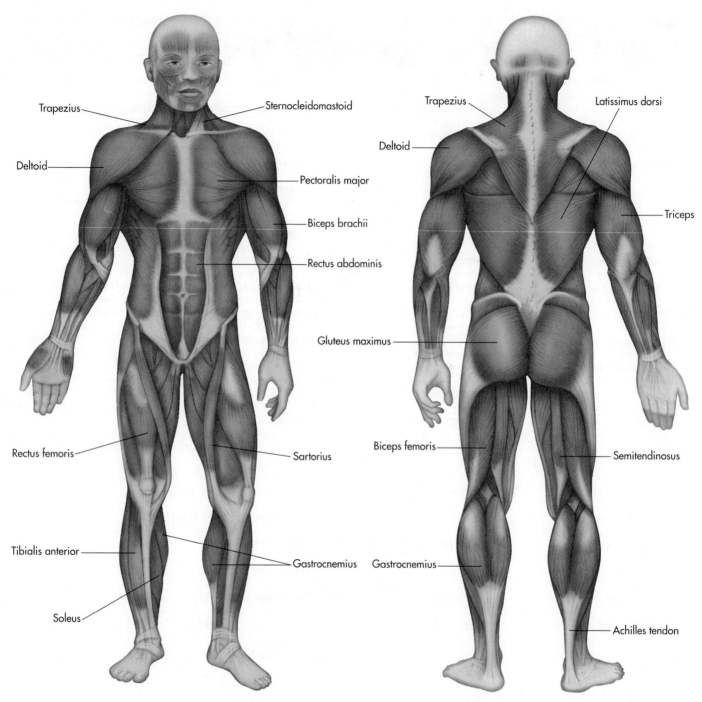

Trapezius

Sternocleidomastoid

Deltoid

Pectoralis major

Biceps brachii

Rectus abdominis

Rectus femoris

Sartorius

Tibialis anterior

Gastrocnemius

Soleus

Trapezius

Latissimus dorsi

Deltoid

Triceps

Gluteus maximus

Biceps femoris

Semitendinosus

Gastrocnemius

Achilles tendon

■ **Figure 7.3** Selected skeletal muscles and the Achilles tendon (anterior and posterior views).

LIFE SPAN CONSIDERATIONS

The movements of a newborn are uncoordinated and random. Muscular development proceeds from head to foot and from the center of the body to the periphery. Head and neck muscles are the first ones that a baby can control. A baby can hold his or her head up before he or she can sit erect.

Muscles have three distinguishable parts: the **body** or main portion, an **origin**, and an **insertion**. The origin is the more fixed attachment of the muscle to the stationary bone and the insertion is the point of attachment of a muscle to the bone that it moves. The means of attachment is a band of connective tissue called a **tendon**, which can vary in length from less than 1 inch to more than 1 foot. Some muscles, such as those in the abdominal region, the dorsal lumbar region, and the palmar region, form attachments using a wide, thin, sheetlike tendon known as an **aponeurosis**.

Skeletal muscles move body parts by pulling from one bone across its joint to another bone, with movement occurring at the diarthrotic (synovial) joint. The types of body movement occurring at the diarthrotic joints are described in Chapter 6, Skeletal System, on page 133.

Muscles and nerves function together as a motor unit. For skeletal muscles to contract, it is necessary to have stimulation by impulses from motor nerves. Skeletal muscles perform in groups and are classified as follows:

- **Antagonist**. Muscle that counteracts the action of another muscle; when one contracts the other relaxes

- **Prime mover or agonist**. Muscle that is primary in a given movement; the movement is produced by its contraction

- **Synergist**. Muscle that acts with another muscle to produce and assist movement

All movement is a result of the contraction of a prime mover (agonist) and the relaxation of the opposing muscle (antagonist). See Figure 7.4 ∎

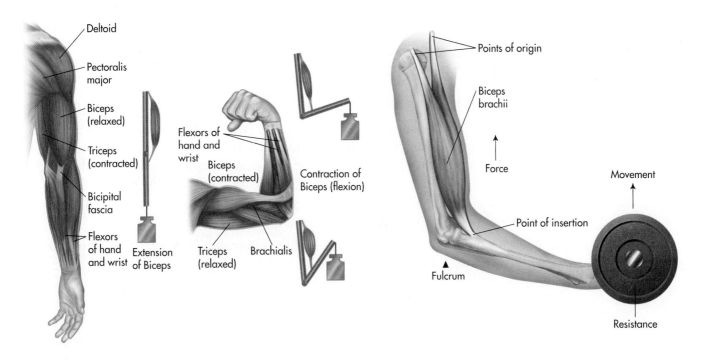

∎ **Figure 7.4** Coordination of antagonist muscles to perform movement.

Smooth Muscle

Also called *involuntary*, *visceral*, or *unstriated*, **smooth muscles** are not controlled by the conscious part of the brain. They are under the control of the autonomic nervous system and, in most cases, produce relatively slow contraction with a greater degree of extensibility. These muscles lack the cross-striped appearance of skeletal muscle and are smooth. Included in this type are the muscles of internal organs of the digestive, respiratory, and urinary tract plus certain muscles of the eye and skin.

Cardiac Muscle

The muscle of the heart (**myocardium**), the **cardiac muscle**, is *involuntary* but *striated* in appearance. It is under the control of the autonomic nervous system and has specialized neuromuscular tissue located within the right atrium. Cardiac muscle differs from the other two muscle types in that contraction can occur even without an initial nervous input. The cells that produce the stimulation for contraction without nervous input are called the **pacemaker cells**. Coordinated contraction of cardiac muscle cells in the heart propel blood from the atria and ventricles to the blood vessels of the circulatory system. Cardiac muscle cells, like all tissues in the body, rely on an ample blood supply to deliver oxygen and nutrients and to remove waste products such as carbon dioxide. The coronary arteries fulfill this function.

LIFE SPAN CONSIDERATIONS

In the older adult, the heart muscle becomes less able to propel the large amount of blood that is needed by the body. This makes a person feel tired more quickly and takes longer for recovery to occur.

FUNCTIONS OF MUSCLES

The following is a list of the primary functions of muscles:

1. Muscles are responsible for movement. The types of movement are locomotion where chemical energy is changed into mechanical energy, propulsion of substances through tubes as in circulation and digestion, and changes in the size of openings as in the contraction and relaxation of the iris of the eye.
2. Muscles help to maintain posture through a continual partial contraction of skeletal muscles. This process is known as **tonicity**.
3. Muscles help to produce heat through the chemical changes involved in muscular action.

Anatomy and Physiology Labeling

Identify the structures shown below by filling in the blanks.

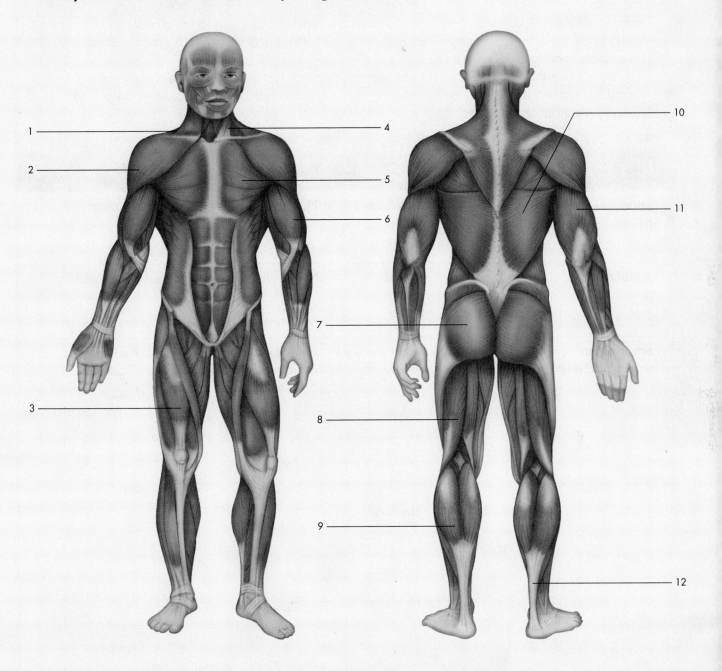

• Building Your Medical Vocabulary •

This section provides the foundation for learning medical terminology. Review the following alphabetized word list. Note how common prefixes and suffixes are repeatedly applied to word roots and combining forms to create different meanings. The word parts are color-coded: prefixes are green, suffixes are blue, **roots/combining forms are red**.

You will find that some terms have not been divided into word parts. These are common words or specialized terms that are included to enhance your medical vocabulary. See Chapter 1, page 7, to review pronunciation guidelines.

MEDICAL WORD	WORD PARTS		DEFINITION
	Part	**Meaning**	
abductor (ăb-dŭk´ tōr)	ab-	away from	Muscle that on contraction draws *away from* the middle
	duct	to lead	
	-or	a doer	
adductor (ă-dŭk´ tōr)	ad-	toward	Muscle that draws a part *toward* the middle
	duct	to lead	
	-or	a doer	
amputation (ăm˝ pū-tā´ shŭn)	amputat	to cut through	Surgical or traumatic removal of a limb, part, or other appendage. See Figure 7.5 ■
	-ion	process	

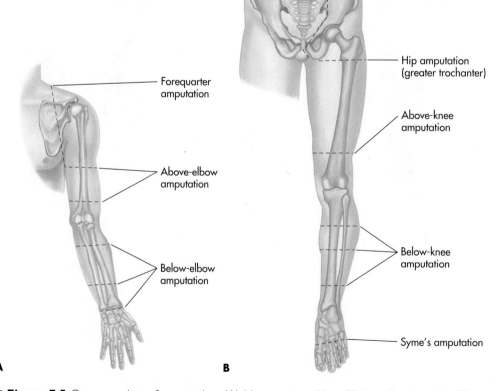

■ **Figure 7.5** Common sites of amputation. (A) Upper extremities. (B) Lower extremities. The surgeon determines the level of amputation based on blood supply and tissue condition.

MEDICAL WORD	WORD PARTS		DEFINITION
	Part	Meaning	
antagonist (ăn-tăg´ ō-nĭst)	ant- agon -ist	against agony, a contest agent	Muscle that counteracts the action of another muscle; when one contracts the other relaxes. See Figure 7.4.
aponeurosis (ăp″ ō-nū-rō´ sĭs)			A strong, flat sheet of fibrous connective tissue that serves as a tendon to attach muscles to bone or as fascia to bind muscles together or to other tissues at their origin or insertion
ataxia (ă-tăks´ ĭ-ă)	a- -taxia	lack of order	Lack of muscular coordination; an inability to coordinate voluntary muscular movements that is symptomatic of some nervous disorders
atonic (ă-tŏn´ ĭk)	a- ton -ic	lack of tone, tension pertaining to	Pertaining to a lack of normal tone or tension; the lack of normal muscle tone
atrophy (ăt´ rō-fē)	a- -trophy	lack of nourishment, development	Literally means *a lack of nourishment;* wasting of muscular tissue that may be caused by lack of use or lack of nerve stimulation of the muscle. *Lipoatrophy* is atrophy of fat tissue. This condition can occur at the site of an insulin and/or corticosteroid injection. It is also known as *lipodystrophy.* See Figure 7.6 ■

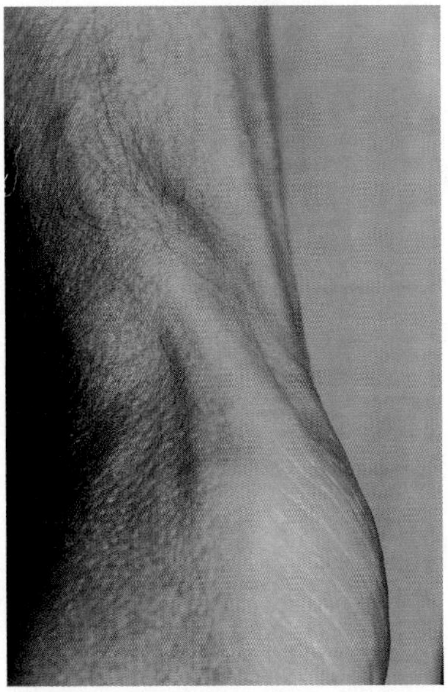

■ **Figure 7.6** Lipoatrophy, wrist.
(Courtesy of Jason L. Smith, MD)

| **biceps** (bī´ sps) | bi-
-ceps | two
head | Muscle with two heads or points of origin |

MEDICAL WORD	WORD PARTS		DEFINITION
	Part	**Meaning**	
brachialgia (brā″ ki-ăl′ jĭ-ă)	brach/i -algia	arm pain	Pain in the arm
bradykinesia (brăd″ ĭ-kĭ-nē′ sĭ-ă)	brady- -kinesia	slow motion	Slowness of motion or movement
clonic (klŏn′ ĭk)	clon -ic	turmoil pertaining to	Pertaining to alternate contraction and relaxation of muscles
contraction (kŏn-trăk′ shŭn)	con- tract -ion	with, together to draw process	Process of drawing up and thickening of a muscle fiber
contracture (kŏn-trăk′ chūr)	con- tract -ure	with, together to draw process	Condition in which a muscle shortens and renders the muscle resistant to the normal stretching process. For example, Dupuytren's contracture is a thickening and tightening of subcutaneous tissue of the palm, causing the ring and little fingers to bend into the palm so that they cannot be extended. See Figure 7.7 ■

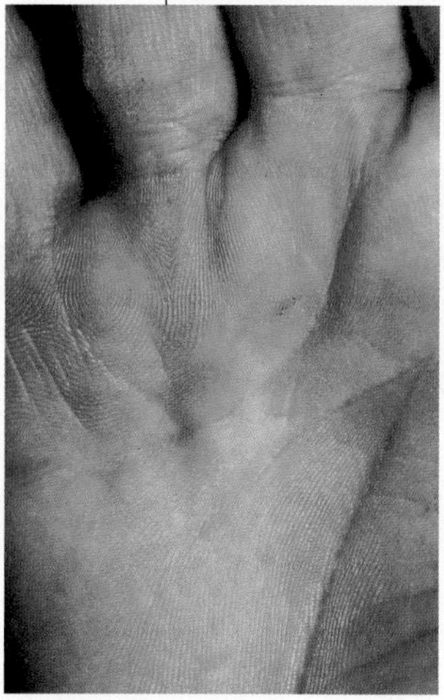

■ **Figure 7.7** Dupuytren's contracture.
(Courtesy of Jason L. Smith, MD)

dactylospasm (dăk′ tĭ-lō-spăzm)	dactyl/o -spasm	finger or toe tension, spasm	Medical term for cramp of a finger or toe

MEDICAL WORD	WORD PARTS		DEFINITION
	Part	Meaning	
dermatomyositis (dĕr″ mă-tō-mī″ ō-sī′ tĭs)	dermat/o my/o(s) -itis	skin muscle inflammation	Chronic, immunological disease with systemic pathology; inflammation of the muscles and the skin; a connective tissue disease characterized by edema, dermatitis, and inflammation of the muscles. See Figure 7.8 ■

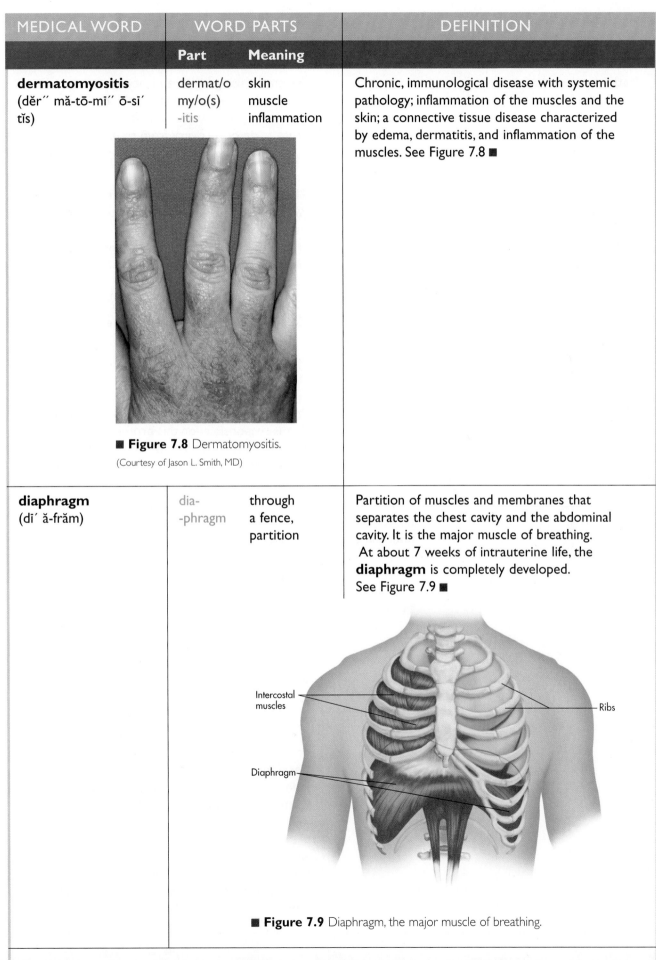

■ **Figure 7.8** Dermatomyositis.
(Courtesy of Jason L. Smith, MD)

| diaphragm (dī′ ă-frăm) | dia- -phragm | through a fence, partition | Partition of muscles and membranes that separates the chest cavity and the abdominal cavity. It is the major muscle of breathing. At about 7 weeks of intrauterine life, the **diaphragm** is completely developed. See Figure 7.9 ■ |

Intercostal muscles

Ribs

Diaphragm

■ **Figure 7.9** Diaphragm, the major muscle of breathing.

MEDICAL WORD	WORD PARTS		DEFINITION
	Part	**Meaning**	
diathermy (dī′ ă-thĕr″ mē)	dia- therm -y	through hot, heat pertaining to	Treatment using high-frequency current to produce heat within a part of the body; used to increase blood flow but should not be used in acute stage of recovery from trauma. Types: **Microwave**. Electromagnetic radiation directed to specified tissues **Short wave**. High-frequency electric current (wavelength of 3–30 m) directed to specified tissues **Ultrasound**. High-frequency sound waves (20,000–10 billion cycles/sec) directed to specified tissues
dystonia (dĭs′ tō′nĭ-ă)	dys- ton -ia	difficult tone, tension condition	Condition of impaired muscle tone
dystrophin (dĭs-trŏf′ ĭn)	dys- troph -in	difficult a turning chemical	Protein found in muscle cells. When the gene that is responsible for this protein is defective and sufficient dystrophin is not produced, muscle wasting occurs. In Duchenne muscular dystrophy, this protein is absent.
dystrophy (dĭs′ trō-fē)	dys- -trophy	difficult nourishment, development	Any condition of abnormal development caused by defective nourishment, often noted by the degeneration of muscles
exercise			Performed activity of the muscles for improvement of health or correction of deformity. Types: **Active**. Muscular contraction and relaxation by patient **Assistive**. Muscular contraction and relaxation with the assistance of a therapist **Isometric**. Active muscular contraction performed against stable resistance, thereby not shortening muscle length **Passive**. Exercise performed by another individual without patient assistance **Range of motion (ROM)**. Movement of each joint through its full range of motion; used to prevent loss of mobility or to regain usage after an injury or fracture **Relief of tension**. Technique used to promote relaxation of the muscles and provide relief from tension

MEDICAL WORD	WORD PARTS		DEFINITION
	Part	**Meaning**	
fascia (făsh´ĭ-ă)	fasc -ia	a band condition	Thin layer of connective tissue covering, supporting, or connecting the muscles or inner organs of the body
fascitis (fă-sī´ tĭs)	fasc -itis	a band inflammation	Inflammation of a fascia
fatigue (fă-tēg´)			State of tiredness occurring in a muscle as a result of repeated contractions
fibromyalgia syndrome (FMS) (fi˝ brō-mī-ăl´ jē-ă sĭn´ drōm)	fibr/o my -algia	fiber muscle pain	Disorder with chronic, widespread musculoskeletal pain and fatigue. Other symptoms include sleep disorders, irritable bowel syndrome, depression, and chronic headaches. Although the exact cause is still unknown, fibromyalgia is often traced to an injury or physical or emotional trauma.

Disorder with chronic, widespread musculoskeletal pain and fatigue. Other symptoms include sleep disorders, irritable bowel syndrome, depression, and chronic headaches. Although the exact cause is still unknown, fibromyalgia is often traced to an injury or physical or emotional trauma.

The American College of Rheumatology (ACR) classifies a patient with fibromyalgia if at least 11 of 18 specific areas of the body (called *trigger points*) are painful under pressure. See Figure 7.10 ■ The location of some of these trigger points includes the inside of the elbow joint, the front of the collarbone, and the base of the skull.

Treatments for fibromyalgia are geared toward improving the quality of sleep, as well as reducing pain.

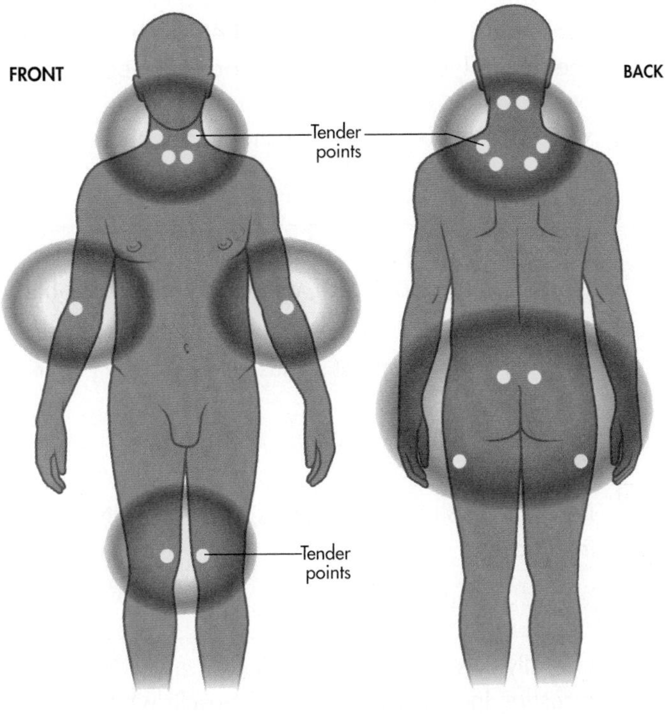

FRONT · BACK · Tender points · Tender points

■ **Figure 7.10** The 18 tender points of fibromyalgia.

fibromyitis (fi˝ brō-mī-i´ tĭs)	fibr/o my -itis	fiber muscle inflammation	Inflammation of muscle and fibrous tissue

MEDICAL WORD	WORD PARTS		DEFINITION
	Part	**Meaning**	
First Aid Treatment— RICE (Rest Ice Compression Elevation)			**Cryotherapy** (use of cold) is the treatment of choice for soft-tissue and muscle injuries. It causes vasoconstriction of blood vessels and is effective in diminishing bleeding and edema. Ice should not be placed directly onto the skin. **Compression** by an elastic bandage is generally determined by the type of injury and physician preference. Some experts disagree on the use of elastic bandages. When used, the bandage should be 3–4 inches wide and applied firmly. Toes or fingers should be periodically checked for blue or white discoloration, indicating that the bandage is too tight. **Elevation** is used to reduce swelling. The injured part should be elevated on two or three pillows.
flaccid (flăk´ sĭd)			Lacking muscle tone; *weak, soft,* and *flabby*
heat			Thermotherapy; treatment using scientific application of heat can be used 48–72 hours after the injury. Types: heating pad, hot water bottle, hot packs, infrared light, and immersion of body part in warm water. Extreme care should be taken when using or applying heat.
hydrotherapy (hĭ-drō-thĕr´ ă-pē)	hydro- -therapy	water treatment	Treatment using scientific application of water; types: hot tub, cold bath, whirlpool, and vapor bath
insertion (ĭn´´ sûr´ shŭn)	in- sert -ion	into to gain process	Point of attachment of a muscle to the part that it moves
intramuscular (IM) (ĭn´´ tră-mŭs´ kū-lər)	intra- muscul -ar	within muscle pertaining to	Pertaining to within a muscle, such as an IM injection
isometric (ī´´ sō-mĕt´ rĭk)	is/o metr -ic	equal to measure pertaining to	Literally means *pertaining to having equal measure;* increasing tension of muscle while maintaining equal length
isotonic (ī´´ sō-tŏn´ ĭk)	is/o ton -ic	equal tone, tension pertaining to	Pertaining to having the same tone or tension

MEDICAL WORD	WORD PARTS		DEFINITION
	Part	Meaning	
levator (lē-vā´ tər)	levat -or	lifter a doer	Muscle that raises or elevates a part
massage (măh-săhzh)			Kneading that applies pressure and friction to external body tissues
muscular dystrophy (MD) (mŭs´ kū-lār dĭs´ trō-fē)			Refers to a group of genetic diseases characterized by progressive weakness and degeneration of the skeletal or voluntary muscles that control movement. The muscles of the heart and some other involuntary muscles are also affected in some forms of MD, and a few forms involve other organs as well. Duchenne muscular dystrophy is the most common form of MD affecting children and myotonic MD is the most common form affecting adults.

LIFE SPAN CONSIDERATIONS

MD can affect people of all ages, with some forms apparent in infancy or childhood and others not appearing until middle age or later. Duchenne muscular dystrophy is an X-linked disorder seen only in males. In this disorder, the protein **dystrophin** is absent from muscle cells, leading to necrosis in muscle fibers and their replacement with connective tissue and fat. There is no specific treatment for any of the forms of MD. Physical therapy to prevent **contractures** (a condition in which shortened muscles around joints cause abnormal and sometimes painful positioning of the joints), **orthoses** (orthopedic appliances used for support), and corrective orthopedic surgery could be needed to improve the quality of life in some cases. Some cases of MD are mild and other cases have marked progressions of muscle weakness, functional disability, and loss of ambulation. See Figure 7.11 ■

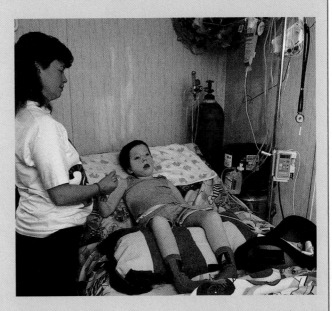

■ **Figure 7.11** This young boy with muscular dystrophy needs to receive tube feedings and home nursing care. He attends school when possible and is able to use an adapted computer.

MEDICAL WORD	WORD PARTS		DEFINITION
	Part	Meaning	

(fyi) The **Gowers' maneuver**, as seen in Figure 7.12 ■, is the use of the upper extremity muscles to raise oneself to a standing position. This is a good indicator of muscle weakness of the legs caused by muscular dystrophy. Early in the diagnostic process, a serum creatine kinase (CK) test, an electromyography (EMG), and a muscle biopsy is ordered.

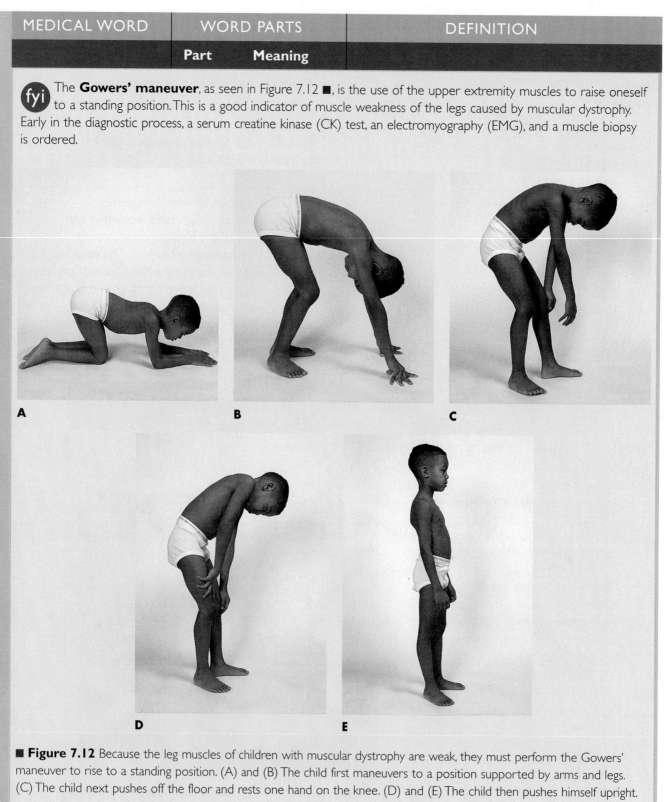

■ **Figure 7.12** Because the leg muscles of children with muscular dystrophy are weak, they must perform the Gowers' maneuver to rise to a standing position. (A) and (B) The child first maneuvers to a position supported by arms and legs. (C) The child next pushes off the floor and rests one hand on the knee. (D) and (E) The child then pushes himself upright.

myalgia (mī-ăl´ jĭ-ă)	my -algia	muscle pain	Pain in the muscle

MEDICAL WORD	WORD PARTS		DEFINITION
	Part	**Meaning**	
myasthenia gravis (MG) (mī-ăs-thē′ nĭ-ă gră vĭs)	my -asthenia gravis	muscle weakness grave	Chronic autoimmune neuromuscular disease characterized by varying degrees of weakness of the skeletal (voluntary) muscles of the body. Its name, which is Latin and Greek in origin, literally means *grave muscle weakness*. The primary symptom is muscle weakness that increases during periods of activity and improves after periods of rest.
myoblast (mī′ ō blăst)	my/o -blast	muscle immature cell, germ cell	Embryonic cell that develops into a cell of muscle fiber
myofibroma (mī″ ō fī-brō′ mă)	my/o fibr -oma	muscle fiber tumor	Tumor that contains muscle and fiber
myograph (mī′ ō-grăf)	my/o -graph	muscle instrument for recording	Instrument used to record muscular contractions
myokinesis (mī″ ō-kĭn-ē′ sĭs)	my/o -kinesis	muscle motion	Muscular motion or activity
myology (mĭ-ŏl ō-jē)	my/o -logy	muscle study of	Study of muscles
myoma (mī-ō′ mă)	my -oma	muscle tumor	Tumor containing muscle tissue
myomalacia (mī″ ō-mă-lā′ sĭ-ă)	my/o -malacia	muscle softening	Softening of muscle tissue
myoparesis (mī″ ō-păr′ ě-sĭs)	my/o -paresis	muscle weakness	Weakness or slight paralysis of a muscle
myopathy (mī-ŏp′ ă-thē)	my/o -pathy	muscle disease	Muscle disease
myoplasty (mī′ ō-plăs″ tē)	my/o -plasty	muscle surgical repair	Surgical repair of a muscle
myorrhaphy (mī-or′ ă-fē)	my/o -rrhaphy	muscle suture	Surgical suture of a muscle wound

MEDICAL WORD	WORD PARTS		DEFINITION
	Part	**Meaning**	
myosarcoma (mǐ″ ō-sar-kō′ mǎ)	my/o sarc -oma	muscle flesh tumor	Malignant tumor derived from muscle tissue
myosclerosis (mǐ″ ō-sklĕr-ō′ sǐs)	my/o scler -osis	muscle hardening condition	Abnormal condition of hardening of muscle
myositis (mǐ″ ō-sī′ tǐs)	my/o (s) -itis	muscle inflammation	Inflammation of muscle tissue, especially skeletal muscles; may be caused by infection, trauma, or parasitic infestation
myospasm (mǐ″ ō-spǎzm)	my/o -spasm	muscle tension, spasm	Spasmodic contraction of a muscle
myotome (mǐ′ ō-tōm)	my/o -tome	muscle instrument to cut	Surgical instrument used to cut muscle
myotomy (mǐ″ ŏt′ ō-mē)	my/o -tomy	muscle incision	Surgical incision into a muscle
neuromuscular (nū″ rō-mǔs′ kū-lǎr)	neur/o muscul -ar	nerve muscle pertaining to	Pertaining to both nerves and muscles
neuromyopathic (nū″ rō-m ǐ″ ō-pǎth′ ǐk)	neur/o my/o path -ic	nerve muscle disease pertaining to	Pertaining to a disease condition involving both nerves and muscles
polyplegia (pŏl″ ē-plē′ jǐ-ǎ)	poly- -plegia	many stroke, paralysis	Paralysis affecting many muscles

MEDICAL WORD	WORD PARTS		DEFINITION
	Part	Meaning	
position			Bodily posture or attitude; the manner in which a patient's body may be arranged for examination. See Table 7.3 ■

TABLE 7.3 Types of Patient Positions

Position	Description
anatomic	Body erect, head facing forward, arms by the sides with palms to the front; used as a standard anatomical position of reference
dorsal recumbent	On back with lower extremities flexed and rotated outward; used in application of obstetric forceps, vaginal and rectal examination, and bimanual palpation
Fowler's	Head of the bed or examining table is raised about 18 inches or 46 cm; patient sitting up with knees also elevated
knee-chest	On knees, thighs upright, head and upper part of chest resting on bed or examining table, arms crossed and above head; used in sigmoidoscopy, displacement of prolapsed uterus, rectal exams, and flushing of intestinal canal
lithotomy	On back with lower extremities flexed and feet placed in stirrups; used in vaginal examination, Pap smear, vaginal operations, and diagnosis and treatment of diseases of the urethra and bladder
orthopneic	Sitting upright or erect; used for patients with dyspnea, shortness of breath (SOB)
prone	Lying face downward; used in examination of the back, injections, and massage
Sims'	Lying on left side, right knee and thigh flexed well up above left leg that is slightly flexed, left arm behind the body, and right arm forward, flexed at elbow; used in examination of rectum, sigmoidoscopy, enema, and intrauterine irrigation after labor
supine	Lying flat on back with face upward and arms at the sides; used in examining the head, neck, chest, abdomen, and extremities and in assessing vital signs
Trendelenburg	Body supine on a bed or examining table that is tilted at about a 45° angle with the head lower than the feet; used to displace abdominal organs during surgery and in treating cardiovascular shock; also called the *shock position*

MEDICAL WORD	WORD PARTS		DEFINITION
	Part	**Meaning**	
prosthesis (prŏs´ thē-sĭs)	prosth/e -sis	an addition condition	Artificial device used to replace an organ or body part, such as a hand, arm, leg, or hip. See Figure 7.13 ■

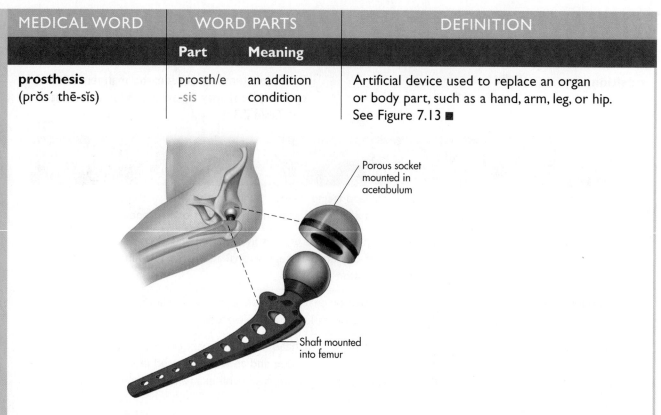

Porous socket mounted in acetabulum

Shaft mounted into femur

■ **Figure 7.13** Total hip prosthesis.

quadriceps (kwŏd´ rĭ-s ĕps)	quadri- -ceps	four head	Muscle that has four heads or points of origin
relaxation (rē-lăk-sā´ shŭn)	relaxat -ion	to loosen process	Process in which a muscle loosens and returns to a resting stage
rhabdomyoma (răb˝ dō-m ī-ō´ mă)	rhabd/o my -oma	rod muscle tumor	Tumor of striated muscle tissue
rheumatism (roo´ mă-tĭzm)	rheumat -ism	discharge condition	General term used to describe conditions characterized by inflammation, soreness, and stiffness of muscles and pain in joints
rigor mortis (rĭg´ ur mōr tĭs)			Stiffness of skeletal muscles seen in death; develops between the 4th and 24th hour after death, then ceases
rotation (rō-tā´ shŭn)	rotat -ion	to turn process	Process of moving a body part around a central axis

MEDICAL WORD	WORD PARTS		DEFINITION
	Part	Meaning	
rotator cuff (rō-tā´ tor kŭf)			Group of muscles and their tendons that act to stabilize the shoulder. The four muscles of the rotator cuff (subscapularis, supraspinatus, infraspinauts, and teres minor), along with the teres major and the deltoid, make up the six **scapulohumeral** (those that connect to the humerus and scapula and act on the glenohumeral joint) muscles of the human body.
sarcolemma (sar˝ kō-lĕm´ ă)	sarc/o lemma	flesh a rind	Plasma membrane surrounding each striated muscle fiber
spasticity (spăs-tĭs´ ĭ-tē)	spastic -ity	convulsive condition	Condition of increased muscular tone causing stiff and awkward movements
sternocleidomastoid (stur˝ nō-klī˝ dō-măs´ toyd)	stern/o cleid/o mast -oid	sternum clavicle breast resemble	Muscle arising from the sternum and clavicle with its insertion in the mastoid process
strain			Excessive, forcible stretching of a muscle or the musculotendinous unit
synergetic (sin˝ ĕr-jĕt´ ĭk)	syn- erget -ic	with, together work pertaining to	Pertaining to certain muscles that work together
synovitis (sĭn˝ o-vī´ tĭs)	synov -itis	synovial membrane inflammation	Inflammation of a synovial membrane

MEDICAL WORD	WORD PARTS		DEFINITION
	Part	**Meaning**	
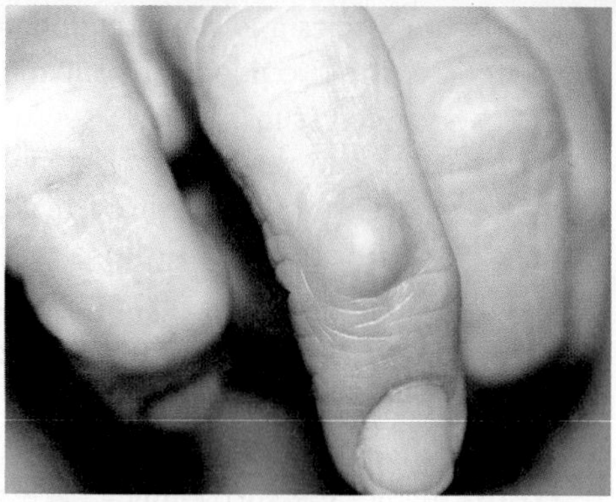 **tendon** (těn´ dŭn)			Band of fibrous connective tissue serving for the attachment of muscles to bones; a giant cell tumor of a tendon sheath is a benign, small, yellow, tumorlike nodule. See Figure 7.14 ■

■ **Figure 7.14** Giant cell tumor of tendon sheath.
(Courtesy of Jason L. Smith, MD)

MEDICAL WORD	WORD PARTS		DEFINITION
	Part	Meaning	
tenodesis (těn-ōd´ ě-sĭs)	ten/o -desis	tendon binding	Surgical binding of a tendon
tenodynia (těn´´ ō-dĭn-ĭ-ă)	ten/o -dynia	tendon pain	Pain in a tendon
tetany (tět´ ă-nē)			Condition characterized by cramps, convulsions, twitching of the muscles, and sharp flexion of the wrist and ankle joints; generally caused by an abnormality in calcium (Ca) metabolism
tonic (tŏn´ ĭk)	ton -ic	tone, tension pertaining to	Pertaining to tone, especially muscular tension
torsion (tor´ shŭn)	tors -ion	twisted process	Process of being twisted
torticollis (tor´´ tĭ-kŏl´ ĭs)	tort/i -collis	twisted neck	Stiff neck caused by spasmodic contraction of the muscles of the neck; *wryneck*
triceps (trī´ sĕps)	tri- -ceps	three head	Muscle having three heads with a single insertion
voluntary (vŏl´ ŭn-tĕr´´ ē)	volunt -ary	will pertaining to	Under the control of one's will

• Drug Highlights •

TYPE OF DRUG	DESCRIPTION AND EXAMPLES
skeletal muscle relaxants	Used to treat painful muscle spasms that can result from strains, sprains, and musculoskeletal trauma or disease. Centrally acting muscle relaxants depress the central nervous system (CNS) and can be administered orally or by injection. The patient must be informed of the sedative effect produced by these drugs. Drowsiness, dizziness, and blurred vision can diminish the patient's ability to drive a vehicle, operate equipment, or climb stairs. EXAMPLES: Lioresal (baclofen), Flexeril (cyclobenzaprine HCl), and Robaxin (methocarbamol)
skeletal muscle stimulants	Used in the treatment of myasthenia gravis, a disease characterized by progressive weakness of skeletal muscles and their rapid fatiguing. Skeletal muscle stimulants inhibit the action of acetylcholinesterase, the enzyme that halts the action of acetylcholine at the neuromuscular junction. By slowing the destruction of acetylcholine, these drugs foster accumulation of higher concentrations of this neurotransmitter and increase the number of interactions between acetylcholine and the available receptors on muscle fibers. EXAMPLES: Tensilon (edrophonium chloride), Prostigmin Bromide (neostigmine bromide), and Mestinon (pyridostigmine bromide)
neuromuscular blocking agents	Used to provide muscle relaxation in patients undergoing surgery and/or electroconvulsive therapy, endotracheal intubation, and to relieve laryngospasm. EXAMPLES: Tracrium (atracurium besylate), Flaxedil (gallamine triethiodide), and Norcuron (vecuronium)
anti-inflammatory agents and analgesics	(See Chapter 6, Skeletal System, Drug Highlights on page 156 for a description of anti-inflammatory agents and analgesics.)

• Diagnostic and Lab Tests •

TEST	DESCRIPTION
aldolase (ALD) blood test (ăl´ dō-lāz)	Test performed on serum that measures ALD enzyme present in skeletal and heart muscle; helpful in the diagnosis of Duchenne's muscular dystrophy before symptoms appear.
calcium blood test (kăl´ sē-ŭm)	Test performed on serum to determine levels of calcium, which is essential for muscular contraction, nerve transmission, and blood clotting.
creatine kinase (CK) (krē´ ă-tĭn kĭn´ āz)	Blood test to determine the level of CK, which is increased in necrosis or atrophy of skeletal muscle, traumatic muscle injury, strenuous exercise, and progressive muscular dystrophy.
electromyography (EMG) (ē-lĕk˝ trō-mī-ŏg´ ră-fē)	Test to measure electrical activity across muscle membranes by means of electrodes attached to a needle that is inserted into the muscle. Electrical activity can be heard over a loudspeaker, viewed on an oscilloscope, or printed on a graph (electromyogram). Abnormal results can indicate myasthenia gravis, amyotrophic lateral sclerosis, muscular dystrophy, peripheral neuropathy, and anterior poliomyelitis.
lactic dehydrogenase (LDH) (lăk´ tĭk dē-hī-drŏj´ ě-nāz)	Blood test to determine the level of LDH enzyme, which is increased in muscular dystrophy, damage to skeletal muscles, after a pulmonary embolism, and during skeletal muscle malignancy.
muscle biopsy	Surgical removal of a small piece of muscle tissue for examination. There are two types. A *needle biopsy* involves inserting a needle into the muscle. When the needle is removed, a small piece of tissue remains in the needle. The tissue is sent to a laboratory for examination. An *open biopsy* involves making a small cut in the skin and into the muscle. The muscle tissue is then removed. A muscle biopsy may be done to identify or detect diseases of the connective tissue and blood vessels (e.g., polyarteritis nodosa); infections that affect the muscles (e.g., trichinosis or toxoplasmosis); muscular disorders such as muscular dystrophy or congenital myopathy and metabolic defects of the muscle.
serum glutamic oxaloacetic transaminase (SGOT) (sē´ rŭm gloo-tăm´ ĭk ŏks˝ ăl-ō-ă-sē´ tĭk trăns ăm´ ĭn-āz)	Blood test to determine the level of SGOT enzyme, which is increased in skeletal muscle damage and muscular dystrophy; test also called *aspartate aminotransferase* (AST).
serum glutamic pyruvic transaminase (SGPT) (sē´ rŭm gloo-tăm´ ĭk pī-roo´ vĭk trăns-ăm´ ĭn-āz)	Blood test to determine the level of SGPT enzyme, which is increased in skeletal muscle damage; test also called *alanine aminotransferase* (ALT).

• Abbreviations •

ABBREVIATION	MEANING
ACR	American College of Rheumatology
AE	above elbow
AK	above knee
ALD	aldolase
ALT	alanine aminotransferase
AST	aspartate aminotransferase
BE	below elbow
BK	below knee
Ca	calcium
CPM	continuous passive motion
DTRs	deep tendon reflexes
EMG	electromyography
FMS	fibromyalgia syndrome
FROM	full range of motion
IM	intramuscular
LDH	lactic dehydrogenase

ABBREVIATION	MEANING
LOM	limitation or loss of motion
MD	muscular dystrophy
MG	myasthenia gravis
MS	musculoskeletal
PM	physical medicine
PMR	physical medicine and rehabilitation
ROM	range of motion
SGOT	serum glutamic oxaloacetic transaminase
SGPT	serum glutamic pyruvic transaminase
sh	shoulder
SOB	shortness of breath
TBW	total body weight
TJ	triceps jerk

and Review • Study and Review • Study and Review
Review • Study and Review • Study and Review • St
w • Study and Review • Study and Review • Study

• Study and Review • Study and Review • Study

Anatomy and Physiology

Write your answers to the following questions.

1. The muscular system is made up of three types of muscle tissue. Name the three types.

    a. _____   **b.** _____

    c. _____

2. Muscles make up approximately _____ percent of a person's body weight.

3. Name the two essential ingredients that are needed for a muscle to perform properly.

    a. _____   **b.** _____

4. Name the two points of attachment for a skeletal muscle.

    a. _____   **b.** _____

5. Skeletal muscle is also known as _____ or _____ .

6. A wide, thin, sheetlike tendon is known as an _____ .

7. Name the three distinguishable parts of a muscle.

    a. _____   **b.** _____

    c. _____

8. Define the following:

    a. Antagonist _____

    b. Prime mover _____

    c. Synergist _____

9. Smooth muscle is also called _____ , _____ , or
_____ .

10. Smooth muscles are found in the internal organs. Name five examples of these locations.

    a. _____   **b.** _____

    c. _____   **d.** _____

    e. _____

11. _____ is the muscle of the heart.

12. Name the three primary functions of the muscular system.

a. _____   **b.** _____

c. _____

Word Parts

PREFIXES

Give the definitions of the following prefixes.

1. a- _____   **2.** ab- _____

3. ad- _____   **4.** ant- _____

5. bi- _____   **6.** brady- _____

7. con- _____   **8.** dia- _____

9. dys- _____   **10.** in- _____

11. intra- _____   **12.** hydro- _____

13. quadri- _____   **14.** syn- _____

15. tri- _____

ROOTS AND COMBINING FORMS

Give the definitions of the following roots and combining forms.

1. agon _____   **2.** brach/i _____

3. cleid/o _____   **4.** amputat _____

5. collis _____   **6.** dactyl/o _____

7. duct _____   **8.** erget _____

9. fasc _____   **10.** dermat/o _____

11. rheumat _____   **12.** fibr _____

13. fibr/o _____   **14.** is/o _____

15. lemma _____   **16.** levat _____

17. prosth/e _____   **18.** mast _____

19. therm _____   **20.** metr _____

21. muscul _____

22. my _____

23. my/o _____

24. my/o(s) _____

25. neur/o _____

26. path _____

27. relaxat _____

28. rhabd/o _____

29. rotat _____

30. troph _____

31. sarc/o _____

32. scler _____

33. sert _____

34. spastic _____

35. stern/o _____

36. teno _____

37. ton _____

38. torti _____

39. tract _____

40. volunt _____

41. synov _____

42. tors _____

SUFFIXES

Give the definitions of the following suffixes.

1. -algia _____

2. -ar _____

3. -ary _____

4. -asthenia _____

5. -blast _____

6. -ceps _____

7. -desis _____

8. -dynia _____

9. -in _____

10. -therapy _____

11. -graph _____

12. -ia _____

13. -ic _____

14. -ion _____

15. -ist _____

16. -itis _____

17. -ity _____

18. -kinesia _____

19. -kinesis _____

20. -logy _____

21. -ure _____

22. -malacia _____

23. -oid _____

24. -oma _____

25. -or _____

26. -osis _____

27. -paresis _____

28. -pathy _____

29. -phragm _____

30. -plasty _____

31. -plegia _____

32. -rrhaphy _____

33. -y _____

34. -spasm _____

35. -taxia _____

36. -tome _____

37. -tomy _____

38. -trophy _____

39. -sis _____

40. -ism _____

Identifying Medical Terms

In the spaces provided, write the medical terms for the following meanings.

1. _____ Pertaining to a lack of normal tone or tension

2. _____ Slowness of motion or movement

3. _____ Medical term for cramp of a finger or toe

4. _____ Any condition of abnormal development caused by defective nourishment, often noted by the degeneration of muscles

5. _____ Pertaining to within a muscle, such as an IM injection

6. _____ Muscle that raises or elevates a part

7. _____ Chronic autoimmune neuromuscular disease characterized by varying degrees of weakness of the skeletal (voluntary) muscles of the body

8. _____ Study of muscles

9. _____ Weakness or slight paralysis of a muscle

10. _____ Surgical repair of a muscle

11. _____ Malignant tumor derived from muscle tissue

12. _____ Surgical incision into a muscle

13. _____ Paralysis affecting many muscles

14. _____ Surgical binding of a tendon

15. _____ Pertaining to certain muscles that work together

16. _____ Muscle having three heads with a single insertion

Spelling

Circle the correct spelling of each medical term.

1. facia / fascia

2. myokinesis / mykinesis

3. dermatomyositis / dermatomyoitis

4. rhadomyoma / rhabdomyoma

5. sarcolemma / sarclemma

6. sterncleidomastoid / sternocleidomastoid

7. dystropin / dystrophin

8. torticollis / torticolis

Matching

Select the appropriate lettered meaning for each of the following words.

_____ **1.** dermatomyositis

_____ **2.** fibromyalgia

_____ **3.** muscular dystrophy

_____ **4.** flaccid

_____ **5.** prosthesis

_____ **6.** rotator cuff

_____ **7.** strain

_____ **8.** tenodynia

_____ **9.** torsion

_____ **10.** voluntary

a. Group of muscles and their tendons that act to stabilize the shoulder

b. Process of being twisted

c. Pain in a tendon

d. Chronic immunological disease with systemic pathology

e. Lacking muscle tone; *weak, soft,* and *flabby*

f. Under the control of one's will

g. Refers to a group of genetic diseases characterized by progressive weakness and degeneration of the skeletal or voluntary muscles that control movement

h. Excessive, forcible stretching of a muscle or the musculotendinous unit

i. A chronic widespread musculoskeletal pain and fatigue disorder

j. Artificial device used to replace an organ or a body part, such as a hand, arm, leg, or hip

k. Pain in a joint

Abbreviations

Place the correct word, phrase, or abbreviation in the space provided.

1. AE _____

2. AST _____

3. calcium_____

4. electromyography _____

5. FROM _____

6. MS _____

7. range of motion _____

8. shoulder _____

9. TBW _____

10. TJ _____

Diagnostic and Laboratory Tests

Select the best answer to each multiple choice question. Circle the letter of your choice.

1. Diagnostic test to help diagnose Duchenne muscular dystrophy before symptoms appear.
   a. creatine kinase
   b. aldolase blood test
   c. calcium blood test
   d. muscle biopsy

2. Test to measure electrical activity across muscle membranes by means of electrodes that are attached to a needle that is inserted into the muscle.
   a. muscle biopsy
   b. lactic dehydrogenase
   c. creatine kinase
   d. electromyography

3. Test that is also called *aspartate aminotransferase*.
   a. lactic dehydrogenase
   b. serum glutamic oxaloacetic transaminase
   c. serum glutamic pyruvic transaminase
   d. creatine kinase

4. Test that is also called *alanine aminotransferase*.
   a. lactic dehydrogenase
   b. serum glutamic oxaloacetic transaminase
   c. serum glutamic pyruvic transaminase
   d. creatine kinase

5. A/an _____ is the surgical removal of a small piece of muscle tissue for examination.
   a. muscle biopsy
   b. electromyography
   c. bone biopsy
   d. electrocardiography

PRACTICAL APPLICATION

MEDICAL RECORD ANALYSIS

This exercise contains information, abbreviations, and medical terminology from an actual medical record or case study that has been adapted for this text. The names and any personal information have been created by the author. Read and study each form or case study and then answers the questions that follow. You may refer to Appendix III, Abbreviations and Symbols, on page A41.

CASE STUDY
DUCHENNE'S MUSCULAR DYSTROPHY

Read the following case study and then answer the questions that follow.

A 3-year-old male child was seen by a physician; the following is a synopsis of the visit.

Present History: The mother states that she noticed that her son has been falling a lot and seems to be very clumsy. She says that he has a waddling gait, is very slow in running and climbing, and walks on his toes. She is most concerned as she is at risk for carrying the gene that causes muscular dystrophy (MD).

Signs and Symptoms: A waddling gait, very slow in running and climbing, walks on his toes, frequent falling, clumsy.

Diagnosis: Duchenne's muscular dystrophy. The diagnosis was determined by the characteristic symptoms, family history, a muscle biopsy, an electromyography (EMG), and an elevated serum creatine kinase (CK) level.

Treatment: Physical therapy, deep breathing exercises to help delay muscular weakness, supportive measures such as splints and braces to help minimize deformities and to preserve mobility. Counseling and referral services are essential. For more information, family may contact the Muscular Dystrophy Association at 3561 E. Sunrise Drive, Tucson, AZ 85718. Telephone: (602) 529-2000 or (800) 572-1717. E-mail: mda@mdausa.org

Case Study Questions

Place the correct answer in the space provided.

1. Signs and symptoms of Duchenne's muscular dystrophy include a _____ gait, frequent falls, clumsiness, slowness in running and climbing, and walking on toes.

2. The diagnosis was determined by the characteristic symptoms, family history, a muscle biopsy, an _____ , and an elevated serum creatine kinase level.

3. As part of the treatment for Duchenne's muscular dystrophy, the use of splints and braces help to (a) _____ and (b) _____ .

4. Define electromyography. _____

_____

5. Define muscle biopsy. _____

_____

PEARSON
mymedicalterminologylab™

MyMedicalTerminologyLab is a premium online homework management system that includes a host of features to help you study. Registered users will find:

- Fun games and activities built within a virtual hospital
- Powerful tools that track and analyze your results—allowing you to create a personalized learning experience
- Videos, flashcards, and audio pronunciations to help enrich your progress
- Streaming lesson presentations and self-paced learning modules
- A space where you and your instructors can view and manage your assignments

8

LEARNING OUTCOMES

On completion of this chapter, you will be able to:

1. Describe the digestive system.

2. Explain the primary functions of the organs of the digestive system.

3. Describe the two sets of teeth with which humans are provided.

4. Identify the three main portions of a tooth.

5. Discuss the accessory organs of the digestive system and state their functions.

6. Analyze, build, spell, and pronounce medical words.

7. Comprehend the drugs highlighted in this chapter.

8. Describe diagnostic and laboratory tests related to the digestive system.

9. Identify and define selected abbreviations.

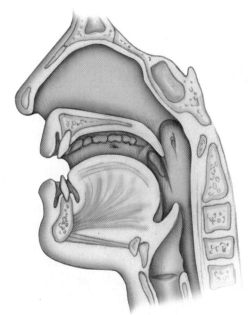

COMBINING FORMS OF THE DIGESTIVE SYSTEM

absorpt/o	to suck in	**gloss/o**	tongue
aden/o	gland	**glyc/o**	sweet, sugar
aliment/o	nourishment	**halit/o**	breath
amyl/o	starch	**hemat/o**	blood
anabol/o	building up	**hemorrh/o**	vein liable to bleed
append/o	appendix	**hepat/o**	liver
appendic/o	appendix	**herni/o**	hernia
bil/i	gall, bile	**ile/o**	ileum
bucc/o	cheek	**labi/o**	lip
catabol/o	a casting down	**lapar/o**	abdomen
celi/o	abdomen, belly	**lingu/o**	tongue
cheil/o	lip	**lip/o**	fat
chol/e	gall, bile	**odont/o**	tooth
choledoch/o	common bile duct	**pancreat/o**	pancreas
cirrh/o	orange-yellow	**pept/o**	to digest
col/o	colon	**pharyng/e**	pharynx
colon/o	colon	**pil/o**	hair
cyst/o	bladder	**prand/i**	meal
dent/o	tooth	**proct/o**	anus and rectum
diverticul/o	diverticula	**pylor/o**	pylorus, gatekeeper
duoden/o	duodenum	**rect/o**	rectum
enter/o	intestine	**sial/o**	saliva, salivary
esophage/o	esophagus	**sigmoid/o**	sigmoid
fibr/o	fibrous tissue	**splen/o**	spleen
gastr/o	stomach	**stomat/o**	mouth
gingiv/o	gums	**verm/i**	worm

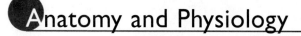natomy and Physiology

A general description of the digestive or gastrointestinal system is that of a continuous tube beginning with the mouth and ending at the anus. This tube is known as the **alimentary canal** and/or **gastrointestinal tract.** It measures about 30 feet in adults and contains both primary and accessory organs for the conversion of food and fluids into a semiliquid that can be absorbed for the body to use.

The three main functions of the digestive system are digestion, absorption, and elimination. **Digestion** is the process by which food is changed in the mouth, stomach, and intestines by chemical, mechanical, and physical action, so that the body can absorb it. Digestive enzymes increase chemical reactions and, in so doing, break down complex nutrients. See further discussion of chemical digestion on page 219. **Absorption** is the process by which nutrient material is taken into the bloodstream or lymph and travels to all cells of the body. Valuable nutrients such as amino acids, glucose, fatty acids, and glycerol can then be utilized for energy, growth, and development of the body. **Elimination** is the

TABLE 8.1 Digestive System at-a-Glance

Organ/Structure	Primary Functions/Description
Mouth	Mechanically breaks food apart by the action of the teeth; moistens and lubricates food with saliva; food formed into a **bolus**, a soft mass of chewed food ready to be swallowed
Teeth	Used in mastication (chewing)
Salivary glands	Secrete saliva to moisten and lubricate food
Pharynx	Common passageway for both respiration and digestion; muscular constrictions move the swallowed bolus into the esophagus
Esophagus	Moves the bolus by peristalsis down the esophagus into the stomach
Stomach	Reduces food to a digestible state; converts the food to a semiliquid state called **chyme**
Small intestine	Digestion and absorption take place chiefly in the small intestine; nutrients are absorbed and transferred to body cells by the circulatory system
Large intestine	Reabsorbs water from the fecal material, stores, and then eliminates waste from the body via the rectum and anus
Liver	Changes glucose to glycogen and stores it until needed; changes glycogen back to glucose; desaturates fats; assists in protein catabolism; manufactures bile, fibrinogen, prothrombin, heparin, and blood proteins; stores vitamins; produces heat; and detoxifies toxins
Gallbladder	Stores and concentrates bile that has been produced by the liver
Pancreas	Secretes pancreatic juice into the small intestine, contains cells that produce digestive enzymes, produces the hormones insulin and glucagon

process whereby the solid waste (end) products of digestion are excreted. Each of the various organs commonly associated with digestion is described in this chapter. See Table 8.1 ■ for the digestive system at-a-glance. The organs of digestion are shown in Figure 8.1 ■

LIFE SPAN CONSIDERATIONS

With aging, the digestive system becomes less motile, as muscle contractions become weaker. Glandular secretions decrease, thus causing a drier mouth and a lower volume of gastric juices. Nutrient absorption is mildly reduced due to **atrophy** of the mucosal lining. The teeth are mechanically worn down with age, and the gums begin to recede from the teeth. There is a loss of taste buds, and food preferences change. Gastric motor activity slows; as a result, gastric emptying is delayed and hunger contractions diminish.

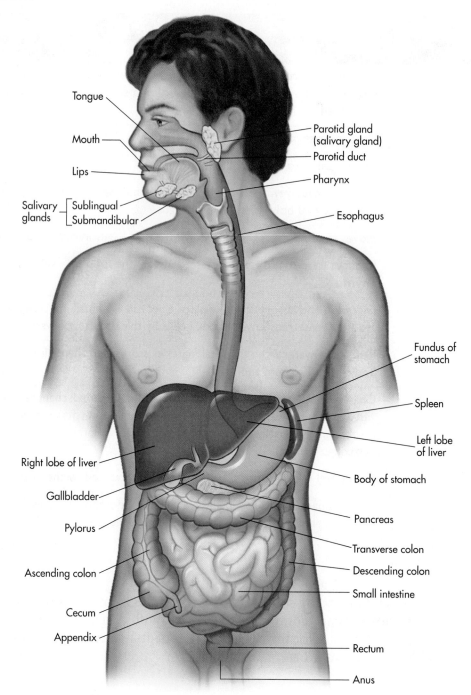

Tongue

Mouth

Lips

Salivary
glands
— Sublingual
— Submandibular

Parotid gland
(salivary gland)

Parotid duct

Pharynx

Esophagus

Fundus of
stomach

Spleen

Left lobe
of liver

Body of stomach

Pancreas

Transverse colon

Descending colon

Small intestine

Rectum

Anus

Right lobe of liver

Gallbladder

Pylorus

Ascending colon

Cecum

Appendix

■ **Figure 8.1** Digestive system.

MOUTH

The **mouth** or oral cavity is formed by the hard and soft palates at the top or roof, the cheeks on the sides, the tongue at the floor, and the lips that frame the opening to the cavity. Contained within are the teeth and salivary glands. The vestibule includes the space between the cheeks and the teeth. The **gingivae** (gums) surround the necks of the teeth. See Figure 8.2A ■ The free portion of the tongue is connected

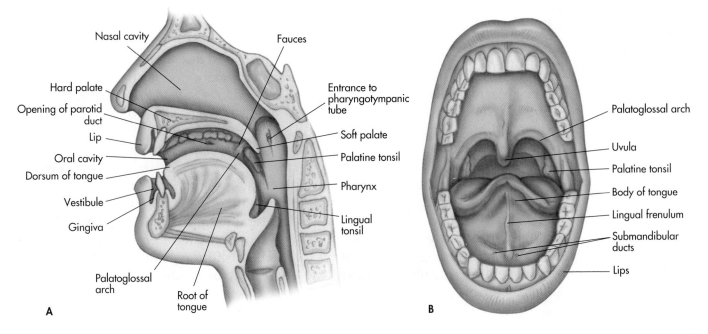

A

B

■ **Figure 8.2** Oral cavity: (A) sagittal section; (B) anterior view as seen through the open mouth.

to the underlying epithelium by a thin fold of mucous membrane, the **lingual frenulum,** which prevents extreme movement of the tongue. See Figure 8.2B ■

The **tongue** is made of skeletal muscle and is covered with mucous membrane. It manipulates food during chewing and assists in swallowing. The tongue can be divided into a blunt rear portion called the **root,** a pointed **tip,** and a central **body.** Located on the surface of the tongue are **papillae** (elevations) and **taste buds** (sweet, salt, sour, and bitter). Three pairs of salivary glands secrete saliva into the oral cavity. The posterior margin of the soft palate supports the dangling uvula and two pairs of muscular pharyngeal arches. On either side, a palatine tonsil lies between an anterior palatoglossal arch and a posterior palatopharyngeal arch. A curving line that connects the palatoglossal arches and uvula forms the boundaries of the fauces, the passageway between the oral cavity and the pharynx. See Figure 8.2A. Digestion begins as food is broken apart by the action of the teeth, moistened and lubricated by saliva, and formed into a bolus. See Figure 8.3 ■

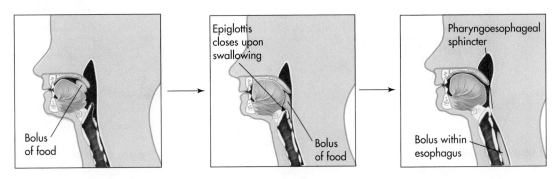

■ **Figure 8.3** Movement of a bolus of food from the mouth to the esophagus. The bolus then travels to the stomach.

TEETH

Human beings are provided two sets of teeth. The 20 **deciduous** teeth, the temporary teeth of the primary dentition, include eight incisors, four canines (cuspids), and eight molars. Deciduous teeth are also referred to as *milk teeth* or *baby teeth*. There are 32 **permanent** or secondary dentition teeth: eight incisors, four canines, eight premolars, and 12 molars. See Figure 8.4 ■

The **incisors** are so named because they present a sharp cutting edge, adapted for biting into food. They form the four front teeth in each dental arch. The **canine** or **cuspid** teeth are larger and stronger than the incisors. Their roots sink deeply into the bones and cause well-marked prominences upon the surface. The **premolars** or **bicuspid** teeth are situated lateral to and behind the canine teeth. The **molar** teeth are the largest of the permanent set, and their broad crowns are adapted for grinding and pounding food. The deciduous teeth are smaller than, but generally resemble in form, the teeth that bear the same names in the permanent set.

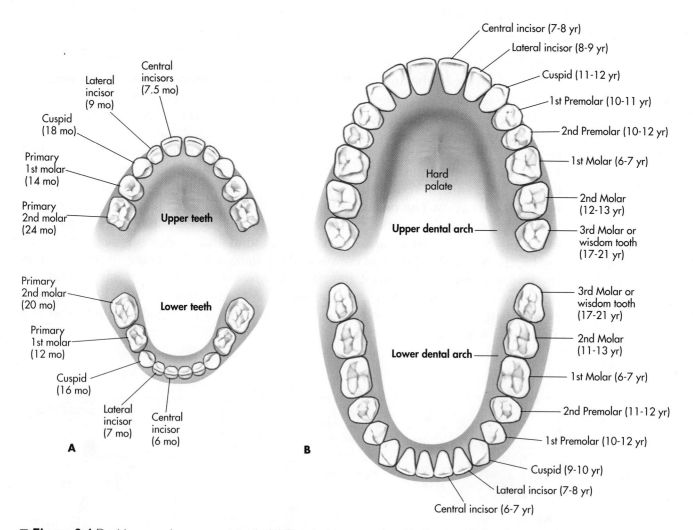

■ **Figure 8.4** Deciduous and permanent teeth. (A) The deciduous teeth, with the age of eruption given in months; (B) the permanent teeth, with the age at eruption given in years.

Each tooth consists of three main portions: the **crown**, projecting above the gum; the **root,** embedded in the alveolus; and the **neck,** the constricted portion between the crown and root. On making a vertical section of a tooth, a cavity will be found in the interior of the crown and the center of each root; it opens by a minute orifice at the extremity of the latter. See Figure 8.5 ■

This cavity is called the **pulp cavity**, which contains the dental pulp, a loose connective tissue richly supplied with vessels and nerves that enter the cavity through the small aperture at the point of each root. The pulp cavity receives blood vessels and nerves from the **root canal**, a narrow tunnel located at the root, or base, of the tooth. Blood vessels and nerves enter the root canal through an opening called the **apical foramen** to supply the pulp cavity.

The root of each tooth sits in a bony socket called an *alveolus*. Collagen fibers of the **periodontal ligament** extend from the dentin of the root to the bone of the alveolus, creating a strong articulation known as a *gomphosis*, which binds the teeth to bony sockets in the maxillary bone and mandible. A layer of **cementum** (a thin layer of bone) covers the dentin of the root, providing protection and firmly anchoring the periodontal ligament.

The solid portion of the tooth consists of the **dentin**, which forms the bulk of the tooth; the **enamel**, which covers the exposed part of the crown and is the hardest and most compact part of a tooth; and the cementum, which is disposed on the surface of the root.

The neck of the tooth marks the boundary between the root and the crown, the exposed portion of the tooth that projects above the soft tissue of the **gingiva**. A shallow groove called the **gingival sulcus** surrounds the neck of each tooth.

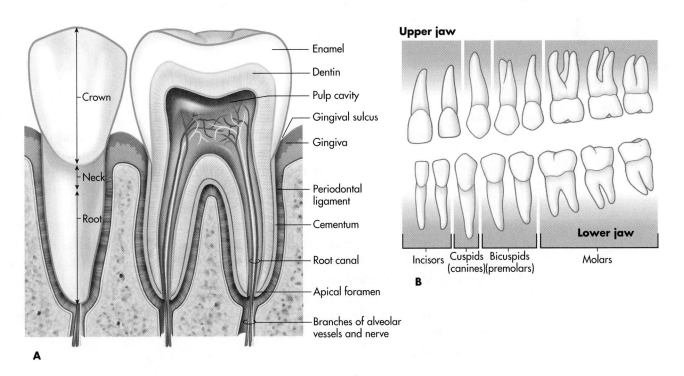

■ **Figure 8.5** Teeth. (A) Diagrammatic section through a typical adult tooth; (B) the adult teeth.

PHARYNX

Just beyond the mouth, at the beginning of the tube leading to the stomach, is the **pharynx**, a musculomembranous tube extending from the base of the skull to the level of the sixth cervical vertebra where it becomes continuous with the esophagus (Figure 8.1). The upper portion, the **nasopharynx**, is above the soft palate. The middle portion, the **oropharynx**, lies between the palate and the hyoid bone and has an opening to the oral cavity. The lowest portion, the **laryngopharynx**, is below the hyoid bone and opens inferiorly to the larynx anteriorly and the esophagus posteriorly.

The pharynx is a common passageway for both respiration and digestion. Both the **larynx**, or voice box, and the esophagus begin in the pharynx. Food that is swallowed passes through the pharynx into the esophagus reflexively. Muscular contractions move the bolus into the esophagus and the **epiglottis** (a flap of tissue) blocks the opening of the larynx, preventing food from entering the airway leading to the trachea (windpipe).

ESOPHAGUS

The **esophagus** is a muscular tube about 10 inches long that leads from the pharynx to the stomach (Figure 8.1). Food and liquids pass down the esophagus and into the stomach. At the junction with the stomach is the lower esophageal or cardiac sphincter. This sphincter relaxes to permit passage of food and then contracts to prevent the backup of stomach contents. Food is carried along the esophagus by a series of wavelike muscular contractions called **peristalsis.**

STOMACH

The **stomach** is a muscular, distensible saclike portion of the alimentary canal between the esophagus and duodenum (see Figure 8.6 ■). The upper region of the stomach is called the *fundus,* the main portion is called the *body,* and the lower region is the *antrum.* There are folds in the mucous membrane lining the stomach called *rugae* that stretch when the stomach fills with food and contain glands that produce digestive juices.

Food and liquids pass from the esophagus into the stomach. Here food is reduced to a digestible state by mechanical churning and the release of chemicals such as hydrochloric acid, digestive hormones, and enzymes. Gastric juices help convert the food to a semiliquid state called chyme, which is passed at intervals through a valve called the pyloric sphincter into the small intestine. An empty stomach has a volume of about 50 mL. Typically after a meal, its capacity can expand to about 1 liter and may expand to hold as much as 4 liters.

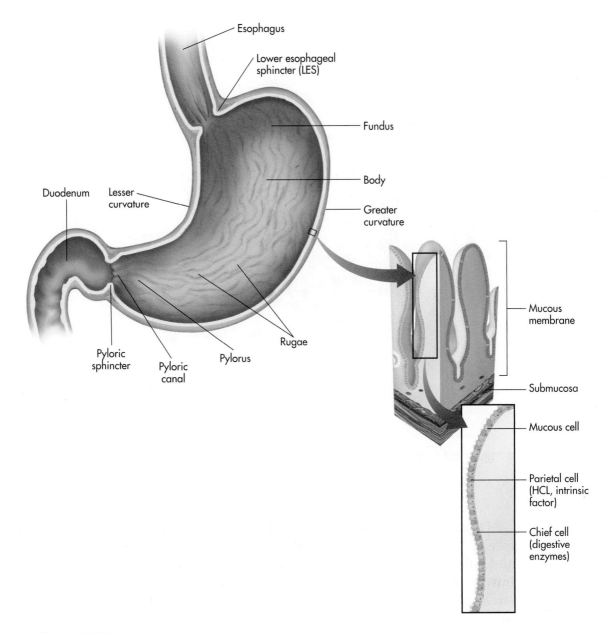

■ Figure 8.6 Stomach.

SMALL INTESTINE

The **small intestine** is about 21 feet long and 1 inch in diameter. It extends from the pyloric sphincter at the base of the stomach to the entrance of the large intestine. The small intestine is divided into three parts: the **duodenum,** the **jejunum,** and the **ileum.** The duodenum is the first 12 inches just beyond the stomach. The jejunum is the next 8 feet or so, and the ileum is the remaining 12 feet of the tube (see Figure 8.7 ■).

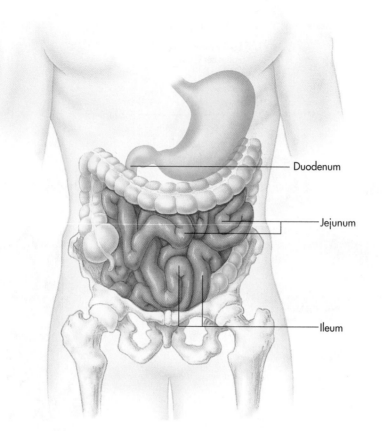

■ **Figure 8.7** Small intestine.

Digestion and absorption take place chiefly in the small intestine. Chyme is received from the stomach through the pylorus and is mixed with bile from the liver and gallbladder along with pancreatic juice from the pancreas. Intestinal villi, the tiny, finger-like projections in the wall of the small intestine, increase the surface area and thus the absorptive area of the intestinal wall, providing more places for food to be absorbed. It is important that food is absorbed at a considerably fast rate so as to allow more food to be absorbed.

Digested nutrients (including sugars and amino acids) pass into the villi through diffusion. Complex proteins are broken down into simple amino acids, complicated sugars are reduced to simple sugars (glucose), and large fat molecules (triglycerides) are broken down to fatty acids and glycerol. Circulating blood then transmits these nutrients to body cells. Enzymes within the villi capillaries collect amino acids and simple sugars, which are taken up by the villi and sent into the bloodstream. Villus lacteals (lymph capillary) collect absorbed lipoproteins and are taken to the rest of the body through the lymph fluid. See Table 8.2 ■ for a general description of chemical digestion.

TABLE 8.2 Components of Chemical Digestion

Digestive Juices and Enzymes	Food Enzyme Digests	Resulting Product
1. Saliva		
a. Ptyalin (salivary amylase)	Starch and sugar	Maltose (a disaccharide, or double sugar)
2. Gastric juice		
a. Rennin	Caseinogen (milk products)	Casein (curds)
b. Pepsin, plus hydrochloric acid (HCl)	Proteins, including casein	Proteoses and peptones (partially digested proteins)
c. Lipase	Emulsified fats (butter, cream)	Fatty acids and glycerol
3. Bile (contains no enzymes)	Large fat droplets (unemulsified fats)	Small fat droplets, or emulsified fats
4. Pancreatic juice		
a. Trypsin (protease)	Proteins	Peptones, peptids, amino acids
b. Steapsin (lipase)	Bile-emulsified fats	Fatty acids and glycerol
c. Amylopsin (pancreatic amylase)	Starch	Maltose
5. Intestinal juice		
a. Erepsin	Partially digested proteins	Amino acids
b. Sucrase	Sucrose (cane sugar)	Glucose and fructose
c. Lactase	Lactose (milk sugar)	Glucose and galactose
d. Maltase	Maltose (malt sugar)	Glucose

LARGE INTESTINE

The **large intestine** is about 5 feet long and $2^1/_2$ inches in diameter. It extends from the ileocecal valve at the small intestine to the anus. The large intestine is divided into the **cecum**, the **colon**, the **rectum**, and the **anal canal**. The cecum is a pouchlike structure forming the beginning of the large intestine. It is about 3 inches long and has the **appendix** attached to it. The colon makes up the bulk of the large intestine and is divided into the ascending colon, the transverse colon, the descending colon, and the sigmoid colon (see Figure 8.8 ■). With digestion and absorption completed in the large intestine, the waste product of digestion (feces, stool) is expelled through the anus during defecation.

LIFE SPAN CONSIDERATIONS

Meconium, the first stool, is a mixture of amniotic fluid and secretions of the intestinal glands. It is thick and sticky, and dark green in color. It is usually passed 8–24 hours following birth. The stool during the first week is loose and greenish-yellow. The stool of a breast-fed baby is bright yellow, soft, and pasty. The stool of a bottle-fed baby is more solid than those of a breast-fed baby, and the color varies from yellow to brown.

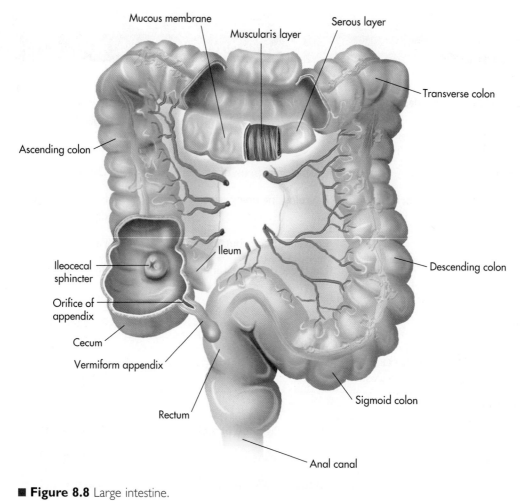

■ **Figure 8.8** Large intestine.

ACCESSORY ORGANS

The salivary glands, the liver, the gallbladder, and the pancreas are not actually part of the digestive tube; however, they are closely related to the digestive process.

Salivary Glands

Located in or near the mouth, the **salivary glands** secrete **saliva** in response to the sight, smell, taste, or mental image of food. Human saliva is composed of 98% water, while the other 2% consists of other compounds such as electrolytes, mucus, antibacterial compounds, and various enzymes that help start the process of digestion. The various salivary glands are the **parotid,** located on either side of the face slightly below the ear; the **submandibular,** located in the floor of the mouth; and the **sublingual,** located below the tongue (see Figure 8.1). All salivary glands secrete through openings (salivary ducts) into the mouth to lubricate food and begin the digestion of carbohydrates. See Figure 8.9 ■

Liver

The largest glandular organ in the body, the **liver** weighs about 3 1/2 lbs and is located in the upper right part of the abdomen (see Figure 8.10 ■). The liver plays an essential role in the normal metabolism of carbohydrates, fats, and proteins. In

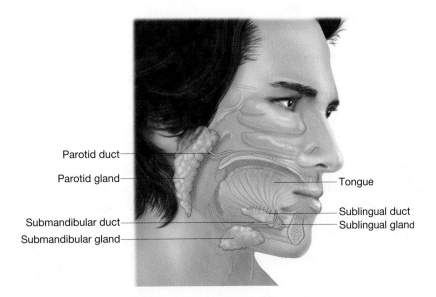

■ Figure 8.9 Salivary glands, salivary ducts, and the tongue.

carbohydrate metabolism, it changes glucose to glycogen and stores the glycogen until needed by body cells. When required, glycogen is converted back to glucose. In fat metabolism, the liver serves as a storage place and acts to desaturate fats before releasing them into the bloodstream. In protein metabolism, the liver acts as a storage place and assists in both protein **anabolism** and **catabolism.**

The liver manufactures the following important substances:

- **Bile.** Digestive juice important in fat emulsification (the breakdown of large fat globules into smaller particles)
- **Fibrinogen** and **prothrombin.** Coagulants essential for blood clotting
- **Heparin.** Anticoagulant that helps to prevent the clotting of blood
- **Blood proteins.** Albumin, gamma globulin

Additionally, the liver stores iron and vitamins B_{12}, A, D, E, and K. It also detoxifies many harmful substances (toxins) such as drugs and alcohol.

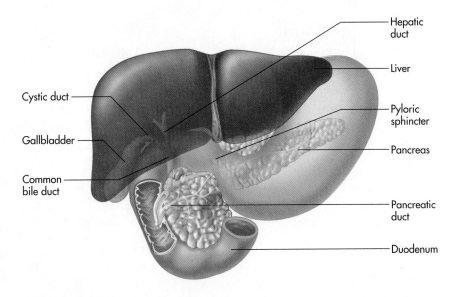

■ Figure 8.10 Liver.

Gallbladder

The **gallbladder** is a membranous sac attached to the liver in which excess bile is stored and concentrated (see Figures 8.1 and 8.10). Bile leaving the gallbladder is 6–10 times as concentrated as that which comes to it from the liver. Concentration is accomplished by reabsorption of water.

Pancreas

The **pancreas** is a large, elongated gland situated behind the stomach and secreting pancreatic juice into the small intestine (see Figures 8.11 ■ and 8.10). The pancreas is 6–9 inches long and contains cells that produce digestive **enzymes.** Other specialized cells in the pancreas secrete the hormones insulin and glucagon directly into the bloodstream. The beta cells of the islets of Langerhans make and release insulin. The alpha cells of the islets of Langerhans synthesize and secrete glucagon.

LIFE SPAN CONSIDERATIONS

Newborns produce very little saliva until they are 3 months of age and swallowing is a reflex action. The infant's stomach is small and empties rapidly. The liver of the newborn is often immature, thereby causing **jaundice**. Fat absorption is poor because of a decreased level of bile production.

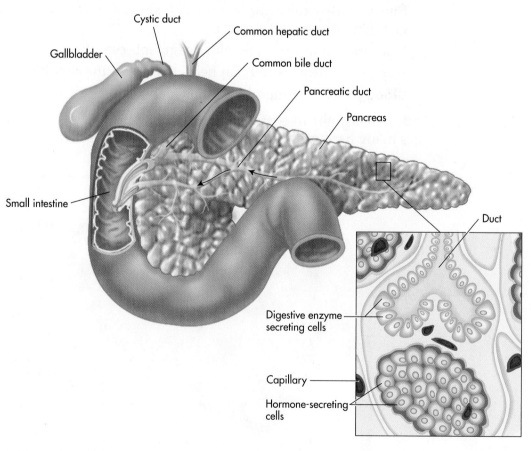

■ **Figure 8.11** Pancreas.

Anatomy and Physiology Labeling

Identify the structures shown below by filling in the blanks.

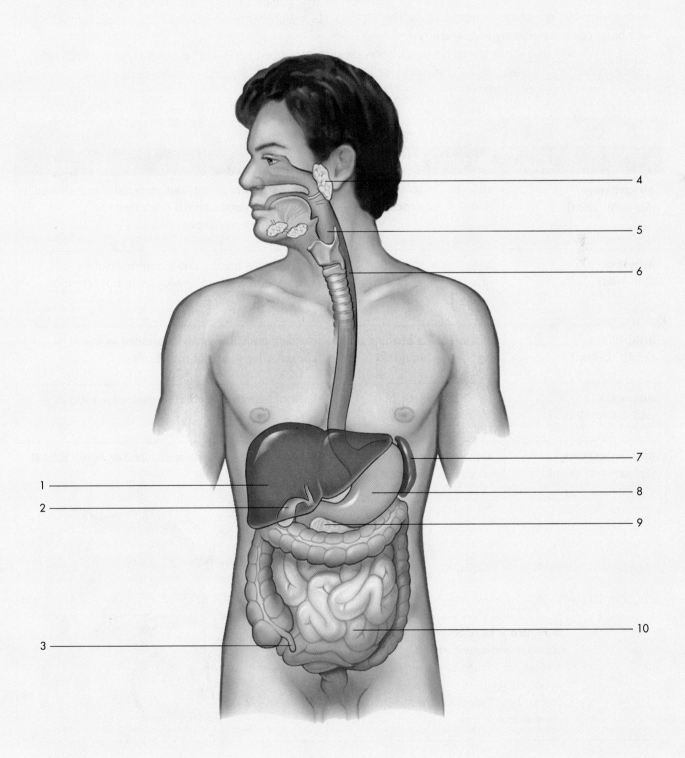

• Building Your Medical Vocabulary •

This section provides the foundation for learning medical terminology. Review the following alphabetized word list. Note how common prefixes and suffixes are repeatedly applied to word roots and combining forms to create different meanings. The word parts are color-coded: prefixes are green, suffixes are blue, roots/combining forms are red.

You will find that some terms have not been divided into word parts. These are common words or specialized terms that are included to enhance your medical vocabulary. See Chapter 1, page 7, to review pronunciation guidelines.

MEDICAL WORD	WORD PARTS		DEFINITION
	Part	Meaning	
absorption (ăb-sōrp´ shŭn)	absorpt -ion	to suck in process	Process by which nutrient material is transferred from the gastrointestinal tract into the bloodstream or lymph
amylase (ăm´ ĭ-lās)	amyl -ase	starch enzyme	Enzyme that breaks down starch. Ptyalin is a salivary amylase and amylopsin is a pancreatic amylase.
anabolism (ă-năb´ ō-lĭzm)	anabol -ism	a building up condition	Building up of the body substance in the constructive phase of metabolism
anorexia (ăn˝ ō-rĕks´ ĭ-ă)	an- -orexia	lack of appetite	Lack of appetite; decreased desire for food
appendectomy (ăp˝ ĕn-děk´ tō-mē)	append -ectomy	appendix surgical excision	Surgical excision of the appendix. See Figure 8.12 ■

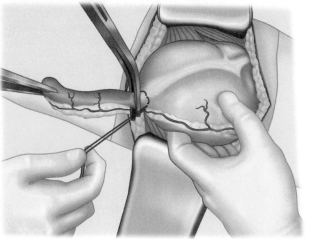

■ **Figure 8.12** Appendectomy. The appendix and cecum are brought through the incision to the surface of the abdomen. The base of the appendix is clamped and ligated, and the appendix is then removed.

MEDICAL WORD	WORD PARTS		DEFINITION
	Part	Meaning	
appendicitis (ă-pĕn″ dĭ-sī′ tĭs)	appendic -itis	appendix inflammation	Inflammation of the appendix. A point of tenderness in acute appendicitis is known as *McBurney's point,* located 1–2 inches above the anterosuperior spine of the ilium on a line between the ilium and the umbilicus. See Figure 8.13 ∎

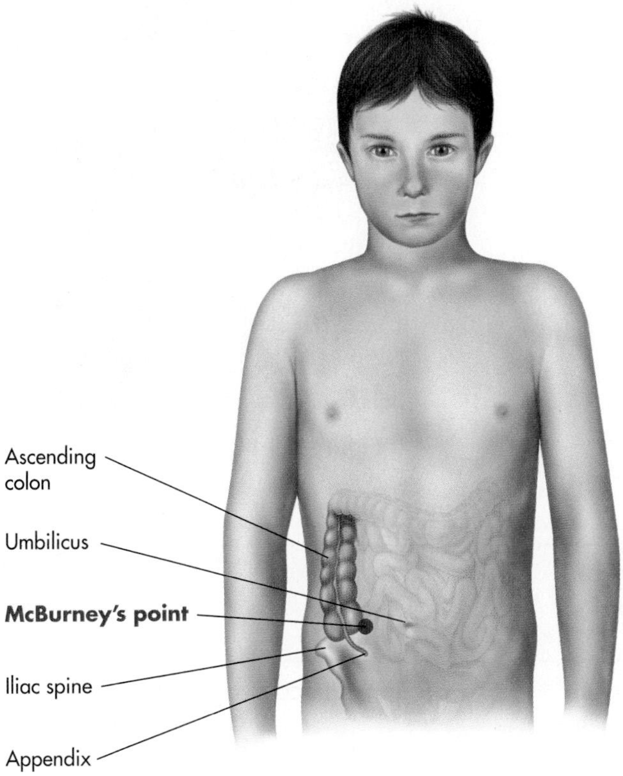

∎ Figure 8.13 McBurney's point is the common location of pain in children and adolescents with appendicitis.

ascites (ă-sī′ tēz)			Significant accumulation of serous fluid in the peritoneal cavity
biliary (bĭl′ ĭ-ār″ ē)	bil/i -ary	gall, bile pertaining to	Pertaining to bile and the gallbladder
bilirubin (bĭl″ ĭ-rōō′ bĭn)			Orange-colored bile pigment produced by the separation of hemoglobin into parts that are excreted by the liver cells

MEDICAL WORD	WORD PARTS		DEFINITION
	Part	**Meaning**	
black hairy tongue			Condition in which the tongue is covered by hairlike papillae entangled with threads produced by *Aspergillus niger* or *Candida albicans* fungi. This unusual condition could be caused by poor oral hygiene and/or overgrowth of fungi due to antibiotic therapy. See Figure 8.14 ■

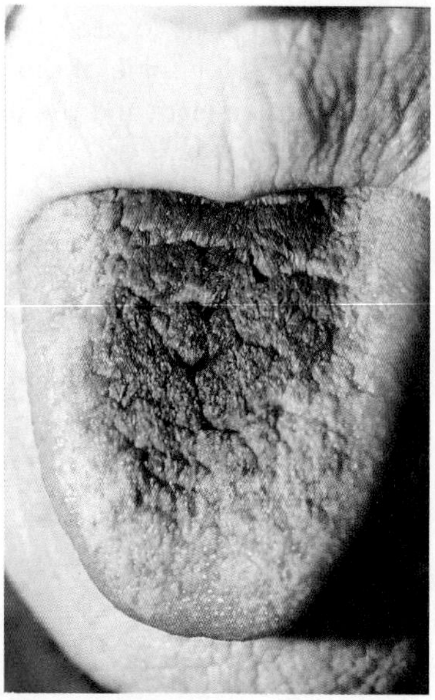

■ **Figure 8.14** Black hairy tongue.
(Courtesy of Jason L. Smith, MD)

MEDICAL WORD	WORD PARTS		DEFINITION
bowel (bou´ əl)			Intestine
buccal (bək´ əl)	bucc -al	cheek pertaining to	Literally means *pertaining to the cheek*; relating to the cheek or mouth
catabolism (kă-tăb´ ō-lĭzm)	catabol -ism	a casting down condition	Literally *a casting down*; in metabolism a breaking of complex substances into more basic elements
celiac (sē´ lĭ-ăk)	celi -ac	abdomen, belly pertaining to	Pertaining to the abdomen
cheilosis (kī-lō´ sĭs)	cheil -osis	lip condition	Abnormal condition of the lip as seen in riboflavin and other B-complex deficiencies

MEDICAL WORD	WORD PARTS		DEFINITION
	Part	Meaning	
cholecystectomy (kō″ lē-sĭs-tĕk′ tō-mē)	chol/e cyst -ectomy	gall, bile bladder surgical excision	Surgical excision of the gallbladder. With laparoscopic cholecystectomy, the gallbladder is removed through a small incision near the navel. *Cholelithiasis* (gallstones) are usually present in the removed gallbladder. See Figure 8.15 ■

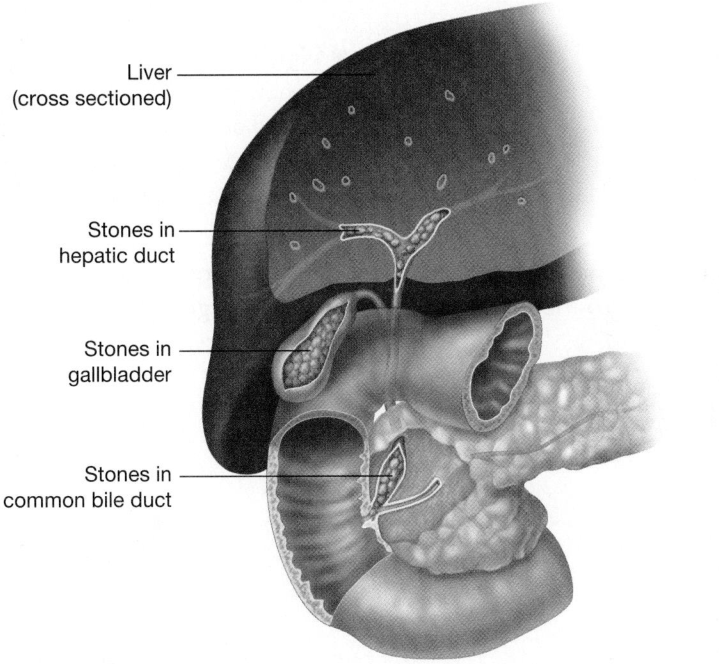

Liver
(cross sectioned)

Stones in
hepatic duct

Stones in
gallbladder

Stones in
common bile duct

■ **Figure 8.15** Gallbladder with gallstones. Note the stones in the hepatic duct, gallbladder, and common bile duct.

MEDICAL WORD	WORD PARTS		DEFINITION
cholecystitis (kō″ lē-sĭs-tī′ tĭs)	chol/e cyst -itis	gall, bile bladder inflammation	Inflammation of the gallbladder
choledochotomy (kō-lĕd″ ō-kŏt′ ō-mē)	chole- doch/o -tomy	common bile duct incision	Surgical incision of the common bile duct
chyle (kīl)			Milky fluid of intestinal digestion composed of lymph and emulsified fats

MEDICAL WORD	WORD PARTS		DEFINITION
	Part	**Meaning**	
cirrhosis (sĭ-rō´ sĭs)	cirrh -osis	orange-yellow condition	Chronic degenerative liver disease characterized by changes in the lobes; parenchymal cells and the lobules are infiltrated with fat (Figure 8.16 ■)

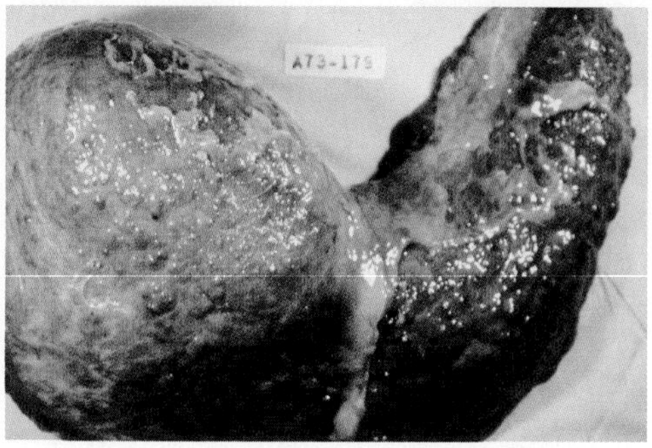

■ **Figure 8.16** The liver in this photograph was from a deceased patient with an advanced state of cirrhosis.
(Source: Pearson Education)

MEDICAL WORD	WORD PARTS		DEFINITION
colectomy (kō-lĕk´ tō-mē)	col -ectomy	colon surgical excision	Surgical excision of part of the colon
colon cancer (kō-lŏn kăn´ ser)			Malignancy of the colon; sometimes called *colorectal cancer* (Figure 8.17 ■)

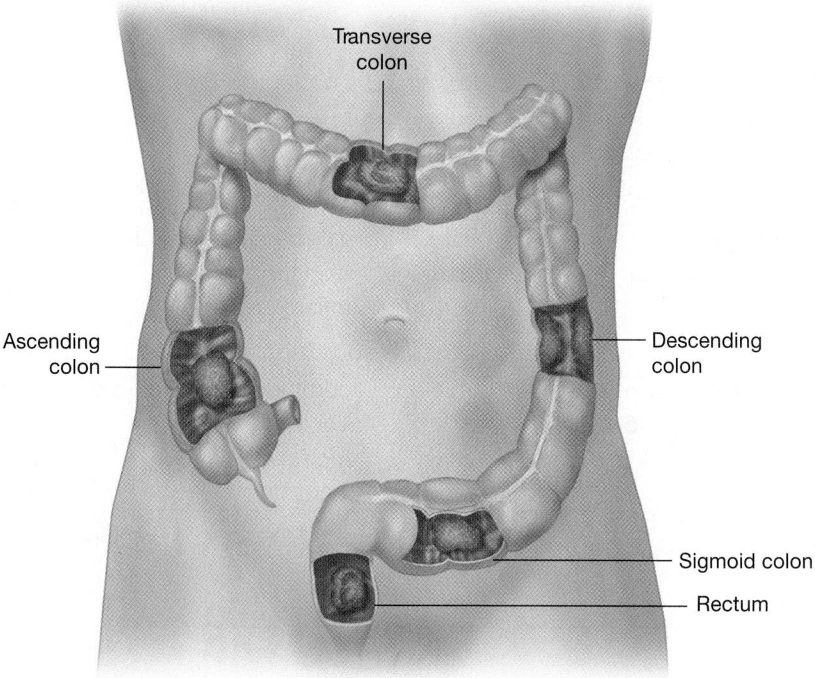

Transverse colon

Ascending colon

Descending colon

Sigmoid colon

Rectum

■ **Figure 8.17**
Common sites of colorectal cancer.

MEDICAL WORD	WORD PARTS		DEFINITION
colonic (kō-lŏn´ ĭk)	colon -ic	colon pertaining to	Pertaining to the colon

MEDICAL WORD	WORD PARTS		DEFINITION
	Part	Meaning	
colonoscope (kō-lŏn´ ŏ-skōp)	colon -scope	colon instrument for examining	Thin, lighted, flexible instrument that is used to view the interior of the colon during a colonoscopy
colonoscopy (kō-lŏn-ŏs´ kō-pē)	colon/o -scopy	colon visual examination, to view, examine	Visual examination of the colon via a colonoscope (Figure 8.18 ■)

Tumor

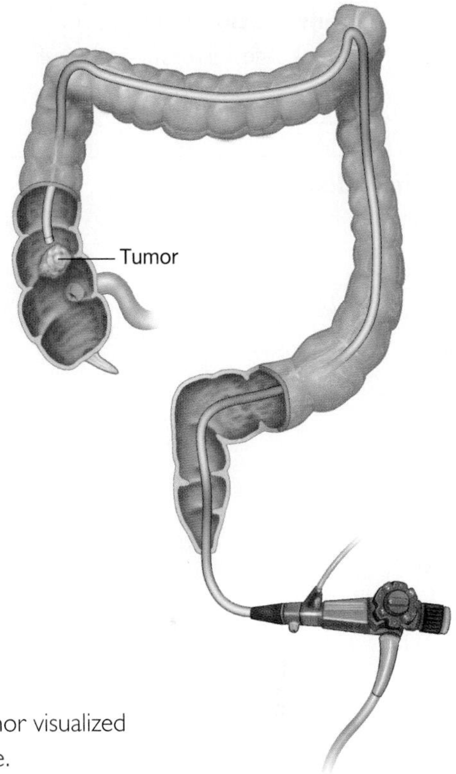

■ **Figure 8.18** Note the tumor visualized with the use of a colonoscope.

colostomy (kō-lŏs´ tō-mē)	col/o -stomy	colon new opening	Literally means *the creation of a new opening into the colon,* performed for the purpose of evacuating the bowel and can be required because of colon cancer, intestinal obstruction, perforation, birth defects, and Crohn's disease. A colostomy can be permanent or temporary. The most common types are transverse, descending, and sigmoid, so named due to the site of the disorder and the location of the stoma. See Figure 8.19 ■

■ **Figure 8.19**
Alternate sites that can be used to create a new opening (-ostomy) in the colon.

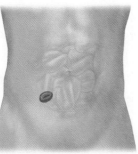
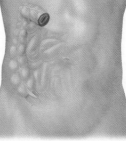
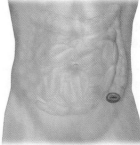

MEDICAL WORD	WORD PARTS		DEFINITION
	Part	**Meaning**	
constipation (kon″ stĭ-pā´ shŭn)	constipat -ion	to press together process	Infrequent passage of unduly hard and dry feces; *difficult defecation*

LIFE SPAN CONSIDERATIONS

Constipation is a frequent problem among older adults. It is believed that constipation is not a normal age-related change but is caused by low fluid intake, dehydration, lack of dietary fiber, inactivity, medicines, depression, and other health-related conditions.

MEDICAL WORD	WORD PARTS		DEFINITION
Crohn's disease (krōnz)			Chronic autoimmune disease that can affect any part of the gastrointestinal tract but most commonly occurs in the ileum (Figure 8.20 ■)

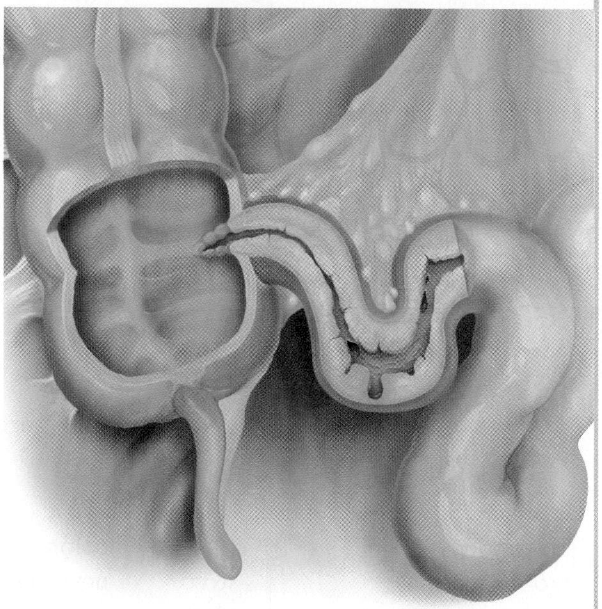

■ **Figure 8.20** Note the thickening of the intestinal wall and the erosion of the inner lining of the ileum, often seen in Crohn's disease.

MEDICAL WORD	WORD PARTS		DEFINITION
defecation (dĕf-ĕ-kā´ shŭn)	defecat -ion	to remove dregs process	Evacuation of the bowel
deglutition (dē″ glōō-tĭsh´ ūn)			Act or process of swallowing
dentalgia (dĕn-tăl´ jĭ-ă)	dent -algia	tooth pain, ache	Pain in a tooth; *toothache*
dentist	dent -ist	tooth one who specializes	One who specializes in dentistry

MEDICAL WORD	WORD PARTS		DEFINITION
	Part	Meaning	
dentition (děn-tǐ´ shŭn)			Type, number, and arrangement of teeth in the dental arch
diarrhea (dī´ ă-rē´ ă)	dia- -rrhea	through flow	Frequent passage of unformed watery stools
digestion (dǐ-jěst´ chŭn)			Process by which food is changed in the mouth, stomach, and intestines by chemical, mechanical, and physical action so that it can be absorbed by the body
diverticulitis (dī´´ věr-tǐk´´ ū-lǐ´ tǐs)	diverticul -itis	diverticula inflammation	Inflammation of the diverticula (pouches in the walls of an organ) in the colon. Symptoms include pain, fever, chills, cramping, bloating, constipation, and diarrhea. Treatment depends on the severity of the condition. See Figure 8.21 ■

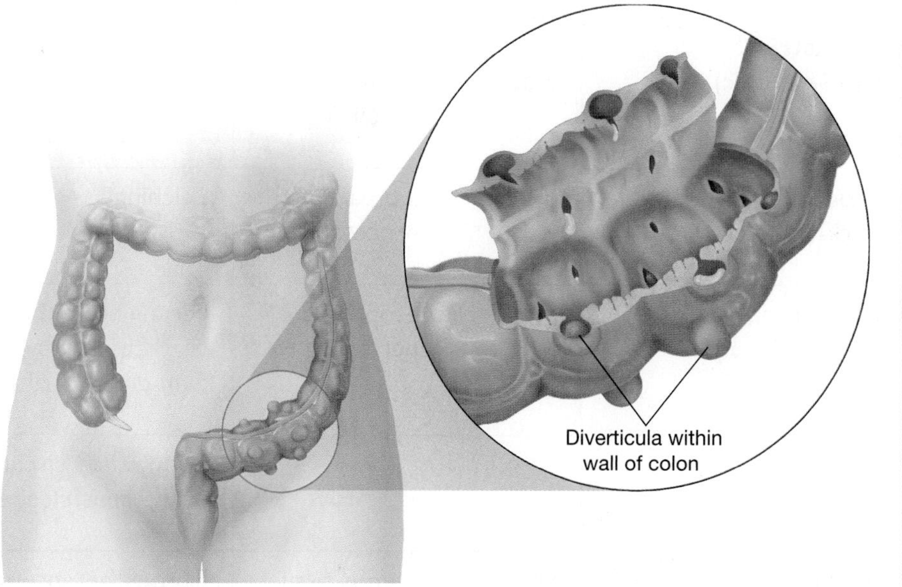

Diverticula within wall of colon

■ **Figure 8.21** Diverticulitis.

MEDICAL WORD	WORD PARTS		DEFINITION
duodenal (dū´´ ō-dē´ năl)	duoden -al	duodenum pertaining to	Pertaining to the duodenum; the first part of the small intestine
dysentery (dǐs´ ěn-těr´´ ē)	dys- enter -y	difficult intestine pertaining to	An intestinal disease characterized by inflammation of the mucous membrane
dyspepsia (dǐs-pěp´ sǐ-ă)	dys- -pepsia	difficult to digest	Difficulty in digestion; *indigestion*

MEDICAL WORD	WORD PARTS		DEFINITION
	Part	**Meaning**	
dysphagia (dĭs-fā´ jĭ-ă)	dys- -phagia	difficult to eat, to swallow	Difficulty in swallowing
emesis (ĕm´ ĕ-sĭs)	eme -sis	to vomit condition	Vomiting
enteric (ĕn-tĕr´ ĭk)	enter -ic	small intestine pertaining to	Pertaining to the small intestine
enteritis (ĕn″ tĕr-i´ tĭs)	enter -itis	small intestine inflammation	Inflammation of the small intestine
enzyme (ĕn´ zīm)			Protein substance capable of causing rapid chemical changes in other substances without being changed itself
epigastric (ĕp´ ĭ-găs´ trĭc)	epi- gastr -ic	above stomach pertaining to	Pertaining to the region above the stomach
eructation (ē-rk-tā´ shŭn)	eructat -ion	a breaking out process	Belching
esophageal (ē-sŏf″ ă-jē´ ăl)	esophage/o -al	esophagus pertaining to	Pertaining to the esophagus. *Note that the suffix begins with a vowel; drop the (o) from the combining form and add -al to form esophageal.*
feces (fē´ sēz)			Body waste discharged from the bowel by way of the anus; *stool, excreta*
fibroma (fĭ-brō´ mă)	fibr -oma	fibrous tissue tumor	Fibrous, encapsulated connective tissue tumor
flatus (flā´ tŭs)			Literally means *a blowing* in Latin; the expelling of gas from the anus. The average person passes 400 to 1200 mL of gas each day.
gastrectomy (găs-trĕk´ tō-mē)	gastr -ectomy	stomach surgical excision	Surgical excision of a part of or the whole stomach
gastric (găs´ trĭk)	gastr -ic	stomach pertaining to	Pertaining to the stomach

MEDICAL WORD	WORD PARTS		DEFINITION
	Part	Meaning	
gastroenterology (găs″ trō-ĕn″ tĕr-ŏl′ ō-jē)	gastr/o enter/o -logy	stomach intestine study of	Literally means *the study of the stomach and the intestines;* study of the entire GI tract from the mouth to the anus
gastroesophageal (găs′ trō ē-sŏf″ ă-jē-ăl)	gastr/o esophage/o -al	stomach esophagus pertaining to	Pertaining to the stomach and esophagus
gastroesophageal reflux disease (GERD) (găs′ trō ē-sŏf″ ă-jē-ăl rē′ flŭcks)			Condition that occurs when the muscle between the esophagus and the stomach, the lower esophageal sphincter, is weak or relaxes inappropriately, allowing the stomach's contents to back up (*reflux*) into the esophagus. Symptoms include heartburn, belching, and regurgitation of food. See Figure 8.22 ■

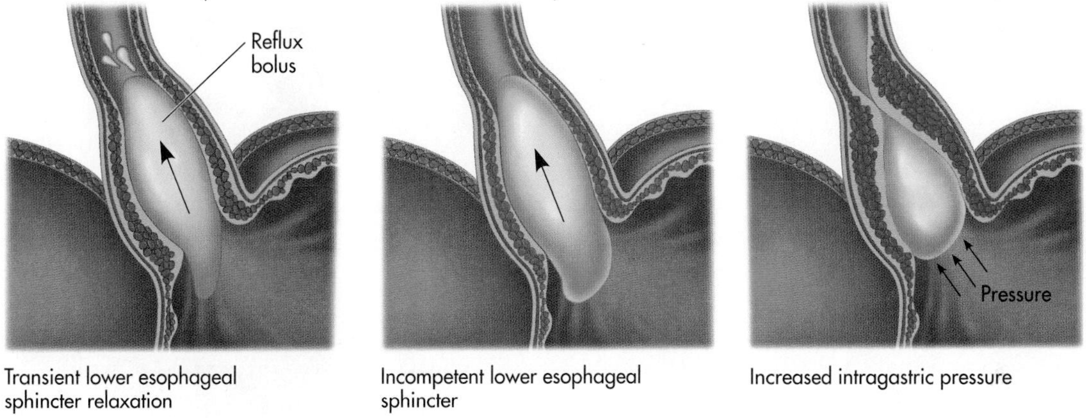

Reflux bolus

Transient lower esophageal sphincter relaxation

Incompetent lower esophageal sphincter

Pressure

Increased intragastric pressure

■ **Figure 8.22** Mechanisms of gastroesophageal reflux.

fyi Dietary and lifestyle choices may contribute to GERD. Studies show that cigarette smoking relaxes the lower esophageal sphincter. Obesity and pregnancy can also cause GERD. Some doctors believe a **hiatal hernia** may weaken the lower esophageal sphincter (LES) and cause reflux.

gavage (gă-văzh′)			To feed liquid or semiliquid food via a tube (stomach or nasogastric)
gingivitis (jĭn″ jĭ-vī′ tĭs)	gingiv -itis	gums inflammation	Inflammation of the gums
glossotomy (glŏ-sŏt′ ō-mē)	gloss/o -tomy	tongue incision	Surgical incision into the tongue

MEDICAL WORD	WORD PARTS		DEFINITION
	Part	**Meaning**	
glycogenesis (glī″ kŏ-jĕn′ ĕ-sĭs)	glyc/o -genesis	sweet, sugar formation, produce	Formation of glycogen from glucose
halitosis (hăl″ ĭ-tō′ sĭs)	halit -osis	breath condition	Bad breath
hematemesis (hĕm″ ăt-ēm′ ĕ-sĭs)	hemat -emesis	blood vomiting	Vomiting of blood
hematochezia (hĕm″ ă-tō-kē′ zē-ă)			Passage of stools that contain red blood
hemorrhoid (hĕm′ ō-royd)	hemorrh -oid	vein liable to bleed resemble	Mass of dilated, tortuous veins in the anorectum; can be internal or external. See Figure 8.23 ■

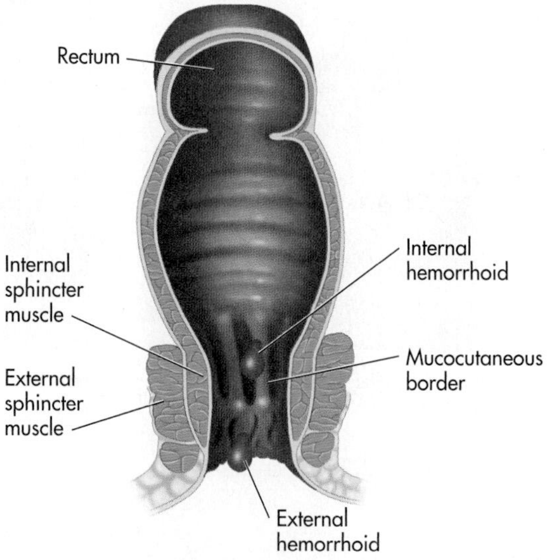

■ **Figure 8.23** Location of internal and external hemorrhoids.

MEDICAL WORD	WORD PARTS		DEFINITION
hepatitis (hĕp″ ă-tī′ tĭs)	hepat -itis	liver inflammation	Inflammation of the liver
hepatoma (hĕp″ ă-tō′ mă)	hepat -oma	liver tumor	Tumor of the liver

MEDICAL WORD	WORD PARTS		DEFINITION
	Part	Meaning	
hernia (hĕr´ nē-ă)			Abnormal protrusion of an organ or a part of an organ through the wall of the body cavity that normally contains it. A *hiatal* hernia occurs when the upper part of the stomach moves up into the chest through a small opening in the diaphragm. An *inguinal* hernia occurs when a loop of intestine enters the inguinal canal, a tubular passage through the lower layers of the abdominal wall. See Figure 8.24 ■

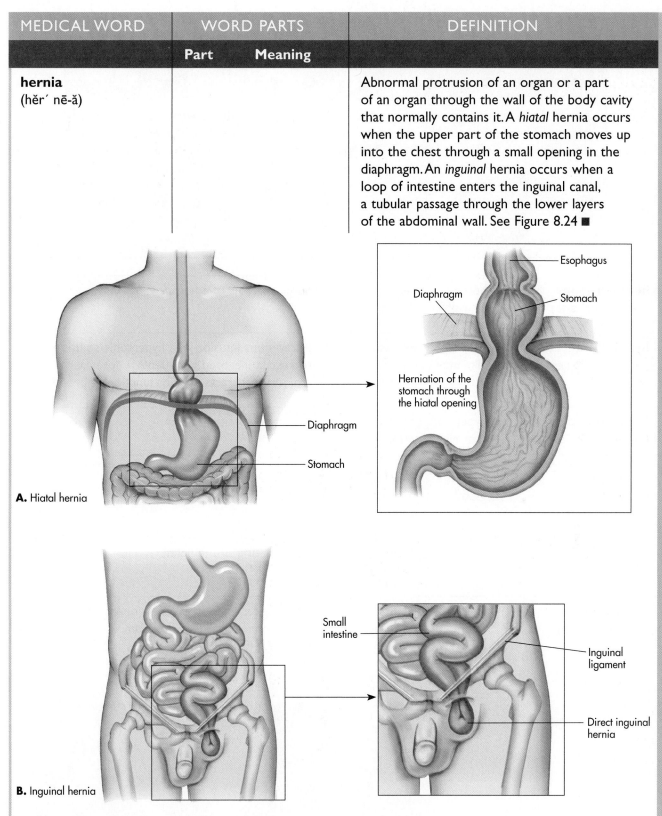

A. Hiatal hernia

B. Inguinal hernia

■ **Figure 8.24** Hernias.

MEDICAL WORD	WORD PARTS		DEFINITION
	Part	Meaning	

Infants and children can also develop inguinal hernias. In these populations, hernias can occur when a portion of the peritoneum (the lining around all of the organs in the abdomen) does not close properly before birth. This causes a small portion of the intestine to push out into the opening (a bulge might be seen in the groin or scrotum). Diagnosis is typically made through a physical examination in which the hernia mass is palpated and increases in size when coughing, bending, lifting, or straining. The hernia (bulge) is not necessarily obvious in infants and children except when the child is crying or coughing. Treatment is usually a **herniorrhaphy**, a hernia repair surgery, in which the hernia is pushed back into the abdominal cavity.

MEDICAL WORD	WORD PARTS		DEFINITION
	Part	Meaning	
herniorrhaphy (hĕr″ nĕ-or′ ă-fē)	herni/o -rrhaphy	hernia suture	Surgical repair of a hernia
hyperalimentation (hī″ pĕr-ăl″ ĭ m ĕn-tā′ shŭn)	hyper- alimentat -ion	excessive nourishment process	Intravenous infusion of a hypertonic solution to sustain life; used in patients whose gastrointestinal tracts are not functioning properly
hyperemesis (hī″ pĕr-ĕm′ ĕ-sĭs)	hyper- -emesis	excessive, above vomiting	Excessive vomiting
hypogastric (hī″ pō-găs′ trĭk)	hypo- gastr -ic	deficient, below stomach pertaining to	Pertaining to below the stomach
ileitis (ĭl″ ē-ī′ tis)	ile -itis	ileum inflammation	Inflammation of the ileum
ileostomy (ĭl″ ē-ŏs′ tō-mē)	ile/o -stomy	ileum new opening	The surgical creation of a new opening through the abdominal wall into the ileum. See Figure 8.25 ■

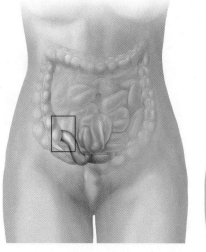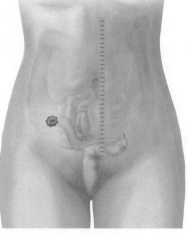

■ **Figure 8.25** Ileostomy. Note that the cecum and colon have been surgically removed.

MEDICAL WORD	WORD PARTS		DEFINITION
	Part	**Meaning**	
irritable bowel syndrome (IBS)			Disorder that interferes with the normal functions of the large intestine (colon); characterized by a group of symptoms, including crampy abdominal pain, bloating, constipation, and diarrhea. One in five Americans has IBS, making it one of the most common disorders diagnosed by doctors.
labial (lā´ bĭ-ăl)	labi -al	lip pertaining to	Pertaining to the lip
laparotomy (lăp˝ ăr-ŏt´ ō-mē)	lapar/o -tomy	abdomen incision	Surgical incision into the abdomen
lavage (lă-văzh´)			To wash out a cavity. Gastric lavage is used to remove or dilute gastric contents in cases of acute poisoning or ingestion of a caustic substance. *Vomiting should not be induced.* A closed system irrigation uses an ordered amount of solution until the desired results are obtained.
laxative (lăk´ să-tĭv)	laxat -ive	to loosen nature of, quality of	Substance that acts to loosen the bowels
lingual (lĭng´ gwal)	lingu -al	tongue pertaining to	Pertaining to the tongue
lipolysis (lĭp-ŏl´ ĭ-sĭs)	lip/o -lysis	fat destruction, to separate	Break down of fat
liver transplant			Surgical process of transferring the liver from a donor to a patient
malabsorption (măl˝ ăb-sōrp´ shŭn)	mal- absorpt -ion	bad to suck in process	An inadequate absorption of nutrients from the intestinal tract
mastication (măs˝ tĭ-kā´ shŭn)	masticat -ion	to chew process	Chewing; the physical breaking up of food and mixing with saliva in the mouth

MEDICAL WORD	WORD PARTS		DEFINITION
	Part	**Meaning**	
melena (mĕl´ ĕ-nă)			Black, tarry feces (stool) that has a distinctive odor and contains digested blood. Usually results from bleeding in the upper GI tract and can be a sign of a peptic ulcer.
mesentery (mĕs´ ĕn-tĕr˝ ē)	mes enter -y	middle small intestine pertaining to	Pertaining to the peritoneal fold encircling the small intestines and connecting the intestines to the posterior abdominal wall
nausea (naw´ sē-ă)			Uncomfortable feeling of the inclination to vomit
pancreas transplant (păn´ krē-ăs trăns plănt)			Surgical process of transferring the pancreas from a donor to a patient
pancreatitis (păn˝ krē-ă-tī´ tĭs)	pancreat -itis	pancreas inflammation	Inflammation of the pancreas
paralytic ileus (păr˝ ă-lĭt´ ĭk ĭl´ ē-ŭs)	paralyt -ic ile -us	to disable; paralysis pertaining to a twisting pertaining to	Paralysis of the intestines that causes distention and symptoms of acute bowel obstruction and prostration
peptic (pĕp´ tĭk)	pept -ic	to digest pertaining to	Pertaining to gastric digestion
peptic ulcer disease (PUD) (pĕp´ tĭk ´əl-sər)	pept -ic	to digest pertaining to	Disease in which an ulcer forms in the mucosal wall of the stomach, the pylorus, the duodenum, or the esophagus. It is referred to as a *gastric, duodenal,* or *esophageal ulcer,* depending on the location. The erosion of the mucosa that characterizes peptic ulcers is often caused by infection with a bacterium called *Helicobacter pylori (H. pylori)*. Approximately 90% of duodenal ulcers and 80% of peptic ulcers are associated with *Helicobacter pylori*. By killing the bacteria with antibiotics, it is estimated that 90% of the ulcers caused by *H. pylori* can be cured. See Figure 8.26 ■

| MEDICAL WORD | WORD PARTS | | DEFINITION |
	Part	Meaning	

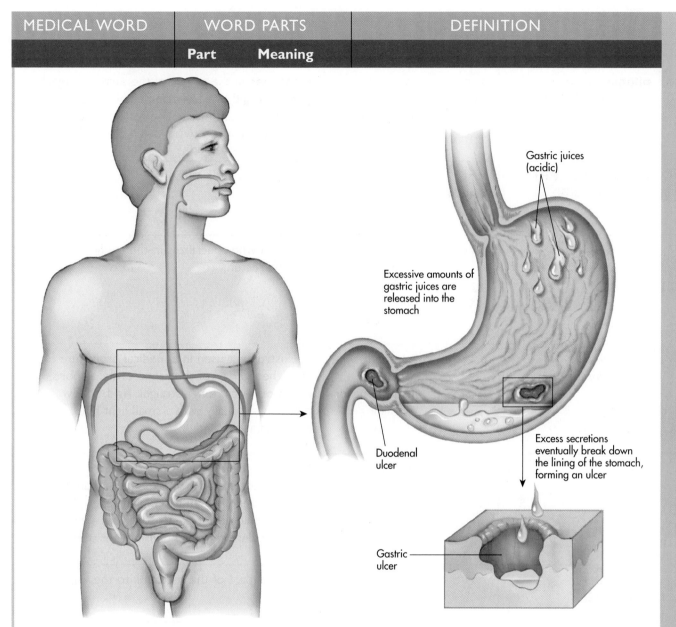

■ **Figure 8.26** Peptic ulcer disease (PUD).

MEDICAL WORD	Part	Meaning	DEFINITION
periodontal (pĕr″ ē-ō-dŏn′ tăl)	peri- odont -al	around tooth pertaining to	Pertaining to the area around the tooth
periodontal disease			Inflammation and degeneration of the gums and surrounding bone, which frequently causes loss of the teeth
peristalsis (pĕr″ ĭ-stăl′ sĭs)	peri- -stalsis	around contraction	Wavelike contraction that occurs involuntarily in hollow tubes of the body, especially the alimentary canal
pharyngeal (făr-ĭn′ jē-ăl)	pharyng/e -al	pharynx pertaining to	Pertaining to the pharynx

MEDICAL WORD	WORD PARTS		DEFINITION
	Part	**Meaning**	
pilonidal cyst (pī″ lō-nī′ dăl sĭst)	pil/o	hair	Closed sac in the crease of the sacrococcygeal region caused by a developmental defect that permits epithelial tissue and hair to be trapped below the skin
	nid	nest	
	-al	pertaining to	
	cyst	sac	
postprandial (PP) (pōst-prăn′ dĭ-ăl)	post-	after	Pertaining to after a meal
	prand/i	meal	
	-al	pertaining to	
proctologist (prŏk-tŏl′ ō-jĭst)	proct/o	anus and rectum	Physician who specializes in the study of the anus and the rectum
	log	study of	
	-ist	one who specializes	
proctoscope (prŏk′ tō-scōp)	proct/o	anus and rectum	An instrument used in a medical procedure to view the interior of the rectal cavity; a short (10 in or 25 cm long), straight, rigid, hollow metal tube, usually with a small light bulb mounted at the end
	-scope	instrument for examining	
pyloric (pī-lōr′ ĭk)	pylor	pylorus, gatekeeper	Pertaining to the gatekeeper, the opening between the stomach and the duodenum. In *pyloric stenosis* seen in an infant, the hypertrophied pyloric muscle causes symptoms of projectile vomiting and visible peristalsis.
	-ic	pertaining to	
rectocele (rĕk′ tō-sēl)	rect/o	rectum	Hernia of part of the rectum into the vagina
	-cele	hernia	
sialadenitis (sī″ ăl-ăd″ ĕ-nī′ tĭs)	sial	saliva	Inflammation of the salivary gland
	aden	gland	
	-itis	inflammation	
sigmoidoscope (sĭg-moy′ dō-skōp)	sigmoid/o	sigmoid	An instrument used in a medical procedure to view the interior of the sigmoid colon
	-scope	instrument for examining	
splenomegaly (splē″ nō-mĕg′ ă-lē)	splen/o	spleen	Enlargement of the spleen
	-megaly	enlargement, large	
stomatitis (stō″ mă-tī′ tĭs)	stomat	mouth	Inflammation of the mouth
	-itis	inflammation	

MEDICAL WORD	WORD PARTS		DEFINITION
	Part	Meaning	
sublingual (sŭb-lĭng′ gwăl)	sub- lingu -al	below tongue pertaining to	Pertaining to below the tongue. See Figure 8.27 ■

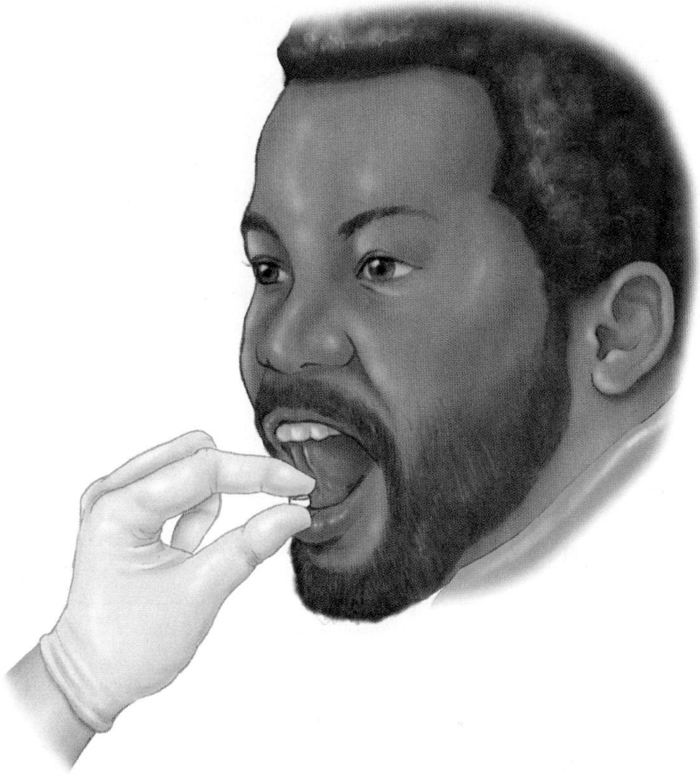

■ **Figure 8.27** Sublingual drug administration.

MEDICAL WORD	WORD PARTS		DEFINITION
ulcer (′əl-sər)			Open lesion or sore of the epidermis or mucous membrane.
ulcerative colitis (ŭl′ sĕr-ă-tĭv kō-lī′ tĭs)			Disease that causes inflammation and ulcers in the lining of the large intestine. The inflammation usually occurs in the rectum and lower part of the colon but can affect the entire colon; also called *colitis* or *proctitis*.
vermiform (vēr′ mĭ-form)	verm/i -form	worm shape	Shaped like a worm; *vermiform appendix*

MEDICAL WORD	WORD PARTS		DEFINITION
	Part	Meaning	
volvulus (vŏl´ vū-lŭs)	volvul	to roll	Twisting of the bowel on itself that causes an obstruction. See Figure 8.28 ∎
	-us	pertaining to	

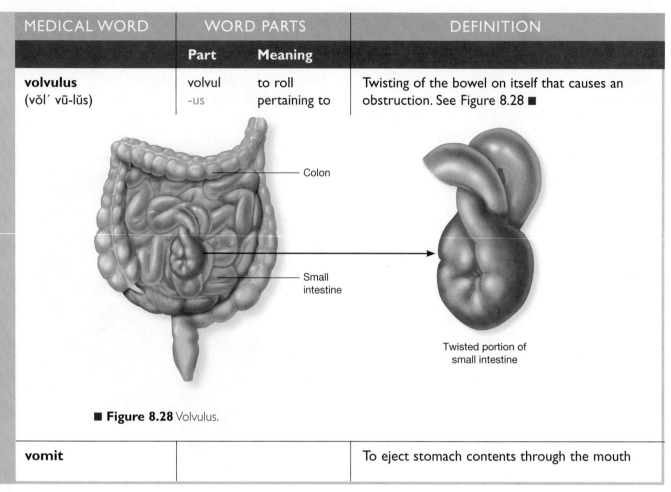

Colon

Small intestine

Twisted portion of small intestine

∎ **Figure 8.28** Volvulus.

vomit			To eject stomach contents through the mouth

• Drug Highlights •

TYPE OF DRUG	DESCRIPTION AND EXAMPLES
antacids	Neutralize hydrochloric acid in the stomach; classified as nonsystemic and systemic.
nonsystemic	EXAMPLES: Amphojel (aluminum hydroxide), Tums (calcium carbonate), Riopan (magaldrate), and Milk of Magnesia (magnesium hydroxide)
systemic	EXAMPLE: sodium bicarbonate
antacid mixtures	Products that combine aluminum (can cause constipation) and/or calcium compounds with magnesium salts (can cause diarrhea). By combining the antacid properties of two single-entity agents, these products provide the antacid action of both yet tend to counter the adverse effects of each other. EXAMPLES: Gaviscon, Gelusil, Maalox Plus, and Mylanta

TYPE OF DRUG	DESCRIPTION AND EXAMPLES
histamine H$_2$-receptor antagonists	Inhibit both daytime and nocturnal basal gastric acid secretion and inhibit gastric acid stimulated by food, histamines, caffeine, insulin, and pentagastrin; used in the treatment of active duodenal ulcer. EXAMPLES: Tagamet (cimetidine), Pepcid (famotidine), Axid (nizatidine), and Zantac (ranitidine)
mucosal protective medications	Medicines that protect the stomach's mucosal lining from acids but do not inhibit the release of acid. EXAMPLES: Carafate (sucralfate) and Cytotec (misoprostol)
gastric acid pump inhibitors (proton-pump inhibitor [PPI])	Antiulcer agents that suppress gastric acid secretion by specific inhibition of the H+/K+ ATPase enzyme at the secretory surface of the gastric parietal cell. Because this enzyme system is regarded as the acid (proton) pump within the gastric mucosa, gastric acid pump inhibitors are so classified because they block the final step of acid production. EXAMPLES: Prilosec (omeprazole), Aciphex (rabeprazole sodium), Prevacid (lansoprazole), and Protonix (pantoprazole)
other ulcer medications	Treatment regimen for active duodenal ulcers associated with *H. pylori* can involve a two- or three-drug program. EXAMPLES: A two-drug program—Biaxin (clarithromycin) and Prilosec (omeprazole); and a three-drug program—Flagyl (metronidazole) and either tetracycline or amoxicillin and Pepto-Bismol *Note: For the treatment to be effective, the patient must complete the full treatment program, which involves taking 15 pills a day for a total of at least 2 weeks.*
laxatives	Used to relieve constipation and to facilitate the passage of feces through the lower gastrointestinal tract. EXAMPLES: Dulcolax (bisacodyl), Milk of Magnesia (magnesium hydroxide), Metamucil (psyllium hydrophilic muciloid), and Ex-Lax (phenolphthalein)
antidiarrheal agents	Used to treat diarrhea. EXAMPLES: Pepto-Bismol (bismuth subsalicylate), Kaopectate (kaolin mixture with pectin), and Imodium (loperamide HCl)

TYPE OF DRUG	DESCRIPTION AND EXAMPLES
antiemetics	Prevent or arrest vomiting; also used in the treatment of vertigo, motion sickness, and nausea. EXAMPLES: Dramamine (dimenhydrinate), Phenergan (promethazine HCl), Tigan (trimethobenzamide HCl), and Transderm Scop (scopolamine)
emetics	Used to induce vomiting in people who have taken an overdose of oral drugs or who have ingested certain poisons. An emetic agent should not be given to a person who is unconscious, in shock, or in a semicomatose state. Emetics are also contraindicated in individuals who have ingested strongly caustic substances, such as lye or acid, because their use could result in additional injury to the person's esophagus. EXAMPLE: Ipecac syrup

• Diagnostic and Lab Tests •

TEST	DESCRIPTION
alcohol toxicology (ethanol and ethyl) (ăl´ kō-hōl tŏks˝ ĭ-kŏl´ ō-jē)	Test performed on blood serum or plasma to determine levels of alcohol. All 50 states and the District of Columbia have laws defining it as a crime to drive with a blood alcohol concentration (BAC) at or above 0.08%. Increased values indicate alcohol consumption that could lead to cirrhosis of the liver, gastritis, malnutrition, vitamin deficiencies, and other gastrointestinal disorders.
ammonia (NH₄) (ă-mō´ nē-ă)	Test performed on blood plasma to determine the level of ammonia (end product of protein breakdown). Increased values can indicate hepatic failure, hepatic encephalopathy, and high protein diet in hepatic failure.
barium enema (BE) (bă´ rē-ŭm ĕn´ ĕ-mă)	Test performed by administering barium (Ba) via the rectum to determine the condition of the colon. X-rays are taken to ascertain the structure and to check the filling of the colon. Abnormal results can indicate cancer of the colon, polyps, fistulas, ulcerative colitis, diverticulitis, hernias, and intus-susception.
bilirubin blood test (total) (bĭl-ĭ-rōō´ bĭn)	Test done on blood serum to determine whether bilirubin is conjugated and excreted in the bile. Abnormal results can indicate obstructive jaundice, hepatitis, and cirrhosis.

TEST	DESCRIPTION
Bravo pH monitor	Test that uses a miniature pH capsule, about the size of a gelcap, which is attached to the wall of the esophagus via an endoscopic procedure. The capsule measures the pH in the esophagus and transmits this information to a receiver worn on the patient's belt or waistband continously for 24–48 hours. The information is uploaded to a computer, which will provide a report for the physician to evaluate. This test is used to diagnose causes of heartburn and provide specific information about gastroesophageal reflux disease (GERD). Several days after the test, the capsule will fall off the wall of the esophagus and pass through the digestive tract and be eliminated via the stool. Bravo is contraindicated in patients with pacemakers, implantable defibrillators, or neurostimulators.
carcinoembryonic antigen (CEA) (kăr″ sĭn-ō-ĕm″ brē-ōn´ ĭk ăn´ tĭ-jĕn)	Test performed on whole blood or plasma to determine the presence of CEA (antigens originally isolated from colon tumors). Increased values can indicate stomach, intestinal, rectal, and various other cancers and conditions. This test is nonspecific and must be combined with other tests for a final diagnosis. It is being used to monitor the course of cancer therapy.
cholangiography (kō-lăn″ jē-ŏg´ ră-fē)	X-ray examination of the common bile duct, cystic duct, and hepatic ducts in which radiopaque dye is injected, and then films are taken. Abnormal results can indicate obstruction, stones, and tumors.
cholecystography (kō″ lē-sĭs-tŏg´ ră-fē)	X-ray examination of the gallbladder in which radiopaque dye is injected, and then films are taken. Abnormal results can indicate cholecystitis, cholelithiasis, and tumors.
colonofiberoscopy (kŏ´ lō-nŏ-fī″ bĕr-ŏs´ kō-pē)	Fiberoptic colonoscopy, a direct visual examination of the colon via a flexible colonoscope; used as a diagnostic aid for removal of foreign bodies, polyps, and tissue. The patient is lightly sedated during the procedure.
colonoscopy (kŏ´ lŏn-ŏs´ kō-pē)	Direct visual examination of the colon via a colonoscope; used to diagnose growths to confirm findings of other tests and to rule out or rule in colon cancer. It can also be used to remove small polyps and to collect tissue samples for analysis. The patient is lightly sedated during the procedure.
endoscopic retrograde cholangiopancreatography (ERCP) (ĕn´ dō-skōp-ĭk rĕt´ rō-grād kō-lăn″ jē-ō-păn″ krē-ă-tŏg´ ră-fē)	X-ray examination of the biliary and pancreatic ducts by injecting a contrast medium, and then films are taken. Abnormal results can indicate fibrosis, biliary or pancreatic cysts, strictures, stones, and chronic pancreatitis.

TEST	DESCRIPTION
esophagogastroduodenal endoscopy (ĕ-sŏf″ ă-gō′ găs″ trō-dū″ ōdē′ năl ĕn-dŏs′kō-pē)	Endoscopic examination of the esophagus, stomach, and small intestine. During the procedure, photographs, biopsy, or brushings may be done.

> **fyi** Upper esophagogastroduodenal endoscopy is considered the reference method of diagnosis of peptic ulcer disease. The diagnosis of *H. pylori* can be made by several methods: The biopsy urease test is a colorimetric test based on the ability of *H. pylori* to produce urease; it provides rapid testing at the time of biopsy. Histological identification of organisms is considered the gold standard of diagnostic tests. Culture of biopsy specimens for *H. pylori*, which requires an experienced laboratory, is necessary when antimicrobial susceptibility testing is desired.

TEST	DESCRIPTION
gamma-glutamyl transferase (GGT) (găm′ ă glōō-tăm′ ĭl trăns′ fĕr-ās)	Test performed on blood serum to determine the level of GGT (enzyme found in the liver, kidney, prostate, heart, and spleen). Increased values can indicate cirrhosis, liver necrosis, hepatitis, alcoholism, neoplasms, acute pancreatitis, acute myocardial infarction, nephrosis, and acute cholecystitis.
gastric analysis (găs′ trĭk ă-năl′ ĭ sĭs)	Test performed to determine quality of secretion, amount of free and combined HCl, and absence or presence of blood, bacteria, bile, and fatty acids. Increased level of HCl can indicate peptic ulcer disease, Zollinger–Ellison syndrome (a condition caused by non-insulin-secreting pancreatic tumors, which secrete excess amounts of gastrin), and hypergastremia. Decreased level of HCl can indicate stomach cancer, pernicious anemia, and atrophic gastritis.
gastrointestinal (GI) series (găs″ trō-ĭn-tes′ tĭn″ ăl)	Fluoroscopic examination of the esophagus, stomach, and small intestine in which barium is given orally and is observed as it flows through the GI system. See Figure 8.29 ■ Abnormal results can indicate esophageal varices, ulcers, gastric polyps, malabsorption syndrome, hiatal hernias, diverticuli, pyloric stenosis, and foreign bodies.

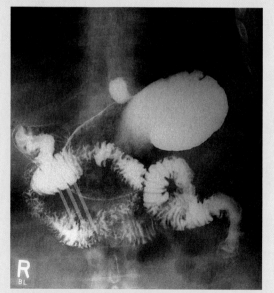

■ **Figure 8.29** Upper GI series.
(Courtesy of Teresa Resch)

TEST	DESCRIPTION
hepatitis-associated antigen (HAA) (hĕp″ ă-tĭ-tĭs ă-sō′ shē-āt′ ĕd ăn′ tĭ-jĕn)	Test performed to determine the presence of the hepatitis B virus.
liver biopsy	Microscopic examination of liver tissue. Abnormal results can indicate cirrhosis, hepatitis, and tumors.
occult blood (ŭ -kŭlt)	Test performed on feces to determine gastrointestinal bleeding that is not visible. Positive results can indicate gastritis, stomach cancer, peptic ulcer, ulcerative colitis, bowel cancer, bleeding esophageal varices, portal hypertension, pancreatitis, and diverticulitis.
ova and parasites (O&P) (o′ vă păr′ ă-sīts)	Test performed on stool to identify ova and parasites. Positive results indicate protozoa infestation.
stool culture	Test performed on stool to identify the presence of organisms.
ultrasonography, gallbladder (ŭl-tră-sŏn-ŏg′ ră-fē)	Test to visualize the gallbladder by using high-frequency sound waves. The echoes are recorded on an oscilloscope and film. See Figure 8.30 ■ Abnormal results can indicate biliary obstruction, cholelithiasis, and acute cholecystitis.

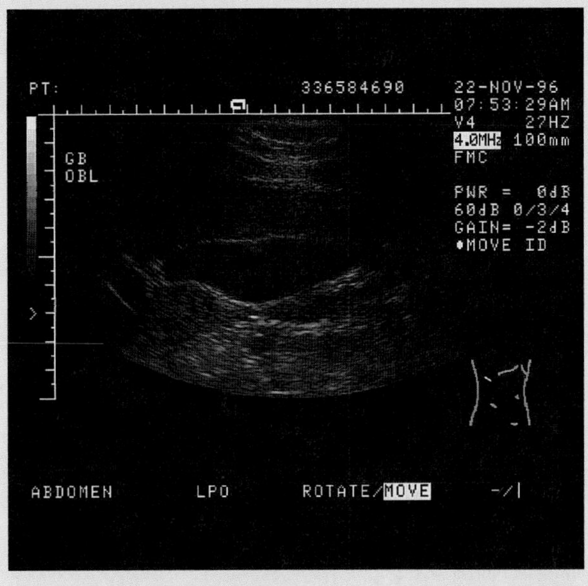

■ **Figure 8.30** Gallbladder ultrasound.
(Courtesy of Teresa Resch)

ultrasonography, liver	Test to visualize the liver by using high-frequency sound waves. The echoes are recorded on an oscilloscope and film. Abnormal results can indicate hepatic tumors, cysts, abscess, and cirrhosis.
upper gastrointestinal fiberoscopy (găs′ trō-ĭn-tĕs′ tĭn″ ăl fĭ′ bĕr-ŏs′ kō-pē)	Direct visual examination of the gastric mucosa via a flexible fiberscope when gastric neoplasm is suspected. Colored photographs or motion pictures can be taken during the procedure.

• Abbreviations •

ABBREVIATION	MEANING	ABBREVIATION	MEANING
ac	before meals (ante cibum)	HBIG	hepatitis B immune globulin
A/G	albumin/globulin (ratio)	HBV	hepatitis B virus
Ba	barium	HCl	hydrochloric acid
BAC	blood alcohol concentration	IBS	irritable bowel syndrome
BE	barium enema	LES	lower esophageal sphincter
BM	bowel movement	MALT	mucosal-associated-lymphoid
BRP	bathroom privileges		type (lymphoma)
BS	bowel sounds	NANBH	non-A, non-B hepatitis virus
CEA	carcinoembryonic antigen	NG	nasogastric (tube)
CHO	carbohydrate	NH$_4$	ammonia
chol	cholesterol	NPO, npo	nothing by mouth
CUC	chronic ulcerative colitis	N&V	nausea and vomiting
E. coli	Escherichia coli	O&P	ova and parasites
ERCP	endoscopic retrograde	pc	after meals (post cibum)
	cholangiopancreatography	PEG	percutaneous endoscopic
GB	gallbladder		gastrostomy
GERD	gastroesophageal reflux disease	PP	postprandial (after meals)
GGT	gamma-glutamyl transferase	PUD	peptic ulcer disease
GI	gastrointestinal	RDA	recommended dietary or daily
GTT	glucose tolerance test		allowance
HAA	hepatitis-associated antigen	TPN	total parenteral nutrition
HAV	hepatitis A virus	UGI	upper gastrointestinal

ly and Review • Study and Review • Study and Revie
Review • Study and Review • Study and Review • St
ew • **Study and Review** • Study and Review • Study

Anatomy and Physiology

Write your answers to the following questions.

1. Name the primary organs commonly associated with digestion.

a. _____   b. _____

c. _____   d. _____

e. _____   f. _____

2. Name four accessory organs of digestion.

a. _____   b. _____

c. _____   d. _____

3. State the three main functions of the digestive system.

a. _____

b. _____

c. _____

4. Define *bolus*. _____

_____

5. Define *peristalsis*. _____

_____

6. _____ and _____ convert the food into a semiliquid state.

7. The _____ is the first portion of the small intestine.

8. Semiliquid food is called _____ .

9. The _____ transports nutrients to body cells.

10. The large intestine can be divided into four distinct sections called the _____ ,

the _____ , the _____ , and the _____ .

11. The _____ is the largest glandular organ in the body.

249

12. State the function of the gallbladder. _____

13. Name an important function of the pancreas. _____

14. State three functions of the liver.

    a. _____   **b.** _____

    c. _____

15. Where does digestion and absorption chiefly take place? _____

16. The salivary glands located in and about the mouth are called the _____ ,

the _____ , and the _____ .

17. Name the two hormones secreted into the bloodstream by the pancreas.

    a. _____   **b.** _____

Word Parts

PREFIXES

Give the definitions of the following prefixes.

1. an- _____   **2.** dys- _____

3. epi- _____   **4.** hyper- _____

5. hypo- _____   **6.** mal- _____

7. peri- _____   **8.** post- _____

9. dia- _____   **10.** sub- _____

ROOTS AND COMBINING FORMS

Give the definitions of the following roots and combining forms.

1. absorpt _____   **2.** aden _____

3. amyl _____   **4.** anabol _____

5. catabol _____   **6.** cirrh _____

7. append _____   **8.** appendic _____

9. bil/i _____   **10.** bucc _____

11. celi _____   **12.** cheil _____

13. chol/e _____   **14.** choledoch/o _____

15. col _____

16. col/o _____

17. colon _____

18. colon/o _____

19. cyst _____

20. dent _____

21. constipat _____

22. diverticul _____

23. duoden _____

24. enter _____

25. defecat _____

26. esophage/o _____

27. gastr _____

28. gastr/o _____

29. gingiv _____

30. gloss/o _____

31. glyc/o _____

32. hemat _____

33. hepat _____

34. hepat/o _____

35. herni/o _____

36. ile _____

37. ile/o _____

38. labi _____

39. lapar/o _____

40. laxat _____

41. lingu _____

42. lip/o _____

43. log _____

44. mes _____

45. pancreat _____

46. pept _____

47. pharyng/e _____

48. prand/i _____

49. eme _____

50. proct/o _____

51. pylor _____

52. rect/o _____

53. sial _____

54. sigmoid/o _____

55. splen/o _____

56. stomat _____

57. tox _____

58. eructat _____

59. verm/i _____

60. halit _____

61. hemorrh _____

62. alimentat _____

63. masticat _____

64. paralyt _____

65. pil/o _____

66. nid _____

67. volvul _____

68. odont _____

SUFFIXES

Give the definitions of the following suffixes.

1. -ac _____

2. -al _____

3. -algia _____

4. -ary _____

5. -ase _____

6. -cele _____

7. -oid _____

8. -sis _____

9. -ectomy _____

10. -emesis _____

11. -form _____

12. -genesis _____

13. -ic _____

14. -in _____

15. -ion _____

16. -ism _____

17. -ist _____

18. -itis _____

19. -ive _____

20. -logy _____

21. -lysis _____

22. -megaly _____

23. -oma _____

24. -orexia _____

25. -osis _____

26. -rrhea _____

27. -pepsia _____

28. -us _____

29. -phagia _____

30. -scope _____

31. -scopy _____

32. -stalsis _____

33. -stomy _____

34. -tomy _____

35. -y _____

36. -rrhaphy _____

Identifying Medical Terms

In the spaces provided, write the medical terms for the following meanings.

1. _____ Enzyme that breaks down starch

2. _____ Building up of the body substance in the constructive phase of metabolism

3. _____ Lack of appetite

4. _____ Surgical excision of the appendix

5. _____ Inflammation of the appendix

6. _____ Pertaining to bile and the gallbladder

7. _____ Pertaining to the abdomen

8. _____ Difficulty in swallowing

9. _____ Inflammation of the liver

10. _____ Surgical repair of a hernia

11. _____ Pertaining to after meals

12. _____ Enlargement of the spleen

13. _____ An instrument used in a medical procedure to view the interior of the sigmoid colon

Spelling

Circle the correct spelling of each medical term.

1. bilery / biliary
2. colonoscopy / colonscopy
3. degulition / deglutition
4. gastroenterology / gastorentreology
5. halitosis / haltosis
6. laxative / laxtive
7. peritalsis / peristalsis
8. salad[e]mitis / sialadenitis
9. periodontal / perodontal
10. vermform / vermiform

Matching

Select the appropriate lettered meaning for each of the following words.

_____ **1.** cirrhosis

_____ **2.** constipation

_____ **3.** diarrhea

_____ **4.** gavage

_____ **5.** hemorrhoid

_____ **6.** hernia

_____ **7.** hyperalimentation

_____ **8.** lavage

_____ **9.** pilonidal cyst

_____ **10.** volvulus

a. To wash out a cavity

b. To feed liquid or semiliquid food via a tube

c. Twisting of the bowel on itself that causes an obstruction

d. Frequent passage of unformed watery stools

e. Chronic degenerative liver disease

f. Infrequent passage of unduly hard and dry feces

g. Closed sac in the crease of the sacrococcygeal region

h. Abnormal protrusion of an organ or a part of an organ through the wall of the body cavity that normally contains it

i. Mass of dilated, tortuous veins in the anorectum

j. Intravenous infusion of a hypertonic solution to sustain life

k. Evacuation of the bowel

Abbreviations

Place the correct word, phrase, or abbreviation in the space provided.

1. before meals _____

2. BM _____

3. BS _____

4. chol _____

5. gallbladder _____

6. hepatitis A virus _____

7. NG _____

8. NPO, npo _____

9. after meals _____

10. total parenteral nutrition _____

Diagnostic and Laboratory Tests

Select the best answer to each multiple-choice question. Circle the letter of your choice.

1. X-ray examination of the common bile duct, cystic duct, and hepatic ducts.
   a. cholangiography
   b. cholecystography
   c. cholangiopancreatography
   d. ultrasonography

2. Direct visual examination of the colon via a flexible colonoscope.
   a. cholangiography
   b. ultrasonography
   c. colonofiberoscopy
   d. cholecystography

3. Fluoroscopic examination of the esophagus, stomach, and small intestine.
   a. barium enema
   b. ultrasonography
   c. cholangiography
   d. gastrointestinal series

4. Endoscopic examination of the esophagus, stomach, and small intestine.
   a. cholangiography
   b. gastroduodenoesophagoscopy
   c. esophagogastroduodenoscopy
   d. gastric analysis

5. Test performed to determine the presence of the hepatitis B virus.
   a. occult blood test
   b. stool culture
   c. hepatic antigen
   d. ova and parasites test

PRACTICAL APPLICATION

MEDICAL RECORD ANALYSIS

The Patient Referral Form is an important part of a patient's chart. As part of your learning process and in preparation for a career in a medical environment, you are to assume the role of a medical employee and use the following information—together with your own input—to complete the Patient Referral Form.

Patient referred to Seymour Butts, MD, Endoscopy Center, 14 Maddox Drive, Rome, GA 30165, phone number (706) 235-3957, fax (706) 235-8877, for a screening colonoscopy on October 17, 2011, at 8:45 A.M. Advise patient to bring a driver, all current medications, driver's license, and proof of insurance.

Referring physician, Angel De'Crohn, MD, Family Practice, 1165 Berry Blvd, Rome, GA 30165, (706) 235-7765, fax (706) 235-6676.

PATIENT REFERRAL FORM

Our practice is affiliated with Mercy Medical Center

Please refer this patient to Mercy Medical Center for any needed surgery or diagnostic procedures so that we can better coordinate this patient's care.

Date: 09/28/11

Patient Name: Ralph J. Starr   DOB: 2/24/43   Phone Number 123-456-7890

Appointment Date: _____   Time: _____

Referred to: _____

_____

For:

_____ Diagnostic Procedure _____

_____ Consultation

_____ Evaluate and treat, initiating appropriate diagnostic
and/or therapeutic services

_____ Report test results to: _____

Reason for referral: _____

Patient Instructions: _____

_____

_____

Referring Physician's Name: _____ Date: _____

Phone #: _____ Fax #: _____

Remit the Record of this Patient's Visit to the Physician Noted Above.

For Office Use Only (appointment made at a time when the patient was not present)

Patient notified of appointment: Date: _____ Initials: _____

Unable to contact patient

Attempts to notify: Date/Time/Initials

1. _____

2. _____

3. _____

Comments: _____

Certified Letter Sent: Date: _____ Initials: _____

Referral Form Questions

Place the correct answer in the space provided.

1. Write in the Appointment Date: _____ and Time: _____

2. The patient was referred to: write in name of physician, center name, and address:

_____

_____

_____

_____

3. The patient was referred for:

_____ Diagnostic Procedure

_____ Screening Colonoscopy

_____ Consultation

_____ Evaluate and treat, initiating appropriate diagnostic and/or therapeutic services

_____ Report test results to: Angel De'Crohn, MD

4. The Patient Instructions were: _____

5. Write in the name of:

Referring Physician: _____

Date: _____

Phone #: _____

Fax #: _____

PEARSON
mymedicalterminologylab

MyMedicalTerminologyLab is a premium online homework management system that includes a host of features to help you study. Registered users will find:

- Fun games and activities built within a virtual hospital
- Powerful tools that track and analyze your results—allowing you to create a personalized learning experience
- Videos, flashcards, and audio pronunciations to help enrich your progress
- Streaming lesson presentations and self-paced learning modules
- A space where you and your instructors can view and manage your assignments

stem • Oncology • Radiology and Nuclear Medicine •
ntal Health • Introduction to Medical Terminology • Suf
• Prefixes • Organization of the Body • Integu ntar
tem • Skeletal System • Muscular System • Di stive S

m • **Cardiovascular System** • Blood and Lymphatic

9

LEARNING OUTCOMES

On completion of this chapter, you will be able to:

1. State the description and primary functions of the organs/structures of the cardiovascular system.

2. Explain the circulation of blood through the chambers of the heart.

3. Identify and locate the commonly used sites for taking a pulse.

4. Explain blood pressure.

5. Analyze, build, spell, and pronounce medical words.

6. Comprehend the drugs highlighted in this chapter.

7. Describe diagnostic and laboratory tests related to the cardiovascular system.

8. Identify and define selected abbreviations.

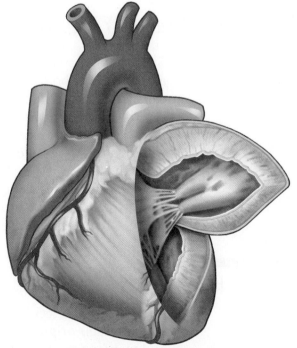

COMBINING FORMS OF THE CARDIOVASCULAR SYSTEM

ang/i	vessel	lun/o	moon
angi/o	vessel	man/o	thin
angin/o	to choke	mitr/o	mitral valve
arter/i	artery	my/o	muscle
arteri/o	artery	occlus/o	to close up
ather/o	fatty substance, porridge	ox/i	oxygen
atri/o	atrium	palpit/o	throbbing
auscultat/o	listen to	pector/o	chest
card/i	heart	phleb/o	vein
cardi/o	heart	phon/o	sound
chol/e	bile	pulmonar/o	lung
circulat/o	circular	rrhythm/o	rhythm
claudicat/o	to limp	scler/o	hardening
corpor/e	body	sept/o	a partition
cyan/o	dark blue	sin/o	a curve
dilat/o	to widen	sphygm/o	pulse
dynam/o	power	sten/o	narrowing
ech/o	reflected sound	steth/o	chest
electr/o	electricity	thromb/o	clot of blood
embol/o	a throwing in	valvul/o	valve
glyc/o	sweet, sugar	vas/o	vessel
hem/o	blood	vascul/o	small vessel
infarct/o	infarct (necrosis of an area)	ven/i	vein
isch/o	to hold back	ventricul/o	ventricle
lipid/o	fat	vers/o	turning

Anatomy and Physiology

The cardiovascular system, also called the *circulatory system,* circulates blood to all parts of the body by the action of the heart. This process provides the body's cells with oxygen and nutritive elements and removes waste materials and carbon dioxide. The heart, a muscular pump, is the central organ of the system. Arteries, veins, and capillaries comprise the network of vessels that transport blood (fluid consisting of blood cells and plasma) throughout the body. Blood flows through the heart, to the lungs, back to the heart, and on to the various body parts. Table 9.1 ■ provides an at-a-glance look at the cardiovascular system. Figure 9.1 ■ shows a schematic overview of the cardiovascular system.

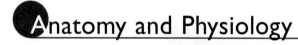

HEART

The **heart** is the center of the cardiovascular system from which the various blood vessels originate and later return. It is slightly larger than a person's fist and weighs approximately 300 g in the average adult. It lies slightly to the left

TABLE 9.1 Cardiovascular System at-a-Glance

Organ/Structure	Primary Functions/Description
Heart	The muscular pump that circulates blood through the heart, the lungs (pulmonary circulation), and the rest of the body (systemic circulation)
Arteries	Branching system of vessels that transports blood from the right and left ventricles of the heart to all body parts; transports blood away from the heart
Veins	Vessels that transport blood from peripheral tissues back to the heart
Capillaries	Microscopic blood vessels that connect arterioles with venules; facilitate passage of life-sustaining fluids containing oxygen and nutrients to cell bodies and the removal of accumulated waste and carbon dioxide
Blood	Fluid consisting of formed elements (erythrocytes, thrombocytes, leukocytes) and plasma. It is a specialized bodily fluid that delivers necessary substances to the body's cells (oxygen, foods, salts, hormones) and transports waste products (carbon dioxide, urea, lactic acid) away from those same cells. Blood is circulated around the body through blood vessels by the pumping action of the heart. See Chapter 10, "Blood and Lymphatic System," for a further discussion of blood.

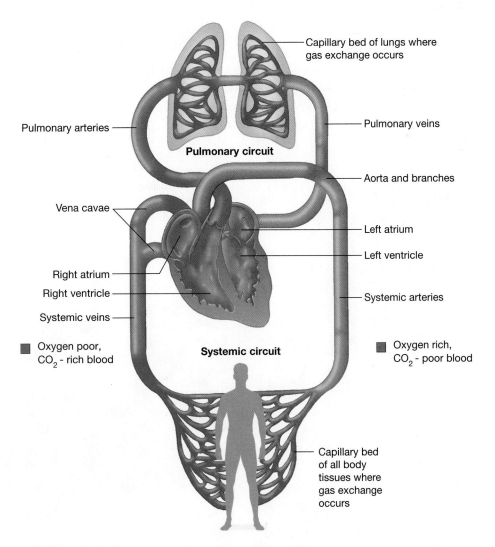

■ **Figure 9.1** Schematic overview of the cardiovascular system.

of the midline of the body, beneath the sternum, and is shaped like an inverted cone with its apex downward (see Figure 9.2 ■). The heart has three layers or linings (see Figure 9.3 ■).

- **Endocardium.** The inner lining of the heart.
- **Myocardium.** The muscular middle layer of the heart.
- **Pericardium.** The outer membranous sac surrounding the heart.

Circulation of Blood through the Chambers of the Heart

The heart is a pump and is divided into the right and left heart by a partition called the **septum**. Each side contains an upper and lower chamber. See Figure 9.4 ■ The **atria**, or upper chambers, are separated by the interatrial septum. The **ventricles**, or lower chambers, are separated by the interventricular septum. The atria receive blood from the various parts of the body. The ventricles pump blood to body parts. Valves control the intake and outflow of blood in the heart chambers. Figure 9.5 ■ shows the functioning of the heart valves and flow of blood through the heart.

Right Atrium

The right upper portion of the heart is called the **right atrium (RA)**. It is a thin-walled space that receives blood from the upper and lower parts of the body (except the lungs). Two large veins, the superior vena cava and inferior vena cava,

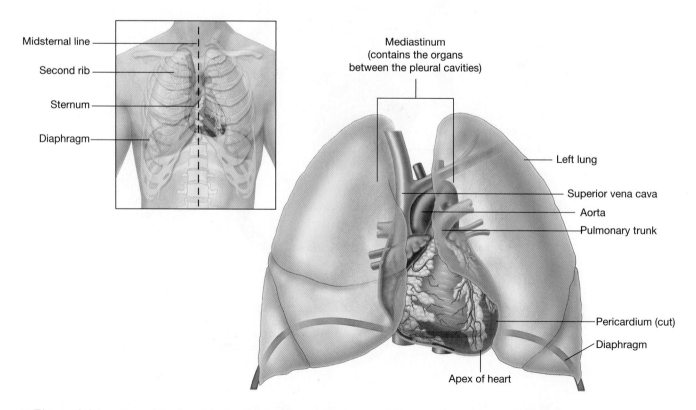

■ **Figure 9.2** Location of the heart in the chest cavity.

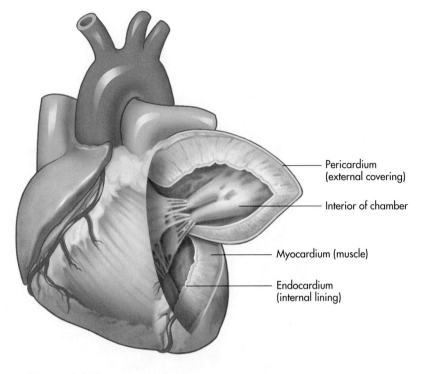

Pericardium (external covering)

Interior of chamber

Myocardium (muscle)

Endocardium (internal lining)

■ **Figure 9.3** Tissues of the heart.

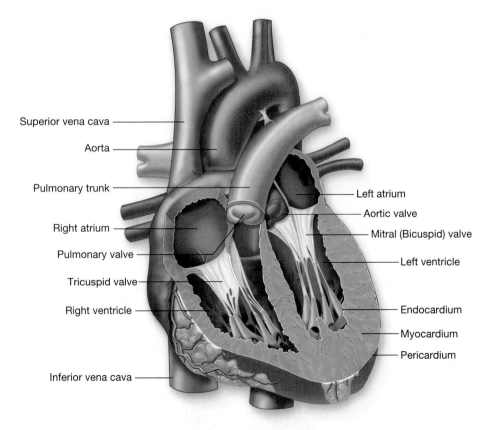

Superior vena cava

Aorta

Pulmonary trunk

Right atrium

Pulmonary valve

Tricuspid valve

Right ventricle

Inferior vena cava

Left atrium

Aortic valve

Mitral (Bicuspid) valve

Left ventricle

Endocardium

Myocardium

Pericardium

■ **Figure 9.4** Interior view of the heart chambers.

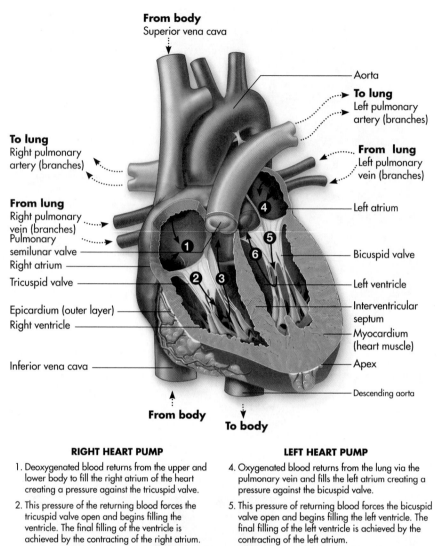

From body
Superior vena cava

Aorta

To lung
Left pulmonary
artery (branches)

To lung
Right pulmonary
artery (branches)

From lung
Left pulmonary
vein (branches)

From lung
Right pulmonary
vein (branches)
Pulmonary
semilunar valve

Left atrium

Right atrium

Bicuspid valve

Tricuspid valve

Left ventricle

Epicardium (outer layer)
Right ventricle

Interventricular
septum

Myocardium
(heart muscle)

Inferior vena cava

Apex

Descending aorta

From body

To body

RIGHT HEART PUMP

1. Deoxygenated blood returns from the upper and lower body to fill the right atrium of the heart creating a pressure against the tricuspid valve.

2. This pressure of the returning blood forces the tricuspid valve open and begins filling the ventricle. The final filling of the ventricle is achieved by the contracting of the right atrium.

3. The right ventricle contracts increasing the internal pressure. This pressure closes the tricuspid valve and forces open the pulmonary semilunar valve thus sending blood toward the lung via the pulmonary artery. This blood will become oxygenated as it travels through the capillary beds of the lung and then return to the left side of the heart.

LEFT HEART PUMP

4. Oxygenated blood returns from the lung via the pulmonary vein and fills the left atrium creating a pressure against the bicuspid valve.

5. This pressure of returning blood forces the bicuspid valve open and begins filling the left ventricle. The final filling of the left ventricle is achieved by the contracting of the left atrium.

6. The left ventricle contracts increasing internal pressure. This pressure closes the bicuspid valve and forces open the aortic valve causing oxygenated blood to flow through the aorta to deliver oxygen throughout the body.

■ **Figure 9.5** The functioning of the heart valves and blood flow.

bring deoxygenated blood into the right atrium. Deoxygeneated blood fills the right atrium before passing through the tricuspid (atrioventricular) valve and into the right ventricle.

Right Ventricle

The right lower portion of the heart is called the **right ventricle (RV)**. It receives blood from the right atrium through the tricuspid valve. When filled, the RV contracts. This creates pressure closing the RA and forcing open the pulmonary (semilunar) valve, sending blood into the left and right pulmonary arteries, which carry it to the lungs. The pulmonary artery is the only artery in the body that carries blood deficient in oxygen. In the lungs, the blood gives up wastes and takes on oxygen as it passes through capillary beds into veins. Oxygenated blood leaves the lungs through the left and right pulmonary veins, which carry it to the heart's left atrium. The pulmonary veins are the only veins in the body that carry oxygen-rich (oxygenated) blood. The circulation of blood through the vessels from the heart to the lungs and then back to the heart again is the pulmonary circulation.

Left Atrium

The left upper portion of the heart is called the **left atrium (LA)**. It receives blood rich in oxygen as it returns from the lungs via the left and right pulmonary veins. As oxygenated blood fills the LA, it creates pressure that forces open the biscuid (mitral) valve and allows the blood to fill the left ventricle.

Left Ventricle

The left lower portion of the heart is called the **left ventricle (LV)**. It receives blood from the left atrium through the biscuid (mitral) valve. When filled, the LV contracts. This creates pressure closing the bicuspid valve and forcing open the aortic valve. The oxygenated blood from the LV flows through the aortic valve and into a large artery known as the **aorta** and from there to all parts of the body (except the lungs) via a branching system of arteries and capillaries.

LIFE SPAN CONSIDERATIONS

Pediatric cardiologists have recognized more than 50 congenital heart defects. If the left side of the heart is not completely separated from the right side, various septal defects develop. If the four chambers of the heart do not occur normally, complex anomalies form, such as tetralogy of Fallot (TOF), a congenital heart condition involving four defects: pulmonary stenosis, ventricular septal defect (VSD), dextroposition of the aorta, and hypertrophy of the right ventricle.

Heart Valves

The **valves** of the heart are located at the entrance and exit of each ventricle and, as you learned in the preceding section, control the flow of blood within the heart. See Figure 9.6 ■

Tricuspid Valve

The **tricuspid** or **right atrioventricular valve** guards the opening between the right atrium and the right ventricle. In a normal state, the tricuspid valve opens to allow the flow of blood into the ventricle and then closes to prevent any backflow of blood.

Pulmonary (*Semilunar*) Valve

The exit point for blood leaving the right ventricle is called the **pulmonary (semilunar) valve**. Located between the right ventricle and the pulmonary artery,

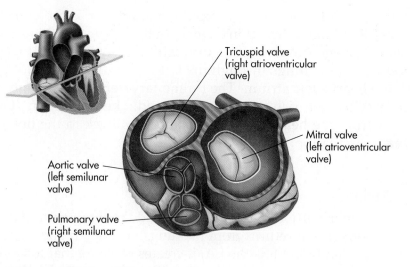

Tricuspid valve
(right atrioventricular
valve)

Mitral valve
(left atrioventricular
valve)

Aortic valve
(left semilunar
valve)

Pulmonary valve
(right semilunar
valve)

■ **Figure 9.6** Valves of the heart.

it allows blood to flow from the right ventricle through the pulmonary artery to the lungs.

Bicuspid or Mitral Valve

The left atrioventricular valve between the left atrium and ventricle is called the **bicuspid** or **mitral valve** (MV). It allows blood to flow to the left ventricle and closes to prevent its return to the left atrium.

Aortic (Semilunar) Valve

Blood exits from the left ventricle through the **aortic (semilunar) valve**. Located between the left ventricle and the aorta, it allows blood to flow into the aorta and prevents its backflow to the ventricle.

Vascular System of the Heart

Due to the membranous lining of the heart (endocardium) and the thickness of the myocardium, the heart has its own vascular system to meet its high oxygen demand. The coronary arteries supply the heart with oxygen-rich blood, and the cardiac veins, draining into the coronary sinus, collect the blood (oxygen poor) and return it to the right atrium (see Figure 9.7 ■).

Conduction System of the Heart

The autonomic nervous system controls the rate and rhythm of the **heartbeat**. It normally is generated by specialized neuromuscular tissue of the heart that is capable of causing cardiac muscle to contract rhythmically. This tissue of the heart comprises the **sinoatrial node**, the **atrioventricular node**, and the **atrioventricular bundle** (see Figure 9.8 ■).

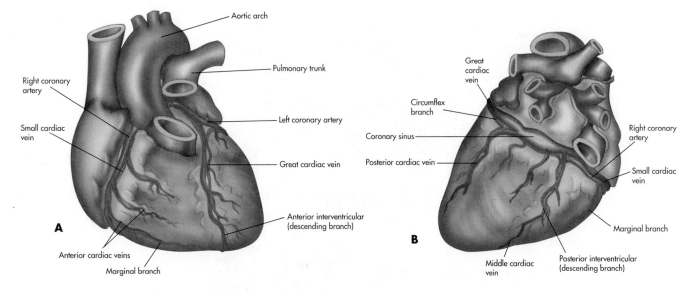

■ Figure 9.7 Coronary circulation. (A) Coronary vessels portraying the complexity and extent of the coronary circulation. (B) Coronary vessels that supply the anterior surface of the heart.

Sinoatrial Node (SA Node)

Called the *pacemaker* of the heart, the **SA node** is located in the upper wall of the right atrium, just below the opening of the superior vena cava. It consists of a dense network of **Purkinje fibers** (*atypical muscle fibers*) considered to be the source of impulses initiating the heartbeat. Electrical impulses discharged by the SA node are distributed to the right and left atria and cause them to contract.

Atrioventricular Node (AV Node)

Located beneath the endocardium of the right atrium, the **AV node** transmits electrical impulses to the bundle of His (*atrioventricular bundle*).

Atrioventricular Bundle (Bundle of His)

The **bundle of His** forms a part of the conduction system of the heart. It is a collection of heart muscle cells specialized for electrical conduction that transmits the electrical impulses from the AV node to the point of the apex of the fascicular branches. The bundle of His branches into the three bundle branches that run along the interventricular septum. The bundles give rise to thin filaments known as Purkinje fibers. These fibers distribute the impulse to the ventricular muscle. Together, the bundle branches and **Purkinje network** comprise the ventricular conduction system.

The average adult heartbeat (*pulse*) is between 60 and 90 beats per minute. The rate of the heartbeat can be affected by emotions, smoking, disease, body size, age, stress, the environment, and many other factors.

The heart's electrical activity can be recorded by an **electrocardiogram (ECG, EKG)**, which provides valuable information in diagnosing cardiac abnormalities,

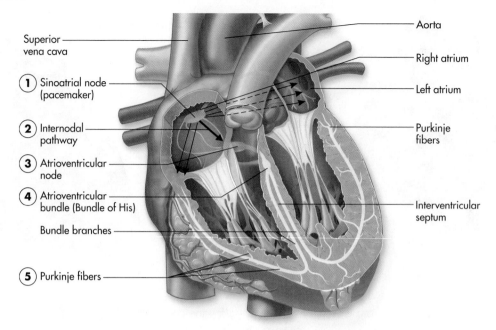

Superior vena cava

Aorta

Right atrium

Left atrium

(1) Sinoatrial node (pacemaker)

(2) Internodal pathway

(3) Atrioventricular node

(4) Atrioventricular bundle (Bundle of His)

Bundle branches

(5) Purkinje fibers

Purkinje fibers

Interventricular septum

1. The sinoatrial (SA) node fires a stimulus across the walls of both left and right atria causing them to contract.

2. The stimulus arrives at the atrioventricular (AV) node.

3. The stimulus is directed to follow the AV bundle (Bundle of His).

4. The stimulus now travels through the apex of the heart through the bundle branches.

5. The Purkinje fibers distribute the stimulus across both ventricles causing ventricular contraction.

■ **Figure 9.8** Conduction system of the heart.

such as myocardial damage and arrhythmias (see Diagnostic and Lab Tests and Figure 9.39 on page 302).

BLOOD VESSELS

There are three main types of blood vessels: arteries, veins, and capillaries. Blood circulates throughout the body through their pathways.

Arteries

The **arteries** constitute a branching system of vessels that transports blood away from the heart to all body parts (see Figure 9.9 ■). In a normal state, arteries are elastic tubes that recoil and carry blood in pulsating waves. All arteries have a pulse, reflecting the rhythmical beating of the heart; however, certain points are commonly used to check the rate, rhythm, and condition of the arterial wall.

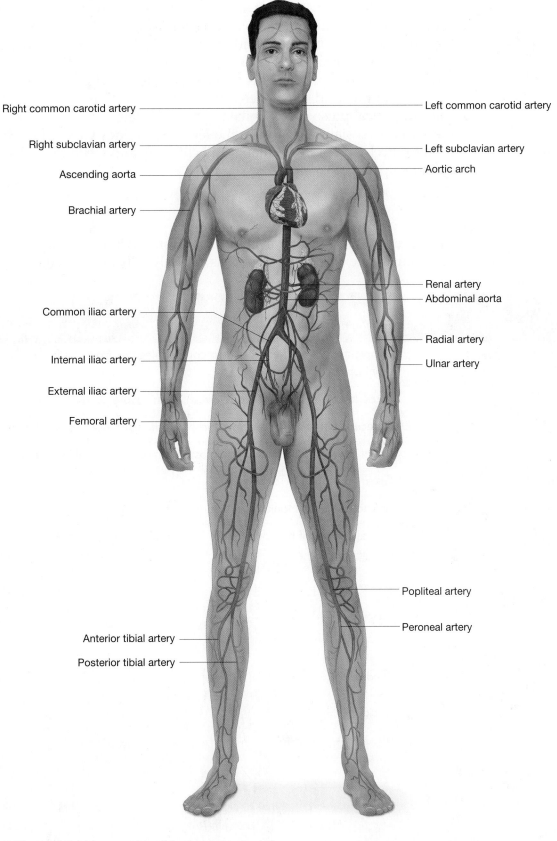

Right common carotid artery

Right subclavian artery

Ascending aorta

Brachial artery

Left common carotid artery

Left subclavian artery

Aortic arch

Renal artery

Abdominal aorta

Common iliac artery

Internal iliac artery

External iliac artery

Femoral artery

Radial artery

Ulnar artery

Popliteal artery

Peroneal artery

Anterior tibial artery

Posterior tibial artery

■ **Figure 9.9** Major arteries of the systemic circulation.

A person's pulse can be felt in a place that allows for an artery to be compressed against a bone. The most commonly used sites for taking a pulse are the radial artery, the brachial artery, and the carotid artery. See Table 9.2 ■ and Figure 9.10 ■ The pulse rate can also be measured by using a stethoscope (*auscultation*) and counting the heartbeat for 1 full minute. This is known as the **apical pulse** and is not taken over an artery, but instead, it is taken over the heart itself. In contrast with other pulse sites, the apical pulse site is unilateral and is located at the apex of the heart or at the fifth intercostal space, just to the left of the midclavicular line. It is commonly used to check pulse rate in infants and children, and when the radial pulse is difficult to palpate (*feel*).

Veins

Veins are the vessels that transport blood from peripheral tissues back to the heart. In a normal state, veins have thin walls and valves that prevent the backflow of blood.

TABLE 9.2 Pulse Checkpoints

Checkpoint	Site/Use
Temporal	Temple area of the head. Used to control bleeding from the head and scalp and to monitor circulation.
Carotid	Neck. In an emergency (*cardiac arrest*), most readily accessible site.
Brachial	Antecubital space of the elbow. Most common site used to check blood pressure.
Radial	Radial (*thumb side*) of the wrist. Most common site for taking a pulse.
Femoral	Groin area. Monitor circulation.
Popliteal	Behind the knee. Monitor circulation.
Dorsalis pedis	Dorsal surface of the foot. Assess peripheral artery disease (PAD).

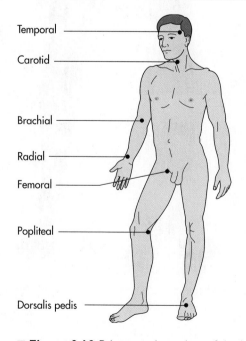

■ **Figure 9.10** Primary pulse points of the body.

The great saphenous vein is the most important superficial vein of the lower limb. The pulmonary veins carry oxygenated blood from the lungs to the heart. The superior and inferior venae cavae carry deoxygenated blood from the upper and lower systemic circulation. See Figure 9.11 ■

Capillaries

The **capillaries** are microscopic blood vessels with single-celled walls that connect **arterioles** (*small arteries*) with **venules** (*small veins*). See Figure 9.12 ■ Blood passing through capillaries gives up the oxygen and nutrients carried to this point by the arteries and picks up waste and carbon dioxide as it enters veins. Veins lead away from the capillaries as tiny vessels and increase in size until they join the superior and inferior vena cavae as they return to the heart. The extremely thin walls of capillaries facilitate passage of oxygen and nutrients to cell bodies and the removal of accumulated waste and carbon dioxide.

Blood Pressure

Blood pressure (BP) is the pressure exerted by the blood on the walls of the arteries. It results from two forces. One is created by the heart as it pumps blood into the arteries and through the circulatory system. The other is the force of the arteries as they resist the blood flow. The higher (systolic) number represents the pressure while the heart contracts to pump blood to the body. The lower (diastolic) number represents the pressure when the heart relaxes between beats. Blood pressure is reported in millimeters of mercury (mmHg) and is measured with a **sphygmomanometer** in concert with a **stethoscope**. See Figure 9.13 ■

The systolic pressure is always stated first. For example, 116/74 (116 over 74); systolic = 116, diastolic = 74. Blood pressure below 120 over 80 mmHg is considered optimal for adults. A systolic pressure of 120–139 mmHg or a diastolic pressure of 80–89 mmHg is considered to be *prehypertension* and needs to be monitored on a regular basis. A blood pressure reading of 140 over 90 or higher is considered elevated (hypertension).

LIFE SPAN CONSIDERATIONS

The **pulse (P)**, **blood pressure (BP)**, and **respiration (R)** vary according to a child's age. A newborn's pulse rate is irregular and rapid, varying from 120 to 140 beats/minute. Blood pressure is low and can vary with the size of the cuff used. The average blood pressure at birth is 80/46. The respirations are approximately 35–50 per minute.

Pulse Pressure

The **pulse pressure** is the difference between the systolic and diastolic readings. This reading indicates the tone of the arterial walls. The normal pulse pressure is found when the systolic pressure is about 40 points higher than the diastolic reading. For example, if the blood pressure is 120/80, the pulse pressure would be 40. A pulse pressure over 50 points or under 30 points is considered abnormal.

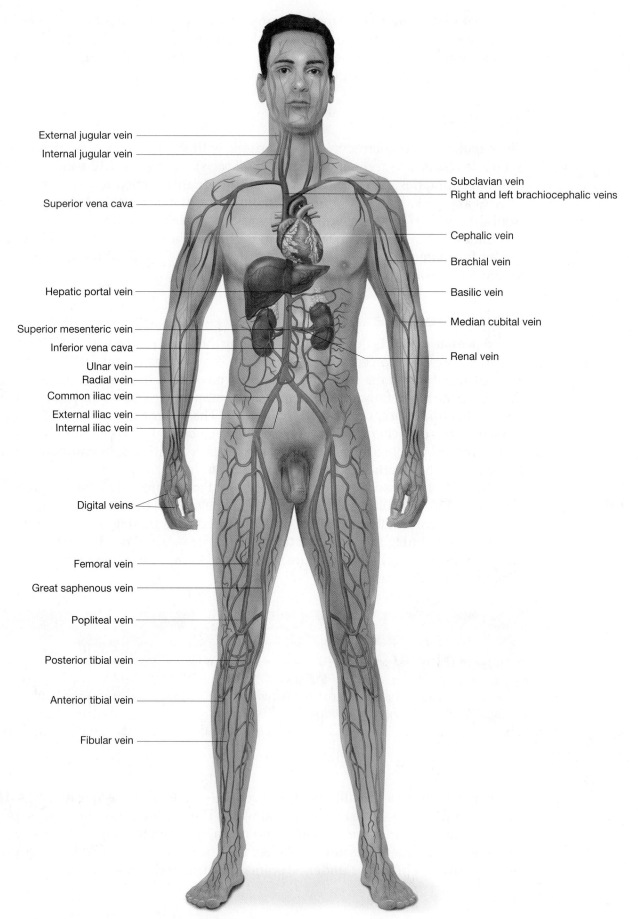

External jugular vein

Internal jugular vein

Superior vena cava

Hepatic portal vein

Superior mesenteric vein

Inferior vena cava

Ulnar vein

Radial vein

Common iliac vein

External iliac vein

Internal iliac vein

Digital veins

Femoral vein

Great saphenous vein

Popliteal vein

Posterior tibial vein

Anterior tibial vein

Fibular vein

Subclavian vein

Right and left brachiocephalic veins

Cephalic vein

Brachial vein

Basilic vein

Median cubital vein

Renal vein

■ **Figure 9.11** Major veins of the systemic circulation.

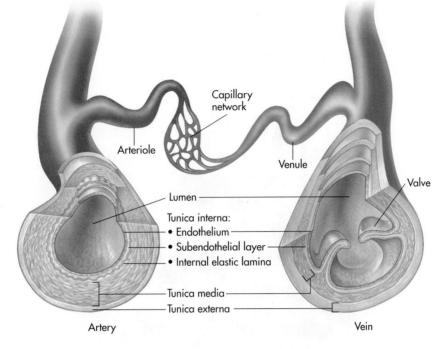

■ **Figure 9.12** Capillaries.

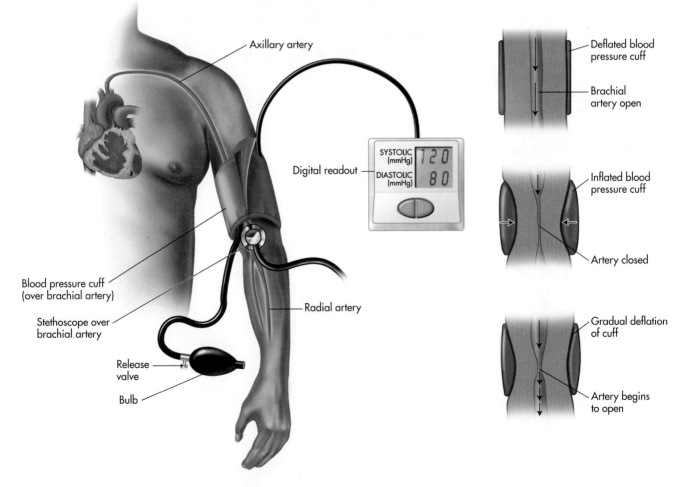

■ **Figure 9.13** Blood pressure measurement.

Anatomy and Physiology Labeling

Identify the structures shown below by filling in the blanks.

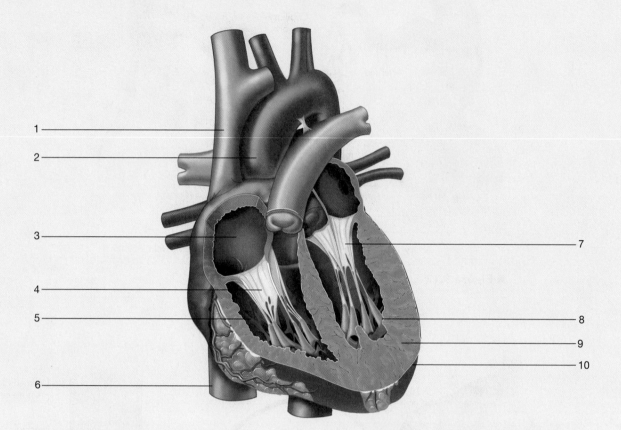

1 _____

2 _____

3 _____

4 _____

5 _____

6 _____

7 _____

8 _____

9 _____

10 _____

• Building Your Medical Vocabulary •

This section provides the foundation for learning medical terminology. Review the following alphabetized word list. Note how common prefixes and suffixes are repeatedly applied to word roots and combining forms to create different meanings. The word parts are color-coded: prefixes are green, suffixes are blue, roots/combining forms are red.

You will find that some terms have not been divided into word parts. These are common words or specialized terms that are included to enhance your medical vocabulary. See Chapter 1, page 7, to review pronunciation guidelines.

MEDICAL WORD	WORD PARTS		DEFINITION
	Part	**Meaning**	
anastomosis (ă-năs″tō-mō′sĭs)	anastom -osis	opening condition	Surgical connection between blood vessels or the joining of one hollow or tubular organ to another
aneurysm (ăn′ ū-rĭzm)			Abnormal widening or ballooning of a portion of an artery due to weakness in the wall of the blood vessel. See Figure 9.14 ■

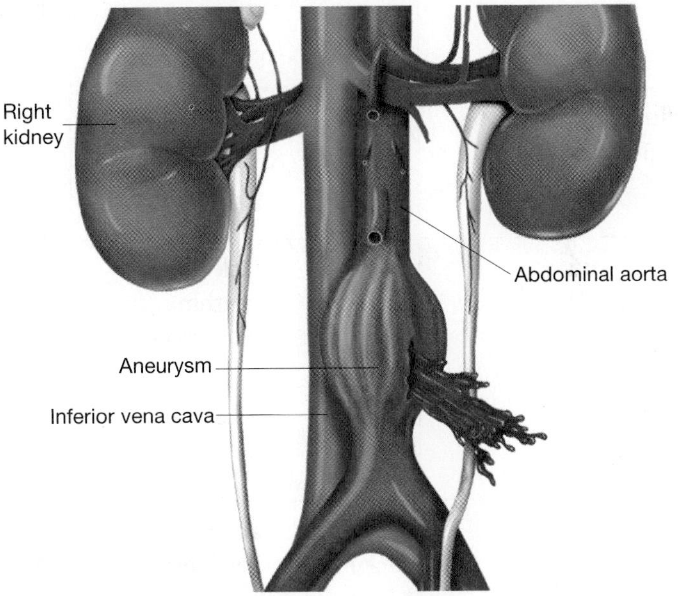

Right kidney

Abdominal aorta

Aneurysm

Inferior vena cava

■ **Figure 9.14** Ruptured abdominal aortic aneurysm.

MEDICAL WORD	WORD PARTS		DEFINITION
angina pectoris (ăn′ jĭ-nă pĕk′ tōr″ĭs)	angin (a) pector -is	to choke chest pertaining to	Chest pain that occurs when diseased blood vessels restrict blood flow to the heart. It is often referred to as *angina*. The pain can radiate to the neck, jaw, or left arm. It is often described as a crushing, burning, or squeezing sensation.
angiocardiography (ACG) (ăn″ jĭ-ō-kăr″ dĭ-ŏg′ ră-fē)	angi/o cardi/o -graphy	vessel heart recording	Video x-ray technique used to follow the passage of blood through the heart and great vessels after an intravenous injection of a radiopaque contrast substance; used to evaluate patient for CV surgery

MEDICAL WORD	WORD PARTS		DEFINITION
	Part	**Meaning**	
angiogram (ăn´jē-ō-grăm)	angi/o -gram	vessel record	X-ray record of the size, shape, and location of the heart and its blood vessels after the introduction of a radiopaque contrast medium
angioma (ăn˝jĭ-ō´mă)	ang/i -oma	vessel tumor	Tumor of a blood vessel. See Figure 9.15 ■ ■ **Figure 9.15** Infarction angioma. (Courtesy of Jason L. Smith, MD)
angioplasty (ăn´jĭ-ō-plăs˝tē)	angi/o -plasty	vessel surgical repair	Surgical repair of a blood vessel(s) or a nonsurgical technique for treating diseased arteries by temporarily inflating a tiny balloon inside an artery
angiostenosis (ăn˝jĭ-ō-stĕ-n ō´sĭs)	angi/o sten -osis	vessel narrowing condition	Pathological condition of the narrowing of a blood vessel
arrhythmia (ă-rĭth´mĭ-ă)	a- rrhythm -ia	lack of rhythm condition	Irregularity or loss of rhythm of the heartbeat; also called *dysrhythmia*
arterial (ăr-tē´rĭ-ăl)	arter/i -al	artery pertaining to	Pertaining to an artery
arteriosclerosis (ăr-tē˝rĭ-ō-sklĕ-rō´sĭs)	arteri/o scler -osis	artery hardening condition	Pathological condition of hardening of arteries. Arteriosclerotic heart disease is hardening of the coronary arteries.

LIFE SPAN CONSIDERATIONS

In some older adults, the heart must work harder to pump blood because of hardening of the arteries (**arteriosclerosis**) and a buildup of fatty plaques (cholesterol deposits and triglycerides) in the arterial walls (**atherosclerosis**). Arteries can gradually become stiff and lose their elastic recoil. The aorta and arteries supplying the heart and brain are generally affected first. **Arteriosclerotic heart disease (ASHD)** occurs when the arterial vessels are marked by thickening, hardening, and loss of elasticity in the arterial walls. Reduced blood flow, elevated blood lipids, and defective endothelial repair that can be seen in aging accelerate the course of cardiovascular disease.

MEDICAL WORD	WORD PARTS		DEFINITION
	Part	**Meaning**	
arteritis (ăr″ tĕ-rī′ tĭs)	arter -itis	artery inflammation	Inflammation of an artery. See Figure 9.16 ■

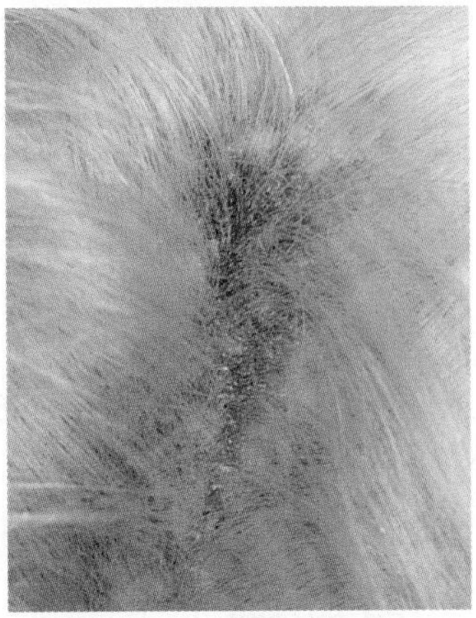

■ **Figure 9.16** Temporal arteritis. (Courtesy of Jason L. Smith, MD)

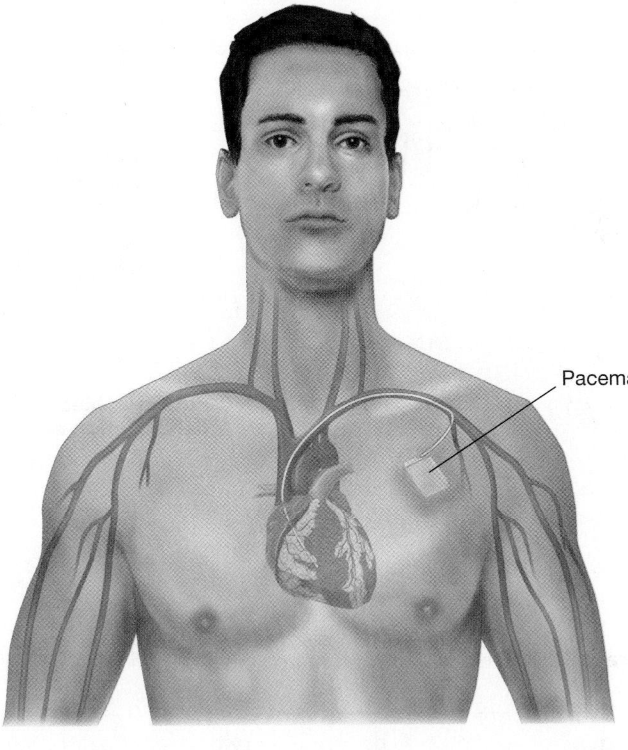

artificial pacemaker			Electronic device that stimulates impulse initiation within the heart. It is a small battery-operated device that helps the heart beat in a regular rhythm. See Figure 9.17 ■

Pacemaker

■ **Figure 9.17** A permanent epicardial pacemaker. The pulse generator can be placed in subcutaneous pockets in the subclavian or abdominal regions.

atheroma (ăth″ ĕr-ō mă)	ather -oma	fatty substance, porridge tumor	Tumor of an artery containing a fatty substance

MEDICAL WORD	WORD PARTS		DEFINITION
	Part	**Meaning**	
atherosclerosis (ăth″ ĕr-ō-sklĕ-rō′ sĭs)	ather/o scler -osis	fatty substance, porridge hardening condition	Pathological condition of the arteries characterized by the buildup of fatty substances (cholesterol deposits and triglycerides) and hardening of the walls
atrioventricular (AV) (ăt″ rĭ-ō-věn-trĭk′ ū-lăr)	atri/o ventricul -ar	atrium ventricle pertaining to	Pertaining to the atrium and the ventricle
auscultation (ŏs″ kool-tā′ shŭn)	auscultat -ion	listen to process	Method of physical assessment using a stethoscope to listen to sounds within the chest, abdomen, and other parts of the body
automated external defibrillator (AED) (aw-tōm′ ăt-ĕd ēx′ těr′ năl dē-fĭb″rĭ-lā′ tor)			Portable automatic device used to restore normal heart rhythm to patients in cardiac arrest. An AED is applied outside the body. It automatically analyzes the patient's heart rhythm and advises the rescuer whether or not a shock is needed to restore a normal heartbeat. If the patient's heart resumes beating normally, the heart has been defibrillated. See Figure 9.18 ■

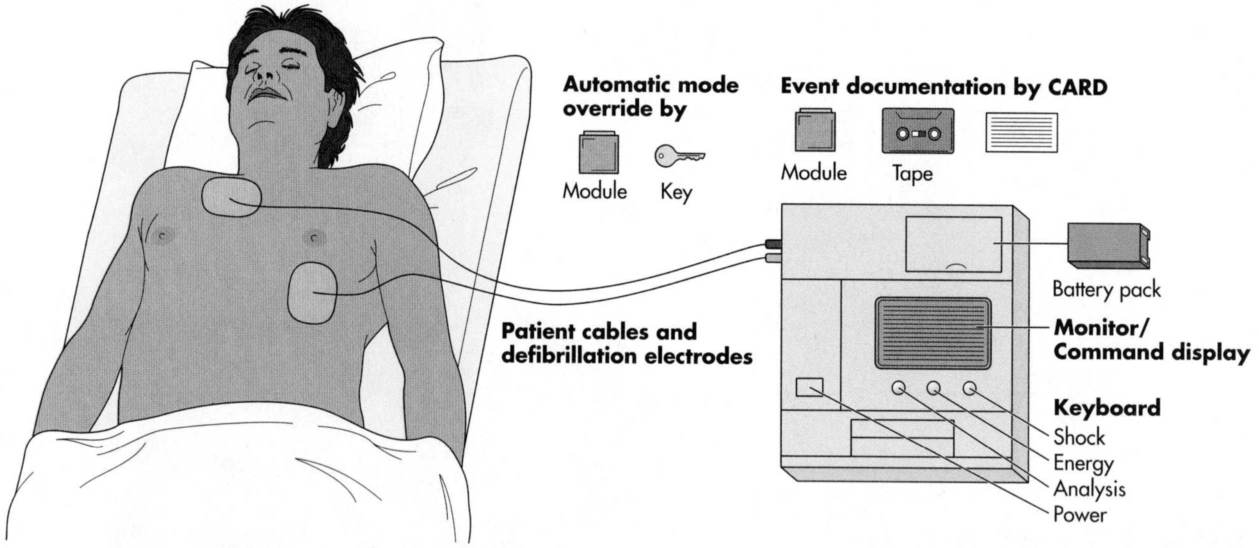

Automatic mode override by
Module   Key

Event documentation by CARD
Module   Tape

Battery pack
Monitor/ Command display
Keyboard
Shock
Energy
Analysis
Power

Patient cables and defibrillation electrodes

■ **Figure 9.18** Schematic of an automated external defibrillator (AED) attached to a patient.

bicuspid (bĭ-kūs′ pĭd)	bi- -cuspid	two point	Valve with two cusps; pertaining to the mitral valve
bradycardia (brăd″ ĭ-kăr′ dĭ-ă)	brady- card -ia	slow heart condition	Abnormally slow heartbeat defined as less than 60 beats per minute

MEDICAL WORD	WORD PARTS		DEFINITION
	Part	**Meaning**	
bruit (brōōt)			Pathological noise; a sound of venous or arterial origin heard on auscultation
cardiac (kăr′ dĭ-ăk)	card/i -ac	heart pertaining to	Pertaining to the heart
cardiac arrest			Loss of effective heart function, which results in cessation of functional circulation. Sudden cardiac arrest (SCA) results in sudden death.
cardiologist (kăr-dē-ŏl′ ō-jĭst)	cardi/o log -ist	heart study of one who specializes	Physician who specializes in the study of the heart
cardiology (kăr″ dĭ-ōl′ ō-jē)	cardi/o -logy	heart study of	Literally means *study of the heart*
cardiomegaly (kăr″ dĭ-ō-mĕg′ ă-lē)	cardi/o -megaly	heart enlargement, large	Enlargement of the heart
cardiometer (kăr″ dĭ-ōm′ ĕ-tĕr)	cardi/o -meter	heart instrument to measure	Instrument used to measure the force of the heart's action
cardiomyopathy (CMP) (kăr″ dē-ō-mī-ŏp′ ă-thē)	cardi/o my/o -pathy	heart muscle disease	Disease of the heart muscle that leads to generalized deterioration of the muscle and its pumping ability. It can be caused by multiple factors including viral infections. See Figure 9.19 ■

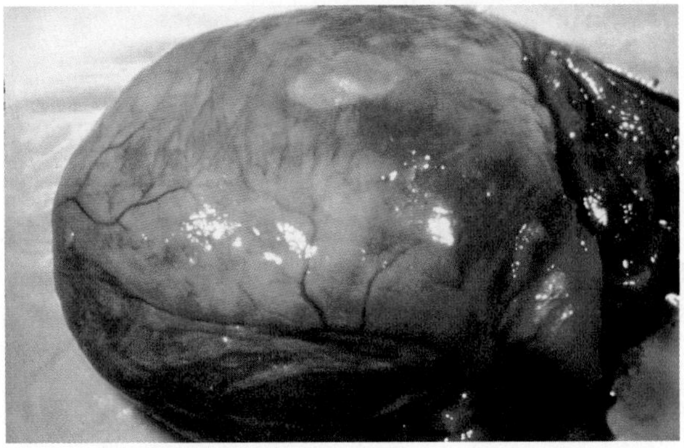

■ **Figure 9.19**
An enlarged heart showing the results of cardiomyopathy.

MEDICAL WORD	WORD PARTS		DEFINITION
	Part	**Meaning**	
cardiopulmonary (kăr″ dĭ-ō-pūl´ mō-nĕr-ē)	cardi/o pulmonar -y	heart lung pertaining to	Pertaining to the heart and lungs (H & L)
cardiotonic (kăr″ dĭ-ō-tŏn´ ĭk)	cardi/o ton -ic	heart tone pertaining to	A class of medication that is used to increase the tone (pumping strength) of the heart
cardiovascular (CV) (kăr″ dĭ-ō-văs´ kū-lar)	cardi/o vascul -ar	heart small vessel pertaining to	Pertaining to the heart and small blood vessels
cardioversion (kăr´ dē-ō-vĕr″ zhūn)	cardi/o vers -ion	heart turning process	Medical procedure used to treat cardiac arrhythmias. An electrical shock is delivered to the heart to restore its normal rhythm. The electrical energy can be delivered externally through electrodes placed on the chest or directly to the heart by placing paddles on the heart during an open chest surgery.
cholesterol (chol) (kō-lĕs´ tĕr-ŏl)	chol/e sterol	bile solid (fat)	A normal soft, waxy substance found among the lipids (fats) in the bloodstream and all body cells. It is the building block of steroid hormones, but it is dangerous when it builds up on arterial walls and can contribute to the risk of coronary heart disease.
circulation (sər″-kyəlā´ shūn)	circulat -ion	circular process	The moving of the blood in the veins and arteries throughout the body
claudication (klaw-dĭ-kā´ shūn)	claudicat -ion	to limp process	Literally means *process of lameness or limping*. It is a dull, cramping pain in the hips, thighs, calves, or buttocks caused by an inadequate supply of oxygen to the muscles, due to narrowed arteries. It is one of the symptoms in peripheral artery disease (PAD).
constriction (kən-strĭk´ shūn)	con- strict -ion	together, with to draw, to bind process	Process of drawing together, as in the narrowing of a vessel

MEDICAL WORD	WORD PARTS		DEFINITION
	Part	Meaning	
coronary artery bypass graft (kŏr´ ō-nă-rē ăr´ tĕr-ē bī´ păs grăft)			Surgical procedure to assist blood flow to the myocardium by using a section of a saphenous vein or internal mammary artery to bypass or reroute blood around an obstructed or occluded coronary artery, thus improving blood flow and oxygen to the heart; sometimes called coronary artery bypass graft (CABG) ("cabbage") (Figure 9.20 ■). Increasing blood flow to the heart muscle can relieve chest pain and reduce the risk of heart attack. A patient may undergo several bypass grafts, depending on how many coronary arteries are blocked.

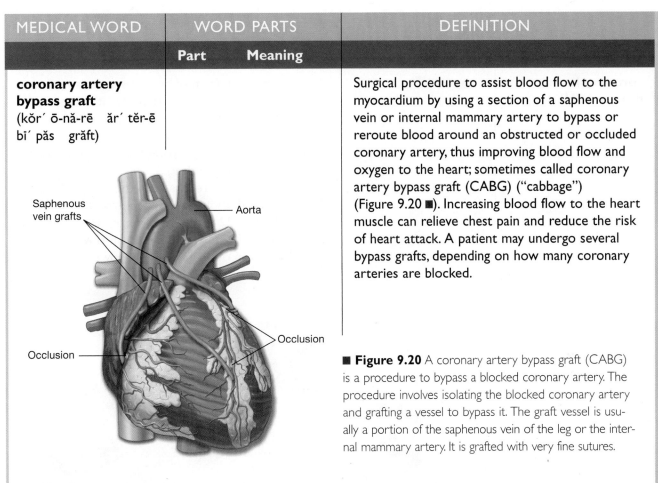

■ **Figure 9.20** A coronary artery bypass graft (CABG) is a procedure to bypass a blocked coronary artery. The procedure involves isolating the blocked coronary artery and grafting a vessel to bypass it. The graft vessel is usually a portion of the saphenous vein of the leg or the internal mammary artery. It is grafted with very fine sutures.

fyi Cardiopulmonary bypass with a pump oxygenator (heart–lung machine) is used for most coronary bypass graft operations. Recently, surgeons have been performing off-pump coronary artery bypass (OPCAB) surgery. In it, the heart continues beating while the bypass graft is sewn in place. In some patients, OPCAB may reduce intraoperative bleeding (and the need for blood transfusion), renal complications, and postoperative neurological deficits (problems after surgery).

MEDICAL WORD	WORD PARTS		DEFINITION
	Part	**Meaning**	
coronary heart disease (CHD)			Most common form of heart disease; also referred to as *coronary artery disease (CAD)*, it is the term for the narrowing of the coronary arteries that supply blood to the heart. It is a progressive disease that increases the risk of myocardial infarction (heart attack) and sudden death. CHD usually results from the buildup of fatty material and plaque (**atherosclerosis**). See Figures 9.21 ■ and 9.22 ■ As the coronary arteries narrow, the flow of blood to the heart can slow or stop. Blockage can occur in one or many coronary arteries.

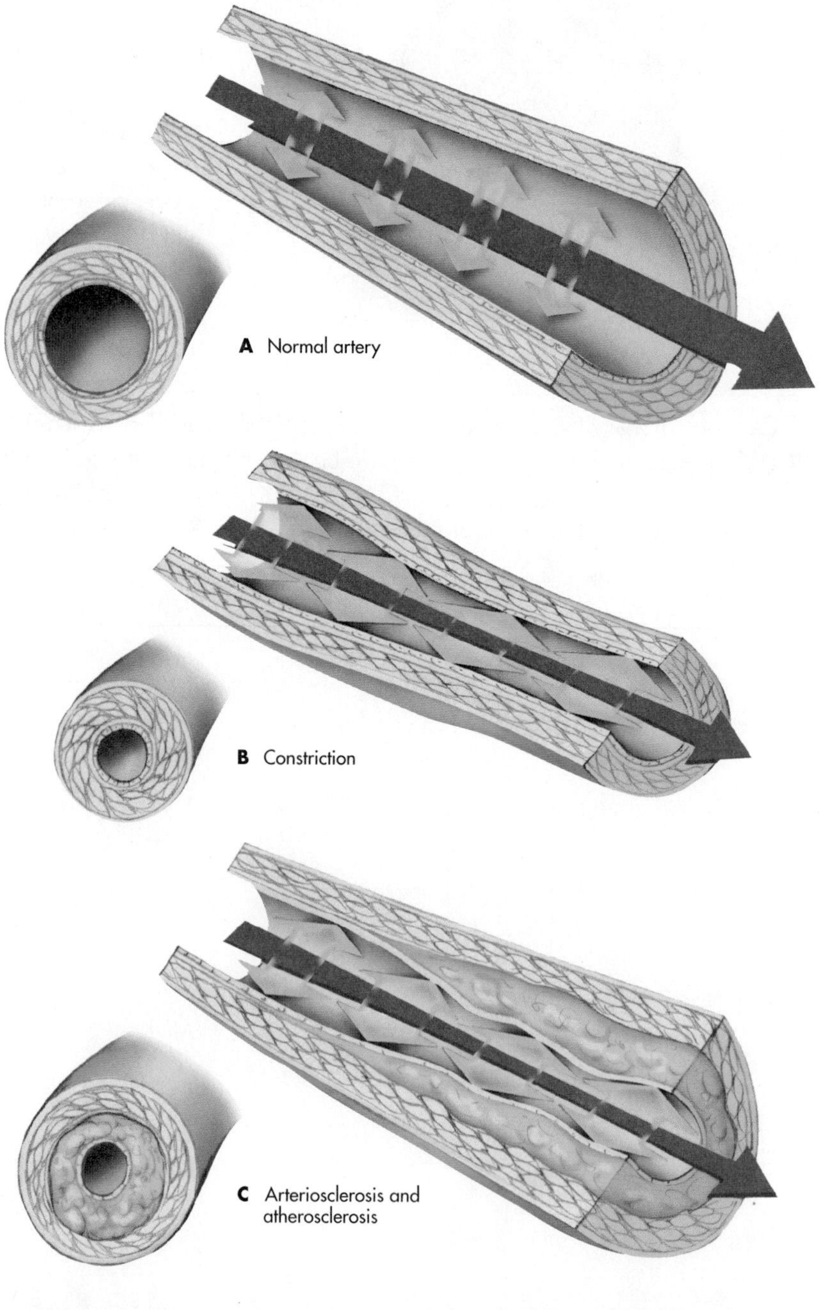

A Normal artery

B Constriction

C Arteriosclerosis and atherosclerosis

■ **Figure 9.21**
Blood vessels:
(A) normal artery,
(B) constriction, and
(C) arteriosclerosis and atherosclerosis.

MEDICAL WORD	WORD PARTS		DEFINITION
	Part	**Meaning**	

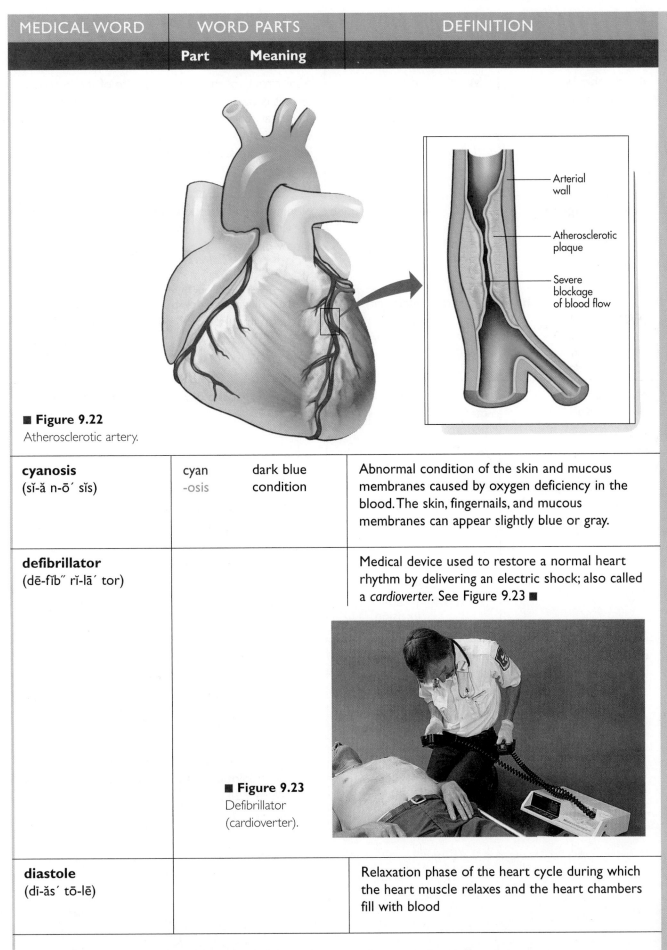

■ **Figure 9.22**
Atherosclerotic artery.

Arterial wall

Atherosclerotic plaque

Severe blockage of blood flow

MEDICAL WORD	WORD PARTS		DEFINITION
cyanosis (sĭ-ă n-ō´ sĭs)	cyan -osis	dark blue condition	Abnormal condition of the skin and mucous membranes caused by oxygen deficiency in the blood. The skin, fingernails, and mucous membranes can appear slightly blue or gray.
defibrillator (dē-fĭb˝ rĭ-lā´ tor)			Medical device used to restore a normal heart rhythm by delivering an electric shock; also called a *cardioverter*. See Figure 9.23 ■

■ **Figure 9.23**
Defibrillator (cardioverter).

MEDICAL WORD	WORD PARTS		DEFINITION
diastole (dī-ăs´ tō-lē)			Relaxation phase of the heart cycle during which the heart muscle relaxes and the heart chambers fill with blood

MEDICAL WORD	WORD PARTS		DEFINITION
	Part	**Meaning**	
dysrhythmia (dĭs-rĭth′ mē-ă)	dys- rhythm -ia	difficult, abnormal rhythm condition	Abnormality of the rhythm or rate of the heartbeat. It is caused by a disturbance of the normal electrical activity within the heart and can be divided into two main groups: **tachycardias** and **bradycardias**. Dysrhythmia is also referred to as an *arrhythmia*.
echocardiography (ECHO) (ĕk″ ō-kăr″ dē-ŏg′ rah-fē)	ech/o cardi/o -graphy	reflected sound heart recording	Noninvasive ultrasound used to evaluate the heart for valvular or structural defects and coronary artery disease
electrocardiograph (ECG, EKG) (ē-lĕk″ trō-kăr′ dĭ-ō-grăf)	electr/o cardi/o -graph	electricity heart instrument for recording	Medical diagnostic device used for recording the electrical impulses of the heart muscle
electrocardio-phonograph (ē-lĕk″ trō-kăr″ dĭ-ō-fō′ nō-grăf)	electr/o cardi/o phon/o -graph	electricity heart sound instrument for recording	Medical diagnostic device used to record heart sounds
embolism (ĕm′ bō-lĭzm)	embol -ism	a throwing in condition	Pathological condition caused by obstruction of a blood vessel by foreign substances or a blood clot
endarterectomy (ĕn″ dăr-tĕr-ĕk′ tō-mē)	end- arter -ectomy	within artery surgical excision	Surgical excision of the inner portion of an artery
endocarditis (ĕn″ dō-kăr-dī′ tĭs)	endo- card -itis	within heart inflammation	Inflammation of the endocardium (inner lining of the heart). It typically occurs when microorganisms, especially bacteria from another part of the body such as the gums/teeth, spread through the bloodstream and affect heart valves and other important structures of the cardiovascular system. Treatments for endocarditis include antibiotics and, in severe cases, surgery. See Figure 9.24 ■

MEDICAL WORD	WORD PARTS		DEFINITION
	Part	**Meaning**	

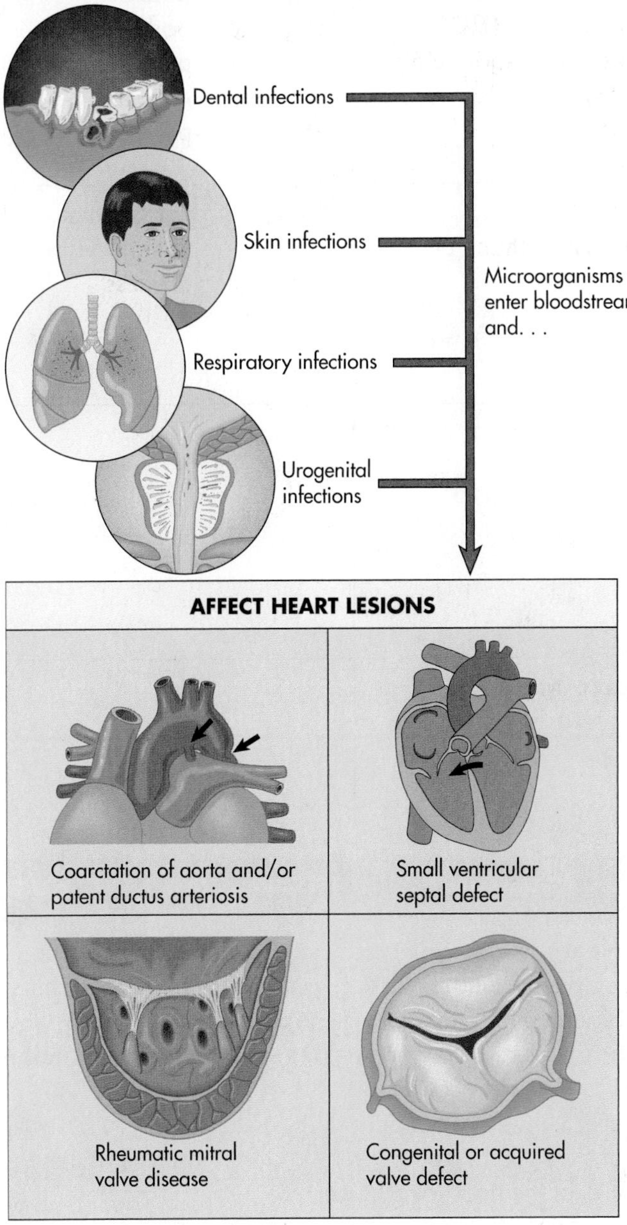

■ **Figure 9.24** How microorganisms enter bloodstream and affect heart lesions, which could result in bacterial endocarditis.

| **endocardium** (ĕn″ dō-kăr′ dē-ūm) | endo-
card/i
-um | within
heart
tissue | Inner lining of the heart |

MEDICAL WORD	WORD PARTS		DEFINITION
	Part	**Meaning**	
extracorporeal circulation (ECC) (ĕks-tră-kor-pōr´ ē-ăl)	extra- corpor/e -al circulat -ion	outside body pertaining to circular process	Pertaining to the circulation of the blood outside the body via a heart–lung machine or in hemodialysis
fibrillation (fī´ brĭl-ā´ shŭn)	fibrillat -ion	fibrils (small fibers) process	Quivering or spontaneous contraction of individual muscle fibers, an abnormal bioelectric potential occurring in neuropathies and myopathies; disorganized pathological rhythm that can lead to death if not immediately corrected
flutter			Pathological rapid heart rate that may cause cardiac output to be decreased. With atrial flutter, the heartbeat is 200 to 400 beats per minute. With ventricular flutter, the heartbeat is 250 beats or more per minute. On an EKG recording, a flutter will demonstrate a "saw-tooth" appearance.
heart failure (HF)			Pathological condition in which the heart loses its ability to pump blood efficiently. Left-sided heart failure is commonly called *congestive heart failure* (CHF).

LIFE SPAN CONSIDERATIONS

Heart failure (HF) is one of the most common types of cardiovascular disease seen in the older adult. It can involve the heart's left side, right side, or both sides. Left-sided failure leads to a backup of blood, which causes a buildup of fluid in the lungs, or **pulmonary edema**, which causes **dyspnea** and shortness of breath. Left-sided heart failure is commonly called **congestive heart failure (CHF).** Right-sided or right ventricular (RV) heart failure usually occurs as a result of left-sided failure. When the left ventricle fails, increased fluid pressure is, in effect, transferred back through the lungs, ultimately damaging the heart's right side. Right-sided failure is a result of a buildup of blood flowing into the right side of the heart, which can lead to enlargement of the liver, distention of the neck veins, and edema of the ankles. See Figure 9.25 ■ for some signs and symptoms of a patient with heart failure.

MEDICAL WORD	WORD PARTS		DEFINITION
	Part	Meaning	

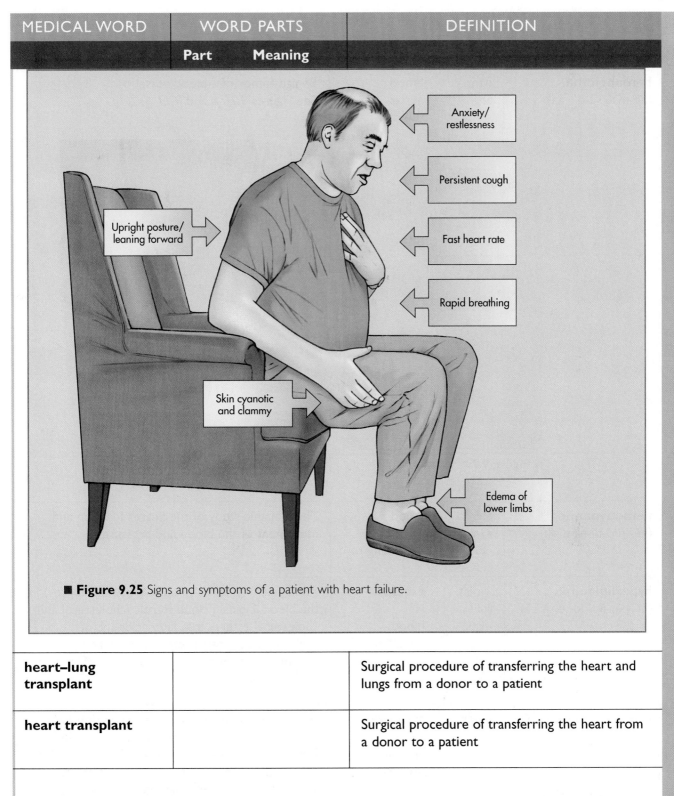

Figure 9.25 Signs and symptoms of a patient with heart failure.

| heart–lung transplant | | | Surgical procedure of transferring the heart and lungs from a donor to a patient |
| heart transplant | | | Surgical procedure of transferring the heart from a donor to a patient |

MEDICAL WORD	WORD PARTS		DEFINITION
	Part	Meaning	
hemangioma (hē-măn″ jĭ-ō′ mă)	hem ang/i -oma	blood vessel tumor	Benign tumor of a blood vessel. See Figures 9.26 ■ and 9.27 ■

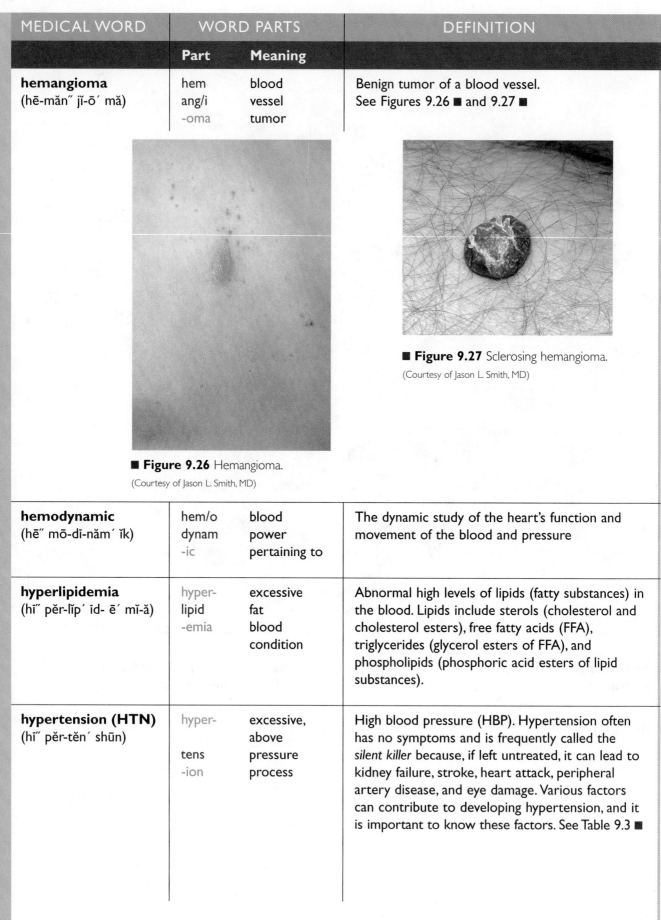

■ **Figure 9.26** Hemangioma.
(Courtesy of Jason L. Smith, MD)

■ **Figure 9.27** Sclerosing hemangioma.
(Courtesy of Jason L. Smith, MD)

MEDICAL WORD	WORD PARTS		DEFINITION
hemodynamic (hē″ mō-dĭ-năm′ ĭk)	hem/o dynam -ic	blood power pertaining to	The dynamic study of the heart's function and movement of the blood and pressure
hyperlipidemia (hī″ pĕr-lĭp′ ĭd- ē′ mĭ-ă)	hyper- lipid -emia	excessive fat blood condition	Abnormal high levels of lipids (fatty substances) in the blood. Lipids include sterols (cholesterol and cholesterol esters), free fatty acids (FFA), triglycerides (glycerol esters of FFA), and phospholipids (phosphoric acid esters of lipid substances).
hypertension (HTN) (hī″ pĕr-tĕn′ shūn)	hyper- tens -ion	excessive, above pressure process	High blood pressure (HBP). Hypertension often has no symptoms and is frequently called the *silent killer* because, if left untreated, it can lead to kidney failure, stroke, heart attack, peripheral artery disease, and eye damage. Various factors can contribute to developing hypertension, and it is important to know these factors. See Table 9.3 ■

MEDICAL WORD	WORD PARTS		DEFINITION
	Part	Meaning	

TABLE 9.3 Factors Contributing to Hypertension

Factors That One Can Control	
Smoking	Avoid the use of tobacco products
Overweight	Maintain a proper weight for age and body size
Lack of exercise	Exercise regularly
Stress	Learn to manage stress
Alcohol	Limit intake of alcohol
Factors That One Cannot Control	
Heredity	Family history of high blood pressure, heart attack, stroke, or diabetes
Race	Incidence of hypertension increases among African Americans
Gender	Chance of developing hypertension increases for males
Age	Likelihood of hypertension increases with age

MEDICAL WORD	Part	Meaning	DEFINITION
hypotension (hī″ pō-těn′ shūn)	hypo- tens -ion	deficient, below pressure process	Low blood pressure
infarction (ĭn-fãrk′ shūn)	infarct -ion	infarct (necrosis of an area) process	Process of development of an infarct, which is death of tissue resulting from obstruction of blood flow
ischemia (ĭs-k ē′ mĭ-ă)	isch -emia	to hold back blood condition	Condition in which there is a lack of oxygen due to decreased blood supply to a part of the body caused by constriction or obstruction of a blood vessel
lipoprotein (lĭp-ō-prō′ tēn)			Fat (*lipid*) and protein molecules that are bound together. They are classified as **VLDL**—very-low-density lipoproteins; **LDL**—low-density lipoproteins; and **HDL**—high-density lipoproteins. High levels of VLDL and LDL are associated with cholesterol and triglyceride deposits in arteries, which could lead to coronary heart disease, hypertension, and atherosclerosis.

MEDICAL WORD	WORD PARTS		DEFINITION
	Part	Meaning	
mitral stenosis (MS) (mī′ trăl stĕ-nō′ sĭs)	mitr -al sten -osis	mitral valve pertaining to narrowing condition	Pathological condition of narrowing of the mitral valve (bicuspid valve)
mitral valve prolapse (MVP) (mī′ trăl vălv prō-lăps′)			Pathological condition that occurs when the leaflets of the mitral valve (bicuspid valve) between the left atrium and left ventricle bulge into the atrium and permit backflow of blood into the atrium. The condition is often associated with progressive mitral regurgitation (blood flows back into the left atrium instead of moving forward into the left ventricle).
murmur (mər′ mər)			An abnormal sound ranging from soft and blowing to loud and booming heard on auscultation of the heart and adjacent large blood vessels. Murmurs range from very faint to very loud. They sometimes sound like a whooshing or swishing noise. Normal heartbeats make a "lub-DUPP" or "lub-DUB" sound. This is the sound of the heart valves closing as blood moves through the heart. Most abnormal murmurs in children are due to congenital heart defects. In adults, abnormal murmurs are most often due to heart valve problems caused by infection, disease, or aging.
myocardial (mī′′ ō-kăr′ dĭ-ăl)	my/o card/i -al	muscle heart pertaining to	Pertaining to the heart muscle (myocardium)
myocardial infarction (MI) (mī′′ ō-kăr′ dē-ăl ĭn-fă rk′ shūn)	my/o card/i -al infarct -ion	muscle heart pertaining to infarct (necrosis of an area) process	Occurs when a focal area of heart muscle dies or is permanently damaged because of an inadequate supply of oxygen to that area; also known as a *heart attack*. The most common symptom of a heart attack is **angina**, which is chest pain often described as a feeling of crushing, pressure, fullness, heaviness, or aching in the center of the chest. Many times people try to ignore the symptoms or say "it's just indigestion." It is imperative to seek medical help immediately. Calling 911 is almost always the fastest way to get lifesaving treatment.
myocarditis (mī′′ ō-kăr-dī′ tĭs)	my/o card -itis	muscle heart inflammation	Inflammation of the heart muscle that is usually caused by viral, bacterial, or fungal infections that reach the heart

MEDICAL WORD	WORD PARTS		DEFINITION
	Part	Meaning	
occlusion (ŏ-kloo´ zhŭn)	occlus -ion	to close up process	A blockage in a vessel, canal, or passage of the body
oximetry (ŏk-sĭm´ ĕ-trē)	ox/i -metry	oxygen measurement	Process of measuring the oxygen saturation of blood. A photoelectric medical device (oximeter) measures oxygen saturation of the blood by recording the amount of light transmitted or reflected by deoxygenated versus oxygenated hemoglobin. A *pulse oximetry* is a noninvasive method of indicating the arterial oxygen saturation of functional hemoglobin. See Figure 9.28 ■

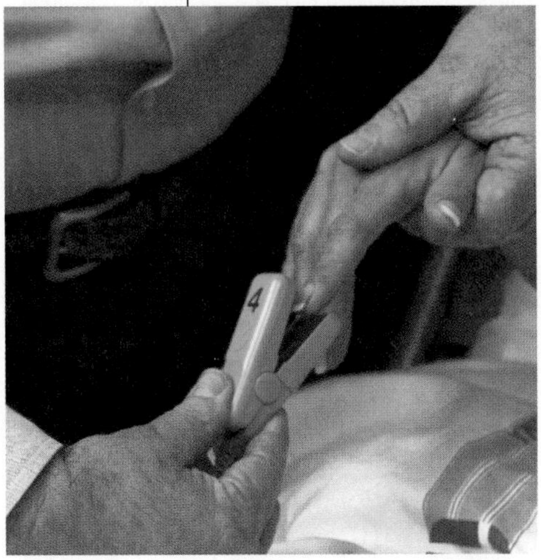

■ **Figure 9.28** Pulse oximetry with the sensor probe applied securely, flush with skin, making sure that both sensor probes are aligned directly opposite each other.

MEDICAL WORD	WORD PARTS		DEFINITION
oxygen (O₂) (ŏk´ sĭ-jĕn)	oxy -gen	sour, sharp, acid formation, produce	Colorless, odorless, tasteless gas essential to respiration in animals
palpitation (păl-pĭ-tā´ shŭn)	palpitat -ion	throbbing process	An abnormal rapid throbbing or fluttering of the heart that is perceptible to the patient and may be felt by the physician during a physical exam
percutaneous transluminal coronary angioplasty (PTCA) (pĕr˝ kū-tā´ nē-ūs trăns-lū´ mĭ-năl kōr´ ō-nă-rē ăn´ jĭ-ō-plăs˝ te)			Use of a balloon-tipped catheter to compress fatty plaques against an artery wall. When successful, the plaques remain compressed, which permits more blood to flow through the artery, therefore providing more oxygen to relieve the symptoms of coronary heart disease. See Figure 9.29 ■

■ **Figure 9.29** Balloon angioplasty. (A) The balloon catheter is threaded into the affected coronary artery. (B) The balloon is positioned across the area of obstruction. (C) The balloon is then inflated, flattening the plaque against the arterial wall. (D) Placque remains flattened after balloon catheter is removed.

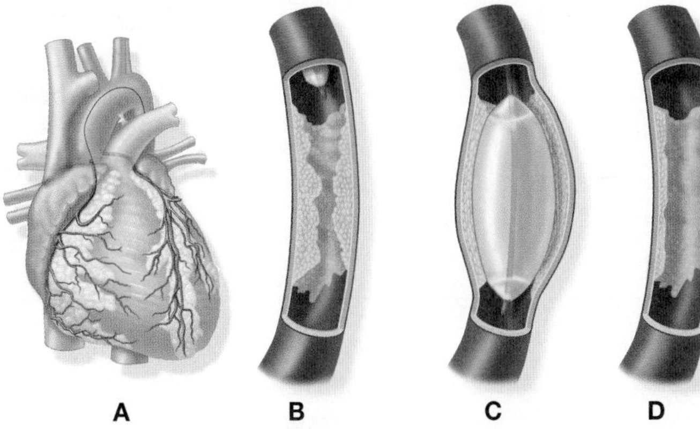

A   B   C   D

MEDICAL WORD	WORD PARTS		DEFINITION
	Part	**Meaning**	
pericardial (pĕr″ ĭ-kăr′ dĭ-ăl)	peri- card/i -al	around heart pertaining to	Pertaining to the pericardium, the sac surrounding the heart
pericardiocentesis (pĕr″ ĭ-kăr″dĭ-ō-sĕn-tē′ sĭs)	peri- cardi/o -centesis	around heart surgical puncture	Surgical procedure to remove fluid from the pericardial sac for therapeutic or diagnostic purposes. See Figure 9.30 ■

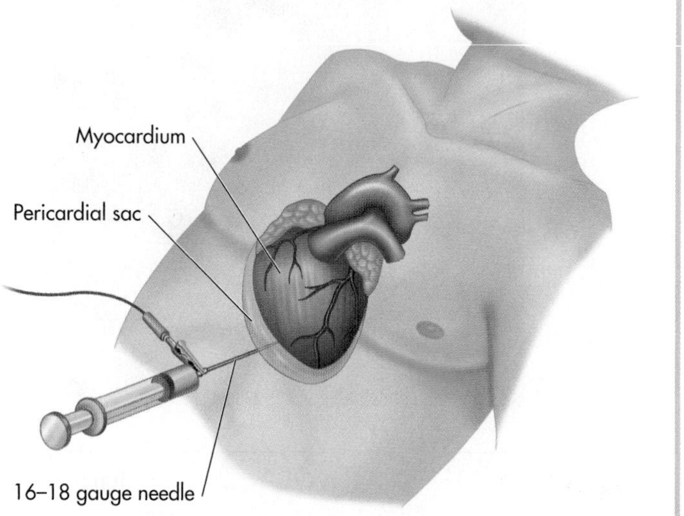

■ **Figure 9.30**
Pericardiocentesis.

Myocardium
Pericardial sac
16–18 gauge needle

| **pericarditis** (pĕr″ ĭ-kăr″ dĭ′tĭs) | peri- card -itis | around heart inflammation | Inflammation of the pericardium (outer membranous sac surrounding the heart) |
| **peripheral artery disease (PAD)** (pər-if′ ər-əl ăr′tĕr-ē) | | | Pathological condition in which fatty deposits build up in the inner linings of the artery walls. These blockages restrict blood circulation, mainly in arteries leading to the kidneys, stomach, arms, legs, and feet. In its early stages, a common symptom is cramping or fatigue in the legs and buttocks during activity. Such cramping subsides when the person stands still. This is called *intermittent claudication*. If left untreated, PAD can progress to *critical limb ischemia* (CLI), which occurs when the oxygenated blood being delivered to the leg is not adequate to keep the tissue alive. An estimated 750,000 people in the United States suffer from CLI. This condition can cause constant pain and even lead to amputation of toes, feet, and/or part of the leg. |

MEDICAL WORD	WORD PARTS		DEFINITION
	Part	Meaning	
phlebitis (flĕ-bī´ tĭs)	phleb -itis	vein inflammation	Literally means inflammation of a vein. There will be redness (erythema), swelling (edema), and pain or burning along the length of the affected vein.
phlebotomy (flĕ-bŏt´ ō-mē)	phleb/o -tomy	vein incision	Medical term used to describe the puncture of a vein to withdraw blood for analysis
Raynaud´s Phenomenon (rā-nōz fĕ-nŏm´ ĕ-nŏn)			Disorder that affects the blood vessels in the fingers and toes; it is characterized by intermittent attacks that cause the blood vessels in the digits to constrict. The cause is believed to be the result of vasospasms that decrease blood supply to the respective regions. Emotional stress and cold are classic triggers of the phenomenon, and discoloration follows a characteristic pattern in time: white, blue, and red. See Figure 9.31 ■

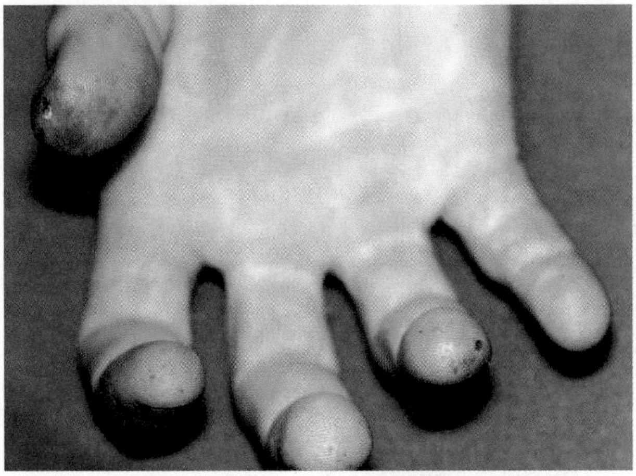

■ **Figure 9.31** Raynaud's phenomenon. Note the discoloration in the thumb and fingers.
(Courtesy of Jason L. Smith, MD)

MEDICAL WORD	WORD PARTS		DEFINITION
rheumatic heart disease (rōō-măt´ĭk)			Pathological condition in which permanent damage to heart valves is a result of a prior episode of rheumatic fever. The heart valve is damaged by a disease process that generally originates with a strep throat caused by streptococcus A bacteria.
semilunar (sĕm˝ ĭ-lū´ năr)	semi- lun -ar	half moon pertaining to	Valves of the aorta and pulmonary artery; shaped like a crescent (half-moon)
septum (sĕp´ tūm)	sept -um	a partition tissue	Wall or partition that divides or separates a body space or cavity

MEDICAL WORD	WORD PARTS		DEFINITION
	Part	Meaning	
shock			A life-threatening condition that occurs when the body is not getting enough blood flow. This can damage multiple organs. Shock requires immediate medical treatment and can get worse very rapidly. In cardiogenic shock, there is failure to maintain the blood supply to the circulatory system and tissues because of inadequate cardiac output. See Figure 9.32 ■

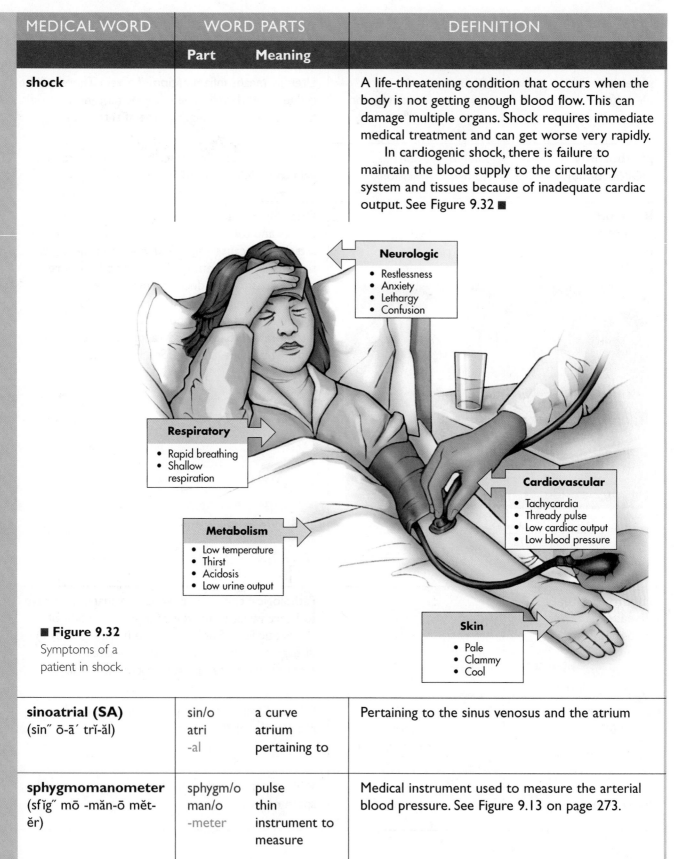

■ **Figure 9.32** Symptoms of a patient in shock.

MEDICAL WORD	WORD PARTS		DEFINITION
sinoatrial (SA) (sĭn″ ō-ā′ trĭ-ăl)	sin/o atri -al	a curve atrium pertaining to	Pertaining to the sinus venosus and the atrium
sphygmomanometer (sfĭg″ mō -măn-ō mĕt-ĕr)	sphygm/o man/o -meter	pulse thin instrument to measure	Medical instrument used to measure the arterial blood pressure. See Figure 9.13 on page 273.

MEDICAL WORD	WORD PARTS		DEFINITION
	Part	**Meaning**	
spider veins			Hemangioma in which numerous telangiectatic vessels radiate from a central point.
stent			Medical device made of expandable, metal mesh that is placed (by using a balloon catheter) at the site of a narrowing artery. The stent is then expanded and left in place to keep the artery open. See Figure 9.33 ■

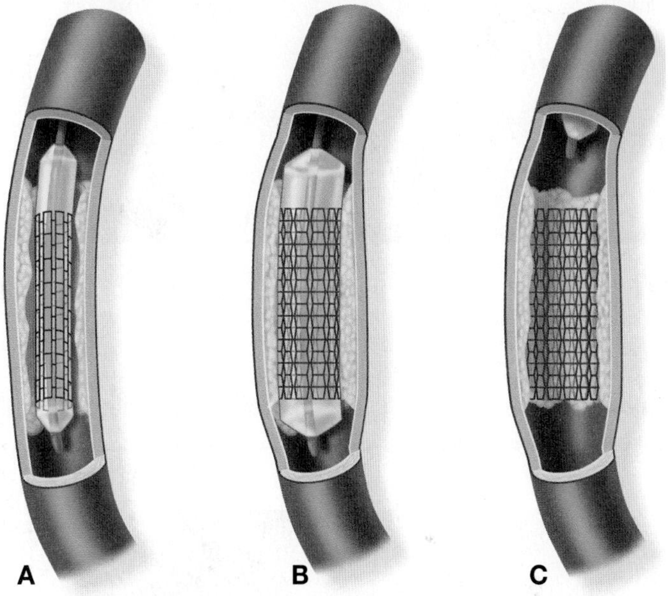

■ **Figure 9.33** Placement of a stent. (A) The stainless steel stent is fitted over a balloon-tipped catheter. (B) The stent is positioned along the blockage and expanded. (C) The balloon is deflated and removed, leaving the stent in place.

A   **B**   **C**

MEDICAL WORD	WORD PARTS		DEFINITION
	Part	**Meaning**	
stethoscope (stĕth´ ō-skōp)	steth/o -scope	chest instrument for examining	Medical instrument used to listen to the normal and pathological sounds of the heart, lungs, and other internal organs
systole (sĭs´ tō-lē)			Contractive phase of the heart cycle during which blood is forced into the systemic circulation via the aorta and the pulmonary circulation via the pulmonary artery
tachycardia (tăk˝ ĭ-kăr´ dĭ-ă)	tachy- card -ia	rapid heart condition	Rapid heartbeat that is over 100 beats per minute

MEDICAL WORD	WORD PARTS		DEFINITION
	Part	**Meaning**	
telangiectasis (tĕl-ăn″ j ĕ-ĕk-tă′ sĭs)	tel ang/i -ectasis	end vessel dilatation	Vascular lesion formed by dilatation of a group of small blood vessels; can appear as a birthmark or be caused by long-term exposure to the sun. See Figure 9.34 ■

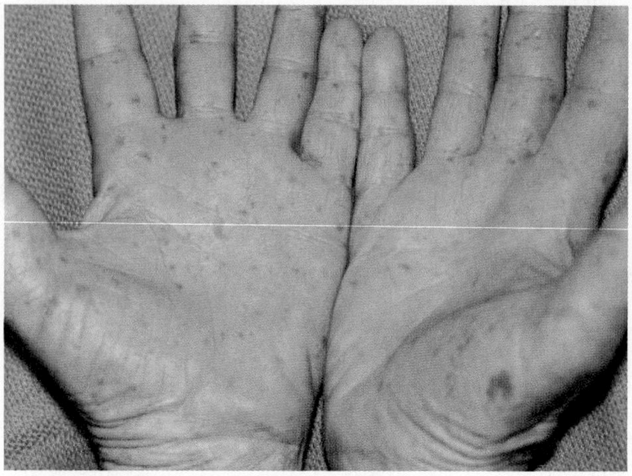

■ **Figure 9.34** Telangiectasis.
(Courtesy of Jason L. Smith, MD)

MEDICAL WORD	WORD PARTS		DEFINITION
thrombophlebitis (thrŏm″ bō-flē-bī′ tĭs)	thromb/o phleb -itis	clot of blood vein inflammation	Inflammation of a vein associated with the formation of a *thrombus* (blood clot). If the clot breaks off and travels to the lungs, it poses a potentially life-threatening condition called pulmonary embolism. See Figure 9.35 ■

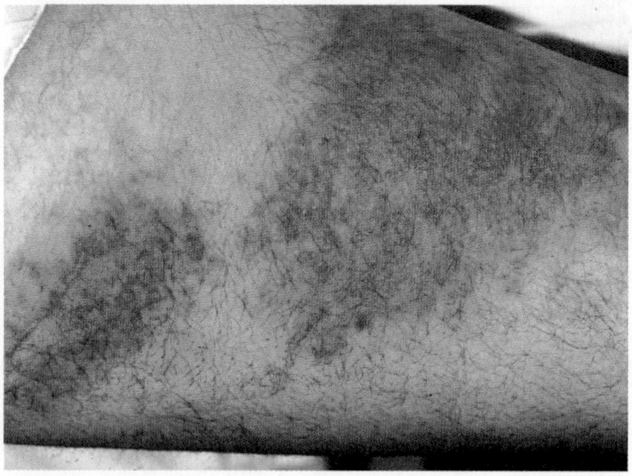

■ **Figure 9.35** Thrombophlebitis.
(Courtesy of Jason L. Smith, MD)

MEDICAL WORD	WORD PARTS		DEFINITION
	Part	**Meaning**	
thrombosis (thrŏm-bō´ sĭs)	thromb -osis	clot of blood condition	A blood clot within the vascular system; *a stationary blood clot.* See Figure 9.36 ■

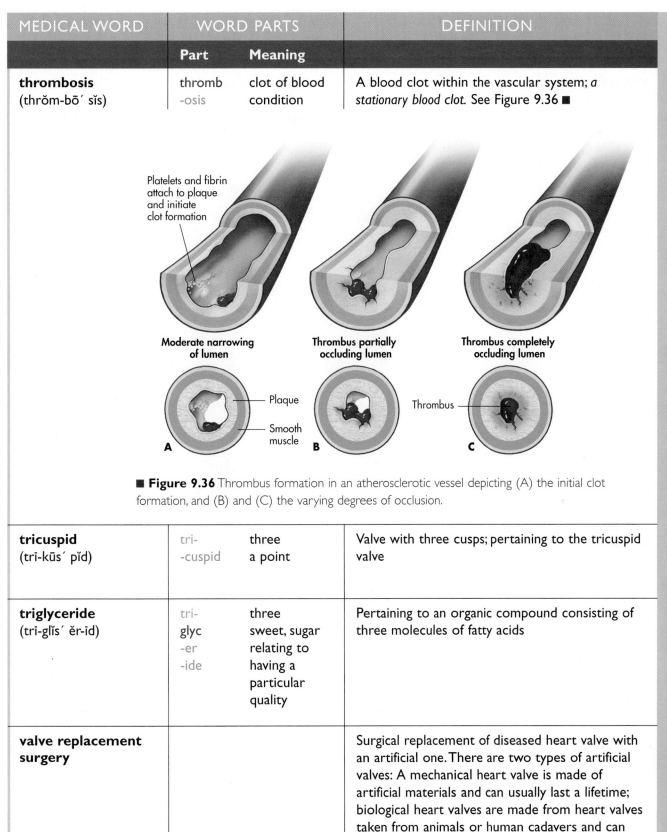

Platelets and fibrin attach to plaque and initiate clot formation

Moderate narrowing of lumen

Thrombus partially occluding lumen

Thrombus completely occluding lumen

Plaque

Smooth muscle

Thrombus

A B C

■ **Figure 9.36** Thrombus formation in an atherosclerotic vessel depicting (A) the initial clot formation, and (B) and (C) the varying degrees of occlusion.

MEDICAL WORD	WORD PARTS		DEFINITION
tricuspid (trī-kūs´ pĭd)	tri- -cuspid	three a point	Valve with three cusps; pertaining to the tricuspid valve
triglyceride (trī-glĭs´ ĕr-īd)	tri- glyc -er -ide	three sweet, sugar relating to having a particular quality	Pertaining to an organic compound consisting of three molecules of fatty acids
valve replacement surgery			Surgical replacement of diseased heart valve with an artificial one. There are two types of artificial valves: A mechanical heart valve is made of artificial materials and can usually last a lifetime; biological heart valves are made from heart valves taken from animals or human cadavers and can wear out over time.
valvuloplasty (văl´ vū-lō-plăs˝ tē)	valvul/o -plasty	valve surgical repair	Surgical repair of a cardiac valve

MEDICAL WORD	WORD PARTS		DEFINITION
	Part	Meaning	
varicose veins (vărʹ ĭ-kōs)			Swollen, dilated, and knotted veins that usually occur in the lower leg(s). They result from a stagnated or sluggish flow of blood in combination with defective valves and weakened walls of the veins. See Figure 9.37 ■

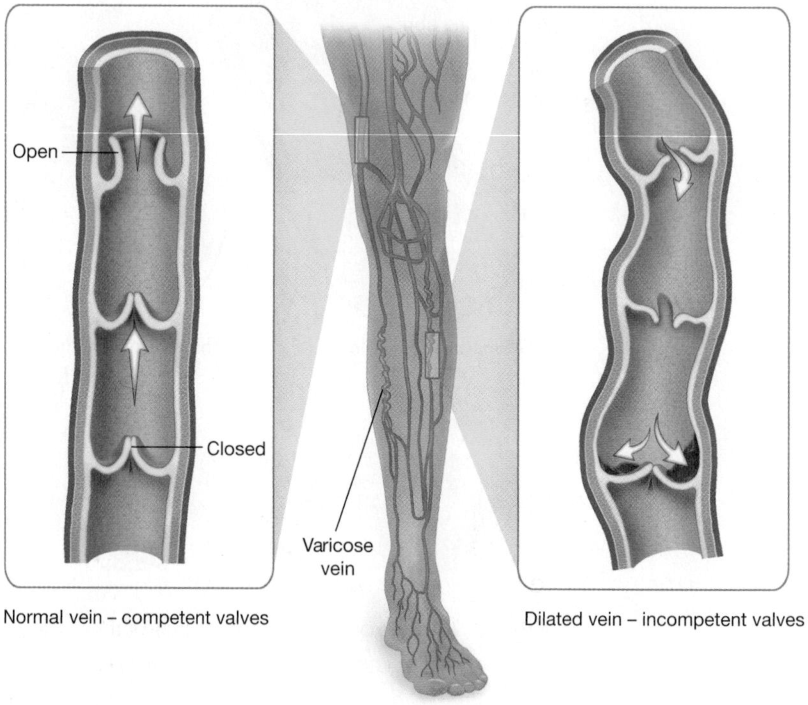

Open
Closed
Varicose vein

Normal vein – competent valves

Dilated vein – incompetent valves

■ **Figure 9.37**
Development of varicose veins.

MEDICAL WORD	WORD PARTS		DEFINITION
	Part	Meaning	
vasoconstrictive (văsʺ ō-kŏn-strĭkʹ tĭv)	vas/o con- strict -ive	vessel together to draw, to bind nature of, quality of	Active narrowing of a blood vessel
vasodilator (văsʺ ō-dī-lāʹ tor)	vas/o dilat -or	vessel to widen one who, a doer	Medicine that acts directly on smooth muscle cells within blood vessels to make them widen (dilate)
vasospasm (vāsʹ ō-spăzm)	vas/o -spasm	vessel contraction, spasm	Spasm of a blood vessel
venipuncture (věnʹ ĭ-pūnkʺ chūr)	ven/i -puncture	vein to pierce	Puncture of a vein for the removal of blood for analysis
ventricular (věn-trĭkʹ ū-lăr)	ventricul -ar	ventricle pertaining to	Pertaining to a cardiac ventricle

• Drug Highlights •

TYPE OF DRUG	DESCRIPTION AND EXAMPLES
digitalis drugs	Strengthen the heart muscle, increase the force and velocity of myocardial systolic contraction, slow the heart rate, and decrease conduction velocity through the atrioventricular (AV) node. These drugs are used in the treatment of congestive heart failure, atrial fibrillation, atrial flutter, and paroxysmal atrial tachycardia. An overdosage of digitalis can cause toxicity. The most common early symptoms of digitalis toxicity are anorexia, nausea, vomiting, and arrhythmias. EXAMPLES: digoxin, Lanoxin (digoxin)
antiarrhythmic agents	Used in the treatment of cardiac arrhythmias (irregular heart rhythms). EXAMPLES: Tambocor (flecainide acetate), Tonocard (tocainide HCl), Inderal (propranolol HCl), Calan (verapamil), and Cordarone and Pacerone (amiodarone)
vasopressors	Cause contraction of the muscles associated with capillaries and arteries, thereby narrowing the space through which the blood circulates. This narrowing results in an elevation of blood pressure. Vasopressors are useful in the treatment of patients suffering from shock. EXAMPLES: Intropin (dopamine HCl), Aramine (metaraminol bitartrate), and Levophed Bitartrate (norepinephrine)
vasodilators	Cause relaxation of blood vessels and lower blood pressure. Coronary vasodilators are used for the treatment of angina pectoris. EXAMPLES: Sorbitrate (isosorbide dinitrate), nitroglycerin, and amyl nitrate
antihypertensive agents	Used in the treatment of hypertension. EXAMPLES: Catapres (clonidine HCl), Lopressor (metoprolol tartrate), Capoten (captopril), and TOPROL–XL (metoprolol succinate)
antihyperlipidemic agents	Used to lower abnormally high blood levels of fatty substances (lipids) when other treatment regimens fail. EXAMPLES: niacin, Mevacor (lovastatin), Lopid (gemfibrozil), Lipitor (atorvastatin calcium), Pravachol (pravastatin), Zocor (simvastatin), Crestor (rosuvastatin calcium), Vytorin (ezetimibe/simvastatin), and Zetia (ezetimibe)
antiplatelet drugs	Help reduce the occurrence of and death from vascular events such as heart attacks and strokes. *Aspirin* is considered to be the reference standard antiplatelet drug and is recommended by the American Heart Association for use in patients with a wide range of cardiovascular disease. Aspirin helps keep platelets from sticking together to form clots. *Plavix (clopidogrel)* is approved by the Food and Drug Administration for many of the same indications as aspirin. It is recommended for patients for whom aspirin fails to achieve a therapeutic benefit.

TYPE OF DRUG	DESCRIPTION AND EXAMPLES
anticoagulants	Act to prevent blood clots from forming. They are known as "blood thinners" and are used in primary and secondary prevention of deep vein thrombosis (DVT), pulmonary embolism (PE), myocardial infarctions (MI), and strokes (CVAs). EXAMPLES: Heplock (heparin), Coumadin, Warfarin (warfarin sodium)
thrombolytic agents	Act to dissolve an existing thrombus when administered soon after its occurrence. They are often referred to as **tissue plasminogen activators** (tPA, TPA) and can reduce the chance of dying after a myocardial infarction by 50%. Unless contraindicated, the drug should be administered within 6 hours of the onset of chest pain. In some hospitals, the time period for administering thrombolytic agents has been extended to 12 and 24 hours. These agents dissolve the clot, reopen the artery, restore blood flow to the heart, and prevent further damage to the myocardium. Bleeding is the most common and potentially serious complication encountered during thrombolytic therapy. Thrombolytic agents are also used in ischemic strokes, deep vein thrombosis, and pulmonary embolism to clear a blocked artery and avoid permanent damage to the perfused tissue. *Note:* Thrombolytic therapy in hemorrhagic strokes is contraindicated, because its use would prolong bleeding into the intracranial space and cause further damage. EXAMPLES: Streptase (streptokinase) and Activase (alteplase)

• Diagnostic and Lab Tests •

TEST	DESCRIPTION
angiography (ăn″ jē-ŏg′ ră-fē)	X-ray recording of a blood vessel after the injection of a radiopaque substance. Used to determine the patency of the blood vessels, organ, or tissue being studied. Types: aortic, cardiac, cerebral, coronary, digital subtraction (use of a computer technique), peripheral, pulmonary, selective, and vertebral.
cardiac catheterization (kăr′ di-ăk kăth″ ĕ-tĕr-ĭ -z ā′ shŭn)	Medical procedure used to diagnose heart disorders. A tiny catheter is inserted into an artery in the arm or leg of the patient and is fed through this artery to the heart. Dye is then pumped through the catheter, enabling the physician to locate by x-ray any blockages in the arteries supplying the heart. See Figure 9.38 ∎

TEST	DESCRIPTION

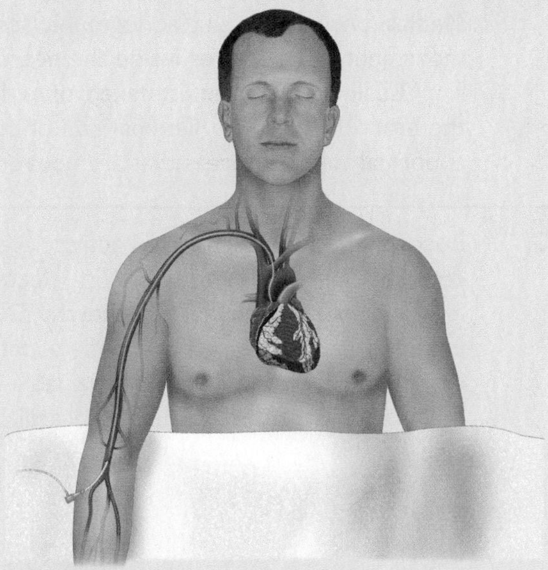

■ **Figure 9.38** Cardiac catheterization.

TEST	DESCRIPTION
cardiac enzymes (kar´ dī-ăk ĕn´-zīmz)	Blood tests performed to determine cardiac damage in an acute myocardial infarction (AMI). Levels begin to rise 6–10 hours after an AMI and peak at 24–48 hours.
alanine aminotransferase (ALT)	
aspartate aminotransferase (AST)	
creatine phosphokinase (CPK)	Used to detect area of damage.
creatine kinase (CK)	Level may be five to eight times normal.
creatine kinase isoenzymes	Used to indicate area of damage; CK-MB heart muscle, CK-MM skeletal muscle, and CK-BB brain
cardiac muscle protein troponins (kăr´ dī-ăk mŭs´əl prō´tēn trō-pə´nənz)	Blood tests performed to determine heart muscle injury (microinfarction) not detected by cardiac enzyme tests. Troponin T (cTnT) and troponin I (cTnI) proteins control the interactions between actin and myosin, which contract or squeeze the heart muscle. Normally the level of cTnT and cTnI in the blood is very low. It increases substantially within several hours (on average 4–6 hours) of muscle damage, so elevated levels can indicate a heart attack, even a mild one. It peaks at 10–24 hours and can be detected for up to 10–14 days.
cholesterol (chol) (kōl-lĕs´ tĕr-ŏl)	Blood test to determine the level of cholesterol in the serum. Elevated levels can indicate an increased risk of coronary heart disease. Any level more than 200 mg/dL is considered too high for heart health.

TEST	DESCRIPTION
echocardiography (ECHO) (ĕk″ ō-kăr″ dē-ŏg′ rah-fē)	Medical procedure using sonographic sound to analyze the size, shape, and movement of structures inside the heart. Usually two echoes are taken: one of the heart at rest and another of the heart under stress. Comparison of the two images helps pinpoint abnormal valves or areas that are not receiving enough blood.
electrocardiogram (ECG, EKG) (ē-lĕk″ trō-kăr′ dĭ-ō-grăm)	Records the heart's electrical activity. A standard electrocardiogram consists of 12 different leads. With electrodes placed on the patient's arms, legs, and six positions on the chest, a 12-lead ECG can be recorded. Six unipolar chest leads record electrical activity of different parts of the heart. An ECG (EKG) provides valuable information in diagnosing cardiac abnormalities, such as myocardial damage and arrhythmias (see Figure 9.39) ▪

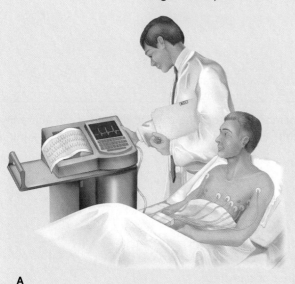

A

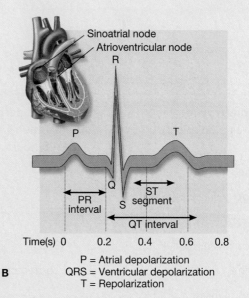

B

P = Atrial depolarization
QRS = Ventricular depolarization
T = Repolarization

Normal sinus rhythm (NSR)

Sinus tachycardia

Sinus arrhythmia

Sinus bradycardia

C

■ **Figure 9.39** An electrocardiogram (ECG, EKG) is a commonly used procedure in which the electrical events associated with the beating of the heart are evaluated. (A) Skin electrodes are applied to the chest-wall, which send electrical signals to a computer that interprets the signals into graph form. (B) Illustration of the electrical events of the heart and a normal ECG/EKG. (C) An electrocardiogram is useful in identifying arrhythmias, as shown here.

TEST	DESCRIPTION
Holter monitor (hōlt ər mŏn´ ĭ–tər)	Portable medical device attached to the patient that is used to record a patient's continuous ECG for 24 hours.
intracardiac electrophysiology study (EPS) (ĭn″ tră-kăr´ dē-ăk ē-lĕk″ trō-fĭz″ ĭ-ŏl´ ō-jē)	Invasive cardiac procedure that involves the placement of catheter-guided electrodes within the heart to evaluate and map the electrical conduction of cardiac arrhythmias.
lactic dehydrogenase (LD or LDH) (lăk´ tĭk dē-hī-drŏj´ ĕ-nās)	Intracellular enzyme present in nearly all metabolizing cells, with the highest concentrations in the heart, skeletal muscles, RBCs, liver, kidney, lung, and brain. When LDH leaks from cardiac cells into the bloodstream, it can be detected and is a good indicator of acute myocardial infarction (AMI). A high serum level occurs 12–24 hours after cardiac injury.
lipid profile (lĭp´ĭd)	Series of blood tests including cholesterol, high-density lipoproteins, low-density lipoproteins, and triglycerides. Used to determine levels of lipids and to assess risk factors of coronary heart disease.
magnetic resonance imaging (MRI) (măg-nĕt´ĭk rĕz´ŏ-năns)	Medical imaging technique that uses a magnet that sets the nuclei of atoms in the heart cells vibrating. The oscillating atoms emit radio signals, which are converted by a computer into either still or moving three-dimensional images. The scan can reveal plaque-filled coronary arteries and the layer of fat that envelopes most hearts. MRI is also an ideal method for scanning children with congenital heart problems. Patients with pacemakers, stents, or other metal implants cannot have MRI. An MRI scan cannot pick up calcium deposits that could signal narrowed vessels.
stress test	A screening test used in evaluating cardiovascular fitness, also called *exercise test, exercise stress test,* or *treadmill test.* The ECG is monitored while the patient is subjected to increasing levels of work using a treadmill or ergometer. It is a common test for diagnosing coronary artery disease, especially in patients who have symptoms of heart disease. The test helps doctors assess blood flow through coronary arteries in response to exercise, usually walking, at varied speeds and for various lengths of time on a treadmill. A stress test can include the use of electrocardiography, echocardiography, and injected radioactive substances.
thallium-201 stress test (thăl ē-ŭm)	X-ray study that follows the path of radioactive thallium carried by the blood into the heart muscle. Damaged or dead muscle can be defined, as can the extent of narrowing in an artery.
triglycerides (trī -glīs´ ĕr-īds)	Blood test to determine the level of triglycerides in the serum. Elevated levels (more than 200 mg/dL) can indicate an increased potential risk of coronary heart disease and diabetes mellitus.

TEST	DESCRIPTION
ultrafast CT scan	Ultrafast CT can take multiple images of the heart within the time of a single heartbeat, thus providing much more detail about the heart's function and structures while greatly decreasing the amount of time required for a study. It can detect very small amounts of calcium within the heart and the coronary arteries. This calcium has been shown to indicate that lesions, which can eventually block off one or more coronary arteries and cause chest pain or even a heart attack, are in the beginning stages of formation. Thus, many physicians are using ultrafast CT scanning as a means to diagnose early coronary artery disease in certain people, especially those who have no symptoms of the disease.
ultrasonography (ŭl-tră-sŏn-ŏg´ră-fē)	Test used to visualize an organ or tissue by using high-frequency sound waves; can be used as a screening test or as a diagnostic tool to determine abnormalities of the aorta, arteries, veins, and the heart.

• Abbreviations •

ABBREVIATION	MEANING
ACG	angiocardiography
AED	automated external defibrillator
AMI	acute myocardial infarction
ASHD	arteriosclerotic heart disease
AST	aspartate aminotransferase
A-V, AV	atrioventricular; arteriovenous
BBB	bundle branch block
BP	blood pressure
CABG	coronary artery bypass graft
CAD	coronary artery disease
CC	cardiac catheterization
CCU	coronary care unit
CHD	coronary heart disease
CHF	congestive heart failure
chol	cholesterol
CK	creatine kinase
CLI	critical limb ischemia
CMP	cardiomyopathy
CO	cardiac output
CPR	cardiopulmonary resuscitation
CV	cardiovascular
CVP	central venous pressure
DVT	deep vein thrombosis
ECC	extracorporeal circulation
ECG, EKG	electrocardiogram
ECHO	echocardiography
EPS	electrophysiology study (intracardiac)
FFA	free fatty acids
FHS	fetal heart sound
HBP	high blood pressure
HDL	high-density lipoprotein
HF	heart failure
Hg	mercury
Hgb	hemoglobin
H&L	heart and lungs
HTN	hypertension

ABBREVIATION	MEANING
IV	intravenous
LA	left atrium
LBBB	left bundle branch block
LD, LDH	lactic dehydrogenase
LDL	low-density lipoprotein
LV	left ventricle
MI	myocardial infarction
MRI	magnetic resonance imaging
MS	mitral stenosis
MV	mitral valve
MVP	mitral valve prolapse
O_2	oxygen
OHS	open heart surgery
OPCAB	off-pump coronary artery bypass surgery
P	pulse
PAD	peripheral artery disease
PAT	paroxysmal atrial tachycardia
PE	pulmonary embolism
PMI	point of maximal impulse
PTCA	percutaneous transluminal coronary angioplasty
PVC	premature ventricular contraction
PVD	peripheral vascular disease
R	respiration
RA	right atrium
RBCs	red blood cells
RV	right ventricle
S-A, SA	sinoatrial (node)
SCA	sudden cardiac arrest
SCD	sudden cardiac death
SOB	shortness of breath
TOF	tetralogy of Fallot
tPA, TPA	tissue plasminogen activator
VLDL	very-low-density lipoprotein
VSD	ventricular septal defect

Anatomy and Physiology

Write your answers to the following questions.

1. The cardiovascular system includes:

   a. _____   b. _____

   c. _____   d. _____

2. Name the three layers of the heart.

   a. _____   b. _____

   c. _____

3. The heart weighs approximately _____ grams.

4. The _____ or upper chambers of the heart are separated by the

   _____ septum.

5. The _____ or lower chambers of the heart are separated by the

   _____ septum.

6. A/An _____ records the heart's electrical activity.

7. The _____ _____ _____ controls

   the heartbeat.

8. The _____ _____ is called the *pacemaker of the heart.*

9. Together, the bundle branches and _____ comprise the ventricular conduction system.

10. Name the three primary pulse points and state their locations on the body.

    a. _____   located _____

    b. _____   located _____

    c. _____   located _____

11. Define the following terms:

    a. *Blood pressure* _____

    b. *Pulse pressure* _____

12. The average adult heart is about the size of a _____ and normally beats at a pulse rate

of _____ to _____ beats per minute.

13. A systolic pressure of _____ to _____ mmHg or a diastolic

pressure of _____ to _____ mmHg is considered

"prehypertension" and needs to be monitored on a regular basis.

14. State the primary function of arteries. _____

_____

_____

15. State the primary function of veins. _____

_____

_____

Word Parts

PREFIXES

Give the definitions of the following prefixes.

1. a- _____ **2.** bi- _____

3. brady- _____ **4.** con- _____

5. end- _____ **6.** endo- _____

7. extra- _____ **8.** hyper- _____

9. hypo- _____ **10.** peri- _____

11. dys- _____ **12.** semi- _____

13. tachy- _____ **14.** tri- _____

ROOTS AND COMBINING FORMS

Give the definitions of the following roots and combining forms.

1. ang/i _____ **2.** angin _____

3. angi/o _____ **4.** anastom _____

5. aort/o _____ **6.** arter _____

7. arter/i _____ **8.** arteri/o _____

9. ather _____

10. ather/o _____

11. atri _____

12. atri/o _____

13. card _____

14. card/i _____

15. cardi/o _____

16. cyan _____

17. auscultat _____

18. dilat _____

19. electr/o _____

20. embol _____

21. glyc _____

22. hem _____

23. isch _____

24. chol/e _____

25. log _____

26. lun _____

27. man/o _____

28. mitr _____

29. my/o _____

30. circulat _____

31. oxy _____

32. phleb _____

33. phleb/o _____

34. phon/o _____

35. pulmonar _____

36. rrhythm _____

37. scler _____

38. sin/o _____

39. sphygm/o _____

40. sten _____

41. steth/o _____

42. strict _____

43. claudicat _____

44. tens _____

45. thromb _____

46. vascul _____

47. vas/o _____

48. ech/o _____

49. ven/i _____

50. corpor/e _____

51. ventricul _____

52. fibrillat _____

53. hem/o _____

54. dynam _____

55. infarct _____

56. occlus _____

57. ox/i _____

58. palpitat _____

59. sept _____

60. tel _____

61. thromb/o _____

62. sterol _____

63. pector _____

64. lipid _____

SUFFIXES

Give the definitions of the following suffixes.

1. -ac _____

2. -al _____

3. -ar _____

4. -gram _____

5. -centesis _____

6. -cuspid _____

7. -metry _____

8. -ectasis _____

9. -ectomy _____

10. -emia _____

11. -er _____

12. -gen _____

13. -graph _____

14. -graphy _____

15. -ia _____

16. -ic _____

17. -ide _____

18. -ion _____

19. -ism _____

20. -ist _____

21. -itis _____

22. -ive _____

23. -logy _____

24. -malacia _____

25. -megaly _____

26. -meter _____

27. -oma _____

28. -or _____

29. -osis _____

30. -pathy _____

31. -plasty _____

32. -puncture _____

33. -scope _____

34. -spasm _____

35. -tomy _____

36. -um _____

37. -y _____

Identifying Medical Terms

In the spaces provided, write the medical terms for the following meanings.

1. _____ Tumor of a blood vessel

2. _____ Video x-ray technique used to evaluate patient for CV surgery

3. _____ Surgical repair of a blood vessel(s)

4. _____ Pathological condition of narrowing of a blood vessel

5. _____ Irregularity or loss (lack of) rhythm of the heartbeat

6. _____ Inflammation of an artery

7. _____ Valve with two cusps; pertaining to the mitral valve

8. _____ Physician who specializes in the study of the heart

9. _____ Enlargement of the heart

10. _____ Pertaining to the heart and lungs

11. _____ Process of drawing together as in the narrowing of a vessel

12. _____ Condition in which a blood clot obstructs a blood vessel

13. _____ Literally means inflammation of a vein

14. _____ Rapid heartbeat

15. _____ Medicine that acts directly on smooth muscles cells within blood vessels to make them widen (dilate)

Spelling

Circle the correct spelling of each medical term.

1. anastomosis / astomosis

2. atherosclerosis / athrosclerosis

3. atriventrcular / atrioventricular

4. endcarditis / endocarditis

5. extracoporal / extracorporeal

6. ischemia / iscemia

7. mycardial / myocardial

8. oxygen / oyxgen

9. phelebitis / phlebitis

10. palpitation / palpitaiton

Matching

Select the appropriate lettered meaning for each of the following words.

_____ 1. cholesterol

_____ 2. claudication

_____ 3. dysrhythmia

_____ 4. diastole

_____ 5. fibrillation

_____ 6. lipoprotein

_____ 7. cardioversion

_____ 8. palpitation

_____ 9. percutaneous transluminal coronary angioplasty

_____ 10. systole

a. Medical procedure used to treat cardiac arrhythmias

b. Quivering of muscle fiber

c. Fat and protein molecules that are bound together

d. A normal soft, waxy substance found among the lipids (fats) in the bloodstream and all body cells

e. Literally means process of lameness, limping

f. An abnormality of the rhythm or rate of the heartbeat

g. Relaxation phase of the heart cycle

h. Contraction phase of the heart cycle

i. An abnormal rapid throbbing or fluttering of the heart

j. Use of a balloon-tipped catheter to compress fatty plaques against an artery wall

k. Process of being closed

Abbreviations

Place the correct word, phrase, or abbreviation in the space provided.

1. acute myocardial infarction _____

2. atrioventricular _____

3. BP _____

4. CAD _____

5. cardiac catheterization _____

6. ECG, EKG _____

7. HDL _____

8. heart and lungs _____

9. MI _____

10. tPA, TPA _____

Diagnostic and Laboratory Tests

Select the best answer to each multiple-choice question. Circle the letter of your choice.

1. _____ is a cardiac procedure that maps the electrical activity of the heart from within the heart itself.
   a. Electrocardiogram
   b. Electrocardiomyogram
   c. Electrophysiology
   d. Cardiac catheterization

2. Blood tests performed to determine cardiac damage in an acute myocardial infarction.
   a. cardiac enzymes
   b. high-density lipoproteins
   c. triglycerides
   d. low-density lipoproteins

3. Method of recording a patient's ECG for 24 hours.
   a. stress test
   b. Holter monitor
   c. ultrasonography
   d. angiography

4. Test used to visualize an organ or tissue by using high-frequency sound waves.
   a. electrophysiology
   b. stress test
   c. ultrasonography
   d. cholesterol

5. X-ray recording of a blood vessel after the injection of a radiopaque contrast medium.
   a. ultrasonography
   b. angiography
   c. stress test
   d. cardiac catheterization

PRACTICAL APPLICATION

SOAP: CHART NOTE ANALYSIS

This exercise will make you aware of the information, abbreviations, and medical terminology typically found in a cardiology patient's chart. Refer to Appendix III, Abbreviations and Symbols, on page A41.

Read the chart note and answer the questions that follow.

GREENLEAF MEDICAL CENTER
420 East First Avenue
Rome, GA 30165
(123) 456-1234

Cardiology Services

Patient: Moore, William T. **Date:** 05/06/20xx **Patient ID:** 32367

Dob: 3/26/1965 **Age:** 47 **Sex:** Male **Allergies:** NKDA

Provider: David R. Briones, MD

S **Subjective:**

Chief Complaint: "Lately I have noticed tightness in my chest during exercise and I feel out of breath. I am real anxious and worried about myself."

47 y/o Caucasian male describes experiencing "tightness" in his chest during a workout session. Noted patient clenching his fist while describing dyspnea (shortness of breath) and how anxious he felt. He denies nausea, vomiting, or radiating pain to his left arm or jaw. The uncomfortable sensation "just went away" after he stopped exercising. He states that he has no prior history of cardiac disease.

O **Objective:**

Vital Signs: **T:** 98.4 F; **P:** 84; **R:** 20; **BP:** 138/90

Ht: 5′ 11″

Wt: 196 lb

General Appearance: Well-developed and muscular. No obvious signs of physical distress noted such as edema, pallor, or diaphoresis. Overall health appears WNL.

Heart: Rate at 84 beats per minute, rhythm regular, no extra sounds, no murmurs.

Lungs: CTA

Abd: Bowel sounds all four quadrants, no masses or tenderness.

MS: Joints and muscles symmetric; no swelling, masses, or deformity; normal spinal curvature. No tenderness to palpation of joints. Full ROM, movement smooth, no crepitant (crackling) sound heard, no tenderness. Muscle strength: able to maintain flexion against resistance and without tenderness.

A **Assessment:**

Chest pain (angina pectoris).

P **Plan:**
1. Schedule patient for an EKG and blood enzyme studies ASAP.
2. Start patient on nitroglycerin (coronary vasodilator) sublingual tablets 0.4 mg prn for chest pain. Instruct patient to seek medical attention immediately if pain is not relieved by nitroglycerin tablets, taken one every 5 minutes over a 15-minute period.
3. To return in 2 weeks for follow-up.
4. Discuss family cardiac history as related to HTN, obesity, diabetes, coronary artery disease, and sudden death of any family member occurring at a young age.
5. Educate patient that angina pectoris occurs due to myocardial ischemia that results when cardiac workload and myocardial oxygen demand exceed the ability of the coronary arteries to supply oxygenated blood. This commonly occurs during exercise or other activity.

Chart Note Questions

Place the correct answer in the space provided.

1. Signs and symptoms of angina pectoris include tightness in the chest, apprehension, and shortness of breath, which is also called _____ .

2. A complete physical, an EKG, and _____ studies are important in determining the diagnosis of angina pectoris.

3. Myocardial ischemia is a result of the body's inability to supply _____ blood.

4. EKG is an abbreviation for _____ .

5. Nitroglycerin is a _____ _____ used to treat angina pectoris.

PEARSON
mymedicalterminologylab

MyMedicalTerminologyLab is a premium online homework management system that includes a host of features to help you study. Registered users will find:

- Fun games and activities built within a virtual hospital
- Powerful tools that track and analyze your results—allowing you to create a personalized learning experience
- Videos, flashcards, and audio pronunciations to help enrich your progress
- Streaming lesson presentations and self-paced learning modules
- A space where you and your instructors can view and manage your assignments

olovy and Nuclear Medicine • Mental Health • Introdu
n to Medical Terminology • Suffixes • Prefixes • Organi
on of the Body • Integumentary System • Skeletal Syste
Muscular System • Digestive System • Cardiovascular S

10

• Blood and Lymphatic System •

LEARNING OUTCOMES

On completion of this chapter, you will be able to:

1. State the description and primary functions of the organs/structures of the blood and lymphatic system.

2. Name the four blood types and their significance in blood typing and blood transfusion.

3. Describe and give the function(s) of the accessory organs of the lymphatic system.

4. Describe the immune system.

5. Explain the immune system's response to foreign substances and the means by which it protects the body.

6. Analyze, build, spell, and pronounce medical words.

7. Comprehend the drugs highlighted in this chapter.

8. Describe diagnostic and laboratory tests related to blood and the lymphatic system.

9. Identify and define selected abbreviations.

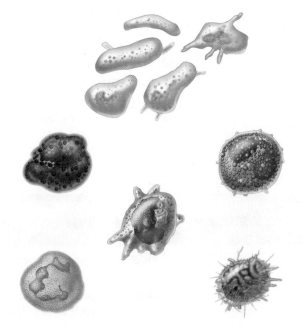

COMBINING FORMS OF THE BLOOD AND LYMPHATIC SYSTEM

aden/o	gland	hem/o	blood
agglutin/o	clumping	immun/o	immunity
all/o	other	leuk/a	white
angi/o	vessel	leuk/o	white
anis/o	unequal	lipid/o	fat
bas/o	base	lymph/o	lymph
calc/o	lime, calcium	macr/o	large
chromat/o	color	neutr/o	neither
coagul/o	clots; to clot	plasm/o	plasma
cyt/o	cell	reticul/o	net
eosin/o	rose-colored	septic/o	putrefying
erythr/o	red	ser/o	whey, serum
fibrin/o	fiber	sider/o	iron
fus/o	to pour	splen/o	spleen
globul/o	globe	thromb/o	clot
glyc/o	sweet, sugar	thym/o	thymus
granul/o	little grain, granular	tonsill/o	tonsil
hemat/o	blood	vascul/o	small vessel

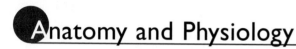natomy and Physiology

Blood and lymph are two of the body's main fluids and are circulated through two separate but interconnected vessel systems. Blood is circulated by the action of the heart, through the circulatory system consisting largely of arteries, veins, and capillaries. Lymph does not actually circulate. It is propelled in one direction, away from its source, through larger lymph vessels, to drain into large veins of the circulatory system located in the upper chest. Numerous valves within the lymph vessels permit one-directional flow, opening and closing as a consequence of pressure caused by the contracting action of muscles on the vessels squeezing the fluid forward.

Table 10.1 ■ provides an at-a-glance look at the blood and lymphatic system.

TABLE 10.1 Blood and Lymphatic System at-a-Glance

Organ/Structure	Primary Functions/Description
Blood	Fluid consisting of formed elements (erythrocytes, thrombocytes, leukocytes) and plasma. It is a specialized bodily fluid that delivers necessary substances to the body's cells (oxygen, foods, salts, hormones) and transports waste products (carbon dioxide, urea, lactic acid) away from those same cells. Blood is circulated around the body through blood vessels by the pumping action of the heart.

TABLE 10.1 Blood and Lymphatic System at-a-Glance *(continued)*

Organ/Structure	Primary Functions/Description
Lymphatic system	Vessel system composed of lymphatic capillaries, lymphatic vessels, lymphatic ducts, and lymph nodes that transport lymph from the tissue to the blood. The three main functions of the lymphatic system are to: 1. Transport proteins and fluids, lost by capillary seepage, back to the bloodstream 2. Protect the body against pathogens by phagocytosis and immune response 3. Serve as a pathway for the absorption of fats from the small intestines into the bloodstream
Spleen	Major site of erythrocyte (red blood cell) destruction; serves as a reservoir for blood; acts as a filter, removing microorganisms from the blood
Tonsils	Filter bacteria and aid in the formation of white blood cells
Thymus	Plays essential role in the formation of antibodies and the development of the immune response in the newborn; manufactures infection-fighting T cells and helps distinguish normal T cells from those that attack the body's own tissue.

BLOOD

Blood is a fluid consisting of formed elements and plasma, both of which are continuously produced by the body for the purpose of transporting respiratory gases (*oxygen and carbon dioxide*), chemical substances (*foods, salts, hormones*), and cells that act to protect the body from foreign substances. The blood volume within an individual depends on body weight. An individual weighing 154 lb (70 kg) has a blood volume of about 5 qt or 5 L.

Formed Elements

The formed elements in blood are the erythrocytes (red blood cells), thrombocytes (platelets), and leukocytes (white blood cells). See Table 10.2 ■ Formed elements constitute about 45% of the total volume of blood. Together, the plasma and formed elements constitute whole blood. These components can be separated for analysis and clinical purposes. See Figure 10.1 ■

TABLE 10.2 Types of Blood Cells and Functions

Blood Cell	Function
Erythrocyte (red blood cell)	Transports oxygen and carbon dioxide
Thrombocyte (platelet)	Clots blood
Leukocyte (white blood cell)	Provides body's main defense against invasion of pathogens
Types of Leukocytes	
Neutrophil	Protects against infection, especially by bacteria; is readily attracted to foreign antigens and destroys them by phagocytosis (engulfing and eating of particulate substances)

TABLE 10.2 Types of Blood Cells and Functions (continued)

Blood Cell	Function
Eosinophil	Destroys parasitic organisms; plays a key role in allergic reactions
Basophil	Plays a key role in releasing histamine and other chemicals that act on blood vessels; essential to nonspecific immune response to inflammation
Monocyte	Provides one of the first lines of defense in the inflammatory process, phagocytosis
Lymphocyte	Provides immune capacity to the body
B lymphocyte	Identifies foreign antigens and differentiates into antibody-producing plasma cells
T lymphocyte	Plays essential role in the specific immune response of the body

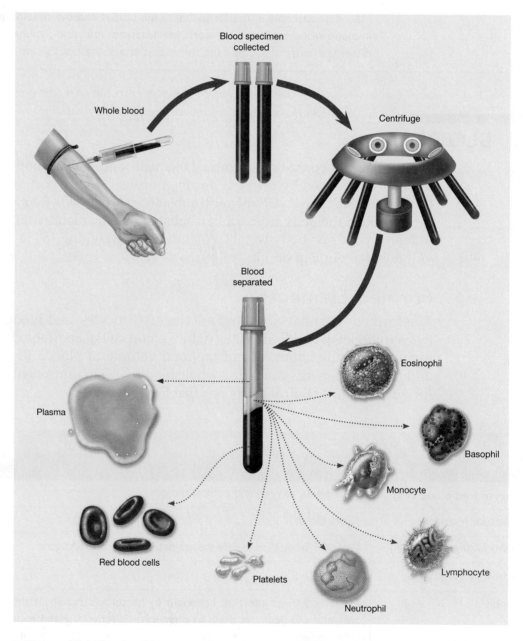

■ **Figure 10.1** Blood and its components.

Erythrocytes

Erythrocytes are commonly called **red blood cells (RBC)**. Mature RBCs are flexible biconcave disks that lack nuclei. They transport oxygen (most of which is bound to hemoglobin contained in the cell) and carbon dioxide. There are approximately 5 million erythrocytes per cubic millimeter of blood, and they have a lifespan of 80–120 days. Erythrocytes are formed in the red bone marrow. See Figure 10.2 ■ and Figure 10.12 on page 334.

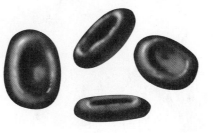

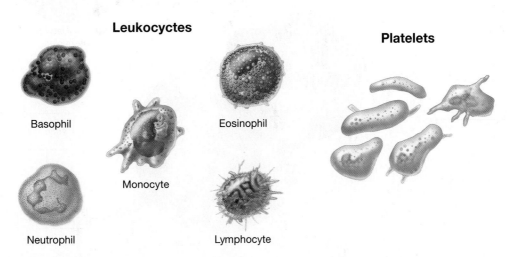

■ **Figure 10.2** Formed elements of blood: erythrocytes, leukocytes (neutrophils, eosinophils, basophils, lymphocytes, and monocytes), and thrombocytes (platelets).

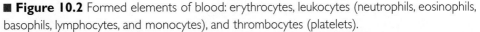

Thrombocytes

Thrombocytes, commonly called *platelets,* are disk-shaped cells about half the size of erythrocytes. See Figure 10.2. They play an important role in the clotting process by releasing *thrombokinase,* which, in the presence of calcium, reacts with *prothrombin* to form *thrombin.* Thrombin (a blood enzyme) converts fibrinogen (a blood protein) into fibrin, an insoluble protein that forms an intricate network of minute thread-like structures called fibrils and causes the blood plasma to coagulate. The blood cells and plasma are enmeshed in the network of fibrils to form the clot.

Coagulation is a complex process by which blood forms clots. See Figure 10.3 ■ It is an important part of hemostasis (the cessation of blood loss from a damaged vessel), wherein a damaged blood vessel wall is covered by a platelet and fibrin-containing clot to stop bleeding and begin repair of the damaged vessel. Disorders of coagulation can lead to an increased risk of bleeding (hemorrhage) or clotting (thrombosis).

Coagulation begins almost instantly after an injury to the blood vessel has damaged the endothelium (lining of the vessel). Exposure of the blood to proteins such as tissue factor initiates changes to blood platelets and the plasma protein fibrinogen, a clotting factor. Platelets immediately form a plug at the site of injury; this is called *primary hemostasis. Secondary hemostasis* occurs simultaneously: Proteins in the blood plasma, called *coagulation factors* or *clotting factors,* respond in a complex cascade to form fibrin strands, which strengthen the platelet plug. This complex process involves several substances—vitamin K, prothrombin, calcium, thrombin, and fibrogen—which all aid in forming fibrin.

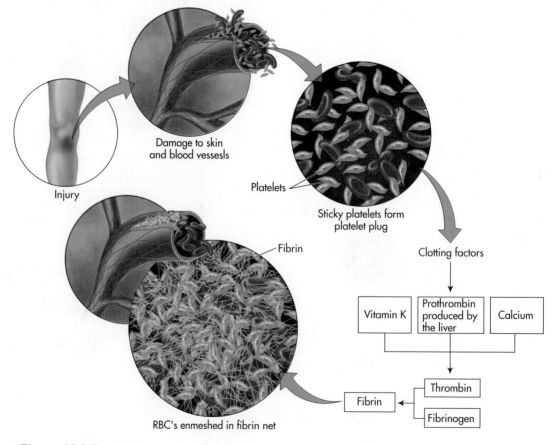

Injury

Damage to skin and blood vessesls

Platelets

Sticky platelets form platelet plug

Clotting factors

Fibrin

| Vitamin K | Prothrombin produced by the liver | Calcium |

Thrombin

Fibrin

Fibrinogen

RBC's enmeshed in fibrin net

■ **Figure 10.3** The clotting process (coagulation).

There are approximately 200,000–500,000 thrombocytes per cubic millimeter of blood. Thrombocytes are fragments of certain giant cells called *megakaryocytes*, which are formed in the red bone marrow.

Leukocytes

Leukocytes, commonly called **white blood cells (WBC),** are sphere-shaped cells containing nuclei of varying shapes and sizes. See Figure 10.2. Leukocytes are the body's main defense against the invasion of **pathogens.** In a normal body state, when pathogens enter the tissue, the leukocytes leave the blood vessels through their walls and move in an amoeba-like motion to the area of infection, where they ingest and destroy the invader. There are approximately 8,000 leukocytes per cubic millimeter of blood. The five types of leukocytes are **neutrophils, eosinophils, basophils, lymphocytes** (lymphs), and **monocytes.**

Neutrophils, eosinophils, basophils, and monocytes contribute to the body's nonspecific defenses. These immune defenses are activated by a variety of stimuli. Lymphocytes are responsible for specific defenses against invading pathogens or foreign proteins. Neutrophils aid in the fight of bacterial infection.

Blood Groups

A number of human blood systems are determined by a series of two or more genes closely linked on a single autosomal chromosome. The **ABO** system, which was discovered in 1901 by Karl Landsteiner, is of great significance in blood typing and blood transfusion. The four blood types identified in this system are types A, B, AB, and O. The differences in human blood are due to the presence or absence of certain protein molecules called *antigens* and *antibodies.* The antigens are located on the surface of the red blood cells, and the antibodies are in the blood plasma. Individuals have different types and combinations of these molecules. Individuals in the A group have the A antigen on the surface of their red blood cells and anti-B antibody in the blood plasma; B group has the B antigen and the anti-A antibody; AB group has both A and B antigens and no anti-A or anti-B antibodies; and group O has neither A or B antigens but has both anti-A and anti-B antibodies. Type AB blood is the universal donor of plasma and the universal recipient of cells, and type O is the universal donor of cells only. See Table 10.3 ■ and Figure 10.4 ■

TABLE 10.3 Blood Groups and Compatibilities

Type	Antigen	Plasma Antibody	Percentage/Population	Compatible Donor Blood Groups	Incompatible Donor Blood Groups
A	A	Anti-B	41	A, O	B, AB
B	B	Anti-A	10	B, O	A, AB
AB	Both A and B	No anti-A or anti-B	4	A, B, AB, O	None
O	No A and B	Both anti-A and anti-B	45	O	A, B, AB

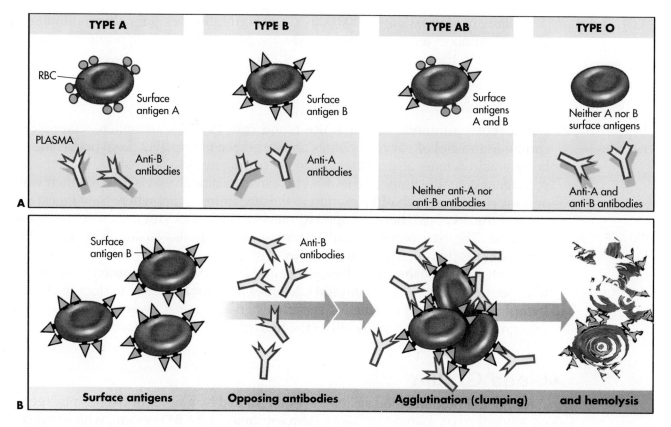

■ **Figure 10.4** Blood-typing and cross-reactions: The blood type depends on the presence of surface antigens (agglutinogens) on RBC surfaces. (A) The plasma antibodies (agglutinins) that will react with foreign surface antigens. (B) In a cross-reaction, antibodies that encounter their target antigens lead to agglutination and hemolysis of the affected RBCs.

Rh Factor

The presence of a substance called an **agglutinogen** in the red blood cells is responsible for what is known as the **Rh factor**. It was first discovered in the blood of the rhesus monkey from which the factor gets its name. About 85% of the population have the Rh factor and are called *Rh positive.* The other 15% lack the Rh factor and are designated *Rh negative.* More than 20 genetically determined blood group systems are known today, but the ABO and Rh systems are the most important ones used for blood transfusions.

For a blood transfusion to be safe and successful, ABO and Rh blood groups of the donor and the recipient must be compatible. If they are not, the red blood cells from the donated blood can agglutinate and cause clogging of blood vessels and slow and/or stop the circulation of blood to various parts of the body. The agglutinated red blood cells can also hemolyze (dissolve or be destroyed), and their contents leak out in the body. This can be very dangerous, even life threatening to the patient. Before blood can be administered to a patient, a type and crossmatch must be performed. This means mixing the donor cells with the recipient's serum and watching for agglutination. If none occurs, the blood is considered compatible. Even though the blood is checked for compatibility, blood transfusion reactions can still occur and usually involve fever and chills. These reactions typically begin during the first 15 minutes of the transfusion. See Table 10.3 for blood group compatibilities.

Plasma

The fluid part of the blood is called **plasma**. Clear and somewhat straw-colored, it comprises about 55% of the total volume of blood and is composed of water (91%) and chemical compounds (9%). Plasma is the circulation medium of blood cells, providing nutritive substances to various body structures and removing waste products of metabolism from body structures. There are four major plasma proteins: **albumin**, **globulin**, **fibrinogen**, and **prothrombin**.

LYMPHATIC SYSTEM

The **lymphatic system** is a vessel system apart from, but connected to, the circulatory system (Figure 10.5 ■). Lymph is a filtrate of blood. The lymphatic system returns fluids from tissue spaces to the bloodstream (Figure 10.6 ■). The lymphatic system is composed of *lymphatic capillaries*, *lymphatic vessels*, *lymphatic ducts*, and *lymph nodes*.

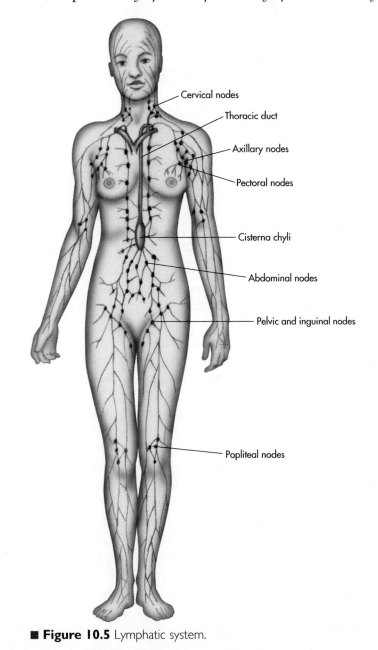

Cervical nodes

Thoracic duct

Axillary nodes

Pectoral nodes

Cisterna chyli

Abdominal nodes

Pelvic and inguinal nodes

Popliteal nodes

■ **Figure 10.5** Lymphatic system.

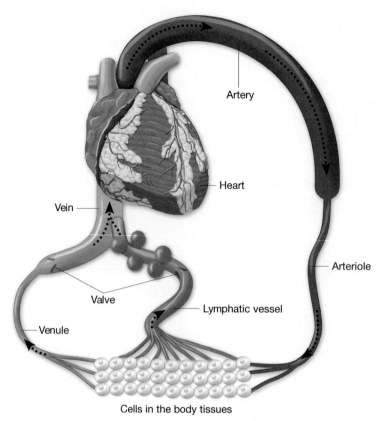

Artery

Heart

Vein

Arteriole

Valve

Lymphatic vessel

Venule

Cells in the body tissues

■ **Figure 10.6** Lymphatic vessels pick up excess tissue fluid, purify it in the lymph nodes, and then return it to the circulatory system.

The system conveys lymph from the tissues to the blood. **Lymph** is a clear, colorless, alkaline fluid that is about 95% water. The principal component of lymph is fluid from plasma that has seeped out of capillary walls into spaces among the body tissues. Lymph contains proteins (serum albumin, serum globulin, serum fibrinogen), salts, organic substances (urea, creatinine, neutral fats, glucose), and water. Cells present are principally lymphocytes, formed in the lymph nodes and other lymphatic tissues. Lymph from the intestines contains fats and other substances absorbed from the intestines.

The lymphatic system can be broadly divided into the conducting system and the lymphoid tissue. The conducting system carries the lymph and consists of tubular vessels that include the lymph capillaries, the lymph vessels, and the right and left thoracic ducts. The lymphoid tissue is primarily involved in immune responses and consists of lymphocytes and other white blood cells enmeshed in connective tissue through which the lymph passes. Regions of the lymphoid tissue that are densely packed with lymphocytes are known as *lymphoid follicles*. Lymphoid tissue can either be structurally well organized as lymph nodes or may consist of loosely organized lymphoid follicles known as the mucosa-associated lymphoid tissue (MALT).

The thymus and the bone marrow constitute the primary lymphoid tissues involved in the production and early selection of lymphocytes. Secondary lymphoid tissue provides the environment for the foreign or altered native molecules (antigens) to interact with the lymphocytes. It is exemplified by the lymph nodes, and the lymphoid follicles in the tonsils and spleen, that are associated with the mucosa-associated lymphoid tissue (MALT).

Review Table 10.1 for an at-a-glance look at the lymphatic system.

ACCESSORY ORGANS

The accessory organs of the lymphatic system includes the spleen, the tonsils, and the thymus. See Figure 10.7 ■ and Table 10.1.

Spleen

The **spleen** is a soft, dark red oval body lying in the upper left quadrant of the abdomen. It is the major site of erythrocyte destruction (old erythrocytes over 80–120 days). It serves as a reservoir for blood. The spleen plays an essential role in the immune response and acts as a filter, removing microorganisms from the blood.

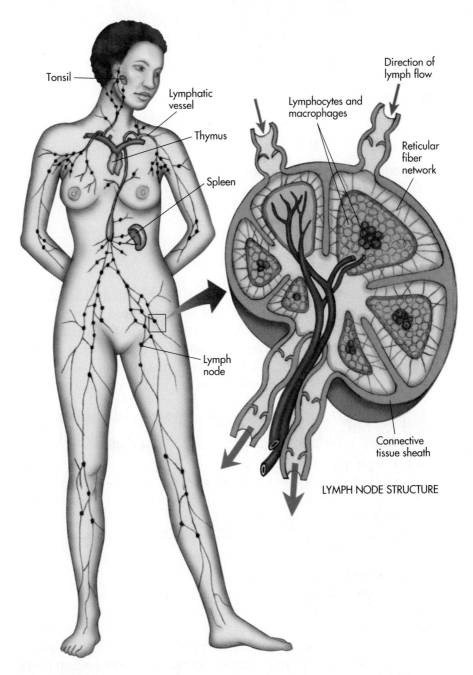

Tonsil

Lymphatic vessel

Thymus

Spleen

Lymph node

Direction of lymph flow

Lymphocytes and macrophages

Reticular fiber network

Connective tissue sheath

LYMPH NODE STRUCTURE

■ **Figure 10.7** Tonsils, lymph nodes, thymus, spleen, and lymphatic vessels with an expanded view of a lymph node.

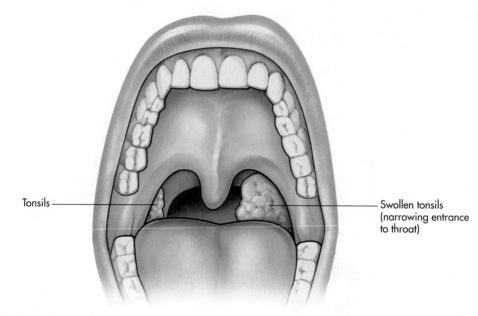

Tonsils

Swollen tonsils
(narrowing entrance
to throat)

■ **Figure 10.8** Tonsils—normal and enlarged.

Tonsils

The **tonsils** are lymphoid masses located in depressions of the mucous membranes of the face and pharynx. They consist of the *palatine tonsil, pharyngeal tonsil* (adenoid), and the *lingual tonsil.* The tonsils filter bacteria and aid in the formation of white blood cells. See Figure 10.8 ■

Thymus

The **thymus** is considered to be one of the endocrine glands, but because of its function and appearance, it is a part of the lymphoid system. Located in the mediastinal cavity, the thymus plays an essential role in the formation of antibodies and the development of the immune response in the newborn. It manufactures infection-fighting **T cells** and helps distinguish normal T cells from those that attack the body's own tissue. T cells are important in the body's cellular immune response.

LIFE SPAN CONSIDERATIONS

The **thymus gland** plays an important role in the development of the immune response in the newborn. At birth, the average weight of the thymus is 10–15 g. It attains a weight of 40 g at puberty, after which it begins to undergo involution, which replaces the thymus with adipose and connective tissue.

IMMUNE SYSTEM

The **immune system** is part of the defense mechanism of the body. It consists of the tissues, organs, and physiological processes used by the body to identify and protect against abnormal cells, foreign substances, and foreign tissue cells that may have been transplanted into the body. Many of these tissues and organs are part of the lymphatic system.

Fortunately, the average, healthy human body is equipped with natural defenses that assist it in fighting off disease and cancer. These natural defenses are intact skin, the cleansing action of the body's secretions (such as tears, mucus), white blood cells, body chemicals (such as hormones, enzymes), and antibodies. As long as the immune system is intact and functioning properly, it can defend the body against invading foreign substances and cancer.

Immunity is the state of being immune to or protected from a disease, especially an infectious disease. This state is usually induced by having been exposed to the antigenic marker of an organism that invades the body or by having been immunized with a vaccine capable of stimulating production of specific antibodies. There are several ways that immunity can be described and some of these ways are described here.

Passive immunity is acquired through transfer of antibodies or activated T-cells from an immune host, and is short lived, usually lasting only a few months; whereas **active immunity** is induced in the host itself by antigen, and lasts much longer, sometimes lifelong. **Humoral immunity** is the aspect of immunity that is mediated by secreted antibodies, whereas the protection provided by **cell-mediated immunity** involves T-lymphocytes alone.

Immune Response

The **immune response** is the reaction of the body to foreign substances and the means by which it protects the body. It is a complex function; the following sections provide an overview of how the immune response works.

The immune response can be described as humoral (pertaining to body fluids) immunity or antibody-mediated immunity and cellular immunity or cell-mediated immunity.

Humoral or Antibody-Mediated Immunity

Humoral immunity or **antibody-mediated immunity** involves the production of plasma lymphocytes (B cells) in response to antigen exposure with subsequent formation of antibodies. Humoral immunity is a major defense against bacterial infections. An **antigen** is any substance to which the immune system can respond. For example, it may be a foreign substance from the environment such as chemicals, bacteria, viruses, or pollen. If the immune system encounters an antigen that is not found on the body's own cells, it will launch an attack against that antigen.

Antibodies are developed in response to a specific antigen. An antibody is also referred to as an *immunoglobulin;* it is a complex glycoprotein produced by B lymphocytes in response to the presence of an antigen. Antibodies neutralize or destroy antigens in several ways. They can initiate destruction of the antigen by activating the complement system, neutralizing toxins released by bacteria, opsonizing (coating) the antigen, or forming a complex to stimulate phagocytosis, promoting antigen clumping or preventing the antigen from adhering to host cells. See Table 10.4 ■ for the five classes of antibodies: IgG, IgM, IgA, IgE, and IgD.

Cellular or Cell-Mediated Immunity

Cellular immunity or cell-mediated immunity involves the production of lymphocytes (T cells) and NK (natural killer) cells that are capable of attacking foreign cells, normal cells infected with viruses, and cancer cells.

Four general phases are associated with the body's immune response to a foreign substance:

TABLE 10.4 Different Classes of Antibodies

Antibody	Functions
IgG	Crosses placenta to provide passive immunity for the newborn; opsonizes (coats) microorganisms to enhance phagocytosis; activates *complement system* (a group of proteins in the blood) *Components of complement are labeled C1–C9. Complement acts by directly killing organisms; by opsonizing an antigen; and by stimulating inflammation and the B-cell-mediated immune response*
IgM	Activates complement; is first antibody produced in response to bacterial and viral infections
IgA	Protects epithelial surfaces; activates complement; is passed to breast-feeding newborn via the colostrum (first milk after birth)
IgE	Responds to allergic reactions and some parasitic infections; triggers mast cells to release histamine, serotonin, kinins, slow-reacting substance of anaphylaxis, and the neutrophil factor, mediators that produce allergic skin reaction, asthma, and hay fever
IgD	Possibly influences B lymphocyte differentiation, but role not clear

1. The first phase recognizes the foreign substance or the invader (enemy).
2. The second phase activates the body's defenses by producing more white blood cells that are designed to seek and destroy the invader(s), especially the macrophages that eat and engulf the foreign substances and lymphocytes, B cells, and T cells (see Table 10.5 ■).
   - T cells of the helper type identify the enemy and rush to the spleen and lymph nodes, where they stimulate the production of other cells to aid in the fight of the foreign substance.
   - T cells of the natural killer (NK) type are large granular lymphocytes that also specialize in killing cells of the body that have been invaded by foreign substances and fighting cells that have turned cancerous.
   - B cells reside in the spleen or lymph nodes and produce antibodies for specific antigens.
3. The third phase is the attack phase during which the preceding defenders of the body produce antibodies and/or seek out to kill and/or remove the foreign invader. They do this by phagocytosis in which the macrophages squeeze out between the cells in the capillaries and crawl into the tissue to the site of the infection. Here they surround and eat the foreign substances that caused the infection. Other white blood cells respond to infection by producing antibodies, which are released into the bloodstream and carried to the site of the infection where they surround and immobilize the invaders. Later, the phagocytes can eat both antibody and invader.
4. The fourth phase is the slowdown phase in which the number of defenders returns to normal, following victory over the foreign invader.

TABLE 10.5 Functions of Lymphocytes

Type of Cell	Functions
T cells (thymus-dependent)	Provide cellular immunity
B cells (bone marrow–derived)	Provide humoral immunity
NK cells (natural killers)	Attack foreign cells, normal cells infected with viruses, and cancer cells

LIFE SPAN CONSIDERATIONS

The immune response declines with age, limiting the body's ability to identify and fight foreign substances such as bacteria and viruses. With aging comes the loss of the thymus cortex, which leads to a reduced production of T lymphocytes, including T cells, natural killer cells, and B lymphocytes. Frequency and severity of infections generally increase in older adults because of a decreased ability of the immune system to respond adequately to invading microorganisms.

Anatomy and Physiology Labeling

Identify the structures shown below by filling in the blanks.

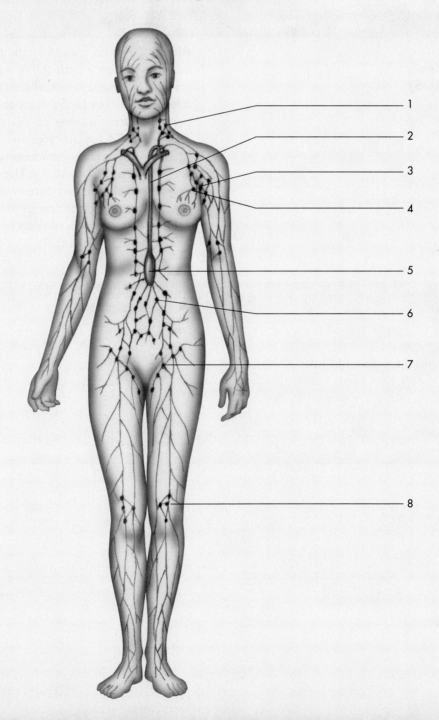

1 _____

2 _____

3 _____

4 _____

5 _____

6 _____

7 _____

8 _____

• Building Your Medical Vocabulary •

This section provides the foundation for learning medical terminology. Review the following alphabetized word list. Note how common prefixes and suffixes are repeatedly applied to word roots and combining forms to create different meanings. The word parts are color-coded: prefixes are green, suffixes are blue, and **roots/combining forms are red.**

You will find that some terms have not been divided into word parts. These are common words or specialized terms that are included to enhance your medical vocabulary. See Chapter 1, page 7, to review pronunciation guidelines.

MEDICAL WORD	WORD PARTS		DEFINITION
	Part	**Meaning**	
acquired immunodeficiency syndrome (AIDS) (ă-kwīrd ĭm″ ū-nō dĕ-fĭsh´ ĕn-sē)			AIDS is a disease caused by the human immunodeficiency virus (HIV), which is transmitted through sexual contact, exposure to infected blood or blood components, and perinatally from mother to infant. The HIV virus invades the T4 lymphocytes and, as the disease progresses, the body's immune system becomes paralyzed. See Figure 10.9 ■ The patient becomes severely weakened and potentially fatal infections can occur. *Pneumocystis carinii* pneumonia (PCP) and Kaposi's sarcoma (KS) account for many of the deaths of AIDS patients.

LIFE SPAN CONSIDERATIONS

One in 10 persons with AIDS is 50 years of age or older. Approximately 4% of all AIDS cases are among those age 65 or older. Immune function diminishes with age and AIDS infection usually progresses more quickly in older adults.

The main form of treatment of AIDS is with antiviral therapy that suppresses the replication of the HIV virus. This treatment involves a combination of several antiretroviral agents, called *highly active antiretroviral therapy (HAART),* and has been highly effective in reducing the number of HIV particles in the bloodstream (as measured by a blood test called the *viral load*). This can help the immune system recover and improve the T cell count.

MEDICAL WORD	WORD PARTS		DEFINITION
	Part	Meaning	

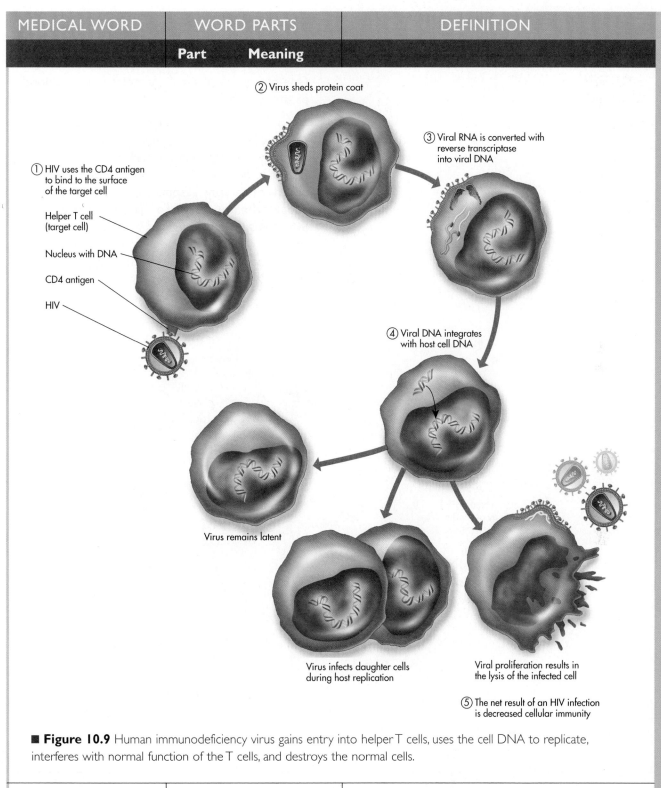

② Virus sheds protein coat

③ Viral RNA is converted with reverse transcriptase into viral DNA

① HIV uses the CD4 antigen to bind to the surface of the target cell

Helper T cell (target cell)

Nucleus with DNA

CD4 antigen

HIV

④ Viral DNA integrates with host cell DNA

Virus remains latent

Virus infects daughter cells during host replication

Viral proliferation results in the lysis of the infected cell

⑤ The net result of an HIV infection is decreased cellular immunity

■ **Figure 10.9** Human immunodeficiency virus gains entry into helper T cells, uses the cell DNA to replicate, interferes with normal function of the T cells, and destroys the normal cells.

agglutination (ă-glōō″ tĭ-nā′ shŭn)	agglutinat -ion	clumping process	Process of clumping together, as of blood cells that are incompatible

MEDICAL WORD	WORD PARTS		DEFINITION
	Part	**Meaning**	
albumin (ăl-bū′ mĭn)			One of a group of simple proteins found in blood plasma and serum
allergy (ăl′ ĕr-jē)	all -ergy	other work	An individual hypersensitivity to a substance that is usually harmless. **Allergic rhinitis** is commonly known as *hay fever*. It is typically caused by the pollens of certain seasonal plants and occurs in people who are allergic to these substances. Symptoms include coughing, headache, sneezing, and itchy nose, mouth, and eyes. See Figure 10.10 ■ This same reaction occurs with allergy to mold, animal dander, dust, and similar inhaled allergens.

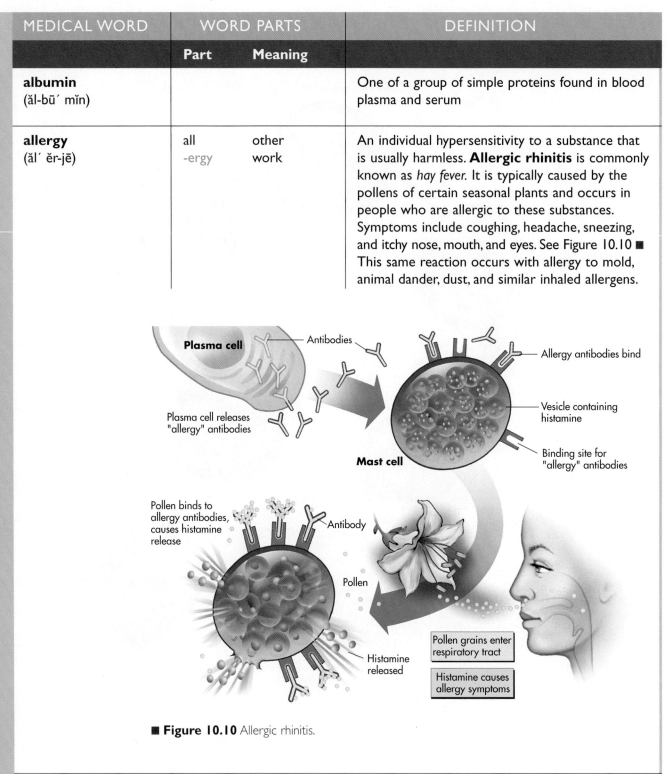

■ **Figure 10.10** Allergic rhinitis.

MEDICAL WORD	WORD PARTS		DEFINITION
	Part	Meaning	
anaphylaxis (ăn″ ă-fĭ-lăk´ sĭs)	ana- -phylaxis	up protection	Unusual or exaggerated allergic reaction to foreign proteins or other substances. It can occur suddenly, be life threatening, and affect the whole body. During an anaphylactic allergic reaction, tissues in different parts of the body release histamine and other substances. This causes constriction of the airways, resulting in wheezing, difficulty breathing, and gastrointestinal symptoms such as abdominal pain, cramps, vomiting, and diarrhea. See Figure 10.11 ■ Anaphylaxis is an emergency condition that requires immediate professional medical attention. Shock can occur as a result of lowered blood pressure and blood volume. Hives and angioedema (hives on the lips, eyelids, throat, and/or tongue) often occur, and angioedema could be severe enough to cause obstruction of the airway. Prolonged anaphylaxis can cause heart arrhythmias.

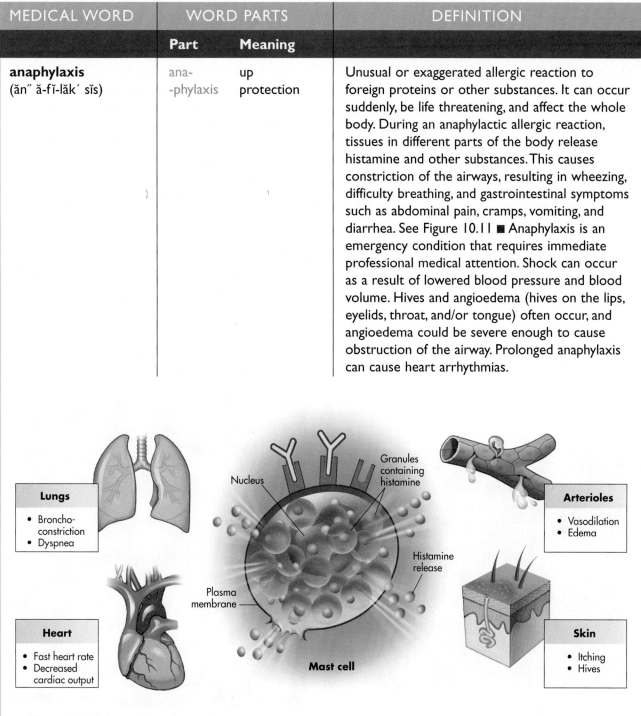

■ **Figure 10.11** Symptoms of anaphylaxis.

MEDICAL WORD	WORD PARTS		DEFINITION
	Part	Meaning	
anemia (ă-nē′ mĭ-ă)	an- -emia	lack of blood condition	Literally *a lack of red blood cells,* it is a reduction in the number of circulating red blood cells, the amount of the hemoglobin, or the volume of packed red cells (hematocrit). A normal red blood cell is biconcave with no nuclei and transports oxygen and carbon dioxide. See Figure 10.12 ■ Symptoms of anemia are due to tissue **hypoxia**, or lack of oxygen. General symptoms include pallor, fatigue, dizziness, headaches, decreased exercise tolerance, tachycardia, and shortness of breath (SOB). There are many types and causes of anemia. Iron-deficiency anemia (see Figure 10.13 ■) occurs when there is an increased iron requirement, impaired absorption of iron, or hemorrhage. Other types of anemias include hemolytic, pernicious, vitamin B_{12} deficiency, folic acid deficiency, sickle cell (see Figure 10.14 ■), and thalassemia.

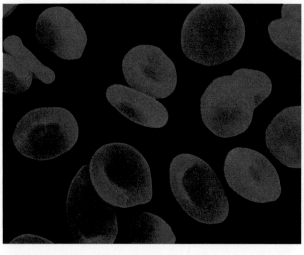

■ **Figure 10.12** Normal red blood cells.

(Source: Dr. Gopal Murti/Science Photo Library/Custom Medical Stock Photo, Inc.)

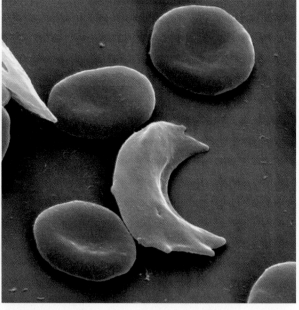

■ **Figure 10.13** Iron deficiency anemia blood cells.

(Source: Oliver Meckes & Nicole Ottawa/Photo Researchers, Inc.)

MEDICAL WORD	WORD PARTS		DEFINITION
	Part	Meaning	

Hemoglobin S and Red Blood Cell Sickling

Sickle cell anemia is caused by an inherited autosomal recessive defect in Hb synthesis. Sickle cell hemoglobin (HbS) differs from normal hemoglobin only in the substitution of the amino acid valine for glutamine in both beta chains of the hemoglobin molecule.

When HbS is oxygenated, it has the same globular shape as normal hemoglobin. However, when HbS loses its oxygen, it becomes insoluble in intracellular fluid and crystallizes into rodlike structures. Clusters of rods form polymers (long chains) that bend the erythrocyte into the characteristic crescent shape of the sickle cell.

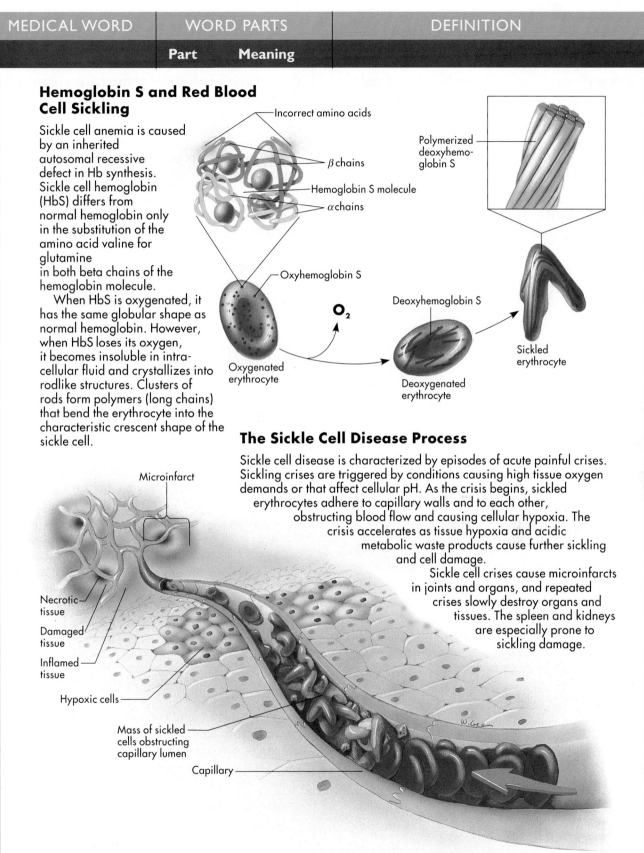

Incorrect amino acids

β chains

Hemoglobin S molecule

α chains

Polymerized deoxyhemo-globin S

Oxyhemoglobin S

Oxygenated erythrocyte

O₂

Deoxyhemoglobin S

Deoxygenated erythrocyte

Sickled erythrocyte

The Sickle Cell Disease Process

Sickle cell disease is characterized by episodes of acute painful crises. Sickling crises are triggered by conditions causing high tissue oxygen demands or that affect cellular pH. As the crisis begins, sickled erythrocytes adhere to capillary walls and to each other, obstructing blood flow and causing cellular hypoxia. The crisis accelerates as tissue hypoxia and acidic metabolic waste products cause further sickling and cell damage.

Sickle cell crises cause microinfarcts in joints and organs, and repeated crises slowly destroy organs and tissues. The spleen and kidneys are especially prone to sickling damage.

Microinfarct

Necrotic tissue

Damaged tissue

Inflamed tissue

Hypoxic cells

Mass of sickled cells obstructing capillary lumen

Capillary

■ **Figure 10.14** Sickle cell anemia. The clinical manifestations of sickle cell anemia result from pathologic changes to structures and systems throughout the body.

MEDICAL WORD	WORD PARTS		DEFINITION
	Part	**Meaning**	
anisocytosis (ăn-ī″ sō-sĭ-tō′ sĭs)	anis/o cyt -osis	unequal cell condition	Condition in which the erythrocytes are unequal in size and shape
antibody (ăn′ tĭ-bŏd″ ē)	anti- -body	against body	Protein substance produced in the body in response to an invading foreign substance (antigen)
anticoagulant (ăn″ tĭ-kō-ăg′ ū-lănt)	anti- coagul -ant	against clots forming	Substance that works against the formation of blood clots; a class of medication used in certain patients to prevent blood from clotting; a chemical compound used in medical equipment, such as test tubes, blood transfusion bags, and renal dialysis equipment. See Drug Highlights.
antigen (ăn′ tĭ-jĕn)	anti- -gen	against formation, produce	Invading foreign substance that induces the formation of antibodies
autoimmune disease (aw″ tō-ĭm-mūn)			Condition in which the body's immune system becomes defective and produces antibodies against itself. Hemolytic anemia, rheumatoid arthritis, myasthenia gravis, and scleroderma are considered to be autoimmune diseases.

LIFE SPAN CONSIDERATIONS

The incidence of **autoimmune diseases** increases with aging, most likely due to a decreased ability of antibodies to differentiate between self and nonself. Failure of the immune response system to recognize mutant, or abnormal, cells could be the reason for the high incidence of cancer associated with increasing age.

MEDICAL WORD	WORD PARTS		DEFINITION
autotransfusion (aw″ tō-trăns-fū′ zhŭn)	auto- trans- fus -ion	self across to pour process	Process of reinfusing a patient's own blood. Methods used include *harvesting* the blood 1–3 weeks before elective surgery; *salvaging* intraoperative blood; and *collecting* blood from trauma or selected surgical patients for reinfusion within 4 hours.
basophil (baso) (bā′ sō-fĭl)	bas/o -phil	base attraction	A white blood cell that has an attraction for a base dye; a circulating granulocyte that is essential to the nonspecific immune response to inflammation because of its role in releasing histamine and other chemicals that act on blood vessels

MEDICAL WORD	WORD PARTS		DEFINITION
	Part	**Meaning**	
blood			Fluid that circulates through the heart, arteries, veins, and capillaries
coagulable (kō-ăg´ ū-lăb-l)	coagul -able	to clot capable	Capable of forming a clot
corpuscle (kŏr´ pŭs-ĕl)			Blood cell
creatinemia (krē˝ ă-tĭn-ē´ mĭ-ă)	creatin -emia	flesh, creatine blood condition	Excess of creatine (nitrogenous compound produced by metabolic processes) in the blood
embolus (ĕm´ bō-lŭs)			Blood clot carried in the bloodstream. A mass of undissolved matter present in a blood or lymphatic vessel and brought there by the blood or lymph current. Emboli can be solid, liquid, or gaseous.
eosinophil (eos, eosin) (ē˝ ŏ-sĭn´ ō-fĭl)	eosin/o -phil	rose-colored attraction	A white blood cell that stains readily with an acid stain; attraction for the rose-colored stain; type of granulocytic white blood cell that destroys parasitic organisms and plays a major role in allergic reactions
erythroblast (ĕ-rĭth´ rō-blăst)	erythr/o -blast	red immature cell, germ cell	Immature red blood cell that is found only in bone marrow and still contains a nucleus
erythrocyte (ĕ-rĭth´ rō-sīt)	erythr/o -cyte	red cell	Mature red blood cell that does not contain a nucleus
erythrocytosis (ĕ-rĭth˝ rō-sī-tō´ sĭs)	erythr/o cyt -osis	red cell condition	Abnormal condition in which there is an increase in production of red blood cells
erythropoiesis (ĕ-rĭth˝ rō-poy-ē´ sĭs)	erythr/o -poiesis	red formation	Formation of red blood cells
erythropoietin (ĕ-rĭth˝ rō-poy´ ĕ-tĭn)	erythr/o poiet -in	red formation chemical	Hormone that stimulates the production of red blood cells
extravasation (ĕks-trä˝ vă-sā´ shŭn)	extra vas(at) -ion	beyond vessel process	Process by which fluids and/or medications (IVs) escape from the blood vessel into surrounding tissue

MEDICAL WORD	WORD PARTS		DEFINITION
	Part	**Meaning**	
fibrin (fī′ brĭn)	fibr -in	fiber chemical	Insoluble protein formed from fibrinogen by the action of thrombin in the blood-clotting process
fibrinogen (fī-brĭn′ ō-gĕn)	fibrin/o -gen	fiber formation, produce	Blood protein converted to fibrin by the action of thrombin in the blood-clotting process
globulin (glŏb′ ū-lĭn)	globul -in	globe chemical	Plasma protein found in body fluids and cells
granulocyte (grăn′ ū-lō-sīt″)	granul/o -cyte	little grain, granular cell	Granular leukocyte (white blood cell containing granules); a polymorphonuclear white blood cell (includes neutrophils, eosinophils, or basophils)
hematocrit **(Hct, HCT)** (hē-măt′ ō-krĭt)	hemat/o -crit	blood to separate	Blood test that separates solids from plasma in the blood by centrifuging the blood sample; the percent of solid components to the plasma (liquid) components of blood and varies with age and gender: men range 40–54%; women range 37–47%; children 35–49%; newborn 49–54%. See Figure 10.1.
hematologist (hē″ mă-tŏl′ ō-jĭst)	hemat/o log -ist	blood study of one who specializes	Literally means *one who specializes in the study of the blood*; physician who specializes in the diagnosis and treatment of blood diseases
hematology (hē″ mă-tŏl′ ō-jē)	hemat/o -logy	blood study of	Literally means *study of the blood*
hematoma (hē″ mă-tō′ mă)	hemat -oma	blood mass, fluid collection	Collection of blood that has escaped from a blood vessel into the surrounding tissues; results from trauma or incomplete hemostasis after surgery. See Figure 10.15 ■

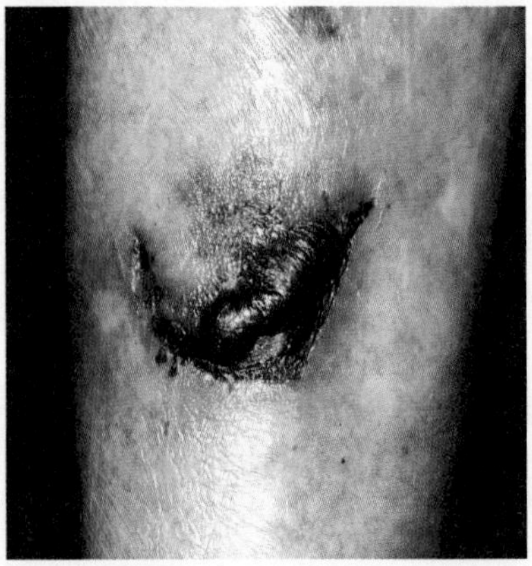

■ **Figure 10.15** Traumatic hematoma.

(Courtesy of Jason L. Smith, MD)

MEDICAL WORD	WORD PARTS		DEFINITION
	Part	**Meaning**	
hemochromatosis (hē″ mō-krō″ mă-tō′ sĭs)	hem/o chromat -osis	blood color condition	Genetic disease condition in which iron is not metabolized properly and accumulates in body tissues. The skin has a bronze hue, the liver becomes enlarged, and diabetes and cardiac failure can occur.
hemoglobin **(Hb, Hgb, HGB)** (hē″ mō-glō′ bĭn)	hem/o -globin	blood globe, protein	Blood protein; the iron-containing pigment of red blood cells that carries oxygen from the lungs to the tissues
hemolysis (hē-mŏl′ ĭ-sĭs)	hem/o -lysis	blood destruction	Destruction of red blood cells
hemophilia (hē″ mō-fĭl′ ĭ-ă)	hem/o -philia	blood attraction	Hereditary blood disease characterized by prolonged coagulation and tendency to bleed
hemorrhage (hĕm′ ĕ-rĭj)	hem/o -rrhage	blood bursting forth	Literally means *bursting forth of blood*; bleeding. See Figure 10.16 ■

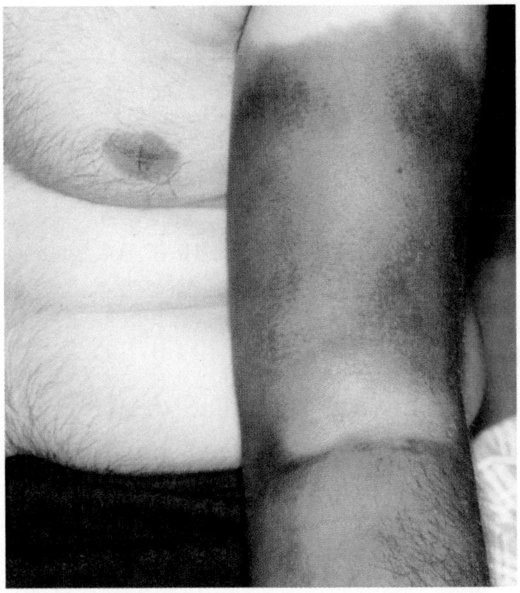

■ **Figure 10.16** Hemorrhage, vein.
(Courtesy of Jason L. Smith, MD)

MEDICAL WORD	WORD PARTS		DEFINITION
	Part	**Meaning**	
hemostasis (hē-mŏs´ tā-sĭs)	hem/o -stasis	blood control, stop, stand still	Control or stopping of bleeding. See Figure 10.17 ■

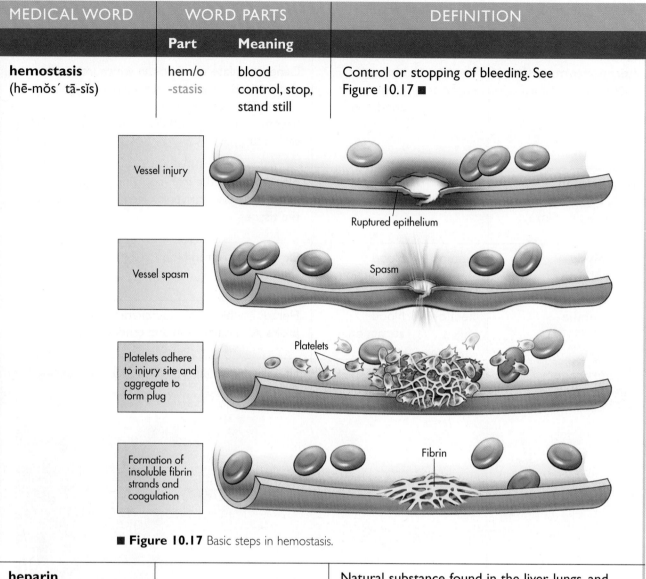

■ **Figure 10.17** Basic steps in hemostasis.

MEDICAL WORD	WORD PARTS		DEFINITION
heparin (hĕp´ ă-rĭn)			Natural substance found in the liver, lungs, and other body tissues that inhibits blood clotting (anticoagulant). As a drug, heparin is used during certain types of surgery and in the treatment of deep venous thrombosis or pulmonary infarction. It can be administered by either subcutaneous or intravenous injection.
hypercalcemia (hī˝ pĕr-kăl-sē´ mĭ-ă)	hyper- calc -emia	excessive lime, calcium blood condition	Pathological condition of excessive amounts of calcium in the blood
hyperglycemia (hī˝ pĕr-glī-sē´ mĭ-ă)	hyper- glyc -emia	excessive sweet, sugar blood condition	Pathological condition of excessive amounts of sugar in the blood
hyperlipidemia (hī˝ pĕr-lĭp-ĭd-ē´ mĭ-ă)	hyper- lipid -emia	excessive fat blood condition	Pathological condition of excessive amounts of lipids (fat) in the blood

MEDICAL WORD	WORD PARTS		DEFINITION
	Part	Meaning	
hypoglycemia (hī″ pō-glī-sē′ mĭ-ă)	hypo- glyc -emia	deficient sweet, sugar blood condition	Condition of deficient amounts of sugar in the blood; low blood sugar
hypoxia (hī″ pŏks′ ē-ă)	hyp- -oxia	deficient oxygen	Deficient amount of oxygen in the blood, cells, and tissues; also known as *anoxia* and *hypoxemia*
immunoglobulin (Ig) (ĭm″ ū-nō-glŏb′ ū-lĭn)	immun/o globul -in	immunity globe chemical	Blood protein capable of acting as an antibody. The five major types are IgA, IgD, IgE, IgG, and IgM.
Kaposi's sarcoma (KS) (kăp′ ō-sēz săr-kō′ mă)			Malignant neoplasm that causes violaceous (violet-colored) vascular lesions and general lymphadenopathy (diseased lymph nodes); it is the most common AIDS-related tumor. See Figure 10.18 ∎
leukapheresis (loo″ kă-fĕ-rē′ sĭs)	leuk/a -pheresis	white removal	Separation of white blood cells from the blood, which are then transfused back into the patient
leukemia (loo-kē′ mē-ă)	leuk -emia	white blood condition	Disease of the blood characterized by overproduction of leukocytes. Common types include chronic lymphocytic leukemia (CLL) and acute lymphocytic leukemia (ALL). CLL is a malignancy (cancer) of the white blood cells (lymphocytes) characterized by a slow, progressive increase of these cells in the blood and the bone marrow. ALL is a cancer of the lymph cells. It is characterized by large numbers of immature white blood cells that resemble lymphoblasts. These cells can be found in the blood, the bone marrow, the lymph nodes, the spleen, and other organs.
leukocyte (loo′ kō-sīt)	leuk/o -cyte	white cell	White blood cell

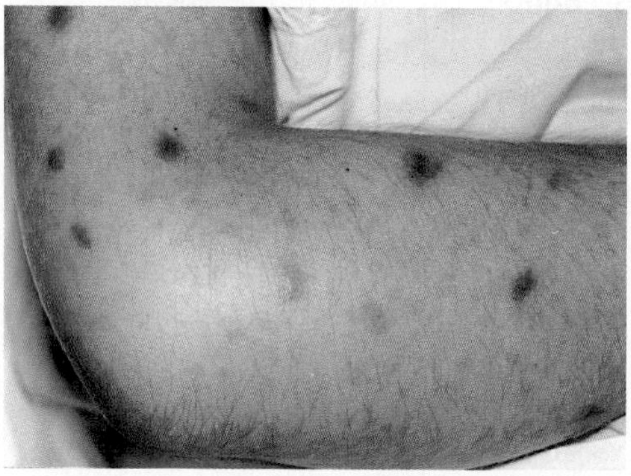

∎ **Figure 10.18**
Kaposi's sarcoma.
(Courtesy of Jason L. Smith, MD)

MEDICAL WORD	WORD PARTS		DEFINITION
	Part	**Meaning**	
leukocytopenia (loo″ kō-sĭ″ tō-pē′ nĭ-ă)	leuk/o cyt/o -penia	white cell lack of	Lack of white blood cells
lymph (lĭmf)			Clear, colorless, alkaline fluid found in the lymphatic vessels
lymphadenitis (lĭm-făd″ ĕn-ī′ tĭs)	lymph aden -itis	lymph gland inflammation	Inflammation of the lymph glands
lymphadenotomy (lĭm-făd″ ĕ-nō tō-mē)	lymph aden/o -tomy	lymph gland incision	Incision into a lymph gland
lymphangiology (lĭm-făn″ jē-ŏl′ ō-jē)	lymph angi/o -logy	lymph vessel study of	Study of the lymphatic vessels
lymphangitis (lĭm″ făn-jī′ tĭs)	lymph ang -itis	lymph vessel inflammation	Inflammation of lymphatic vessels. See Figure 10.19 ■

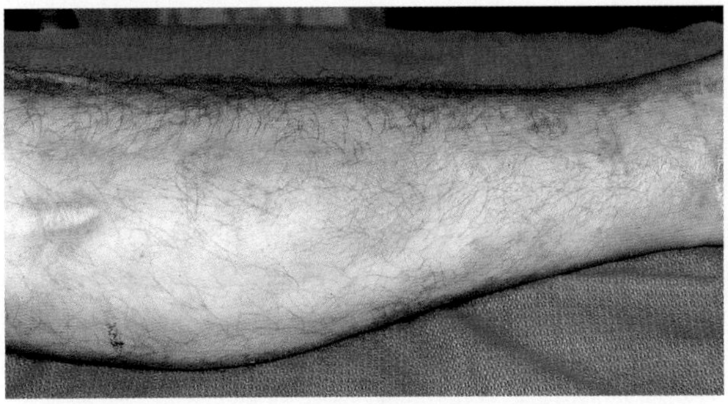

■ **Figure 10.19**
Lymphangitis.
(Courtesy of Jason L. Smith, MD)

MEDICAL WORD	WORD PARTS		DEFINITION
lymphedema (lĭmf-ĕ-dē′ mă)	lymph -edema	lymph swelling	Abnormal accumulation of lymph in the interstitial spaces. See Figure 10.20 ■

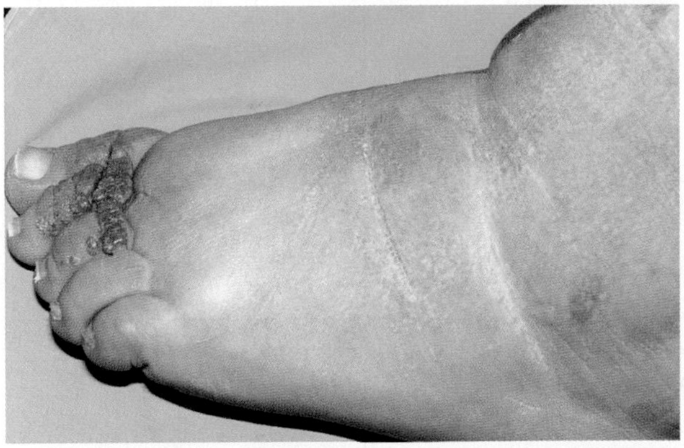

■ **Figure 10.20**
Chronic lymphedema.
(Courtesy of Jason L. Smith, MD)

MEDICAL WORD	WORD PARTS		DEFINITION
	Part	Meaning	
lymphoma (lĭm-fō´ mă)	lymph -oma	lymph mass, fluid collection	Lymphoid neoplasm, usually malignant. See Figures 10.21 ■ and 10.22 ■ Lymphomas are identified as Hodgkin's disease or non-Hodgkin's lymphomas. Radiation therapy is the primary treatment for early-stage Hodgkin's disease.

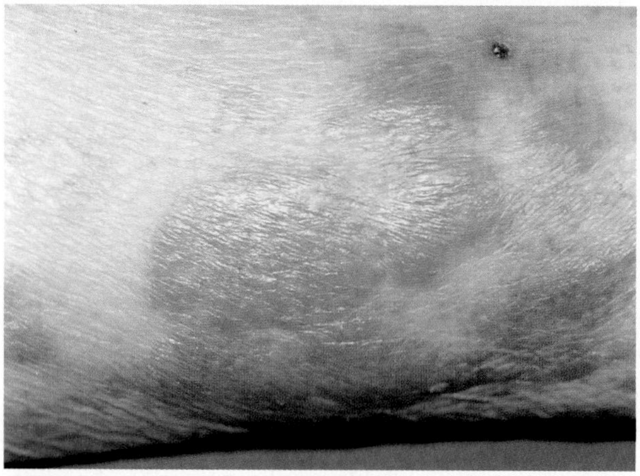

■ **Figure 10.21** Lymphoma.
(Courtesy of Jason L. Smith, MD)

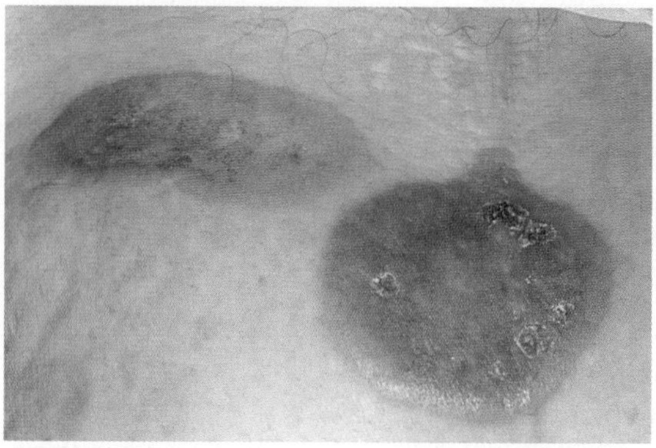

■ **Figure 10.22** Cutaneous T cell lymphoma.
(Courtesy of Jason L. Smith, MD)

lymphostasis (lĭm-fō´ stā-sĭs)	lymph/o -stasis	lymph control, stop, stand still	Control or stopping of the flow of lymph
macrocyte (măk´ rō-sīt)	macr/o -cyte	large cell	Abnormally large erythrocyte
monocyte (mono) (mŏn´ ō-sīt)	mono- -cyte	one cell	Largest leukocyte, which has one nucleus
mononucleosis (mŏn″ ō-nū″ klē-ō´ sĭs)	mono- nucle -osis	one kernel, nucleus condition	Condition of excessive amounts of mononuclear leukocytes in the blood. See Figure 10.23 ■

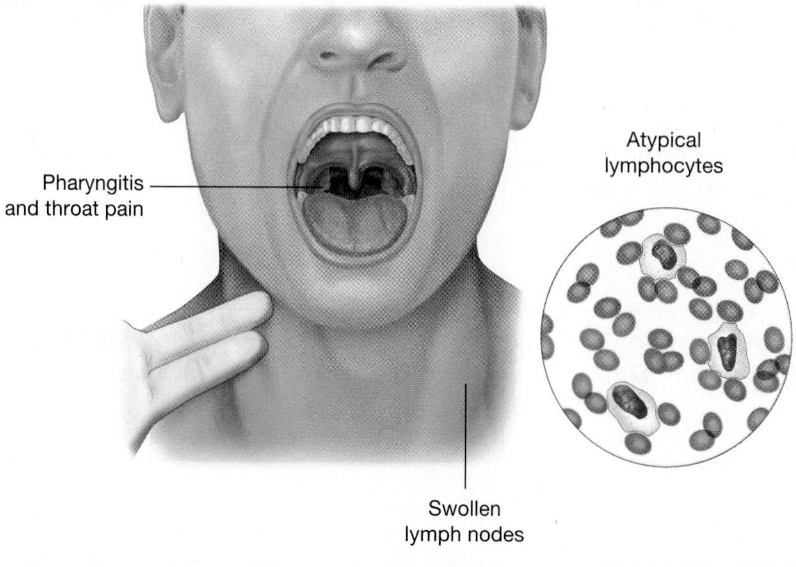

■ **Figure 10.23** Mononucleosis is caused by the Epstein–Barr virus. Symptoms of the infectious disease are swollen palatine tonsils (pharyngitis), swollen cervical lymph nodes (lymphadenopathy), high fever, and a blood sample that shows atypical lymphocytes.

Pharyngitis and throat pain

Atypical lymphocytes

Swollen lymph nodes

MEDICAL WORD	WORD PARTS		DEFINITION
	Part	**Meaning**	
neutrophil (nū´ trō-fĭl)	neutr/o -phil	neither attraction	Leukocyte that stains with neutral dyes
opportunistic infection (ŏp″ ŏr-too-nĭs´ tĭk)			Protozoal (PCP or toxoplasmosis), fungal/yeast (candidiasis), viral (herpes simplex), or bacterial (TB) infection that occurs when the immune system is compromised. AIDS patients are very vulnerable to these types of infections.
pancytopenia (păn″ sĭ-tō-pē´ nĭ-ă)	pan- cyt/o -penia	all cell lack of	Literally means *lack of the cellular elements of the blood*
phagocytosis (făg″ ō-sī-tō´ sĭs)	phag/o cyt -osis	eat, engulf cell condition	Engulfing and eating of particulate substances such as bacteria, protozoa, cells and cell debris, dust particles, and colloids by phagocytes (leukocytes or macrophages)
plasma (plăz´ ma)			Fluid part of the blood
plasmapheresis (plăz″ mă-fĕr-ē´ sĭs)	plasma -pheresis	a thing formed, plasma removal	Removal of blood from the body and centrifuging it to separate the plasma from the blood and reinfusing the cellular elements back into the patient
Pneumocystis carinii (nū″ mō-sĭs´ tĭs kă-rī´ nē-ĭ)			Protozoan that causes *Pneumocystis carinii* pneumonia
***Pneumocystis carinii* pneumonia (PCP)**			Opportunistic infection that is prevalent in AIDS patients; has high mortality rate if not treated
polycythemia (pŏl″ ē-sī-thē´ mĭ-ă)	poly- cyt hem -ia	many cell blood condition	Increased number of red blood cells
prothrombin (prō-thrŏm´ bĭn)	pro- thromb -in	before clot chemical	Chemical substance that interacts with calcium salts to produce thrombin

MEDICAL WORD	WORD PARTS		DEFINITION
	Part	Meaning	
radioimmunoassay (RIA) (rā″ dē-ō-ĭm″ ū-nō-ăs′ā)			Method of determining the concentration of protein-bound hormones in the blood plasma
reticulocyte (rĕ-tĭk′ ū-lō-sīt)	reticul/o -cyte	net cell	Red blood cell containing a network of granules; the last immature stage of a red blood cell
retrovirus (rĕt″ rō-vī′ rŭs)			Virus that contains a unique enzyme called *reverse transcriptase* that allows it to replicate within new host cells. HIV is a retrovirus; once it enters the cell, it can replicate and kill the cells, some lymphocytes directly, and disrupt the functioning of the remaining CD4 cells.

fyi Although the HIV virus can remain inactive in infected cells for years, antibodies are produced to its proteins, a process known as **seroconversion**. These antibodies are usually detectable 6 weeks to 6 months after the initial infection. Helper T or CD4 cells are the primary cells infected by HIV; these cells are involved in cellular immunity and the body's immune response in fighting off infection and disease. The loss of these CD4 cells leads to immunodeficiencies and developing opportunistic infections. A normal CD4 lymphocyte count is 1,000–1,300 cells/mm^3. It is not uncommon for an HIV-infected person's count to be 180 cells/mm^3.

MEDICAL WORD	WORD PARTS		DEFINITION
septicemia (sĕp″ tĭ-sē′ mĭ-ă)	septic -emia	putrefying blood condition	Pathological condition in which bacteria are present in the blood
seroculture (sē′ rō-kŭl″ chūr)	ser/o -culture	whey, serum cultivation	Bacterial culture of blood
serum (sē′ rŭm)	ser(a) -um	whey, serum tissue	Blood serum is the clear, thin, and sticky fluid part of the blood that remains after blood clots; any clear watery fluid that has been separated from its more solid elements, such as the exudates from a blister
sideropenia (sĭd″ ĕr-ō-pē′ nĭ-ă)	sider/o -penia	iron lack of	Lack of iron in the blood
splenomegaly (splē″ nō-mĕg′ ă-lē)	splen/o -megaly	spleen enlargement	Abnormal enlargement of the spleen
stem cell			A bone marrow cell that gives rise to different types of blood cells
thalassemia (thăl-ă-sē′ mĭ-ă)	thalass -emia	sea blood condition	Hereditary anemias occurring in populations bordering the Mediterranean Sea and in Southeast Asia

MEDICAL WORD	WORD PARTS		DEFINITION
	Part	Meaning	
thrombectomy (thrŏm-bĕk´ tō-mē)	thromb -ectomy	clot surgical excision	Surgical excision of a blood clot
thrombin (thrŏm´ bĭn)	thromb -in	clot chemical	Blood enzyme that converts fibrinogen into fibrin
thrombocyte (thrŏm´ bō-sīt)	thromb/o -cyte	clot cell	Clotting cell; *a blood platelet*
thromboplastin (thrŏm″ bō-plăs´ tĭn)	thromb/o plast -in	clot a developing chemical	Essential factor in the production of thrombin and blood clotting
thrombosis (thrŏm-bō´ sĭs)	thromb -osis	clot condition	Formation, development, or existence of a blood clot (thrombus) within the vascular system. In venous thrombosis (thrombophlebitis), a thrombus forms on the wall of a vein, accompanied by inflammation and obstructed blood flow. Thrombi can form in either superficial or deep veins. Deep vein thrombosis (DVT) is generally a complication of hospitalization, surgery, and immobilization. See Figure 10.24 ■

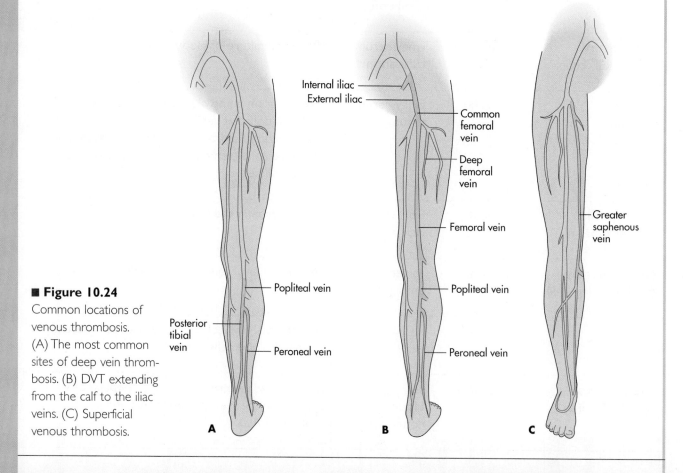

■ **Figure 10.24**
Common locations of venous thrombosis. (A) The most common sites of deep vein thrombosis. (B) DVT extending from the calf to the iliac veins. (C) Superficial venous thrombosis.

MEDICAL WORD	WORD PARTS		DEFINITION
	Part	**Meaning**	
thymoma (thĭ-mō´ mă)	thym -oma	thymus mass, fluid collection	Tumor of the thymus
tonsillectomy (tŏn″ sĭl-ĕk´ tō-mē)	tonsill -ectomy	tonsil surgical excision	Surgical excision of the tonsil. *Note that the root tonsill has two l's for tonsil. This is to form the correct spelling of the word tonsillectomy or other such words that relate to the tonsil.*
transfusion (trăns-fū″ zhŭn)	trans- fus -ion	across to pour process	Process by which blood is transferred from one individual to the vein of another
vasculitis (văs″ kŭ-lī´ tĭs)	vascul -itis	small vessel inflammation	Inflammation of a lymph or blood vessel. See Figure 10.25 ■

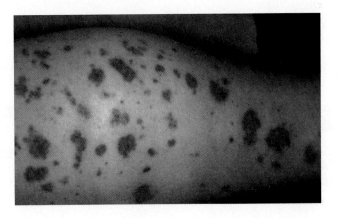

■ **Figure 10.25** Vasculitis.
(Courtesy of Jason L. Smith, MD)

• Drug Highlights •

TYPE OF DRUG	DESCRIPTION AND EXAMPLES
anticoagulants	Used in inhibiting or preventing a blood clot formation. Hemorrhage can occur at almost any site in patients on anticoagulant therapy. EXAMPLES: heparin sodium, Coumadin (warfarin sodium), and Lovenox (enoxaparin)
hemostatic agents	Used to control bleeding; can be administered systemically or topically. EXAMPLES: Amicar (aminocaproic acid) and vitamin K

TYPE OF DRUG	DESCRIPTION AND EXAMPLES
antianemic agents (*irons*)	Used to treat iron-deficiency anemia. Oral iron preparations interfere with the absorption of oral tetracycline antibiotics. These products should not be taken within 2 hours of each other. EXAMPLES: Oral iron supplements (ferrous sulfate); prescription IV medications Infed (iron dextran) and Venofer (iron sucrose)
epoetin alfa (*EPO, Procrit*)	Genetically engineered hemopoietin that stimulates the production of red blood cells. It is a recombinant version of erythropoietin and is indicated for treating anemia in patients with chronic renal failure and HIV-infected patients taking zidovudine (AZT).
other agents	Agents used in treating folic acid deficiency including Folvite (folic acid). Agents used in treating vitamin B_{12} deficiency include vitamin B_{12} (cyanocobalamin) injection.

• Diagnostic and Lab Tests •

TEST	DESCRIPTION
antinuclear antibodies (ANA) (ăn″ tĭ-nū´ klē-ăr ăn´ tĭ-bŏd″ ēs)	Blood test to identify antigen–antibody reactions. ANA antibodies are present in a number of autoimmune diseases (e.g., lupus).
bleeding time	Puncture of the earlobe or forearm to determine the time required for blood to stop flowing. With the Duke method (earlobe), 1–3 minutes is the normal time, and with the Ivy (forearm), 1–9 minutes is the normal time for the flow of blood to cease. Times longer than these can indicate thrombocytopenia, aplastic anemia, leukemia, decreased platelet count, hemophilia, and potential hemorrhage. Anticoagulant drugs delay the bleeding time.
blood typing (ABO groups and Rh factor)	Blood test to determine an individual's blood type (A, B, AB, and O) and Rh factor (can be negative [Rh–] or positive [Rh +]).
bone marrow aspiration (ăs-pĭ-rā´ shŭn)	Removal of bone marrow for examination; can be performed to determine aplastic anemia, leukemia, certain cancers, and polycythemia.
CD4 cell count	Most widely used serum blood test to monitor the progress of AIDS. CD4 count of less than $200/mm^3$ confirms AIDS diagnosis. CD4 is a protein on the surface of cells that normally helps the body's immune system fight disease. The HIV attaches itself to the protein to attack WBC, causing a failure of the patient's defense system.

TEST	DESCRIPTION
complete blood count (CBC)	Blood test that includes a hematocrit, hemoglobin, red and white blood cell count, and differential; usually part of a complete physical examination and a good indicator of hematological system.
enzyme-linked immunosorbent assay (ELISA) (ĕn´zīm-līnk´ĕd ĭm˝ū-nō- sŏr-bĕnt´ ă-sā)	Most widely used screening test for HIV. The latest generation of ELISA tests are 99.5% sensitive to HIV. Occasionally, the ELISA test will be positive for a patient without symptoms of AIDS from a low-risk group. Because this result is likely to be a false positive, the ELISA must be repeated *on the same sample of the patient's blood.* If the second ELISA is positive, the result should be confirmed by the Western blot test.
hematocrit (Hct, HCT) (hē-măt´ ō-krĭt)	Blood test performed on whole blood to determine the percentage of red blood cells in the total blood volume.
hemoglobin (Hb, Hgb, HGB) (hē˝ mō-glō´ bĭn)	Blood test to determine the amount of iron-containing pigment of the red blood cells.
immunoglobulins (Ig) (ĭm˝ ŭ-nō-glŏb´ ū-lĭns)	Serum blood test to determine the presence of IgA, IgD, IgE, IgG, and/or IgM. Lymphocytes and plasma cells produce immunoglobulins in response to antigen exposure. Increased and/or decreased values can indicate certain disease conditions.
partial thromboplastin time (PTT) (păr´ shāl thrŏm˝ bō-plăs´ tĭn)	Test performed on blood plasma to determine how long it takes for fibrin clots to form; used to regulate heparin dosage and to detect clotting disorders.
platelet count (plāt´ lĕt)	Test performed on whole blood to determine the number of thrombocytes present. Increased and/or decreased amounts can indicate certain disease conditions.
prothrombin time (PT) (prō-thrŏm´ bĭn)	Test performed on blood plasma to determine the time needed for oxalated plasma to clot; used to regulate anticoagulant drug therapy and to detect clotting disorders.
red blood count (RBC)	Test performed on whole blood to determine the number of erythrocytes present. Increased and/or decreased amounts can indicate certain disease conditions.
sedimentation rate (ESR) (sĕd˝ -ĭmĕn-tā´ shŭn)	Blood test to determine the rate at which red blood cells settle in a long, narrow tube. The distance the RBCs settle in 1 hour is the rate. Higher or lower rate can indicate certain disease conditions.
viral load	Blood test that measures the amount of HIV in the blood. Results can range from 50 to more than 1 million copies per milliliter (mL) of blood. Two tests that are used to measure viral load are bDNA and PCR.

TEST	DESCRIPTION
western blot test or immunoblot test (ĭm″ū-nō-blōt)	Used as a reference procedure to confirm the diagnosis of AIDS. In Western blot testing, HIV antigen is purified by electrophoresis (large protein molecules are suspended in a gel and separated from one another by running an electric current through the gel). If antibodies to HIV are present, a detectable antigen–antibody response occurs and a positive result is noted.
white blood count (WBC)	Blood test to determine the number of leukocytes present. Increased level indicates infection and/or inflammation and leukemia. Decreased level indicates aplastic anemia, pernicious anemia, and malaria.

• Abbreviations •

ABBREVIATION	MEANING	ABBREVIATION	MEANING
ABO	blood groups	**Ig**	immunoglobulin
AIDS	acquired immunodeficiency syndrome	**IV**	intravenous
ALL	acute lymphocytic leukemia	**KS**	Kaposi's sarcoma
ANA	antinuclear antibodies	**lymphs**	lymphocytes
AZT	zidovudine	**MALT**	mucosa-associated lymphoid tissue
baso	basophil	**mL**	milliliter
CBC	complete blood count	**mono**	monocyte
CLL	chronic lymphocytic leukemia	**NK**	natural killer (cells)
CPR	cardiopulmonary resuscitation	**PCP**	*Pneumocystis carinii* pneumonia
diff	differential count	**PT**	prothrombin time
DVT	deep vein thrombosis	**PTT**	partial thromboplastin time
ELISA	enzyme-linked immunosorbent assay	**RBC**	red blood cell (count)
eos, eosin	eosinophil	**Rh**	Rhesus (factor)
HAART	highly active antiretroviral therapy	**RIA**	radioimmunoassay
Hb, Hgb, HGB	hemoglobin	**SOB**	shortness of breath
Hct, HCT	hematocrit	**TB**	tuberculosis
HIV	human immunodeficiency virus	**WBC**	white blood cell (count)

Anatomy and Physiology

Write your answers to the following questions.

1. Name the three formed elements of blood.

   a. _____   b. _____

   c. _____

2. State the function of erythrocytes. _____

   _____

   _____

3. There are approximately _____ million erythrocytes per cubic millimeter of blood.

4. The life span of an erythrocyte is _____ .

5. State the function of leukocytes. _____

6. There are approximately _____ thousand leukocytes per cubic millimeter of blood.

7. Name the five types of leukocytes.

   a. _____   b. _____

   c. _____   d. _____

   e. _____

8. State the function of thrombocytes. _____

9. There are approximately _____ thrombocytes per cubic millimeter of blood.

10. Name the four blood types.

    a. _____   b. _____

    c. _____   d. _____

11. State the three main functions of the lymphatic system.

    a. _____

    b. _____

    c. _____

351

12. Name the three accessory organs of the lymphatic system.

a. _____

b. _____

c. _____

Word Parts

PREFIXES

Give the definitions of the following prefixes.

1. an- _____   **2.** anti- _____

3. auto- _____   **4.** ana- _____

5. extra- _____   **6.** hyper- _____

7. hypo- _____   **8.** mono- _____

9. pan- _____   **10.** poly- _____

11. pro- _____   **12.** trans- _____

13. hyp- _____

ROOTS AND COMBINING FORMS

Give the definitions of the following roots and combining forms.

1. aden _____   **2.** aden/o _____

3. agglutinat _____   **4.** all _____

5. angi/o _____   **6.** anis/o _____

7. bas/o _____   **8.** calc _____

9. chromat _____   **10.** fus _____

11. coagul _____   **12.** creatin _____

13. cyt _____   **14.** hem _____

15. cyt/o _____   **16.** eosin/o _____

17. erythr/o _____   **18.** globul _____

19. granul/o _____   **20.** hemat _____

21. hemat/o _____   **22.** hem/o _____

23. leuk _____   **24.** leuk/o _____

25. lipid _____

26. log _____

27. lymph _____

28. lymph/o _____

29. macr/o _____

30. neutr/o _____

31. nucle _____

32. phag/o _____

33. plasma _____

34. reticul/o _____

35. septic _____

36. ser/o _____

37. sider/o _____

38. fibr _____

39. splen/o _____

40. thalass _____

41. thromb _____

42. thromb/o _____

43. thym _____

44. fibrin/o _____

45. tonsill _____

46. poiet _____

47. immun/o _____

48. ang _____

49. ser (a) _____

50. plast _____

51. vas (at) _____

52. vascul _____

SUFFIXES

Give the definitions of the following suffixes.

1. -able _____

2. -ant _____

3. -blast _____

4. -body _____

5. -edema _____

6. -crit _____

7. -culture _____

8. -cyte _____

9. -ectomy _____

10. -emia _____

11. -ergy _____

12. -gen _____

13. -phylaxis _____

14. -globin _____

15. -um _____

16. -ic _____

17. -in _____

18. -ion _____

19. -ist _____

20. -itis _____

21. -logy _____

22. -lysis _____

23. -megaly _____

24. -oma _____

25. -osis _____

26. -penia _____

27. -pheresis _____

28. -phil _____

29. -philia _____

30. -poiesis _____

31. -rrhage _____

32. -stasis _____

33. -tomy _____

34. -ia _____

35. —oxia _____

Identifying Medical Terms

In the spaces provided, write the medical terms for the following meanings.

1. _____ Process of clumping together, as of blood cells that are incompatible

2. _____ An individual hypersensitivity to a substance that is usually harmless

3. _____ Protein substance produced in the body in response to an invading foreign substance

4. _____ Substance that works against the formation of blood clots

5. _____ Invading foreign substance that induces the formation of antibodies

6. _____ A white blood cell that has an attraction for a base dye

7. _____ Capable of forming a clot

8. _____ Excess of creatine in the blood

9. _____ A white blood cell that readily stains with the acid stain

10. _____ Granular leukocyte

11. _____ Literally means one who specializes in the study of the blood

12. _____ Blood protein; the iron-containing pigment of red blood cells

13. _____ Pathological condition of excessive amounts of sugar in the blood

14. _____ Pathological condition of excessive amounts of lipids (fat) in the blood

15. _____ White blood cell

16. _____ Control or stopping of the flow of lymph

17. _____ Condition of excessive amounts of mononuclear leukocytes in the blood

18. _____ Chemical substance that interacts with calcium salts to produce thrombin

19. _____ Abnormal enlargement of the spleen

20. _____ Clotting cell; blood platelet

Spelling

Circle the correct spelling of each medical term.

1. allregy / allergy

2. cretinemia / creatinemia

3. extravasation / etravasation

4. erythrocytosis / erythcytosis

5. thrombplastin / thromboplastin

6. hemacrit / hematocrit

7. hemorrhage / hemorhage

8. leukemia / lukemia

9. lymphadnotomy / lymphadenotomy

10. anaphylaxis / anphylaxis

Matching

Select the appropriate lettered meaning for each of the following words.

_____ 1. autotransfusion

_____ 2. erythrocyte

_____ 3. erythropoietin

_____ 4. extravasation

_____ 5. hemorrhage

_____ 6. immunoglobulin

_____ 7. hemochromatosis

_____ 8. radioimmunoassay

_____ 9. reticulocyte

_____10. thrombectomy

a. Method of determining the concentration of protein-bound hormones in the blood plasma

b. Genetic disease condition in which iron is not metabolized properly and accumulates in body tissues

c. Blood protein capable of acting as an antibody

d. Mature red blood cell that does not contain a nucleus

e. Hormone that stimulates the production of red blood cells

f. Bleeding

g. Process by which fluids and/or medications escape from the blood vessel into surrounding tissue

h. Process of reinfusing a patient's own blood

i. Surgical excision of a blood clot

j. Red blood cell containing a network of granules

k. White blood cell

Abbreviations

Place the correct word, phrase, or abbreviation in the space provided.

1. acquired immunodeficiency syndrome _____

2. body systems isolation _____

3. CML _____

4. hemoglobin _____

5. Hct _____

6. human immunodeficiency virus _____

7. PCP _____

8. PT _____

9. RBC _____

10. radioimmunoassay _____

Diagnostic and Laboratory Tests

Select the best answer to each multiple-choice question. Circle the letter of your choice.

1. Blood test to identify antigen–antibody reactions.
   - **a.** sedimentation rate
   - **b.** hematocrit
   - **c.** immunoglobulins
   - **d.** antinuclear antibodies

2. Blood test that includes a hematocrit, hemoglobin, red and white blood cell count, and differential.
   - **a.** blood typing
   - **b.** sedimentation rate
   - **c.** CBC
   - **d.** Hb, Hgb

3. Blood test performed on whole blood to determine the percentage of red blood cells in the total blood volume.
   - **a.** RBC
   - **b.** WBC
   - **c.** Hct
   - **d.** PTT

4. Blood test to determine the number of leukocytes present.
   - **a.** RBC
   - **b.** WBC
   - **c.** Hct
   - **d.** PTT

5. Puncture of the earlobe or forearm to determine the time required for blood to stop flowing.
   - **a.** bleeding time
   - **b.** platelet count
   - **c.** prothrombin time
   - **d.** PTT

PRACTICAL APPLICATION

MEDICAL RECORD ANALYSIS

This exercise contains information, abbreviations, and medical terminology from an actual medical record or case study that has been adapted for this text. The names and any personal information have been created by the author. Read and study each form or case study and then answer the questions that follow. You may refer to Appendix III, Abbreviations and Symbols, on page A41.

Harbin Clinic Hematology
2324 Shorter Avenue
Rome, GA 30165
555-1234

Patient: Sanchez, Carlos
    100 Main Street
    Cedar Bluff, AL 35959

Age/DOB 42 yrs 19-Feb-1968
Home: (256) 123-4567

Results

Lab Accession # 0010871292009
Ordering Provider: Mann, Keith
Performing Location: Main Harbin Clinic

Collected: 4/20/xx   10:38:00 AM
Resulted: 4/20/xx   10:20:00 AM
Verified By: Mann, Keith
Auto Verify: N
Stage: Final

CBC WITH AUTO DIFF

Test	Result	Units	Flag	Reference Range
WBC	7.9	$\times 10^3/\mu L$		4.0–10.0
RBC	4.44	$\times 10^3/\mu L$		3.80–5.80
HGB	14.4	g/dl		11.5–16.0
HCT	41.9	%		37.0–47.0
MCV	94.0	fL		80.0–100
MCH	32.4	pg	H	27.0–32.0
MCHC	34.3	g/dl		32.0–36.0
RDW	12.6	%		11.0–16.0
PLATELETS	248	$\times 10^3/\mu L$		115–436
MPV	8.8	fL		6.0–11.0
NEUT%	56.3	%		37.0–80.0
LYMPH%	32.4	%		10.0–50.0
MONO%	8.2	%		0.1–10.0
EOS%	1.6	%		0.1–6.0
BASO%	1.5	%		0.0–3.0

Test	Result	Units	Flag	Reference Range
NEUT#	4.5	×10³/μL		2.9–6.2
LYMPH#	2.6	×10³/μL		0.8–3.9
MONO#	0.7	×10³/μL		0.0–1.2
EOS#	0.1	×10³/μL		0.0–0.6
BASO#	0.1	×10³/μL		0.1–0.3

Medical Record Questions

Place the correct answer in the space provided.

1. What does the abbreviation *CBC* mean? _____

2. What does the abbreviation *diff* mean? _____

3. Which one of the test results was flagged high?_____

4. What is the normal range for white blood cells? _____

5. What is the normal range for red blood cells?_____

PEARSON
mymedicalterminologylab

MyMedicalTerminologyLab is a premium online homework management system that includes a host of features to help you study. Registered users will find:

- Fun games and activities built within a virtual hospital

- Powerful tools that track and analyze your results—allowing you to create a personalized learning experience

- Videos, flashcards, and audio pronunciations to help enrich your progress

- Streaming lesson presentations and self-paced learning modules

- A space where you and your instructors can view and manage your assignments

ental Health • Introduction to Medical Terminology • S
xes • Prefixes • Organization of the Body • Integument
System • Skeletal System • Muscular System • Digestiv
tem • Cardiovascular System • Blood and Lymphatic S

m • **Respiratory System** • Urinary System • Endoc

LEARNING OUTCOMES

On completion of this chapter, you will
be able to:

1. Describe respiration.

2. State the description and primary functions
   of the organs/structures of the respiratory
   system.

3. Define terms that physiologists and
   respiratory specialists use to describe the
   volume of air exchanged in breathing.

4. Analyze, build, spell, and pronounce medical
   words.

5. Comprehend the drugs highlighted in this
   chapter.

6. Describe diagnostic and laboratory tests
   related to the respiratory system.

7. Identify and define selected abbreviations.

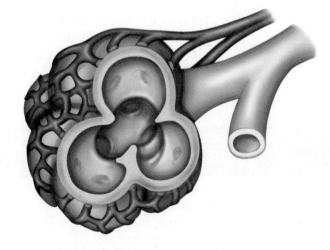

COMBINING FORMS OF THE RESPIRATORY SYSTEM

alveol/o	small, hollow air sac	orth/o	straight
anthrac/o	coal	ox/o	oxygen
aspirat/o	to draw in	palat/o	palate
atel/o	imperfect	pector/o	breast, chest
bronch/i	bronchi	pharyng/o	pharynx, throat
bronch/o	bronchi	pleur/o	pleura
bronchiol/o	bronchiole	pneum/o	air
cheil/o	lip	pneumon/o	lung
con/i	dust	pulmon/o	lung
cyan/o	dark blue	py/o	pus
cyst/o	sac	respirat/o	breathing
diaphragmat/o	diaphragm, partition	rhin/o	nose
fibr/o	fiber	rhonch/o	snore
halat/o	breathe	sarc/o	flesh
hem/o	blood	spir/o	breath
laryng/e	larynx, voice box	thel/i	nipple
laryng/o	larynx, voice box	thorac/o	chest
lob/o	lobe	tonsill/o	tonsil, almond
mes/o	middle	trach/e	trachea
nas/o	nose	trache/o	trachea
olfact/o	smell	tubercul/o	a little swelling
or/o	mouth	ventilat/o	to air

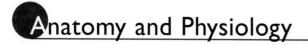Anatomy and Physiology

The respiratory system consists of the nose, pharynx, larynx, trachea, bronchi, and lungs. Its primary function is to furnish oxygen (O_2) for individual tissue cells to use and to take away their gaseous waste product, carbon dioxide (CO_2). See Figure 11.1 ■ This process is accomplished through the act of **respiration (R)**, which consists of external and internal processes. **External respiration** is the process by which the lungs are ventilated and oxygen and carbon dioxide are exchanged between the air in the lungs and the blood within capillaries of the alveoli. **Internal respiration** is the process by which oxygen and carbon dioxide are exchanged between the blood in tissue capillaries and the cells of the body. Table 11.1 ■ provides an at-a-glance look at the respiratory system.

TABLE 11.1 Respiratory System at-a-Glance

Organ/Structure	Primary Functions/Description
Nose	Serves as an air passageway; warms and moistens inhaled air; its cilia and mucous membrane trap dust, pollen, bacteria, and other foreign matter; contains special smell receptor cells (nerve cells), which assist in distinguishing various smells; contributes to phonation and the quality of voice
Pharynx	Serves as a passageway for air and for food; contributes to phonation as a chamber where the sound is able to resonate

TABLE 11.1 Respiratory System at-a-Glance *(continued)*	
Organ/Structure	**Primary Functions/Description**
Larynx	Produces vocal sounds. High notes are formed by short, tense vocal cords. Low notes are produced by long, relaxed vocal cords. The nose, mouth, pharynx, and bony sinuses aid in phonation and the tone that is produced to give each person a distinctive sound.
Trachea	Provides an open passageway for air to and from the lungs
Bronchi	Provide a passageway for air to and from the lungs
Lungs	Bring air into intimate contact with blood so that oxygen and carbon dioxide can be exchanged in the alveoli

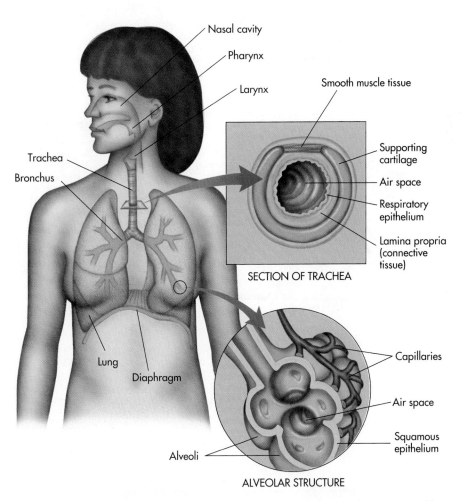

■ **Figure 11.1** The respiratory system: nasal cavity, pharynx, larynx, trachea, bronchus, and lung with expanded views of the trachea and alveolar structure.

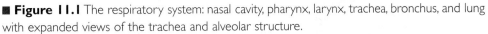

NOSE

The **nose** is the projection in the center of the face; it consists of an external and internal portion. The *external portion* is a triangle of cartilage and bone that is covered with skin and lined with mucous membrane. The external entrance of the nose is known as the **nostrils** or **anterior nares**. The *internal portion* of the nose is divided into two chambers by a partition, the **septum**, separating it into a right and a left cavity. These cavities are divided into three air passages: the *superior, middle,* and *inferior conchae.* These passages lead to the pharynx and are connected with the paranasal sinuses by openings, with the ears by the eustachian tube, and with the region of the eyes by the nasolacrimal ducts. See Figure 11.2 ■

The nose is lined with mucous membrane, which is covered with **cilia** (hairlike processes). The nose plays an important role in the sense of smell. Smell receptor cells are located in the upper part of the nasal cavity. These cells are special nerve cells that have cilia. The cilia of each cell are sensitive to different chemicals and, when stimulated, create a nerve impulse that is sent to the nerve cells of the olfactory bulb, which lies inside the skull just above the nose. The olfactory nerves carry the nerve impulse from the olfactory bulb directly to the brain, where it is perceived as a smell.

The nasal mucosa produces about 946 mL or 1 qt of mucus per day. Four pairs of paranasal sinuses drain into the nose. These are the *frontal, maxillary, ethmoidal,* and *sphenoidal* sinuses. See Figure 11.3 ■ The *palatine bones* and *maxillae* separate the nasal cavities from the mouth cavity.

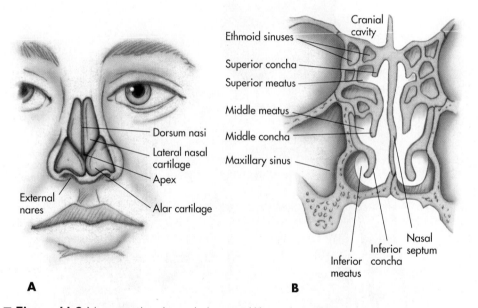

A **B**

■ **Figure 11.2** Nose, nasal cavity, and pharynx: (A) nasal cartilages and external structure; (B) meatus and positions of the entrance to the ethmoid and maxillary sinuses.

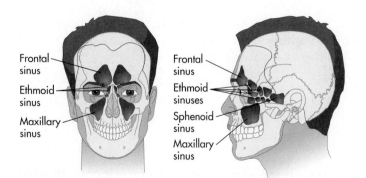

■ **Figure 11.3** Paranasal sinuses.

PHARYNX

The **pharynx** is a musculomembranous tube about 5 inches long that extends from the base of the skull, lies anterior to the cervical vertebrae, and becomes continuous with the esophagus. It is divided into three portions: the *nasopharynx* located behind the nose, the *oropharynx* located behind the mouth, and the *laryngopharynx* located behind the larynx. Seven openings are found in the pharynx: two openings from the eustachian tubes, two openings from the posterior nares into the nasopharynx, the fauces or opening from the mouth into the oropharynx, and the openings from the larynx and the esophagus into the laryngopharynx. See Figure 11.4 ■ Associated with the pharynx are three pairs of lymphoid tissues, which are the **tonsils**. The nasopharynx contains the *adenoids* or *pharyngeal* tonsils. The oropharynx contains the *faucial* or *palatine* tonsils and the *lingual* tonsils. The tonsils are accessory organs of the lymphatic system and aid in filtering bacteria and other foreign substances from the circulating lymph in the head and neck region.

LARYNX

The **larynx** or voicebox is a structure made of muscle and cartilage and lined with mucous membrane. It is the enlarged upper end of the trachea below the root of the tongue and hyoid bone. See Figures 11.1 and 11.4.

The cavity of the larynx contains a pair of *ventricular folds* (false vocal cords) and a pair of vocal folds or true vocal cords. The cavity is divided into three regions: vestibule, ventricle, and entrance to the glottis. The **glottis** is a narrow slit at the opening between the true vocal folds.

Cartilages of the Larynx

The larynx is composed of nine cartilages bound together by muscles and ligaments. The three unpaired cartilages, each of which is described in the following sections, are the *thyroid, cricoid,* and *epiglottis,* and the three paired cartilages are the *arytenoid, cuneiform,* and *corniculate.*

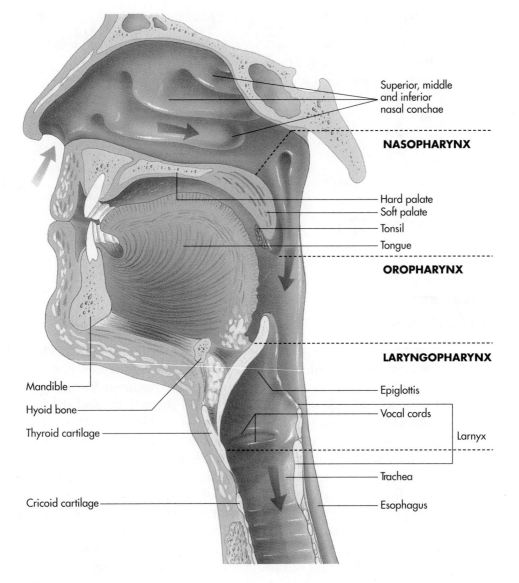

■ **Figure 11.4** Sagittal section of the nasal cavity and pharynx.

Thyroid Cartilage

The **thyroid cartilage** is the largest cartilage in the larynx and forms the structure commonly called the *Adam's apple.* This structure is usually larger and more prominent in men than in women and contributes to the deeper male voice.

Epiglottis

The **epiglottis** covers the entrance of the larynx. During swallowing, it acts as a lid to prevent aspiration of food into the trachea. When the epiglottis fails to cover the entrance to the larynx, food or liquid intended for the esophagus can enter the trachea, causing irritation, coughing, or, in extreme cases, choking.

Cricoid Cartilage

The **cricoid cartilage** is the lowermost cartilage of the larynx. It is shaped like a signet ring with the broad portion being posterior and the anterior portion forming the arch and resembling the ring's band.

TRACHEA

The **trachea** or *windpipe* is a semi-cylindrical cartilaginous tube that is the air passageway extending from the pharynx and larynx to the main bronchi. It is about 1 inch wide and $4^1/_2$ inches (11.3 cm) long. It is composed of smooth muscle that is reinforced at the front and sides by C-shaped rings of cartilage. The mucous membrane lining the trachea contains cilia, which sweep foreign matter out of the passageway. The trachea provides an open passageway for air to and from the lungs. See Figure 11.1.

BRONCHI

The **bronchi** are the two main branches of the trachea, which provide the passageway for air to the lungs. The trachea divides into the **right bronchus** and the **left bronchus**. The right bronchus is larger and extends down in a more vertical direction than the left bronchus. When a foreign body is inhaled or aspirated, it more frequently lodges in the right bronchus or enters the right lung. Each bronchus enters the lung at a depression, the **hilum**. The bronchi then subdivide into the bronchial tree composed of smaller bronchi, bronchioles, and alveolar ducts. The bronchial tree terminates in the *alveoli*, which are tiny air sacs supporting a network of capillaries from pulmonary blood vessels. The function of the bronchi is to provide an open passageway for air to and from the lungs. See Figure 11.1.

LUNGS

The two **lungs** are conical-shaped spongy organs of respiration. They lie on both sides of the heart within the pleural cavity of the thorax. They occupy a large portion of the thoracic cavity and are enclosed in the **pleura**, a serous membrane composed of several layers. The six layers of the pleura are the *costal, parietal, pericardiaca, phrenica, pulmonalis,* and *visceral.* The *parietal pleura* extends from the roots of the lungs and lines the walls of the thorax and the superior surface of the diaphragm. The *visceral pleura* covers the surface of the lungs and enters into and lines the interlobar fissures. The pleural cavity is a space between the parietal and visceral pleura and contains a serous fluid that lubricates and prevents friction caused by the rubbing together of the two layers. The thoracic cavity is separated from the abdominal cavity by a musculomembranous wall, the **diaphragm**. The central portion of the thoracic cavity, between the lungs, is a space called the **mediastinum**, containing the heart and other structures.

LIFE SPAN CONSIDERATIONS

With advancing age, the respiratory system is vulnerable to injuries caused by infections, environmental pollutants, and allergic reactions. The number of cilia decline in number as one grows older. At the same time, the number of mucus-producing cells may increase, resulting in mucus clogging the airways.

Another change that can occur is in the composition of the connective tissues of the lungs and chest. The lungs become stiffer, respiratory muscle strength and endurance diminishes, and the chest wall becomes more rigid. Total lung capacity is relatively constant across the life span but vital capacity (volume of air that can be exhaled after a maximal inspiration) decreases because the residual volume increases (amount of air remaining in the lungs after maximal expiration).

The lungs consist of elastic tissue filled with interlacing networks of tubes and sacs that carry air and with blood vessels carrying blood. The broad inferior surface of the lung is the **base**, which rests on the diaphragm, while the **apex**, or pointed upper margin, rises from 2.5 to 5.0 cm above the sternal end of the first rib. The lungs are divided into **lobes**, with the right lung having three lobes and the left lung having two lobes. The left lung has an indentation, the **cardiac depression**, for the normal placement of the heart. In an average adult male, the right lung weighs approximately 625 g and the left about 570 g. In an average adult male, the total lung capacity (TLC) is 3.6–9.4 L, whereas in an average adult female it is 2.5–6.9 L. The lungs contain around 300 million **alveoli**, which are the air cells where the exchange of oxygen and carbon dioxide takes place. The main function of the lungs is to bring air into intimate contact with blood so that oxygen and carbon dioxide can be exchanged in the alveoli. See Figure 11.5 ■

LIFE SPAN CONSIDERATIONS

At 12 weeks' gestation, the lungs of the fetus have a definite shape. At 20 weeks, the cellular structure of the alveoli is complete; the fetus is able to suck its thumb and swallow amniotic fluid. At 24 weeks, the nostrils open and respiratory movements occur. At 26–32 weeks, **surfactant** (a substance formed in the lung that regulates the amount of surface tension of the fluid lining the alveoli) is produced. In preterm infants, the lack of surfactant contributes to infant respiratory distress syndrome (IRDS), previously called hyaline membrane disease (HMD). It is also called neonatal respiratory distress syndrome or respiratory distress syndrome (RDS) of the newborn.

During fetal life, gaseous exchange occurs at the placental interface. The lungs do not function until birth.

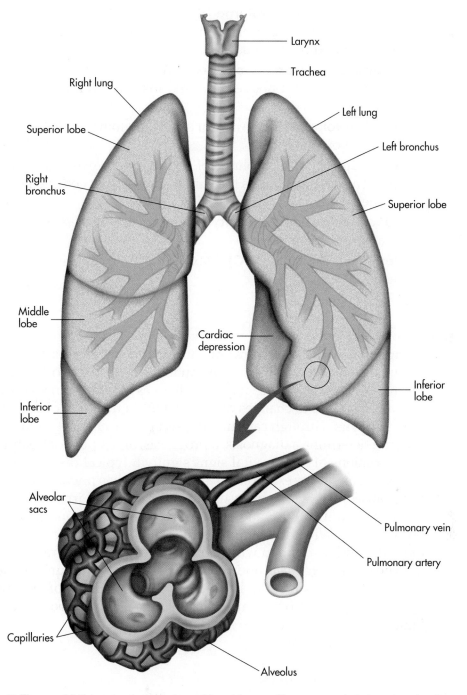

■ **Figure 11.5** Larynx, trachea, bronchi, and lungs with an expanded view showing the structures of an alveolus and the pulmonary blood vessels.

RESPIRATION

Volume

The following terms are used by physiologists and respiratory specialists to describe the volume of air exchanged in breathing:

Tidal volume (TV). Amount of air in a single inspiration and expiration. In the average adult male, about 500 mL of air enters the respiratory tract during normal quiet breathing.

Expiratory reserve volume (ERV). Amount of air that can be forcibly expired after a normal quiet respiration. This is also called the *supplemental air* and measures approximately 1000–1200 mL.

Inspiratory reserve volume (IRV). Amount of air that can be forcibly inspired over and above a normal inspiration and measures approximately 3600 mL.

Residual volume (RV). Amount of air remaining in the lungs after maximal expiration, about 1500 mL.

Vital capacity (VC). Volume of air that can be exhaled after a maximal inspiration. This amount equals the sum of the tidal air, complemental air, and the supplemental air.

Functional residual capacity. Volume of air that remains in the lungs at the end of a normal expiration.

Total lung capacity (TLC). Maximal volume of air in the lungs after a maximal inspiration.

Vital Function of Respiration

Temperature, pulse, respiration, and **blood pressure** are the vital signs that are essential elements for determining an individual's state of health. A deviation from normal of one or all of the vital signs denotes a state of illness. Evaluation of an individual's response to changes occurring within the body can be measured by taking the vital signs. Through careful analysis of these changes in the vital signs, a physician can determine a diagnosis, a prognosis, and a plan of treatment for the patient. The variations of certain vital signs signify a typical disease process and its stages of development. For example, in a patient who has pneumonia (inflammation of the lung caused by bacteria, viruses, fungi, or chemical irritants), the temperature can be elevated to 101–106°F, and pulse and respiration can increase to almost twice their normal rates. When the temperature falls, the patient will perspire profusely and the pulse and respiration will begin to return to normal rates.

The *medulla oblongata* and the *pons*, two of the structures of the brainstem, regulate and control respiration. The rate, rhythm, and depth of respiration are controlled by nerve impulses from the medulla oblongata and the pons via the spinal cord. See Figure 11.6 ■

Respiratory Rate

Individuals of different ages breathe at different respiratory rates. The **respiratory rate** is regulated by the respiratory center located in the medulla oblongata. The following are respiratory rates for some different age groups:

Newborn	30–80 per minute
1st year	20–40 per minute
5th year	20–25 per minute
15th year	15–20 per minute
Adult	12–20 per minute

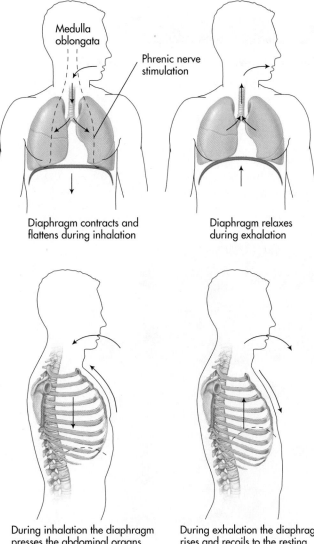

Medulla oblongata

Phrenic nerve stimulation

Diaphragm contracts and flattens during inhalation

Diaphragm relaxes during exhalation

During inhalation the diaphragm presses the abdominal organs forward and downward

During exhalation the diaphragm rises and recoils to the resting position

■ **Figure 11.6** The process of respiration.

Anatomy and Physiology Labeling

Identify the structures shown below by filling in the blanks.

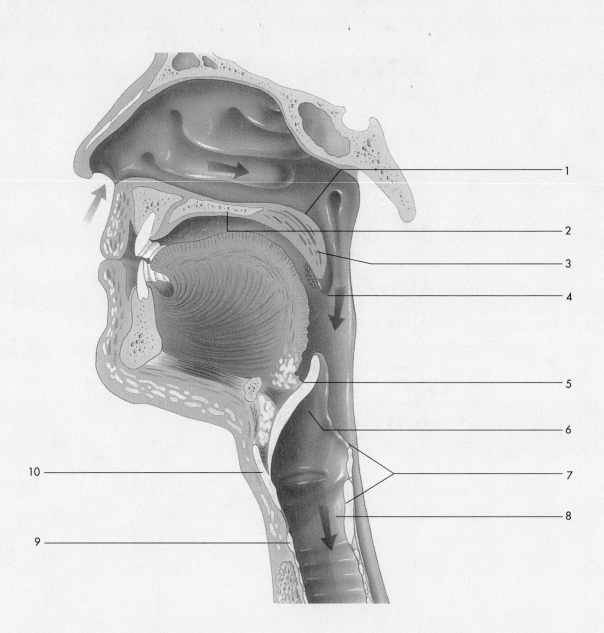

1 _____

2 _____

3 _____

4 _____

5 _____

6 _____

7 _____

8 _____

9 _____

10 _____

• Building Your Medical Vocabulary •

This section provides the foundation for learning medical terminology. Review the following alphabetized word list. Note how common prefixes and suffixes are repeatedly applied to word roots and combining forms to create different meanings. The word parts are color-coded: prefixes are green, suffixes are blue, roots/combining forms are red.

You will find that some terms have not been divided into word parts. These are common words or specialized terms that are included to enhance your medical vocabulary. See Chapter 1, page 7, to review pronunciation guidelines.

MEDICAL WORD	WORD PARTS		DEFINITION
	Part	**Meaning**	
alveolus (ăl-vē′ ō-lŭs)	alveoli -us	small, hollow air sac pertaining to	Pertaining to a small air sac in the lungs
anthracosis (ăn″ thră-kō′ sĭs)	anthrac -osis	coal condition	Lung condition caused by inhalation of coal dust and silica; also called *black lung*
apnea (ăp′-nĕă)	a- -pnea	lack of breathing	Temporary cessation of breathing. **Sleep apnea** is a temporary cessation of breathing during sleep. To be so classified, the apnea must last for at least 10 seconds and occur 30 or more times during a 7-hour period of sleep. Sleep apnea is classified according to the mechanisms involved. **Obstructive apnea** is caused by obstruction to the upper airway. **Central apnea** is marked by absence of respiratory muscle activity.
asphyxia (ăs-fĭk′ sĭ-ă)	a- sphyx -ia	lack of pulse condition	Emergency condition in which there is a depletion of oxygen in the blood with an increase of carbon dioxide in the blood and tissues; symptoms include dyspnea, cyanosis, tachycardia, impairment of senses, and, in extreme cases, convulsions, unconsciousness, and death. Some of the more common causes include drowning, electrical shock, aspiration of vomitus, lodging of a foreign body in the respiratory tract, inhalation of toxic gas or smoke, and poisoning. Artificial ventilation and oxygen should be administered ASAP.
aspiration (ăs″ pĭ-rā′ shŭn)	aspirat -ion	to draw in process	The act of drawing in or out by suction using a device such as a syringe or needle; the process of drawing foreign bodies, such as food, liquid, or other substances, into the nose, throat, or lungs on inspiration

MEDICAL WORD	WORD PARTS		DEFINITION
	Part	**Meaning**	
asthma (ăz´ mă)			Disease of the bronchi characterized by wheezing, dyspnea, and a feeling of constriction in the chest. See Figure 11.7 ■ Inflammation of the airways causes airflow into and out of the lungs to be restricted. During an asthma attack, the muscles of the bronchial tree constrict and the linings of the air passages swell, reducing airflow and producing the characteristic wheezing sound. See Figure 11.8 ■ See the FYI box for asthma triggers.

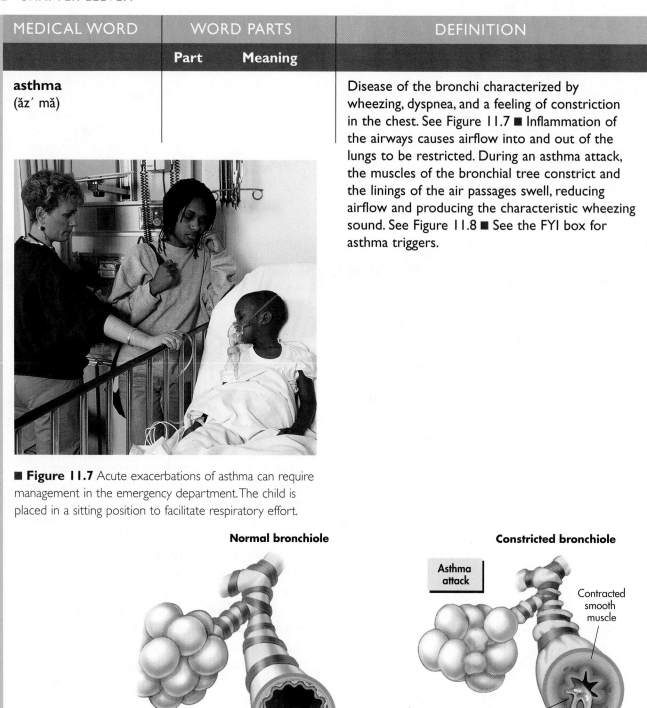

■ **Figure 11.7** Acute exacerbations of asthma can require management in the emergency department. The child is placed in a sitting position to facilitate respiratory effort.

Normal bronchiole

Constricted bronchiole

Asthma attack

Contracted smooth muscle

Mucous membrane

Smooth muscle

Swollen mucous membrane

Excessive mucus secretion

A

B

■ **Figure 11.8** Changes in bronchioles during an asthma attack: (A) normal bronchiole and (B) in asthma attack.

MEDICAL WORD	WORD PARTS		DEFINITION
	Part	Meaning	

In asthma-prone individuals, symptoms can be triggered by inhaled allergens, such as pet dander, dust mites, cockroach allergens, molds, or pollens. A variety of other situations can also trigger symptoms, including respiratory infections, exercise, cold air, tobacco smoke and other pollutants, stress, and food or drug allergies. Figure 11.9 ■, from the American Lung Association, shows what can trigger an asthmatic episode.

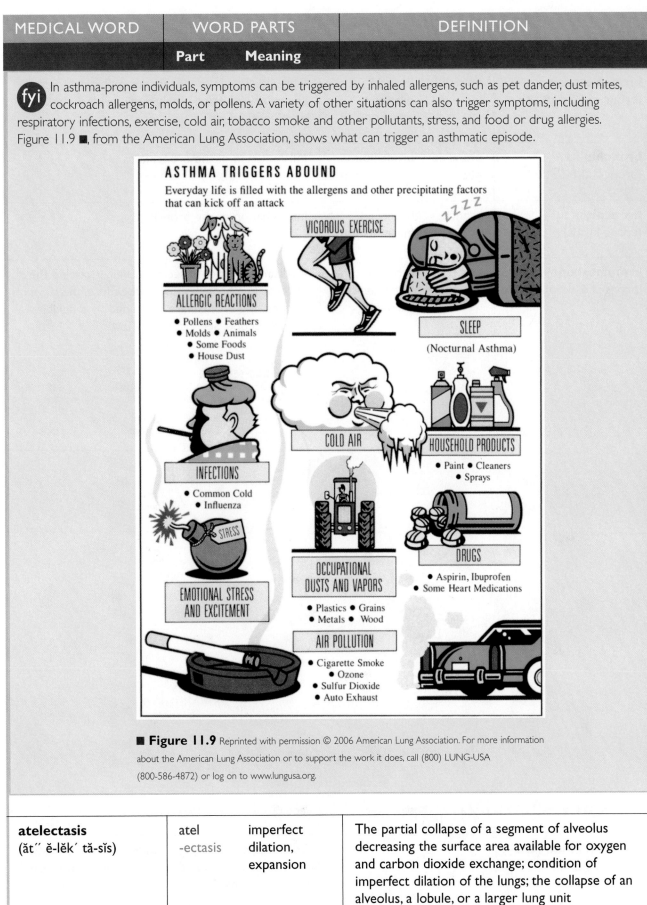

■ **Figure 11.9** Reprinted with permission © 2006 American Lung Association. For more information about the American Lung Association or to support the work it does, call (800) LUNG-USA (800-586-4872) or log on to www.lungusa.org.

MEDICAL WORD	WORD PARTS		DEFINITION
atelectasis (ăt″ ĕ-lĕk′ tă-sĭs)	atel -ectasis	imperfect dilation, expansion	The partial collapse of a segment of alveolus decreasing the surface area available for oxygen and carbon dioxide exchange; condition of imperfect dilation of the lungs; the collapse of an alveolus, a lobule, or a larger lung unit

MEDICAL WORD	WORD PARTS		DEFINITION
	Part	**Meaning**	
bronchiectasis (brŏng″ kĭ-ĕk′ tă-sĭs)	bronch/i -ectasis	bronchi dilation, expansion	Chronic dilation of a bronchus or bronchi, with a secondary infection that usually involves the lower portion of a lung
bronchiolitis (brŏng″ kĭ-ō-lī′ tĭs)	bronchiol -itis	bronchiole inflammation	Inflammation of the bronchioles
bronchitis (brŏng-kī′ tĭs)	bronch -itis	bronchi Inflammation	Inflammation of the bronchi
bronchoscope (brŏng′ kō-skōp)	bronch/o -scope	bronchi instrument for examining	Medical instrument used to visually examine the bronchi. In a bronchoscopy procedure, the larynx, trachea, and bronchi are examined by a flexible bronchoscope. See Figure 11.10 ■

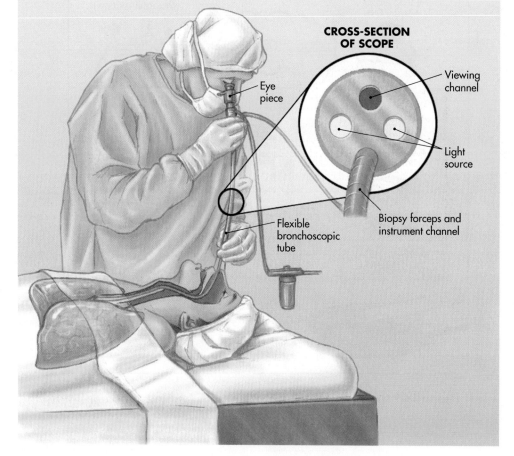

■ **Figure 11.10** Use of a bronchoscope during a bronchoscopy to visualize the bronchus.

carbon dioxide (CO₂) (kăr bən dī-ŏk′ sīd)			Colorless, odorless gas produced by the oxidation of carbon; it is a waste gas from metabolism that needs to be exhaled

MEDICAL WORD	WORD PARTS		DEFINITION
	Part	**Meaning**	
Cheyne–Stokes respiration (chān´–stōks´ rĕs˝ pĭr-ā´ shŭn)			Rhythmic cycle of breathing with a gradual increase in respiration followed by apnea (which may last from 10 to 60 sec), then a repeat of the same cycle
cough (kawf)			Sudden, forceful expulsion of air from the lungs; an essential protective response that clears irritants, secretions, or foreign objects from the trachea, bronchi, and/or lungs
croup (croop)			Acute respiratory disease (ARD) characterized by obstruction of the larynx, a barking cough, dyspnea, hoarseness, and stridor. See Figure 11.11 ■

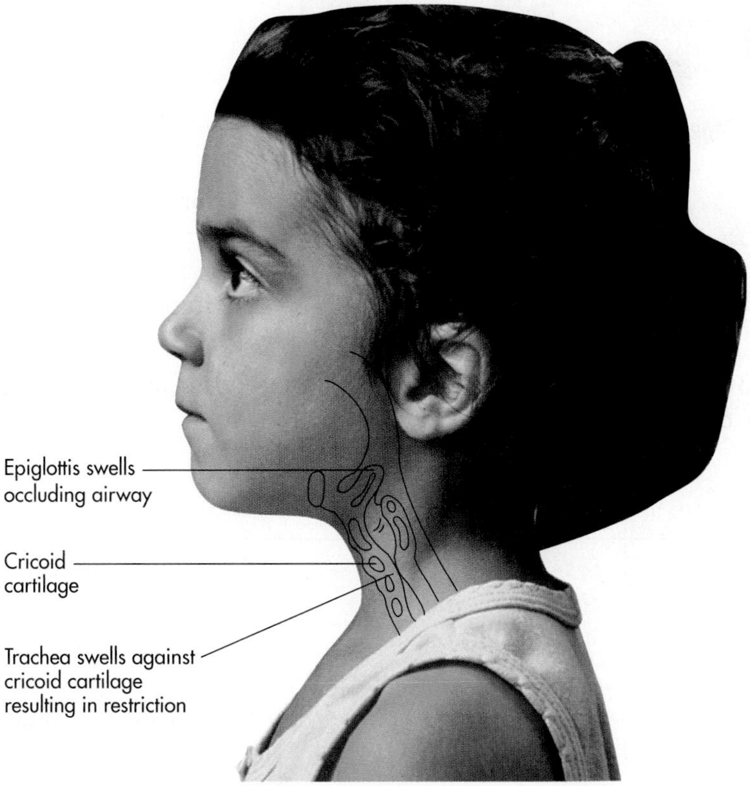

Epiglottis swells occluding airway

Cricoid cartilage

Trachea swells against cricoid cartilage resulting in restriction

■ **Figure 11.11** Two important changes occur in the upper airway in croup: The epiglottis swells, thereby occluding the airway, and the trachea swells against the cricoid cartilage, causing restriction.

MEDICAL WORD	WORD PARTS		DEFINITION
cyanosis (sī˝ ăn-ō´ -sĭs)	cyan	dark blue	Abnormal condition of the skin and mucous membrane caused by oxygen deficiency in the blood. The skin, fingernails, and mucous membranes can appear slightly bluish or grayish.
	-osis	condition	

MEDICAL WORD	WORD PARTS		DEFINITION
	Part	**Meaning**	
cystic fibrosis (CF) (sĭs´ tĭk fĭ-brō´ sĭs)	cyst -ic fibr -osis	sac pertaining to fiber condition	Inherited disease that affects the entire body, causing progressive disability and often early death. The name *cystic fibrosis* refers to the characteristic scarring (fibrosis) and cyst formation within the pancreas. Cystic fibrosis may be diagnosed by many different categories of testing, including newborn screening, sweat testing, or genetic testing. The gene responsible for this condition has been identified, and persons carrying the gene can be determined through genetic testing. See Figure 11.12 ■
diaphragmatocele (dī´´ ă-frăg-măt´ ō-sēl)	diaphrag- mat/o -cele	diaphragm, partition hernia, tumor, swelling	Hernia of the diaphragm
dysphonia (dĭs-fō´ nĭ-ă)	dys- phon -ia	difficult voice condition	Condition of difficulty in speaking; *hoarseness*
dyspnea (dĭsp-nē´ ă)	dys -pnea	difficult breathing	Literally means *difficulty in breathing*
emphysema (ĕm´´ fĭ-sē´ mă)			Chronic pulmonary disease in which the alveoli become distended and the alveolar walls become damaged or destroyed, making it difficult to exhale air from the lungs. It is included in a group of diseases called chronic obstructive pulmonary disease, or COPD. The primary cause of emphysema is the smoking of cigarettes. See Figure 11.13 ■

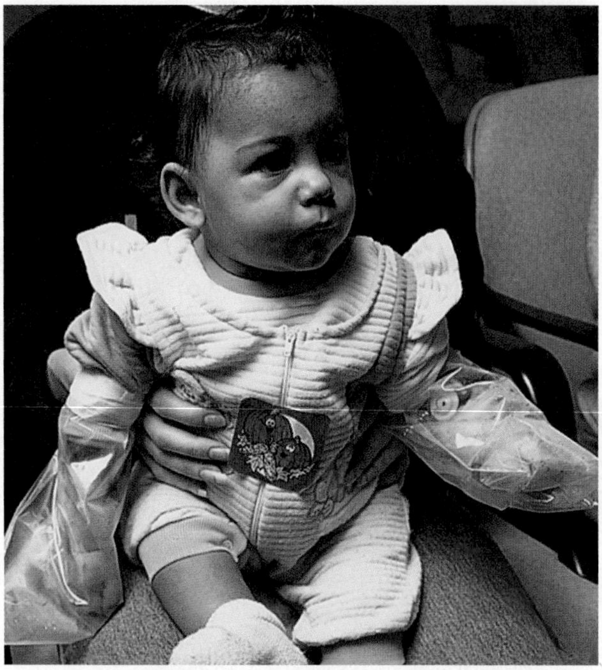

■ **Figure 11.12** Evaluation of a child for cystic fibrosis with a sweat chloride test. Sweat is being collected under the wrappings for later analysis of the amount of sodium and chloride.

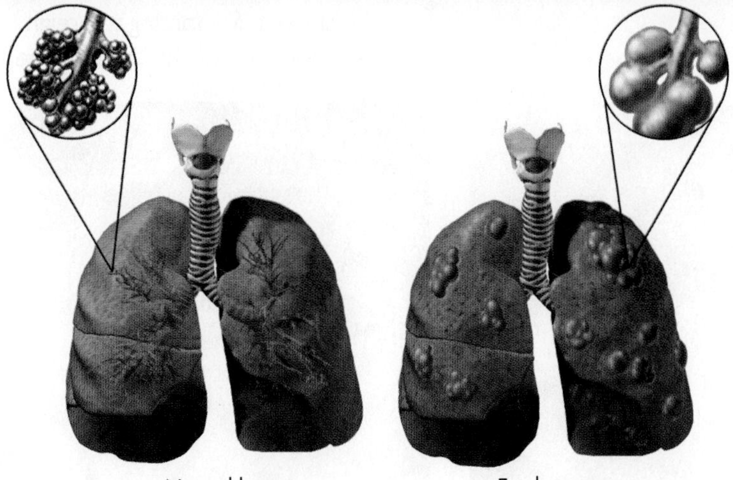

MEDICAL WORD	WORD PARTS		DEFINITION
	Part	**Meaning**	

■ **Figure 11.13** Normal lung and one with emphysema.

MEDICAL WORD	WORD PARTS		DEFINITION
	Part	Meaning	
empyema (ĕm″ pĭ-ē´ mă)			Pus in a body cavity, especially the pleural cavity
endotracheal (ET) (ĕn″ dō-trā´ kē-ăl)	endo- trach/e -al	within trachea pertaining to	Within the trachea. An endotracheal tube is used in general anesthesia, intensive care, and emergency medicine for airway management, mechanical ventilation, and as an alternative route for the administration of medicines when an intravenous (IV) infusion line cannot be established.
epistaxis (ĕp″ ĭ-stăk´ sĭs)	epi- -staxis	upon dripping	Nosebleed; usually results from traumatic or spontaneous rupture of blood vessels in the mucous membranes of the nose
eupnea (ūp-nē´ ă)	eu- -pnea	good, normal breathing	Good or normal breathing
exhalation (ĕks″ hə-lā´ shŭn)	ex- halat -ion	out breathe process	Process of breathing out
expectoration (ĕk-spĕk″ tə´ rā´ shŭn)	ex- pector (at) -ion	out breast, chest process	Process of coughing up and spitting out material (sputum) from the lungs, bronchi, and trachea

MEDICAL WORD	WORD PARTS		DEFINITION
	Part	Meaning	
Heimlich maneuver (hīm´ lĭk mă-nōō´ văr)			Technique for forcing a foreign body (usually a bolus of food) out of the trachea. See Figure 11.14 ■

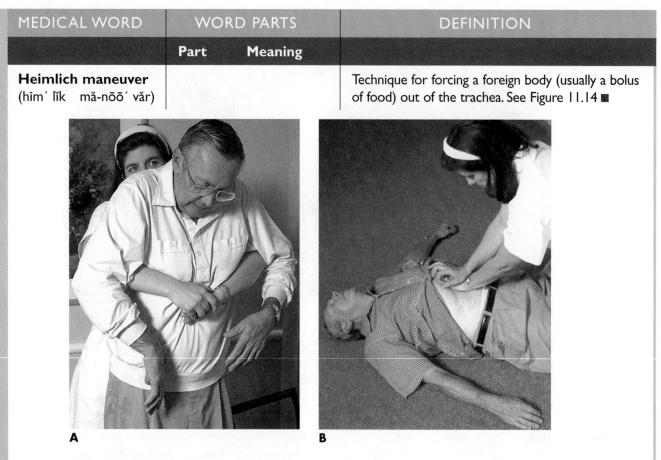

A **B**

■ **Figure 11.14** Administration of abdominal thrusts (the Heimlich maneuver) to (A) a conscious victim and (B) an unconscious victim.

MEDICAL WORD	WORD PARTS		DEFINITION
	Part	Meaning	
hemoptysis (hē-mŏp´ tĭ-sĭs)	hem/o -ptysis	blood to spit	Spitting up blood
hyperpnea (hī´´ pĕrp-nē´ ă)	hyper- -pnea	excessive breathing	Excessive or rapid breathing
hyperventilation (hī´´ pĕr-vĕn´´ tĭ-lā´ shŭn)	hyper- ventilat -ion	excessive to air process	Process of excessive ventilating, thereby increasing the air in the lungs beyond the normal limit
hypoxia (hĭ-pŏks´ ĭ-ă)	hyp- ox -ia	below, deficient oxygen condition	Condition of deficient amounts of oxygen in the inspired air
influenza (ĭn´´ floo-ĕn´ ză)			Acute, contagious respiratory infection caused by a virus. Onset is usually sudden, and symptoms are fever, chills, headache, myalgia, cough, and sore throat.
inhalation (ĭn´´ hă-lă´ shŭn)	in- halat -ion	in breathe process	Process of breathing in

MEDICAL WORD	WORD PARTS		DEFINITION
	Part	**Meaning**	
laryngeal (lăr-ĭn´ jĭ-ăl)	laryng/e -al	larynx, voice box pertaining to	Pertaining to the larynx (voice box)
laryngitis (lăr˝ ĭn-jī´ tĭs)	laryng -itis	larynx, voice box inflammation	Inflammation of the larynx (voice box). See Figure 11.15 ■

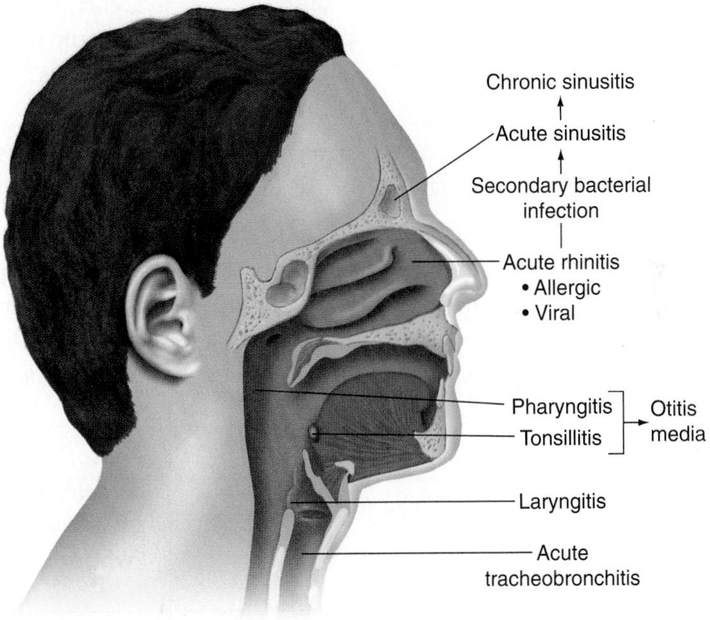

■ **Figure 11.15** Paranasal sinuses are part of the upper respiratory system. From here, infections can spread via the nasopharynx to the middle ear or bronchi. Note locations of laryngitis, pharyngitis, sinusitis, and tonsillitis.

MEDICAL WORD	WORD PARTS		DEFINITION
laryngoscope (lăr-ĭn´ gō-skōp)	laryng/o -scope	larynx, voice box instrument for examining	Medical instrument used to visually examine the larynx (voice box). The procedure using a laryngoscope is known as laryngoscopy.
Legionnaire's disease (lē jə naerz´)			Severe pulmonary pneumonia caused by *Legionella pneumophilia*
lobectomy (lō-běk´ tō-mē)	lob -ectomy	lobe surgical excision	Surgical excision of a lobe of any organ or gland, such as the lung
mesothelioma (měs˝ ō-thē˝ lĭ-ō´ mă)	mes/o thel/i -oma	middle nipple tumor	Malignant tumor of mesothelium (serous membrane of the pleura) caused by the inhalation of asbestos

MEDICAL WORD	WORD PARTS		DEFINITION
	Part	**Meaning**	
nasopharyngitis (nā″ zō-făr′ ĭn-jī′ tĭs)	nas/o pharyng -itis	nose pharynx, throat inflammation	Inflammation of the nose and pharynx (throat)
olfaction (ŏl-făk′ shŭn)	olfact -ion	smell process	Process of smelling
oropharynx (or″ ō-făr′ ĭnks)	or/o pharynx	mouth pharynx, throat	Central portion of the throat that lies between the soft palate and upper portion of the epiglottis
orthopnea (or″ thŏp-nē′ ă)	orth/o -pnea	straight breathing	Inability to breathe unless in an upright or straight position
palatopharyngo-plasty (păl″ ăt-ō-făr″ ĭn′ gō-plăs″ tē)	palat/o pharyng/o -plasty	palate pharynx, throat surgical repair	Type of surgery that relieves snoring and sleep apnea by removing the uvula and the tonsils and reshaping the lining at the back of the throat to enlarge the air passageway
pertussis (pĕr-tŭs′ ĭs)			Acute, infectious disease caused by the bacterium *Bordetella pertussis;* characterized by a peculiar paroxysmal cough ending in a "crowing" or "whooping" sound; also called *whooping cough*
pharyngitis (făr″ ĭn-jī′ tĭs)	pharyng -itis	pharynx, throat inflammation	Inflammation of the pharynx (throat). See Figure 11.15.
pleurisy (ploo′ rĭsē)			Inflammation of the pleura caused by injury, infection, or a tumor. The inflamed pleural layers rub against each other every time the lungs expand to breathe in air. This can cause sharp pain with breathing (also called pleuritic chest pain).
pleuritis (ploo-rī′ tĭs)	pleur -itis	pleura inflammation	Inflammation of the pleura
pleurodynia (ploo″ rō-dĭn′ ĭ-ă)	pleur/o -dynia	pleura pain	Pain in the pleura
pneumoconiosis (nū″ mō-kō″ nĭ-ō′ sĭs)	pneum/o con/i -osis	lung, air dust condition	Abnormal condition of the lung caused by the inhalation of dust particles such as coal dust (*anthracosis*), stone dust (*chalicosis*), iron dust (*siderosis*), asbestos (*asbestosis*), and quartz (*silica*) dust (*silicosis*). Fiberotic tissue surrounding the alveoli limit their ability to stretch, thereby restricting the intake of air.

MEDICAL WORD	WORD PARTS		DEFINITION
	Part	**Meaning**	
pneumonia (nū-mō´ nǐ-ă)	pneumon -ia	lung, air condition	Inflammation of the lung caused by bacteria, viruses, fungi, or chemical irritants. See Figure 11.16 ■ Pneumonia affects 3–4 million people each year in the United States. Symptoms include a cough with greenish mucus or puslike sputum, chills, fever, fatigue, chest pain, and muscle aches. Initial diagnosis is made through auscultation of the chest with a stethoscope. In patients with pneumonia, rales and other abnormal breathing sounds can be heard. Tests that are used to confirm the diagnosis include a chest x-ray (see Figure 11.17 ■) and a sputum culture.

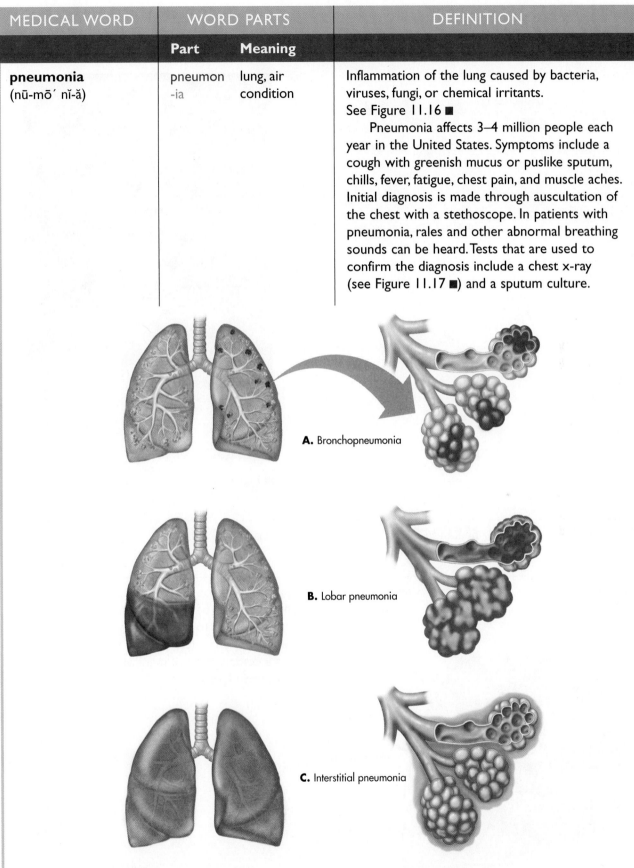

A. Bronchopneumonia

B. Lobar pneumonia

C. Interstitial pneumonia

■ **Figure 11.16** (A) Bronchopneumonia with localized pattern. (B) Lobar pneumonia with a diffuse pattern within the lung lobe. (C) Interstitial pneumonia is typically diffuse and bilateral.

MEDICAL WORD	WORD PARTS		DEFINITION
	Part	**Meaning**	

LIFE SPAN CONSIDERATIONS

In adults, bacteria are the most common causes of pneumonia, and of these, *Streptococcus pneumoniae* (pneumococcus) is the most common. Bacterial pneumonias tend to be the most serious. In some people, particularly older adults and those who are debilitated, pneumonia can follow influenza.

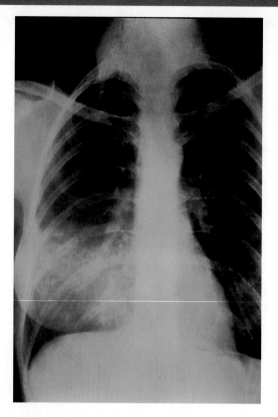

■ **Figure 11.17** Lobar pneumonia.
(Source: Photo Researchers, Inc.)

pneumonitis (nū″ mō-nī′ tĭs)	pneumon -itis	lung inflammation	Inflammation of the lung
pneumothorax (nū″ mō-thō′ răks)	pneum/o thorax	air chest	A pathological condition in which there is a collection of air between the chest wall and lungs, causing the lung to collapse. It may occur spontaneously or after physical trauma to the chest or as a complication of medical treatment. See Figure 11.18 ■

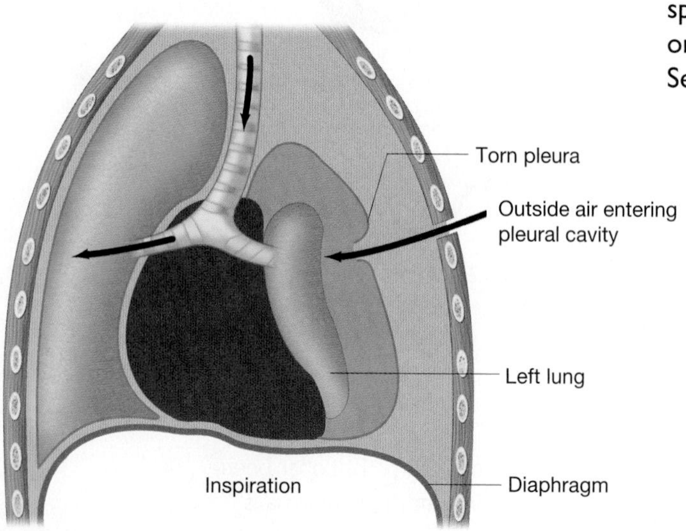

Torn pleura
Outside air entering pleural cavity
Left lung
Inspiration
Diaphragm

■ **Figure 11.18** Pneumothorax (sucking chest wound).

MEDICAL WORD	WORD PARTS		DEFINITION
	Part	**Meaning**	
polyp (pŏl´ ĭp)			Tumor with a stem; can occur where there are mucous membranes, such as the nose, ears, mouth, uterus, and intestines
pulmonectomy (pŭl″ mō-něk´ tō-mē)	pulmon -ectomy	lung surgical excision	Surgical excision of the lung or a part of a lung
pyothorax (pī″ ō-thō´ răks)	py/o thorax	pus chest	Pus in the chest cavity
rale			Abnormal sound heard on auscultation of the chest; a crackling, rattling, or bubbling sound
respirator (rĕs´ pĭ-rā″ tor)	respirat -or	breathing a doer	Medical device used to assist in breathing; type of machine used for prolonged artificial respiration
respiratory distress syndrome (RDS) (rĕs´ pĭ-ră-tō″ rē)			Condition that can occur in a premature infant in which the lungs are not matured to the point of manufacturing lecithin, a pulmonary surfactant, resulting in collapse of the alveoli, which leads to cyanosis and hypoxia; also called *hyaline membrane disease (HMD)*
respiratory syncytial virus (RSV) infection (sĭn″sĭ´ shăl)			Most common cause of bronchiolitis and pneumonia among infants and children under 1 year of age. Illness begins with fever, runny nose, cough, and sometimes wheezing. Most children recover from illness in 8–15 days. It is contagious and is spread from respiratory secretions through close contact with infected persons or contact with contaminated surfaces or objects.
rhinoplasty (rī´ nō-plăs″ tē)	rhin/o -plasty	nose surgical repair	Surgical repair of the nose
rhinorrhea (rī″ nō-rē´ ă)	rhin/o -rrhea	nose flow, discharge	Discharge from the nose
rhinovirus (rī″ nō-vī´ rŭs)	rhin/o vir -us	nose virus pertaining to	One of a subgroup of viruses that cause the common cold (*coryza*) in humans

MEDICAL WORD	WORD PARTS		DEFINITION
	Part	Meaning	
rhonchus (rŏng´ kŭs)	rhonch -us	snore pertaining to	Rale or rattling sound in the throat or bronchial tubes caused by a partial obstruction
sarcoidosis (sar˝ koyd-ō´ sĭs)	sarc -oid -osis	flesh resemble condition	Chronic granulomatous condition that can involve almost any organ system of the body, usually the lungs, causing dyspnea on exertion
severe acute respiratory syndrome (SARS)			Contagious viral respiratory infection that was first described in February 2003; serious form of pneumonia resulting in acute respiratory distress and sometimes death
sinusitis (sī˝ nūs-ī´ tĭs)	sinus -itis	a curve, hollow inflammation	Inflammation of a sinus. See Figure 11.15 on page 379.
spirometer (spī-rŏm´ ĕt-ĕr)	spir/o -meter	breath instrument to measure	Medical instrument used to measure lung volume during inspiration and expiration
sputum (spū´ tŭm)			Substance coughed up from the lungs; can be watery, thick, purulent, clear, or bloody and can contain microorganisms
stridor (strī´ dōr)			High-pitched sound caused by partial obstruction of the air passageway
tachypnea (tăk˝ ĭp-nē´ ă)	tachy- -pnea	rapid breathing	Rapid breathing
thoracocentesis (thō˝ răk-ō-sĕn-tē´ sĭs)	thorac/o -centesis	chest surgical puncture	Surgical puncture of the chest wall for removal of fluid; also called *thoracentesis*. Can be used in pleurisy to remove excess fluid that has accumulated in the chest cavity. See Figure 11.19 ■

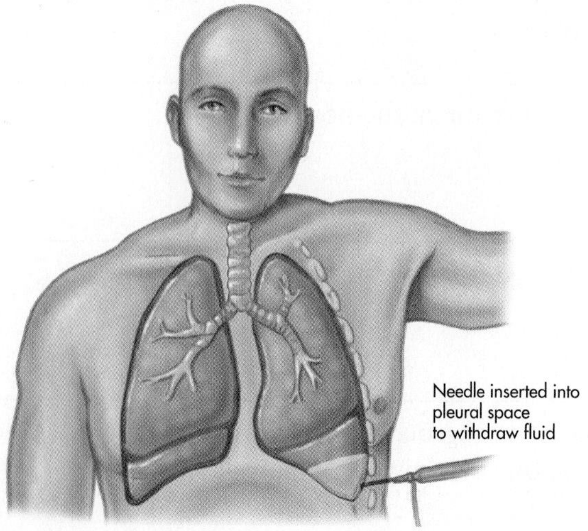

Needle inserted into pleural space to withdraw fluid

■ **Figure 11.19** Thoracocentesis (thoracentesis).

MEDICAL WORD	WORD PARTS		DEFINITION
	Part	**Meaning**	
thoracoplasty (thō′ră-kō-plăs″ tē)	thorac/o -plasty	chest surgical repair	Surgical repair of the chest wall
thoracotomy (thō″răk-ŏt′ō-mē)	thorac/o -tomy	chest incision	Incision into the chest wall
tonsillectomy (tŏn″sĭl-ĕk′tō-mē)	tonsil -ectomy	almond, tonsil surgical excision	Surgical excision of the tonsils
tonsillitis (tŏn″sĭl-ī′tĭs)	tonsil -itis	almond, tonsil inflammation	Inflammation of the tonsils. See Figure 11.15 on page 379.
tracheal (trā′kē-ăl)	trach/e -al	trachea, windpipe pertaining to	Pertaining to the trachea (windpipe)
trachealgia (trā″kē-ăl′jĭ-ă)	trach/e -algia	trachea, windpipe pain	Pain in the trachea (windpipe)
tracheolaryngotomy (trā″kē-ō-lăr″ĭn-gŏt′ō-mē)	trache/o laryng/o -tomy	trachea, windpipe larynx, voice box incision	Incision into the larynx (voice box) and trachea (windpipe)
tracheostomy (trā″kē-ŏs′tō-mē)	trache/o -stomy	trachea, windpipe new opening	New opening into the trachea (windpipe). See Figure 11.20 ■

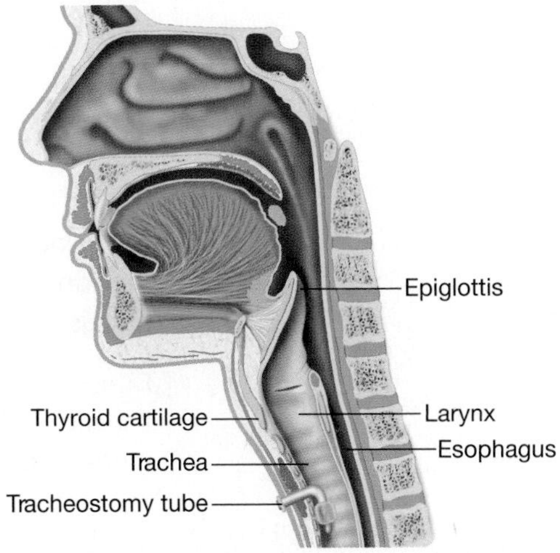

■ **Figure 11.20** Tracheostomy tube in place.

MEDICAL WORD	WORD PARTS		DEFINITION
	Part	Meaning	
tuberculosis (TB) (tū-běr″ kū-lō´ sĭs)	tubercul -osis	a little swelling condition	Infectious disease caused by the tubercle bacillus, *Mycobacterium tuberculosis*. TB can be diagnosed with a positive sputum culture indicating *Mycobacterium tuberculosis* and a chest x-ray revealing lesions in the lung.

fyi The development of drug-resistant strains of bacteria is one of the most alarming trends in health care. The problem is particularly serious with regard to TB bacteria that have developed strains resistant to treatment with one of each of the major tuberculosis medications. Even more dangerous are strains that are resistant to at least two anti-TB drugs, leading to a condition called **multidrug-resistant TB (MDR TB)**. This can develop when people either do not complete the entire course of medication or fail to take their medications as prescribed, when health care professionals prescribe the wrong kinds of treatment, or when the drug supply is inconsistent—a particular problem in impoverished or war-torn areas. People with untreated MDR TB are highly contagious. Although MDR TB can be treated successfully, it is much more difficult to combat than regular tuberculosis and requires long-term therapy—up to 2 years—with drugs that can cause serious side effects.

For more information on tuberculosis, go to the Centers for Disease Control and Prevention (CDC) website: www.cdc.gov or call (800) 458-5231.

wheeze (hwēz)			A high-pitched whistling sound caused by constriction of the air passageway associated with an asthma attack

• Drug Highlights •

TYPE OF DRUG	DESCRIPTION AND EXAMPLES
antihistamines	Act to counter the effects of histamine by blocking histamine 1 (H_1) receptors. They are used to treat allergy symptoms, prevent or control motion sickness, and in combination with cold remedies to decrease mucus secretion and produce bedtime sedation. See Figure 11.21 ■ EXAMPLES: Benadryl (diphenhydramine HCl), Dimetane (brompheniramine maleate), Allegra (fexofenadine), Claritin (loratadine), and Zyrtec (cetirizine)

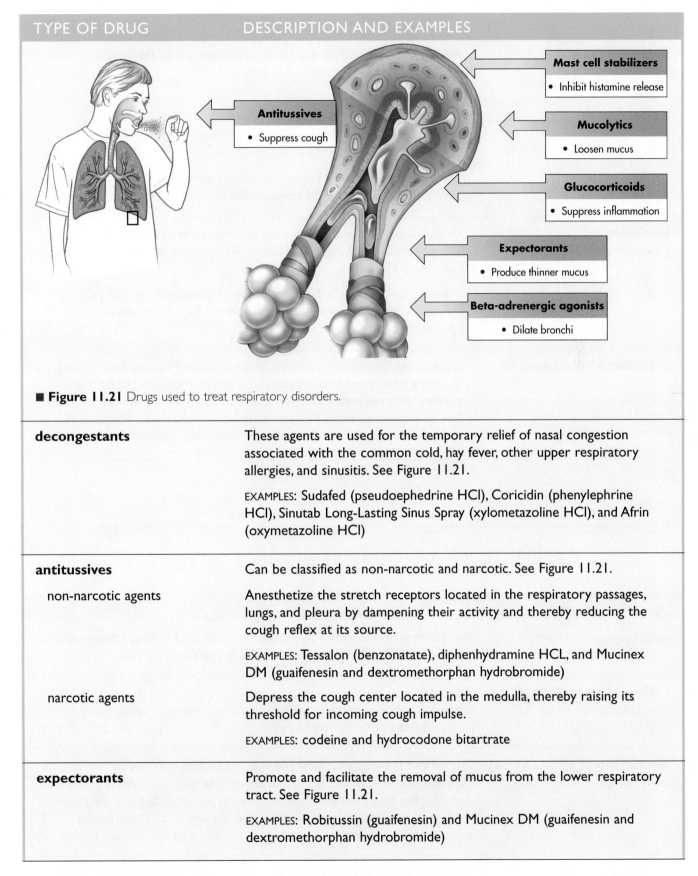

| TYPE OF DRUG | DESCRIPTION AND EXAMPLES |

Mast cell stabilizers
- Inhibit histamine release

Antitussives
- Suppress cough

Mucolytics
- Loosen mucus

Glucocorticoids
- Suppress inflammation

Expectorants
- Produce thinner mucus

Beta-adrenergic agonists
- Dilate bronchi

■ **Figure 11.21** Drugs used to treat respiratory disorders.

decongestants	These agents are used for the temporary relief of nasal congestion associated with the common cold, hay fever, other upper respiratory allergies, and sinusitis. See Figure 11.21. EXAMPLES: Sudafed (pseudoephedrine HCl), Coricidin (phenylephrine HCl), Sinutab Long-Lasting Sinus Spray (xylometazoline HCl), and Afrin (oxymetazoline HCl)
antitussives	Can be classified as non-narcotic and narcotic. See Figure 11.21.
non-narcotic agents	Anesthetize the stretch receptors located in the respiratory passages, lungs, and pleura by dampening their activity and thereby reducing the cough reflex at its source. EXAMPLES: Tessalon (benzonatate), diphenhydramine HCL, and Mucinex DM (guaifenesin and dextromethorphan hydrobromide)
narcotic agents	Depress the cough center located in the medulla, thereby raising its threshold for incoming cough impulse. EXAMPLES: codeine and hydrocodone bitartrate
expectorants	Promote and facilitate the removal of mucus from the lower respiratory tract. See Figure 11.21. EXAMPLES: Robitussin (guaifenesin) and Mucinex DM (guaifenesin and dextromethorphan hydrobromide)

TYPE OF DRUG	DESCRIPTION AND EXAMPLES
mucolytics	Break chemical bonds in mucus, thereby lowering its thickness. See Figure 11.21. EXAMPLE: acetylcysteine
bronchodilators	Used to improve pulmonary airflow by dilating air passages. See Figure 11.21. EXAMPLES: Proventil HFA (albuterol sulfate), ephedrine sulfate, aminophylline, and Theo-24 (theophylline)
inhalational glucocorticoids	Used in the treatment of bronchial asthma and in seasonal or perennial allergic conditions when other forms of treatment are not effective. See Figure 11.21. EXAMPLES: Beconase AQ (beclomethasone dipropionate monohydrate), Azmacort (triamcinolone acetonide), Flovent HFA (fluticasone propionate), and Aerobid (flunisolide)
antituberculosis agents	Used in the long-term treatment of tuberculosis (9 months to 1 year). They are often used in combination of two or more drugs and the primary drug regimen for active tuberculosis combines the drugs Myambutol (ethambutol HCl), isoniazid, Rifadin, Rimactane (rifampin), pyrazenamide, or Rifater (isoniazid, pyrazinamide, rifampin)

• Diagnostic and Lab Tests •

TEST	DESCRIPTION
acid-fast bacilli (AFB) (ăs ĭd-fãst″ bă-sĭl′ĭ)	Test performed on sputum to detect the presence of *Mycobacterium tuberculosis,* an acid-fast bacilli. Positive results indicate tuberculosis.
antistreptolysin O (ASO) (ăn″ tĭ-strĕp-tŏl′ ĭ-sĭn)	Test performed on blood serum to detect the presence of streptolysin enzyme O, which is secreted by beta-hemolytic streptococcus. Positive results indicate streptococcal infection.
arterial blood gases (ABGs) (ăr-tē′ rē-ăl)	Test measures the acidity (pH) and the levels of oxygen and carbon dioxide in the blood. This test is used to check how well the lungs are able to move oxygen into the blood and remove carbon dioxide from the blood. Important in determining respiratory acidosis and/or alkalosis, metabolic acidosis, and/or alkalosis.
bronchoscopy (brŏng-kŏs′ kō-pē)	Visual examination of the larynx, trachea, and bronchi via a flexible bronchoscope. With the use of biopsy forceps, tissues and secretions can be removed for further analysis.

TEST	DESCRIPTION
culture, sputum (spū tŭm)	Examination of the sputum to determine the presence of pathogenic microorganisms. Abnormal results can indicate tuberculosis, bronchitis, pneumonia, bronchiectasis, and other infectious respiratory diseases (RD).
culture, throat	Test that identifies the presence of pathogenic microorganisms in the throat, especially beta-hemolytic streptococci.
laryngoscopy (lăr″ ĭn-gŏs′ kō-pē)	Visual examination of the larynx via a laryngoscope.
nasopharyngography (nā″ zō-făr-ĭn-ŏg′ ră-fē)	X-ray examination of the nasopharynx.
pulmonary function test (pŭl′ mō-nĕ-rē)	Series of tests performed to determine the diffusion of oxygen and carbon dioxide across the cell membrane in the lungs, including tidal volume (TV), vital capacity (VC), expiratory reserve volume (ERV), inspiratory capacity (IC), residual volume (RV), forced inspiratory volume (FIV), functional residual capacity (FRC), maximal voluntary ventilation (MVV), total lung capacity (TLC), and flow volume loop (F-V loop). Abnormal results can indicate various respiratory diseases and conditions.
rhinoscopy (rī-nŏs′ kō-pē)	Visual examination of the nasal passages.

• Abbreviations •

ABBREVIATION	MEANING	ABBREVIATION	MEANING
ABGs	arterial blood gases	IRV	inspiratory reserve volume
AFB	acid-fast bacilli	IV	intravenous
AIDS	acquired immunodeficiency syndrome	MBC	maximal breathing capacity
		MV	minute volume
ARD	acute respiratory disease	MVV	maximal voluntary ventilation
ARDS	adult respiratory distress syndrome	NSAIDs	nonsteroidal anti-inflammatory drugs
ASO	antistreptolysin O	O_2	oxygen
CF	cystic fibrosis	PE	pulmonary embolism
CO_2	carbon dioxide	PEEP	positive end-expiratory pressure
COLD	chronic obstructive lung disease		
COPD	chronic obstructive pulmonary disease	PND	postnasal drip, paroxysmal nocturnal dyspnea
CXR	chest x-ray	PPD	purified protein derivative
ENT	ear, nose, throat (otorhinolaryngology)	R	respiration
		RD	respiratory disease
ERV	expiratory reserve volume	RDS	respiratory distress syndrome
ET	endotracheal		
FEF	forced expiratory flow	RSV	respiratory syncytial virus
FEV	forced expiratory volume	RV	residual volume
FIV	forced inspiratory volume	SARS	severe acute respiratory syndrome
FRC	functional residual capacity		
F-V loop	flow volume loop	SIDS	sudden infant death syndrome
HBOT	hyperbaric oxygen therapy		
HIV	human immunodeficiency virus	SOB	shortness of breath
HMD	hyaline membrane disease	T & A	tonsillectomy and adenoidectomy
IC	inspiratory capacity		
IPPB	intermittent positive-pressure breathing	TLC	total lung capacity
		TV	tidal volume
IRDS	infant respiratory distress syndrome	URI	upper respiratory infection
		VC	vital capacity

Study and Review • Study and Review • Study and Review
Review • Study and Review • Study and Review • St
ew • Study and Review • Study and Review • Study

Anatomy and Physiology

Write your answers to the following questions.

1. List the organs of the respiratory system.

a. _____   b. _____

c. _____   d. _____

e. _____   f. _____

2. State the primary function of the respiratory system. _____

_____

_____

3. Define *external respiration*. _____

4. Define *internal respiration*. _____

5. List the five functions of the nose.

a. _____

b. _____

c. _____

d. _____

e. _____

6. List the three functions of the pharynx.

a. _____

b. _____

c. _____

7. State the function of the epiglottis. _____

8. Define *glottis*. _____

9. State the function of the larynx. _____

10. State the function of the trachea. _____

11. State the function of the bronchi. _____

12. Give a brief description of the lungs. _____

_____

13. Define *pleura*. _____

14. The thoracic cavity is separated from the abdominal cavity by a musculomembranous wall commonly known as

the _____

15. The central portion of the thoracic cavity between the lungs is a space called the_____

16. The right lung has _____ lobes and the left lung has _____

lobes.

17. The air cells of the lungs are the _____

18. State the main function of the lungs. _____

_____

19. The vital signs, which are essential elements for determining an individual's state of health, are

_____, _____,

_____, and _____.

20. Define the following terms:

    a. *Tidal volume* _____   **b.** *Residual volume* _____

    c. *Vital capacity* _____

21. The _____ _____ and the _____ of

the central nervous system regulate and control respiration.

22. The respiratory rate for a newborn is _____ to _____ breaths

per minute.

23. The respiratory rate for an adult is _____ to _____

breaths per minute.

Word Parts

PREFIXES

Give the definitions of the following prefixes.

    1. a- _____   **2.** epi- _____

    3. dys- _____   **4.** endo- _____

5. eu- _____

6. ex- _____

7. hyp- _____

8. hyper- _____

9. in- _____

10. tachy- _____

ROOTS AND COMBINING FORMS

Give the definitions of the following roots and combining forms

1. aspirat _____

2. alveol _____

3. anthrac _____

4. atel _____

5. bronch _____

6. bronch/i _____

7. bronchiol _____

8. bronch/o _____

9. con/i _____

10. cyan _____

11. halat _____

12. hem/o _____

13. laryng _____

14. larynge _____

15. laryng/o _____

16. lob _____

17. cyst _____

18. fibr _____

19. nas/o _____

20. orth/o _____

21. mes/o _____

22. tubercul _____

23. palat/o _____

24. pector (at) _____

25. pharyng _____

26. pharyng/o _____

27. thel/i _____

28. phragmat/o _____

29. pleur _____

30. pleura _____

31. pleur/o _____

32. pneum/o _____

33. pneumon _____

34. pulm/o _____

35. pulmon/o _____

36. py/o _____

37. rhin/o _____

38. sinus _____

39. spir/o _____

40. respirat _____

41. thorac/o _____

42. ventilat _____

43. tonsill _____

44. trach/e _____

45. trache/o _____   **46.** rhonch _____

47. sarc _____   **48.** diaphragmat/o _____

SUFFIXES

Give the definitions of the following suffixes.

1. -al _____   **2.** -algia _____

3. -cele _____   **4.** -centesis _____

5. -dynia _____   **6.** -ectasis _____

7. -ectomy _____   **8.** -ic _____

9. -ia _____   **10.** -ion _____

11. -itis _____   **12.** -meter _____

13. -osis _____   **14.** -oma _____

15. -staxis _____   **16.** -plasty _____

17. -or _____   **18.** -pnea _____

19. -ptysis _____   **20.** -rrhea _____

21. -scope _____   **22.** -stomy _____

23. -tomy _____   **24.** -us _____

Identifying Medical Terms

In the spaces provided, write the medical terms for the following meanings.

1. _____ Pertaining to a small air sac in the lungs

2. _____ Chronic dilation of a bronchus or bronchi

3. _____ Inflammation of the bronchi

4. _____ Condition of difficulty in speaking

5. _____ Good or normal breathing

6. _____ Spitting up blood

7. _____ Process of breathing in

8. _____ Inflammation of the larynx

9. _____ A collection of air between the chest wall and lungs

10. _____ Surgical repair of the nose

11. _____ Discharge from the nose

12. _____ Inflammation of a sinus

Spelling

Circle the correct spelling of each medical term.

1. bronchoscope / bronchscope

2. diaphramatcele / diaphragmatocele

3. expectoration / expectorion

4. laryngeal / laryngal

5. orthopnea / orthpnea

6. pleuritis / peluritis

7. pulmonectomy / plumonectomy

8. rhoncus / rhonchus

9. tachypnea / trachypnea

10. trachial / tracheal

Matching

Select the appropriate lettered meaning for each of the following words.

_____ 1. cough

_____ 2. cystic fibrosis

_____ 3. influenza

_____ 4. inhalation

_____ 5. olfaction

_____ 6. pleurodynia

_____ 7. rhinovirus

_____ 8. sputum

_____ 9. tachypnea

_____ 10. thoracocentesis

a. Substance coughed up from the lungs

b. Pain in the pleura

c. Process of smelling

d. One of a subgroup of viruses that causes the common cold in humans

e. Rapid breathing

f. Process of breathing in

g. Surgical puncture of the chest wall for removal of fluid

h. Sudden, forceful expulsion of air from the lungs

i. Inherited disease that affects the pancreas, respiratory system, and sweat glands

j. Slow breathing

k. Acute, contagious respiratory infection caused by a virus

Abbreviations

Place the correct word, phrase, or abbreviation in the space provided.

1. acid-fast bacilli _____

2. CF _____

3. chest x-ray _____

4. chronic obstructive lung disease _____

5. ET _____

6. PND _____

7. respiration _____

8. SIDS _____

9. shortness of breath _____

10. TB _____

Diagnostic and Laboratory Tests

Select the best answer to each multiple-choice question. Circle the letter of your choice.

1. Test performed on sputum to detect the presence of *Mycobacterium tuberculosis*.
   - **a.** antistreptolysin O
   - **b.** acid-fast bacilli
   - **c.** pulmonary function test
   - **d.** bronchoscopy

2. Visual examination of the nasal passages.
   - **a.** bronchoscopy
   - **b.** laryngoscopy
   - **c.** rhinoscopy
   - **d.** nasopharyngography

3. _____ is/are important in determining respiratory acidosis and/or alkalosis, metabolic acidosis, and/or alkalosis.
   - **a.** Acid-fast bacilli
   - **b.** Antistreptolysin O
   - **c.** Arterial blood gases
   - **d.** Pulmonary function test

4. Series of tests to determine the diffusion of oxygen and carbon dioxide across the cell membrane in the lungs.
   - **a.** acid-fast bacilli
   - **b.** antistreptolysin O
   - **c.** arterial blood gases
   - **d.** pulmonary function test

5. Visual examination of the larynx, trachea, and bronchi via a flexible scope.
   - **a.** bronchoscopy
   - **b.** laryngoscopy
   - **c.** nasopharyngography
   - **d.** rhinoscopy

PRACTICAL APPLICATION

MEDICAL RECORD ANALYSIS

This exercise contains information, abbreviations, and medical terminology from an actual medical record or case study that has been adapted for this text. The names and any personal information have been created by the author. Read and study each form or case study and then answer the questions that follow. You may refer to Appendix III, Abbreviations and Symbols, on page A41.

GOODWILL HEALTH CLINIC
1001 Evergreen Park Drive
Lakeland, FL 33813
(123) 456-7890

Progress Note
_____

Wilmer Sanchez, Patient # 8234

Thursday, February 25, 20xx

Subjective:
The patient presents today for re-evaluation.

Wilmer Sanchez is a 28-year-old male migrant worker seen in the Lakeland, FL, office. Patient presents with a history of pulmonary tuberculosis and returns for a check of his sputum and a liver function test. He has been taking isoniazid, rifampin, and ethambutol for 4 months. He states that since he has been taking his medicine, he is feeling better.

Objective:
The patient appears to be in no apparent distress. The patient's mood and affect appeared normal throughout the visit. Afebrile, P 72, R 18, BP 118/64, Wt 143. No rales noted upon auscultation. Occasional cough, nonproductive.

Assessment:
Apparent state of health improved over the last 4 months. Patient has gained 3 lbs.

Patient is following medication regimen and does participate in the DOT system, which is documented in his record.

Plan:
Send to lab for a sputum culture and liver function test.

Schedule a return visit for 2 weeks.

Medical Record Questions

Place the correct answer in the space provided.

1. Define *rale*. _____

2. What does the abbreviation *DOT* mean? _____

3. Define *afebrile*. _____

4. Did this patient seem anxious? _____

5. What type of cough did this patient have? _____

PEARSON
mymedicalterminologylab™

MyMedicalTerminologyLab is a premium online homework management system that includes a host of features to help you study. Registered users will find:

- Fun games and activities built within a virtual hospital

- Powerful tools that track and analyze your results—allowing you to create a personalized learning experience

- Videos, flashcards, and audio pronunciations to help enrich your progress

- Streaming lesson presentations and self-paced learning modules

- A space where you and your instructors can view and manage your assignments

LEARNING OUTCOMES

On completion of this chapter, you will
be able to:

1. Describe the urinary system and explain its
   vital function.

2. State the descriptions and primary functions
   of the organs/structures of the urinary
   system.

3. Define urinalysis and state its significance.

4. Identify normal and abnormal constituents of
   urine.

5. Analyze, build, spell, and pronounce medical
   words.

6. Comprehend the drugs highlighted in this
   chapter.

7. Describe diagnostic and laboratory tests
   related to the urinary system.

8. Identify and define selected abbreviations.

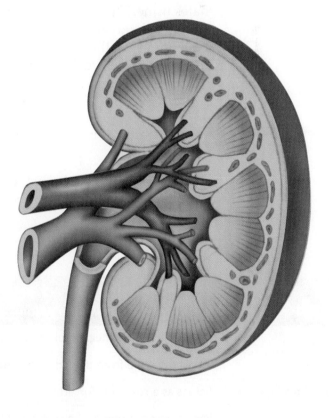

COMBINING FORMS OF THE URINARY SYSTEM

albumin/o	protein	micturit/o	to urinate
bacter/i	bacteria	nephr/o	kidney
calc/i	calcium	noct/o	night
col/o	colon	perine/o	perineum
corpor/e	body	periton/e	peritoneum
cutan/e	skin	py/o	pus
cyst/o	bladder	pyel/o	renal pelvis
excret/o	sifted out	ren/o	kidney
glomerul/o	glomerulus, little ball	scler/o	hardening
glycos/o	glucose, sugar	son/o	sound
hem/o	blood	ur/o	urine, urinate, urination
hemat/o	blood	ureter/o	ureter
keton/o	ketone	urethr/o	urethra
lith/o	stone	urin/o	urine
meat/o	passage		

Anatomy and Physiology

The urinary system consists of two kidneys, two ureters, one bladder, and one urethra (see Figure 12.1 ■). It is also called the excretory, genitourinary (GU), or urogenital (UG) system and is the organ system that produces, stores, and eliminates urine. The vital function of the urinary system is to extract certain wastes from the bloodstream, convert these materials to urine, transport the urine from the kidneys via the ureters to the bladder, and eliminate it (void) at appropriate intervals via the urethra. Through this vital function, homeostasis of body fluids is maintained. Table 12.1 ■ provides an at-a-glance look at the urinary system.

KIDNEYS

The **kidneys** are purplish-brown, bean-shaped organs located behind the abdominal cavity (*retroperitoneal area*) on either side of the spine between thoracic vertebrae (T 12)

TABLE 12.1 Urinary System at-a-Glance

Organ/Structure	Primary Functions/Description
Kidneys	Produce urine and help regulate and control body fluids
Ureters	Transport urine from the kidneys to the bladder
Urinary bladder	Serves as a reservoir for urine
Urethra	Passageway of urine to the outside of the body; in the male conveys both urine and semen

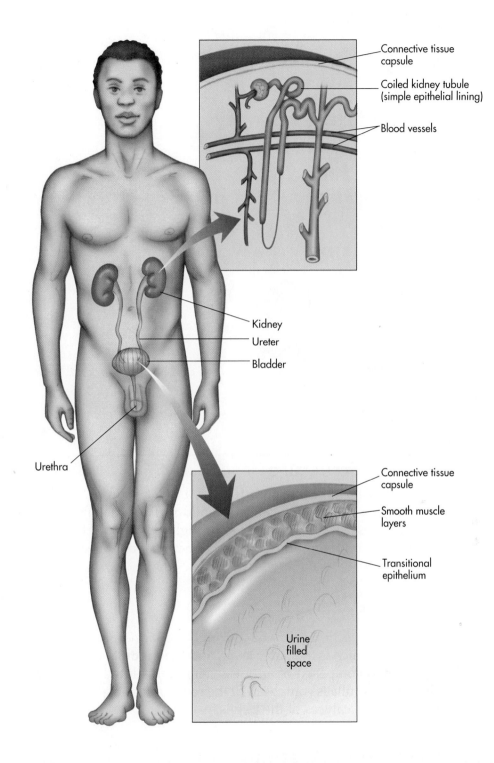

Connective tissue capsule

Coiled kidney tubule (simple epithelial lining)

Blood vessels

Kidney

Ureter

Bladder

Urethra

Connective tissue capsule

Smooth muscle layers

Transitional epithelium

Urine filled space

■ **Figure 12.1** The urinary system: kidneys, ureters, bladder, and urethra with expanded view of a nephron and the urine-filled space within a bladder.

and the lumbar region (Figure 12.2 ■). Each kidney is surrounded by three capsules; the **true capsule**, the **perirenal fat**, and the **renal fascia.** The true capsule is a smooth, fibrous connective membrane that loosely adheres to the surface of the kidney. The perirenal fat is the adipose capsule that embeds each kidney in fatty tissue. The renal fascia is a sheath of fibrous tissue that helps to anchor the kidney to the surrounding structures and helps to maintain its normal position.

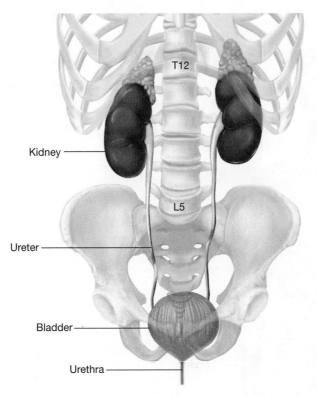

T12

Kidney

L5

Ureter

Bladder

Urethra

■ **Figure 12.2** Position of the urinary organs.

External Structure

Each kidney has a *concave* border and a *convex* border. The center of the concave border opens into a notch called the **hilum.** The renal artery and vein, nerves, and lymphatic vessels enter and leave through the hilum. The ureter enters the kidney through the hilum into a saclike collecting portion called the *renal pelvis.* See Figure 12.3 ■

Internal Structure

When a cross-section is made through the kidney, two distinct areas can be seen: the **cortex**, which is the outer layer, and the **medulla** or inner portion (Figure 12.3). The cortex is composed of arteries, veins, convoluted tubules, and glomerular capsules. The medulla is composed of the renal pyramids, conelike masses with papillae projecting into calyces of the pelvis.

Microscopic Anatomy

Microscopic examination of the kidney reveals about 1 million **nephrons**, which are the structural and functional units of the organ (Figure 12.3). Each nephron consists of a **renal corpuscle** and **tubule.** The renal corpuscle or malpighian body consists of a **glomerulus**, a tuft of blood vessels surrounded by the Bowman's capsule. The **Bowman's capsule** is a cup-like sac at the beginning of the tubular component of a nephron in the kidney that performs the first step in the filtration of blood to form urine. Extending from each Bowman's capsule is a tubule consisting of the proximal convoluted portion, the loop of Henle, and a distal convoluted portion that opens into a collecting duct.

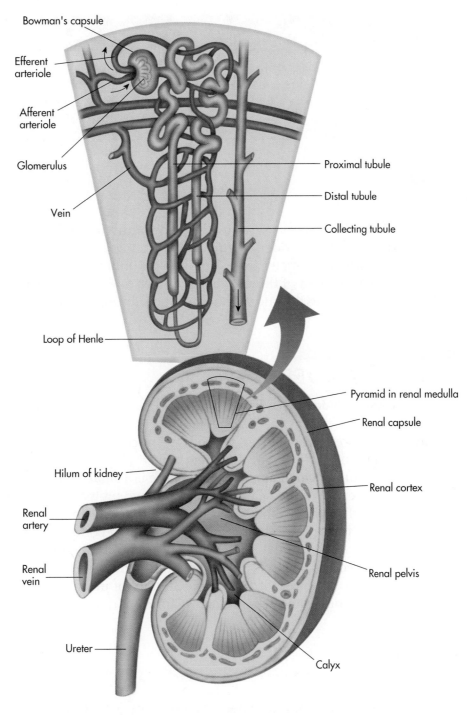

Bowman's capsule

Efferent arteriole

Afferent arteriole

Glomerulus

Vein

Loop of Henle

Proximal tubule

Distal tubule

Collecting tubule

Pyramid in renal medulla

Renal capsule

Hilum of kidney

Renal cortex

Renal artery

Renal vein

Renal pelvis

Ureter

Calyx

■ **Figure 12.3** Kidney with an expanded view of a nephron.

Nephron

The vital function of the **nephron** is to regulate, control, and then remove the waste products of metabolism from the blood plasma. These waste products are urea, uric acid, and creatinine, as well as any excess sodium, chloride, and potassium ions and ketone bodies. The nephron plays a vital role in the maintenance of normal fluid balance in the body by regulated reabsorption of water and selected electrolytes back into the blood. Approximately 1000–1200 milliliters (mL) of blood flows through the kidney per minute. At a rate of 1000 mL of blood per minute, about 1.5 million mL flows through the kidney in each 24-hour day.

LIFE SPAN CONSIDERATIONS

At 10 weeks' gestation, urine forms and enters the bladder of the fetus. At about the third month the fetal kidneys begin to secrete urine. The amount increases gradually as the fetus matures. The newborn's kidneys are immature and lack the ability to concentrate urine. Glomerular filtration and reabsorption are relatively low until the child is 1 or 2 years of age.

URETERS

Each kidney has a **ureter**. They are narrow, muscular tubes that drain urine from the kidneys to the bladder (Figure 12.1). They are from 28 to 34 centimeters (cm) long and vary in diameter from 1 millimeter (mm) to 1 centimeter (cm). The walls of the ureters consist of three layers: an inner coat of mucous membrane, a middle coat of smooth muscle, and an outer coat of fibrous tissue.

URINARY BLADDER

The **urinary bladder** (see Figures 12.1 and 12.2) is the muscular, membranous sac that serves as a reservoir for urine. It is located in the anterior portion of the pelvic cavity and consists of a lower portion, the **neck**, which is continuous with the urethra, and an upper portion, the **apex**, which is connected with the umbilicus by the median umbilical ligament. The **trigone** is a small triangular area near the base of the bladder between the openings of the two ureters and the opening of the urethra. The wall of the bladder consists of four layers: an inner layer of epithelium, a muscular coat of smooth muscle, an outer layer composed of longitudinal muscle (*detrusor urinae*), and a fibrous layer. An empty bladder feels firm as the muscular wall becomes thick. As the bladder fills with urine, the muscular wall becomes thinner and distends according to the amount of urine present. Normally, urine is formed continously and when there is sufficient quantity the need to void occurs.

URETHRA

The **urethra** is the musculomembranous tube extending from the bladder to the outside of the body. The external urinary opening is the **urinary meatus.** The male urethra is approximately 20 cm long and is divided into three sections: *prostatic, membranous,* and *penile.* It conveys both urine and semen out of the body. The female urethra is approximately 3 cm long. The urinary meatus is situated between the clitoris and the opening of the vagina. The female urethra conveys urine out of the body. See Figure 12.4 ■

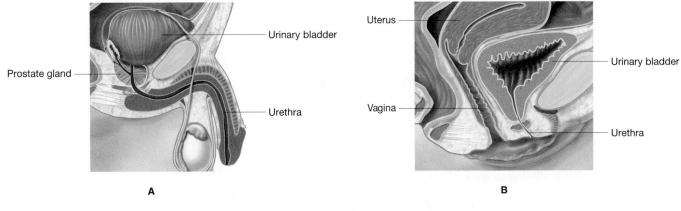

■ Figure 12.4 (A) The male urethra. (B) The female urethra.

LIFE SPAN CONSIDERATIONS

Urinary tract infections (UTIs) are common in children. The microorganisms *Escherichia coli, Klebsiella,* and *Proteus* cause most urinary tract infections seen in children. The signs and symptoms of a urinary tract infection are age related. Infants can experience fever, weight loss, nausea and vomiting, increased urination, foul-smelling urine, persistent diaper rash, and failure to thrive. Older children can have frequent and/or painful urination, abdominal pain, hematuria, fever, chills, and bed-wetting episodes in a trained child.

URINE

Urine is formed by the process of *filtration* and *reabsorption* in the nephron. It consists of 95% water and 5% solid substances. It is secreted by the kidneys and transported by the ureters to the bladder, where it is stored before being discharged from the body via the urethra. See Figure 12.5 ■

An average normal adult feels the need to void when the bladder contains around 300–350 mL of urine. An average of 1000–1500 mL of urine is voided daily. Normal urine is clear and yellow to amber in color and has a faintly aromatic odor, a specific gravity of 1.003–1.030, and a slightly acid pH (hydrogen ion concentration).

LIFE SPAN CONSIDERATIONS

Changes noted in the urinary system of the older adult are loss of muscle tone in the ureters, bladder, and urethra. Bladder capacity can be reduced by half, and the older adult could have to make frequent trips to the bathroom. **Urge incontinence** (or the inability to retain urine voluntarily) is a concern for older adults. There is a leakage of urine due to bladder muscles that contract inappropriately. Often these contractions occur regardless of the amount of urine that is in the bladder. Causes of urge incontinence can include bladder infection, inflammation, cancer, stones, other forms of outlet obstruction, neurological diseases, or injuries. In men, urge incontinence can be caused by benign prostatic hyperplasia (BPH) or prostate cancer. In most cases of urge incontinence, no specific cause can be identified. Although urge incontinence may occur in anyone at any age, it is more common in women and older adults.

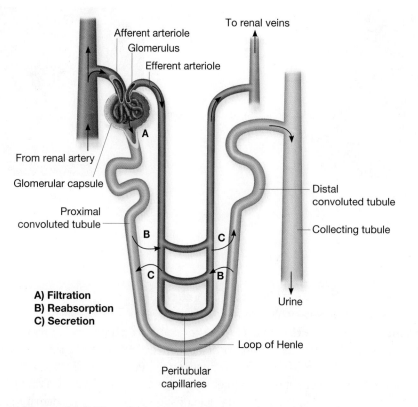

Afferent arteriole
Glomerulus
Efferent arteriole
To renal veins
From renal artery
Glomerular capsule
Proximal convoluted tubule
Distal convoluted tubule
Collecting tubule
Urine
Loop of Henle
Peritubular capillaries

A) Filtration
B) Reabsorption
C) Secretion

■ **Figure 12.5** Sites of tubular reabsorption and secretion.

Urinalysis

Urinalysis (UA) is a laboratory test that evaluates the physical, chemical, and microscopic properties of urine. A freshly voided urine specimen provides for more accurate test results. A urine sample that is left standing for an extended period of time will deteriorate. If the urinalysis cannot be performed on the specimen within 1 hour of the time voided, it should be refrigerated, with the time of collection written on the label of the container. Urine should be collected in a clean, dry, disposable container. When a bacteriological culture is to be done on urine, the specimen is collected by **catheterization.** A urinary catheterization is the process of introducing a catheter through the urethra into the bladder for withdrawal of urine. This is a sterile procedure and performed by individuals trained and skilled in the proper technique.

Urinalysis is a valuable diagnostic tool. Abnormal conditions or diseases can be quickly and easily detected because of the fact that the physical and chemical constituents of normal urine are constant. See Table 12.2 ■

TABLE 12.2 Normal and Abnormal Constituents of Urine

Constituent	Normal	Abnormal/Significance
Color	Yellow to amber	Red or reddish—presence of hemoglobin Orange—due to Pyridium (a drug used to treat the discomfort of a urinary tract infection Greenish-brown or black—caused by bile pigments. *The color of urine darkens upon standing.*
Appearance	Clear	Milky—fat globules, pus, bacteria Smoky—blood cells Hazy—refrigeration
Reaction	Between 4.6 and 8.0 pH, with an average of 6.0	High acidity—diabetic acidosis, fever, dehydration Alkaline—urinary tract infection, renal failure
Specific gravity (sp. gr.)	Between 1.003 and 1.030	Low (1.001–1.002)—diabetes insipidus High (over 1.030)—diabetes mellitus, hepatic disease, congestive heart failure
Odor	Faintly aromatic	Fruity sweet—acetone, associated with diabetes mellitus Unpleasant—decomposition of drugs, foods, alcohol
Quantity	Around 1000–1500 mL per day	High—diabetes mellitus, diabetes insipidus, nervousness, diuretics, excessive intake Low—acute nephritis, heart disease, diarrhea, vomiting None—uremia, renal failure
Protein	Negative	Positive—renal disease, pyelonephritis
Glucose	Negative	Positive—diabetes mellitus
Ketones	Negative	Positive—uncontrolled diabetes mellitus, high-protein, low-carbohydrate diet, starvation
Bilirubin	Negative	Positive—liver disease, biliary obstruction, congestive heart failure
Blood	Negative	Positive—renal disease, trauma
Nitrites	Negative	Positive—bacteriuria
Urobilinogen	0.1–1.0	Absent—biliary obstruction Reduced—antibiotic therapy Increased—early warning of hepatic or hemolytic disease

Anatomy and Physiology Labeling

Identify the structures shown below by filling in the blanks.

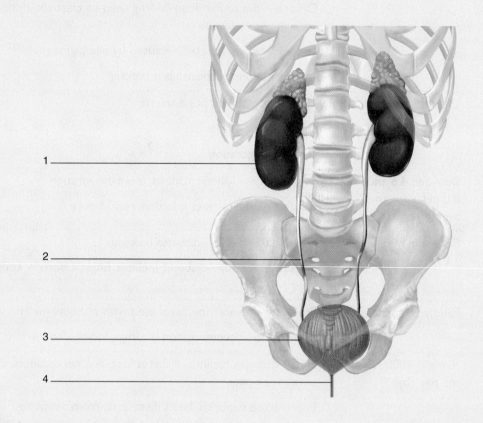

1 _____

2 _____

3 _____

4 _____

• Building Your Medical Vocabulary •

This section provides the foundation for learning medical terminology. Review the following alphabetized word list. Note how common prefixes and suffixes are repeatedly applied to word roots and combining forms to create different meanings. The word parts are color-coded: prefixes are green, suffixes are blue, **roots/combining forms are red.**

You will find that some terms have not been divided into word parts. These are common words or specialized terms that are included to enhance your medical vocabulary. See Chapter 1, page 7, to review pronunciation guidelines.

MEDICAL WORD	WORD PARTS		DEFINITION
	Part	**Meaning**	
albuminuria (ăl-bū″ mĭn-oo′ rĭ-ă)	albumin -uria	protein urine	Indicates the presence of serum protein in the urine. Albumin is the major protein in blood plasma. When detected in urine (*albuminuria*), it may indicate a leak in the glomerular membrane, which allows albumin to enter the renal tubule and pass into the urine.
antidiuretic (ăn″ tĭ-dī″ ū-rĕt′ ĭk)	anti- di(a)- uret -ic	against complete, through urine pertaining to	Pertaining to a medication that decreases urine production and secretion
anuria (ăn-ū′ rĭ-ă)	an- -uria	without urine	Literally means *without the formation of urine;* lack of urine production
bacteriuria (băk-tē″ rĭ-ū′ rĭ-ă)	bacter/i -uria	bacteria urine	Presence of bacteria in the urine
calciuria (kăl″ sĭ-ū′ rĭ-ă)	calc/i -uria	calcium urine	Presence of calcium in the urine
calculus (kăl′ kū-lŭs)			Pebble; any abnormal concretion (*stone*); plural: calculi. See Figure 12.6 ■

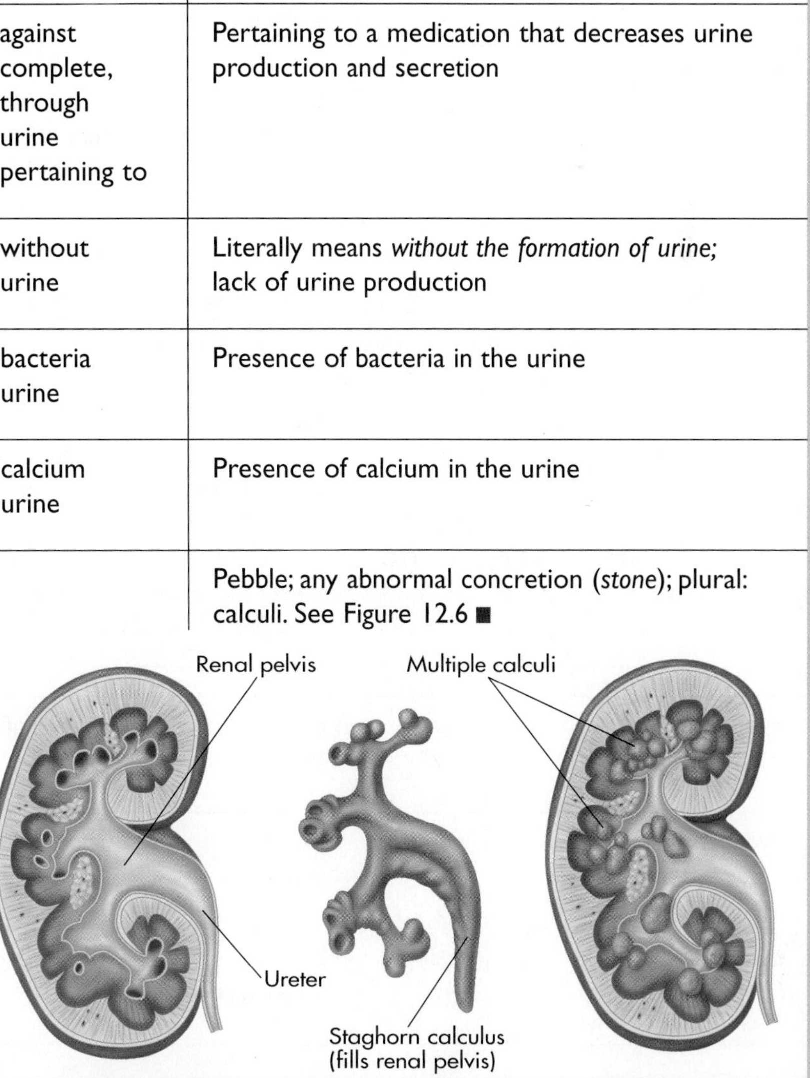

Renal pelvis

Multiple calculi

Ureter

Staghorn calculus (fills renal pelvis)

■ **Figure 12.6** Urinary calculi.

MEDICAL WORD	WORD PARTS		DEFINITION
	Part	Meaning	
catheter (kăth´ ĕ-tĕr)			Tube of elastic, elastic web, rubber, glass, metal, or plastic that is inserted into a body cavity to remove fluid or to inject fluid. See Figure 12.7 ■ ■ **Figure 12.7** Closed urinary drainage system. Urine being measured after it leaves patient's body via catheter.
cystectomy (sĭs-tĕk´ tō-mē)	cyst -ectomy	bladder surgical excision	Surgical excision of the bladder or part of the bladder
cystitis (sĭs-tī´ tĭs)	cyst -itis	bladder inflammation	Inflammation of the bladder, usually occurring secondarily to ascending urinary tract infections. More than 85% of cases of cystitis are caused by *Escherichia coli*, a bacillus found in the lower gastrointestinal tract.

LIFE SPAN CONSIDERATIONS

Cystitis is very common and occurs in more than 6 million Americans a year. It frequently affects sexually active women ages 20–50 but can also occur in those who are not sexually active or in young girls and older adults. Females are more prone to cystitis because of their shorter urethra (bacteria do not have to travel as far to enter the bladder) and because of the short distance between the opening of the urethra and the anus.

Interstitial cystitis (IC) is a painful inflammation of the bladder wall. Approximately 450,000 people suffer from this condition and, of those, 90% are women. Symptoms can vary from mild to severe. The cause is unknown, and IC does not respond well to antibiotic therapy.

MEDICAL WORD	WORD PARTS		DEFINITION
cystocele (sĭs´ tō-sēl)	cyst/o -cele	bladder hernia	Hernia of the bladder that protrudes into the vagina
cystodynia (sĭs˝ tō-dĭn´ ĭ-ă)	cyst/o -dynia	bladder pain	Pain in the bladder; commonly called *cystalgia*
cystogram (sĭs´ tō-grăm)	cyst/o -gram	bladder a mark, record	X-ray record of the bladder

MEDICAL WORD	WORD PARTS		DEFINITION
	Part	**Meaning**	
cystolithectomy (sĭs″ tō-lĭ-thĕk′ tō-mē)	cyst/o -lith -ectomy	bladder stone surgical excision	Surgical excision of a stone from the bladder
cystoscope (sĭst′ ō-skōp)	cyst/o -scope	bladder instrument for examining	Medical instrument used for visual examination of the bladder
dialysis (dī-ăl′ ĭ-sĭs)	dia- -lysis	complete, through destruction, to separate	Medical procedure to separate waste material from the blood and to maintain fluid, electrolyte, and acid–base balance in impaired kidney function or in the absence of the kidney. The two main types of dialysis, hemodialysis (HD) and peritoneal dialysis (PD), remove wastes and excess water from the blood in different ways.
diuresis (dī″ ū-rē′ sĭs)	di(a)- ur -esis	complete, through urinate condition	Pathological condition of increased or excessive flow of urine; occurs in conditions such as diabetes mellitus, diabetes insipidus, and acute renal failure. Diuretics can also produce diuresis.
dysuria (dĭs-ū′ rĭ-ă)	dys- -uria	difficult, painful urine	Difficult or painful urination
edema (ĕ-dē′ mă)			Pathological condition in which the body tissues contain an accumulation of fluid
enuresis (ĕn″ ū-rē′ sĭs)	en- ur -esis	within urinate condition	Condition of involuntary emission of urine; *bedwetting*
excretory (ĕks′ krə-tō-rē)	excretor -y	sifted out pertaining to	Pertaining to the elimination of waste products from the body
extracorporeal shock wave lithotriptor (ESWL) (ĕks″ tră-kor-por′ ē-ăl lĭth′ ō-trĭp″ tor)	extra- corpor/e -al	outside, beyond body pertaining to	Medical device used to crush kidney stones (*renal calculi*). The patient is sedated and immersed in a water bath while shock waves pound the stones until they crumble into small pieces. These pieces are intended to be flushed out with urine. See Figure 12.8 ∎

MEDICAL WORD	WORD PARTS		DEFINITION
	Part	Meaning	

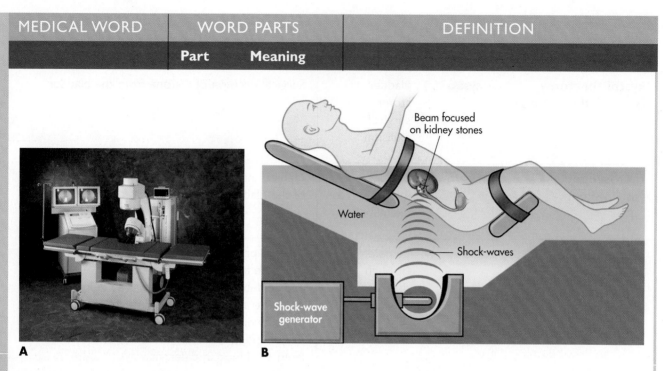

■ **Figure 12.8** (A) Dornier Compact Delta® lithotripsy system. Acoustic shock waves generated by the shock-wave generator travel through soft tissue to shatter the renal stone into fragments, which are then eliminated in the urine. (B) Illustration of water immersion lithotripsy procedure.

(Source: Courtesy of Dornier Medical Products, Inc.)

| **glomerular** (glō-měr´ ū-lăr) | glomerul | glomerulus, little ball | Literally means *pertaining to the glomerulus*; a tuft of blood vessels located within the Bownam's capsule that permit a greater surface area for filtration. See Figure 12.9 ■ |
| | -ar | pertaining to | |

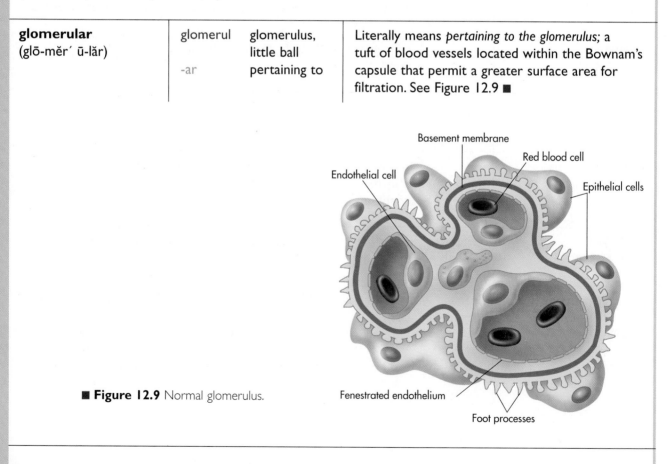

■ **Figure 12.9** Normal glomerulus.

MEDICAL WORD	WORD PARTS		DEFINITION
	Part	**Meaning**	
glomerulitis (glō-měr″ ū-lī′ tǐs)	glomerul/o -itis	glomerulus, little ball inflammation	Inflammation of the renal glomeruli
glomerulonephritis (glō-měr″ ū-lō-ně-frī′ tǐs)	glomerul/o nephr -itis	glomerulus, little ball kidney inflammation	Inflammation of the kidney involving primarily the glomeruli. There are three types: acute glomeru-lonephritis (AGN), chronic glomerulonephritis (CGN), and subacute glomerulonephritis. See Figure 12.10 ■

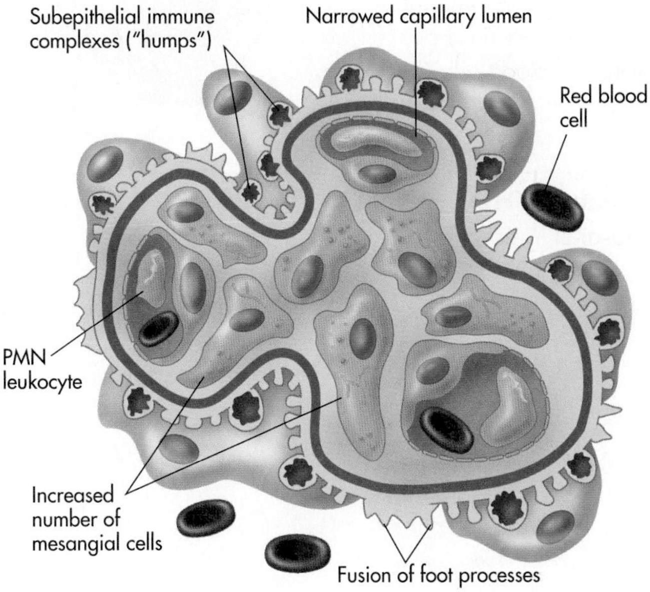

■ **Figure 12.10** Acute glomerulonephritis.

glycosuria (glī″ kō-soo′ rǐ-ă)	glycos -uria	glucose, sugar urine	Presence of glucose in the urine
hematuria (hē″ mă-tū′ rǐ-ă)	hemat -uria	blood urine	Presence of red blood cells (erythrocytes) in the urine. In microscopic hematuria, the urine appears normal to the naked eye, but examination with a microscope shows a high number of RBCs. Gross hematuria can be seen with the naked eye—the urine is red or the color of cola. If white blood cells are found in addition to red blood cells, then it is a sign of urinary tract infection. See Figure 12.11 ■

MEDICAL WORD	WORD PARTS		DEFINITION
	Part	**Meaning**	

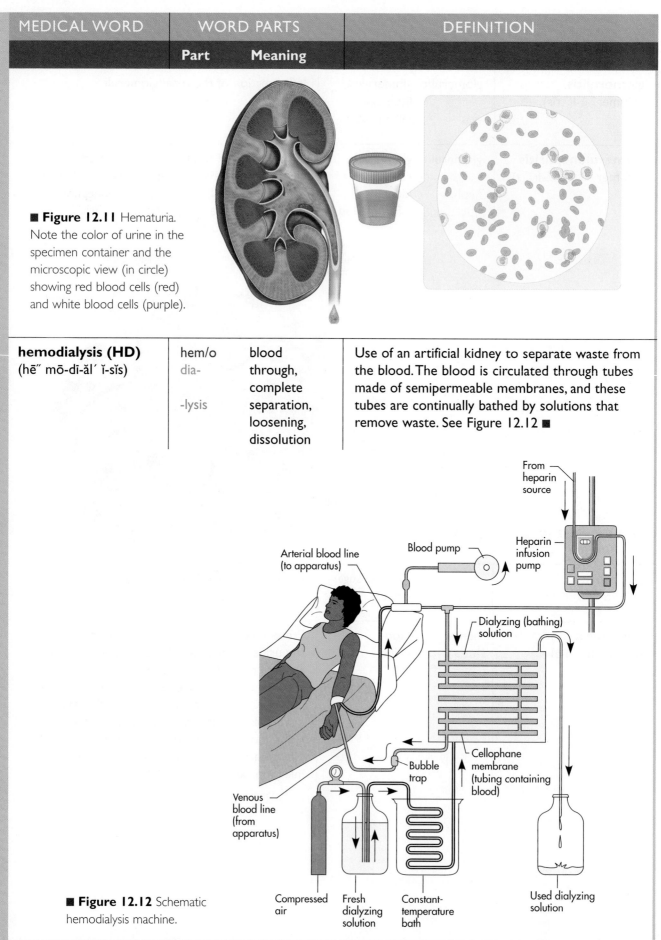

■ **Figure 12.11** Hematuria. Note the color of urine in the specimen container and the microscopic view (in circle) showing red blood cells (red) and white blood cells (purple).

| **hemodialysis (HD)** (hē″ mō-dī-ăl′ ĭ-sĭs) | hem/o dia- -lysis | blood through, complete separation, loosening, dissolution | Use of an artificial kidney to separate waste from the blood. The blood is circulated through tubes made of semipermeable membranes, and these tubes are continually bathed by solutions that remove waste. See Figure 12.12 ■ |

■ **Figure 12.12** Schematic hemodialysis machine.

MEDICAL WORD	WORD PARTS		DEFINITION
	Part	Meaning	
hydronephrosis (hī″ drō-něf-rō′ sĭs)	hydro- nephr -osis	water kidney condition	Pathological condition in which urine collects in the renal pelvis because of an obstructed outflow, thereby forming distention and damage to the kidney; can be caused by renal calculi, tumor, or hyperplasia of the prostate gland. See Figure 12.13 ■

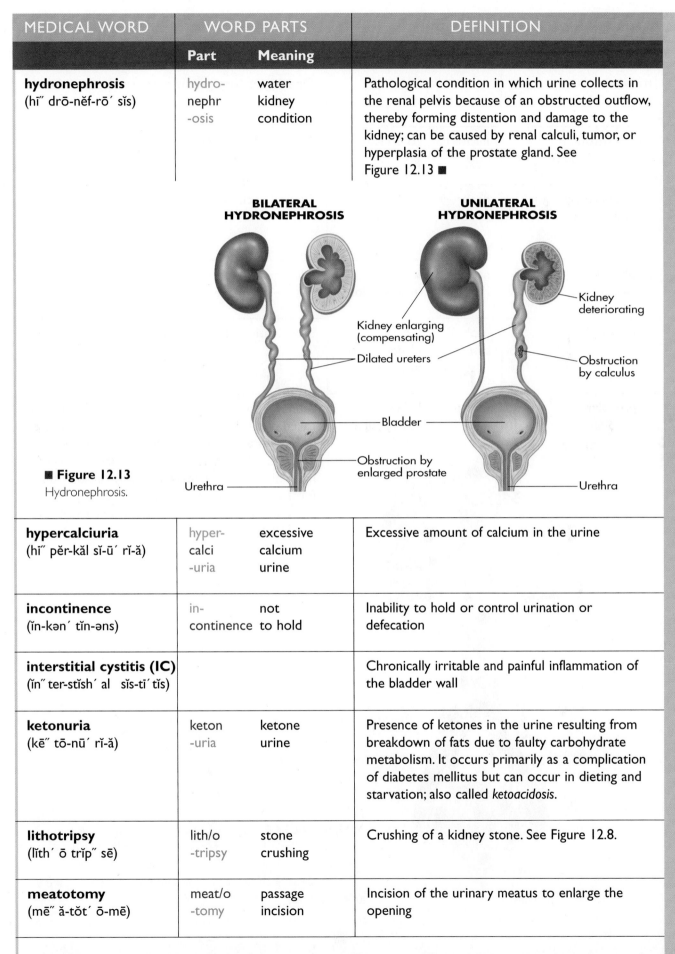

■ Figure 12.13
Hydronephrosis.

hypercalciuria (hī″ pĕr-kăl sĭ-ū′ rĭ-ă)	hyper- calci -uria	excessive calcium urine	Excessive amount of calcium in the urine
incontinence (ĭn-kən′ tĭn-əns)	in- continence	not to hold	Inability to hold or control urination or defecation
interstitial cystitis (IC) (ĭn″ ter-stĭsh′ al sĭs-tī′ tĭs)			Chronically irritable and painful inflammation of the bladder wall
ketonuria (kē″ tō-nū′ rĭ-ă)	keton -uria	ketone urine	Presence of ketones in the urine resulting from breakdown of fats due to faulty carbohydrate metabolism. It occurs primarily as a complication of diabetes mellitus but can occur in dieting and starvation; also called *ketoacidosis*.
lithotripsy (lĭth′ ō trĭp″ sē)	lith/o -tripsy	stone crushing	Crushing of a kidney stone. See Figure 12.8.
meatotomy (mē″ ă-tŏt′ ō-mē)	meat/o -tomy	passage incision	Incision of the urinary meatus to enlarge the opening

MEDICAL WORD	WORD PARTS		DEFINITION
	Part	Meaning	
meatus (mē-ā´ tŭs)			Opening or passage; the external opening of the urethra
micturition (mĭk´ tū-rĭ´ shŭn)	micturit -ion	to urinate process	Process of urination
nephrectomy (nĕ-frĕk´ tō-mē)	nephr -ectomy	kidney surgical excision	Surgical excision of a kidney.
nephritis (nĕf-rī´ tĭs)	nephr -itis	kidney inflammation	Inflammation of the kidney
nephrocystitis (nĕf´ rō-sĭs´ tĭ´ tĭs)	nephr/o cyst -itis	kidney bladder inflammation	Inflammation of the bladder and the kidney
nephrolith (nĕf´ rō-lĭth)	nephr/o -lith	kidney stone, calculus	Kidney stone; usually deposits of mineral salts, called *calculi,* in the kidney. These stones can pass into the ureter, irritate kidney tissue, and block urine flow. Kidney stones occur when the urine has a high level of minerals (usually calcium) that form stones. A condition characterized by the presence of a kidney stone is called *nephrolithiasis.* See Figure 12.14 ■

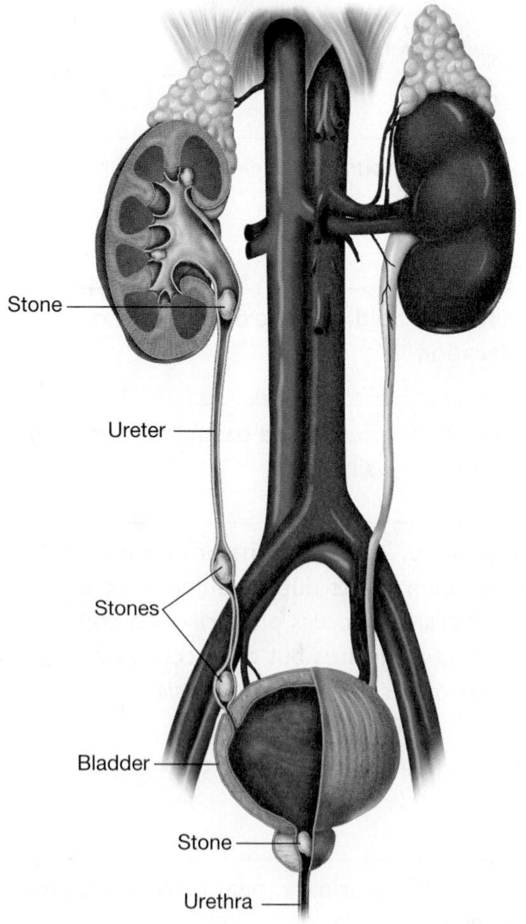

Stone
Ureter
Stones
Bladder
Stone
Urethra

■ **Figure 12.14** Renal calculi (stones) can form in several areas within the urinary tract. When they form in the kidney, they usually arise within the renal pelvis, forming the condition called nephrolithiasis. Stones can also form obstructions in the ureter, bladder, or urethra.

MEDICAL WORD	WORD PARTS		DEFINITION
	Part	Meaning	

fyi Kidney stones are common and painful disorders of the urinary tract. Men tend to be affected more frequently than women. Most kidney stones pass out of the body without any intervention, but stones that cause lasting symptoms or other complications should be treated. Two treatment techniques used are **extracorporeal shock wave lithotripsy (ESWL)** (see Figure 12.8 on page 412) or **percutaneous ultrasonic lithotripsy (PUL)** (see Figure 12.15 on page 418).

Usually, the first symptom of a kidney stone is extreme pain, which begins suddenly when a stone moves in the urinary tract, causing irritation or blockage. A sharp, cramping pain in the back and side in the area of the kidney or in the lower abdomen is felt; nausea and vomiting may occur. If the stone is too large to pass easily, pain continues, and blood may appear in the urine.

MEDICAL WORD	Part	Meaning	DEFINITION
nephrology (ně-frŏl´ ō-jē)	nephr/o -logy	kidney study of	Literally means *study of the kidney*; study of kidney function as well as diagnosis and treatment of renal diseases
nephroma (ně-frō´ mǎ)	nephr -oma	kidney tumor	Kidney tumor
nephron (něf´ rŏn)			Basic structural and functional unit of the kidney
nephropathy (nē-frŏp´ ǎ-thē)	nephr/o -pathy	kidney disease	Pathological disease of the kidney
nephrosclerosis (něf´ rō-sklē-rō´ sĭs)	nephr/o scler -osis	kidney hardening condition	Condition of hardening of the kidney
nocturia (nŏk-tū´ rĭ-ǎ)	noct -uria	night urine	Urination during the night
oliguria (ŏl-ĭg-ū´ rĭ-ǎ)	olig- -uria	scanty urine	Scanty, decreased amount of urine. The decreased production of urine may be a sign of dehydration, renal failure, hypovolemic shock, multiple organ dysfunction syndrome, or urinary obstruction/urinary retention. It can be contrasted with anuria, which represents a more complete suppression of urination.

MEDICAL WORD	WORD PARTS		DEFINITION
	Part	**Meaning**	
percutaneous ultrasonic lithotripsy (PUL) (pĕr″ kū-tā′ nē-ŭs) ŭl-tră-sōn′ ĭk lĭth′ ō-trĭp″ sē)	per- cutan/e -ous ultra- son -ic lith/o -tripsy	through skin pertaining to beyond sound pertaining to stone crushing	Crushing of a kidney stone by using ultrasound. This is an invasive surgical procedure performed by using a nephroscope or fluoroscopy. See Figure 12.15 ∎

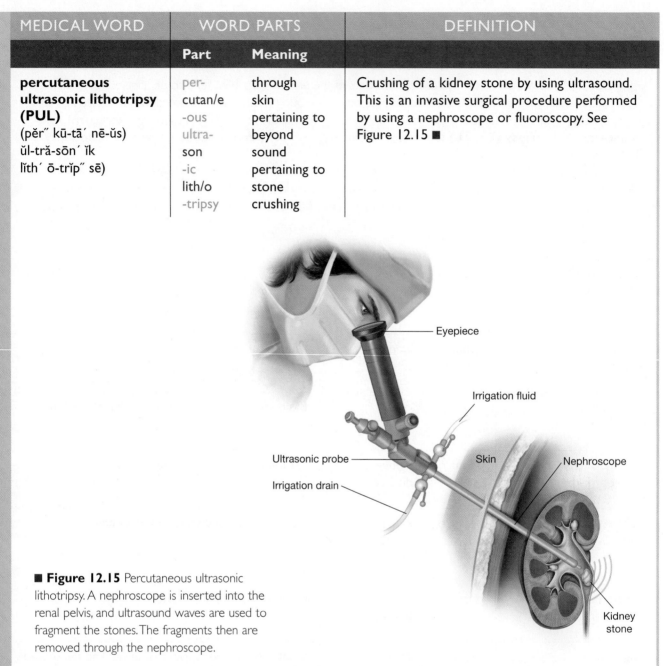

Eyepiece

Irrigation fluid

Ultrasonic probe

Skin

Nephroscope

Irrigation drain

Kidney stone

∎ **Figure 12.15** Percutaneous ultrasonic lithotripsy. A nephroscope is inserted into the renal pelvis, and ultrasound waves are used to fragment the stones. The fragments then are removed through the nephroscope.

MEDICAL WORD	WORD PARTS		DEFINITION
peritoneal dialysis (PD) (pĕr″ ĭ-tō-nē′ ăl dī-ăl′ ĭ-sĭs)	periton/e -al dia- -lysis	peritoneum pertaining to complete, through to separate	Separation of waste from the blood by using a peritoneal catheter and dialysis. Fluid is introduced into the peritoneal cavity, and wastes from the blood pass into this fluid. The fluid and waste are then removed from the body. Types of peritoneal dialysis are IPD—intermittent and CAPD—continuous ambulatory. See Figure 12.16 ∎

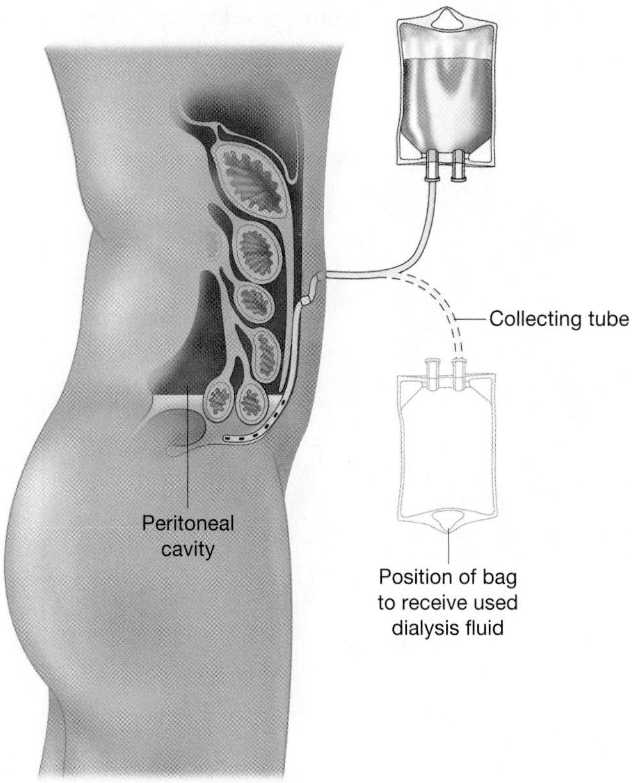

MEDICAL WORD	WORD PARTS		DEFINITION
	Part	Meaning	

■ **Figure 12.16** Peritoneal dialysis.

MEDICAL WORD	WORD PARTS		DEFINITION
	Part	Meaning	
periurethral (pĕr″ ĭ-ū-rē´ thrăl)	peri- urethr -al	around urethra pertaining to	Literally means *pertaining to around the urethra;* the immediate area surrounding the urethra
polyuria (pŏl″ ē-ū´ rĭ-ă)	poly- -uria	excessive urine	Literally means *excessive secretion and discharge of urine;* frequent urination; occurs in diabetes mellitus, chronic nephritis, and nephrosclerosis, and can be induced with diuretics and following excessive intake of liquids
pyelocystitis (pī″ ĕ-lō-sĭs-tī´ tĭs)	pyel/o cyst -itis	renal pelvis bladder inflammation	Inflammation of the bladder and renal pelvis
pyelolithotomy (pī″ ĕ-lō-lĭth-ŏt´ ō-mē)	pyel/o lith/o -tomy	renal pelvis stone incision	Surgical incision into the renal pelvis for removal of a stone

MEDICAL WORD	WORD PARTS		DEFINITION
	Part	**Meaning**	
pyelonephritis (pī″ ě-lō-ně-frī′ tĭs)	pyel/o nephr -itis	renal pelvis kidney inflammation	Inflammation of the kidney and renal pelvis. It is usually caused by bacteria entering the kidneys from the bladder. *Escherichia coli* is a bacillus that is normally found in the large intestine. These infections usually spread from the genital area through the ureters to the bladder. See Figure 12.17 ∎

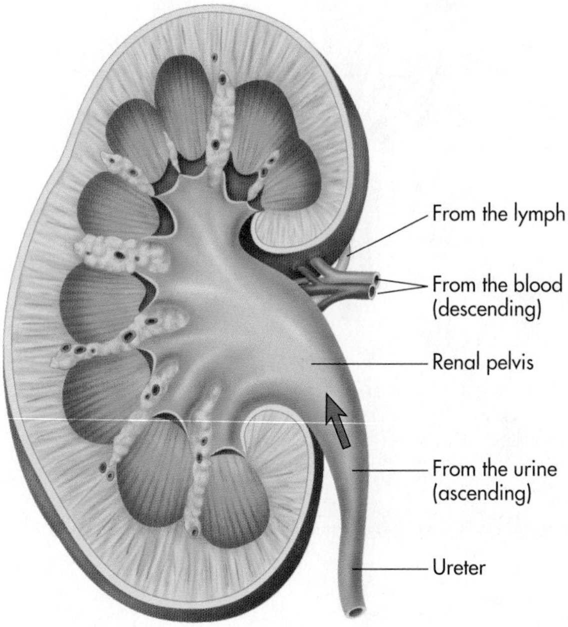

■ **Figure 12.17** Routes of infection for pyelonephritis.

Labels: From the lymph; From the blood (descending); Renal pelvis; From the urine (ascending); Ureter

pyuria (pī-ū′ rĭ-ă)	py -uria	pus urine	Pus in the urine
renal (rē′ năl)	ren -al	kidney pertaining to	Pertaining to the kidney
renal colic (kŏl′ ĭk)			Sharp, severe pain in the lower back over the kidney, radiating forward into the groin. It usually accompanies forcible dilation of a ureter, followed by spasm as a stone is lodged or passed through it.
renal failure			Pathological failure of the kidney to function. There are two types of renal (kidney) failure: acute and chronic. **Acute renal failure (ARF)** occurs when the filtering function of the kidneys changes so that the kidneys are not able to maintain healthy body function. People who have preexisting kidney disease or damage are at higher risk for acute renal failure. Some common symptoms of acute renal failure include excess fluid in the abdomen (ascites) and swelling of the extremities (edema).

MEDICAL WORD	WORD PARTS		DEFINITION
	Part	**Meaning**	
urethralgia (ū-rē-thrăl´ jĭ-ă)	urethr -algia	urethra pain	Pain in the urethra
urethral stricture (ū-rē´ thrăl strĭk´ chŭr)	urethr -al strict -ure	urethra pertaining to to tighten, contraction process	Narrowing or constriction of the urethra
urethroperineal (ū-rē˝ thrō-pĕr˝ ĭ nē´ ăl)	urethr/o perine -al	urethra perineum pertaining to	Pertaining to the urethra and perineum
urgency			Sudden need to void, urinate
uric acid (ū´ rĭk)			End product of purine metabolism; common component of urinary and renal stones
urinal (ū´ rĭn-ăl)	urin -al	urine pertaining to	Container, toilet, or bathroom fixture into which one urinates
urinalysis (UA) (ū´ rĭ-năl´ ĭ-sĭs)	urin a- -lysis	urine apart destruction, to separate	Analysis of urine; separating of the urine for examination to determine the presence of abnormal elements; a laboratory test that evaluates the physical, chemical, and microscopic properties of urine
urination (ū˝ rĭ-nā´ shŭn)	urinat -ion	urine process	Process of voiding urine
urine (ū´ rĭn)			Fluid secreted by the kidneys, transported by the ureters, stored in the bladder, and voided through the urethra.

MEDICAL WORD	WORD PARTS		DEFINITION
	Part	**Meaning**	
urinometer (ū″ rĭ-nŏm´ ĕ-tĕr)	urin/o -meter	urine instrument	Medical instrument used to measure the specific gravity of urine. See Figure 12.19 ■

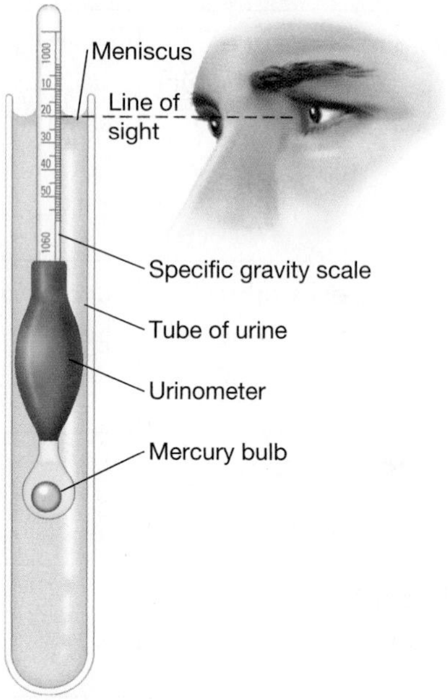

■ **Figure 12.19** Urinometer. In this procedure, a urine sample and urinometer are placed within a tube, and the liquid level is compared to the scale. The procedure provides information on the concentration of solids within a urine sample.

MEDICAL WORD	WORD PARTS		DEFINITION
urobilin (ū″ rō-bī´ lĭn)	ur/o bil -in	urination bile chemical	Brown pigment formed by the oxidation of urobilinogen; may be formed in the urine after exposure to air
urochrome (ū´ rō-krōm)			Pigment that gives urine the normal yellow color
urologist (ū-rŏl´ ō-jĭst)	ur/o log -ist	urination study of one who specializes	Literally means *a physician who specializes in the study of the urinary system*
urology (ū-rŏl´ ō-jē)	ur/o -logy	urination study of	Literally means *study of the urinary system*
void			To empty the bladder

• Drug Highlights •

TYPE OF DRUG	DESCRIPTION AND EXAMPLES
diuretics	Decrease in reabsorption of sodium chloride by the kidneys, thereby increasing the amount of salt and water excreted in the urine. This action reduces the amount of fluid retained in the body and prevents edema. Diuretics are classified according to site and mechanism of action.
thiazide	Appears to act by inhibiting sodium and chloride reabsorption in the early portion of the distal tubule. EXAMPLES: Diuril (chlorothiazide), HydroDiuril (hydrochlorothiazide), and Lozol (indapamide)
loop	Acts by inhibiting the reabsorption of sodium and chloride in the ascending loop of Henle. EXAMPLES: Bumex (bumetanide) and Lasix (furosemide)
potassium sparing	Acts by inhibiting the exchange of sodium for potassium in the distal tubule; inhibits potassium excretion. EXAMPLES: Aldactone (spironolactone) and Dyrenium (triamterene)
osmotic	Capable of being filtered by the glomerulus but has a limited capability of being reabsorbed into the bloodstream. EXAMPLE: Osmitrol (mannitol)
carbonic anhydrase inhibitor	Acts to increase the excretion of bicarbonate (HCO_3) ion, which carries out sodium (Na), water (H_2O), and potassium (K). EXAMPLE: Diamox (acetazolamide)
urinary tract antibacterials	Sulfonamides are generally the drugs of choice for treating acute, uncomplicated urinary tract infections, especially those caused by *Escherichia coli* and *Proteus mirabilis* bacterial strains. They exert a bacteriostatic effect against a wide range of gram-positive and gram-negative microorganisms. EXAMPLES: Gantrisin (sulfisoxazole), Microsulfon (sulfadiazine), and Bactrim and Septra, which are mixtures of trimethoprim and sulfamethoxazole
urinary tract antiseptics	May inhibit the growth of microorganisms by bactericidal, bacteriostatic, anti-infective, and/or antibacterial action. EXAMPLES: NegGram (nalidixic acid), Furadantin and Macrodantin (nitrofurantoin), methenamine hippurate, and Cipro (ciprofloxacin HCl)

TYPE OF DRUG	DESCRIPTION AND EXAMPLES
other drugs	Treat disorders of the lower urinary tract by either stimulating or inhibiting smooth muscle activity, thereby improving urinary bladder functions. These functions are the storage of urine and its subsequent excretion from the body. EXAMPLES: Urispas (flavoxate HCl) and Urecholine (bethanechol chloride)
Rimso-50 (dimethyl sulfoxide)	Used in the treatment of interstitial cystitis.
Pyridium (phenazopyridine HCl)	Analgesic, anesthetic action on the urinary tract mucosa, used to treat the discomfort of a urinary tract infection. Causes the urine to turn an orange color and can stain clothing. The patient should be informed of this.
Urispas (flavoxate HCl)	Reduces dysuria, nocturia, and urinary frequency.
Tofranil (imipramine HCl)	Treats nocturnal enuresis in children.
Ditropan XL (oxybutynin chloride)	Relaxes the muscles in the bladder, thereby decreasing the occurrence of wetting accidents.
Detrol (tolterodine tartrate)	Helps control involuntary contractions of the bladder muscle.

• Diagnostic and Lab Tests •

TEST	DESCRIPTION
blood urea nitrogen (BUN) (ū-rē´ ă nĭ´ trō-jĕn)	Blood test to determine the amount of urea excreted by the kidneys. Abnormal results indicate renal dysfunction.
creatinine (krē´ ă-tĭn ēn)	Blood test to determine the amount of creatinine present. Abnormal results indicate renal dysfunction.
creatinine clearance (krē´ ă-tĭn ēn)	Urine test to determine the glomerular filtration rate (GFR). Abnormal results indicate renal dysfunction.
culture, urine	Urine test to determine the presence of microorganisms. Abnormal results indicate urinary tract infection.
cystoscopy (cysto) (sĭs-tŏs´ kə-pē)	Visual examination of the bladder and urethra via a lighted cystoscope. Abnormal results can indicate the presence of renal calculi, a tumor, prostatic hyperplasia, and/or bleeding.

TEST	DESCRIPTION
intravenous pyelography (pyelogram) (IVP) (ĭn-tră-vē′ nŭs pī′′ ĕ-lŏg′ ră-fē)	Test to visualize the kidneys, ureters, and bladder. A radiopaque substance is intravenously injected, and x-rays are taken. Abnormal results can indicate renal calculi, kidney or bladder tumors, and kidney disease.
kidney, ureter, bladder (KUB)	With the patient supine a flat-plate x-ray is taken of the abdomen to indicate the size and position of the kidneys, ureters, and bladder.
renal biopsy	Removal of tissue from the kidney. Abnormal results can indicate kidney cancer, kidney transplant rejection, and glomerulonephritis.
retrograde pyelography (RP) (rĕt′rō-grād)	X-ray recording of the kidneys, ureters, and bladder following the injection of a contrast medium backward through a urinary catheter into the ureters and the calyces of the pelves of the kidneys. Useful in locating urinary stones and obstructions. See Figure 12.20 ■

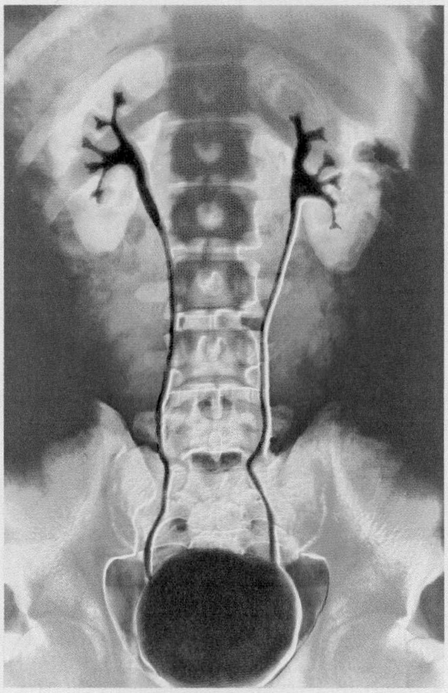

■ **Figure 12.20** Retrograde pyelography (RP). Note the contrasting of the renal calyces, ureters, and bladder following an injection of a contrast medium.

TEST	DESCRIPTION
Ultrasonography, kidneys (ŭl-tră-sŏn-ŏg′ ră-fē)	Use of high-frequency sound waves to visualize the kidneys. The sound waves (echoes) are recorded on an oscilloscope and film. Abnormal results can indicate kidney tumors, cysts, abscess, and kidney disease.

• Abbreviations •

ABBREVIATION	MEANING	ABBREVIATION	MEANING
AGN	acute glomerulonephritis	IPD	intermittent peritoneal dialysis
ARF	acute renal failure	IVP	intravenous pyelogram
BUN	blood urea nitrogen	K	potassium
CAPD	continuous ambulatory peritoneal dialysis	KUB	kidney, ureter, bladder
CGN	chronic glomerulonephritis	LOC	level of consciousness
CLIA	clinical laboratory improvement amendments	mL	milliliter
		mm	millimeter
cm	centimeter	Na	sodium
CRF	chronic renal failure	NaCl	sodium chloride
cysto	cystoscopy	NH$_3$	ammonia
ESRD	end-stage renal disease	PD	peritoneal dialysis
ESWL	extracorporeal shock wave lithotripsy	pH	hydrogen ion concentration
		PKU	phenylketonuria
GFR	glomerular filtration rate	PUL	percutaneous ultrasonic lithotripsy
GU	genitourinary		
H	hydrogen	RP	retrograde pyelography
HCO$_3$	bicarbonate	sp. gr.	specific gravity
HD	hemodialysis	UA	urinalysis
H$_2$O	water	UG	urogenital
IC	interstitial cystitis	UTI	urinary tract infection

Anatomy and Physiology

Write your answers to the following questions.

1. List the organs of the urinary system.

a. _____   **b.** _____

c. _____   **d.** _____

2. State the vital function of the urinary system. _____

_____

3. Define *hilum.*_____

4. Define *renal pelvis.* _____

5. The medulla is the _____ portion of the kidney.

6. Define *nephron.* _____

7. Each nephron consists of a _____ _____ and a _____ .

8. The malpighian corpuscle consists of _____ and _____

_____ .

9. Urine is formed by the process of _____ and _____ in the

nephron.

10. An average of _____ to _____ mL of urine is voided daily.

11. Describe the ureters and state their function. _____

_____

12. Describe the urinary bladder and state its function. _____

_____

13. The external urinary opening is the _____ .

14. Define *urinalysis.* _____

_____

15. Give the normal constituents for the physical examination of urine.

    a. Color _____   **b.** Appearance _____

    c. Reaction _____   **d.** Specific gravity _____

    e. Odor _____   **f.** Quantity _____

16. A urine that has a fruity, sweet odor can indicate _____

_____

17. Under chemical examination, the presence of protein in urine is an important sign of

_____.

Word Parts

PREFIXES

Give the definitions of the following prefixes.

    1. an- _____   **2.** anti- _____

    3. di(a)- _____   **4.** dia- _____

    5. dys- _____   **6.** en- _____

    7. hydro- _____   **8.** extra- _____

    9. in- _____   **10.** olig- _____

    11. per- _____   **12.** ultra- _____

    13. poly- _____

ROOTS AND COMBINING FORMS

Give the definitions of the following roots and combining forms.

    1. excretor _____   **2.** albumin _____

    3. bacter/i _____   **4.** bil _____

    5. calc/i _____   **6.** col/ o _____

    7. continence _____   **8.** cyst _____

    9. corpor/e _____   **10.** cyst/o _____

    11. cutan/e _____   **12.** glomerul _____

    13. glomerul/o _____   **14.** glycos _____

15. hemat _____

16. keton _____

17. lith/o _____

18. log _____

19. hem/o _____

20. meat/o _____

21. micturit _____

22. nephr _____

23. nephr/o _____

24. noct _____

25. periton/e _____

26. perine _____

27. son _____

28. strict _____

29. py _____

30. pyel/o _____

31. ren _____

32. scler _____

33. trigon _____

34. ur _____

35. uret _____

36. ureter/o _____

37. urethr _____

38. urethr/o _____

39. urin _____

40. urinat _____

41. urin/o _____

42. ur/o _____

SUFFIXES

Give the definitions of the following suffixes.

1. -al _____

2. -algia _____

3. -ar _____

4. -cele _____

5. -dynia _____

6. -y _____

7. -ous _____

8. -ectomy _____

9. -emia _____

10. -gram _____

11. -ic _____

12. -in _____

13. -ion _____

14. -ist _____

15. -itis _____

16. -lith _____

17. -logy _____

18. -lysis _____

19. -tripsy _____

20. -ure _____

21. -meter _____

22. -oma _____

23. -osis _____   **24.** -pathy _____

25. -plasty _____   **26.** -scope _____

27. -esis _____   **28.** -stomy _____

29. -tomy _____   **30.** -uria _____

Identifying Medical Terms

In the spaces provided, write the medical terms for the following meanings.

1. _____ Pertaining to a medication that decreases urine production and secretion

2. _____ Surgical excision of the bladder or part of the bladder

3. _____ Inflammation of the bladder

4. _____ Difficult or painful urination

5. _____ Inflammation of the renal glomeruli

6. _____ Excessive amount of calcium in the urine

7. _____ Process of urinating

8. _____ Kidney stone

9. _____ Pertaining to around the urethra

10. _____ Pus in the urine

11. _____ Disease of the ureter

12. _____ Pain in the urethra

13. _____ Physician who specializes in the study of the urinary system

Spelling

Cirlce the correct spelling of each medical term.

1. excreteory / excretory   2. euresis / enuresis

3. glycosuria / glycouria   4. hematuria / hemauria

5. incontence / incontinence   6. nephrcysitis / nephrocystitis

7. nocuria / nocturia   8. ureteroplasty / ueteroplasty

9. urinalysis / urinalsis   10. urbilin/ urobilin

Matching

Select the appropriate lettered meaning for each of the following words.

_____ **1.** lithotriptor

_____ **2.** hemodialysis

_____ **3.** lithotripsy

_____ **4.** peritoneal dialysis

_____ **5.** renal colic

_____ **6.** urethral stricture

_____ **7.** urgency

_____ **8.** urination

_____ **9.** urochrome

_____ **10.** urinometer

a. Sharp, severe pain in the lower back over the kidney radiating forward into the groin caused by blockage during the passage of a stone

b. Crushing of a kidney stone

c. Process of voiding urine

d. Medical device used to crush kidney stones

e. Use of an artificial kidney to separate waste from the blood

f. Separation of waste from the blood by using a peritoneal catheter and dialysis

g. Narrowing or constriction of the urethra

h. Pigment that gives urine its normal yellow color

i. Medical instrument used to measure the specific gravity of urine

j. Sudden need to void, urinate

k. Analysis of urine

Abbreviations

Place the correct word, phrase, or abbreviation in the space provided.

1. acute renal failure _____

2. BUN _____

3. chronic renal failure _____

4. cysto _____

5. GU _____

6. HD _____

7. intravenous pyelogram _____

8. PD _____

9. pH _____

10. urinalysis _____

Diagnostic and Laboratory Tests

Select the best answer to each multiple-choice question. Circle the letter of your choice.

1. Urine test to determine the glomerular filtration rate.
   - **a.** BUN
   - **b.** creatinine
   - **c.** creatinine clearance
   - **d.** KUB

2. Urine test to determine the presence of microorganisms.
   - **a.** BUN
   - **b.** creatinine
   - **c.** urine culture
   - **d.** KUB

3. Test to visualize the kidneys, ureters, and bladder.
   - **a.** cystoscopy
   - **b.** intravenous pyelography
   - **c.** KUB
   - **d.** renal biopsy

4. Use of high-frequency sound waves to visualize the kidneys.
   - **a.** retrograde pyelography
   - **b.** intravenous pyelography
   - **c.** ultrasonography
   - **d.** cystoscopy

5. Flat-plate x-ray of the abdomen to indicate the size and position of the kidneys, ureters, and bladder.
   - **a.** cystoscopy
   - **b.** KUB
   - **c.** BUN
   - **d.** retrograde pyelography

PRACTICAL APPLICATION

MEDICAL RECORD ANALYSIS

This exercise contains information, abbreviations, and medical terminology from an actual medical record or case study that has been adapted for this text. The names and any personal information are made up by the author. Read and study each form or case study and then answer the questions that follow. You may refer to Appendix III, Abbreviations and Symbols, on page A41.

Note: Congress passed the Clinical Laboratory Improvement Amendments (CLIA) in 1988, establishing quality standards for all laboratory testing to ensure the accuracy, reliability, and timeliness of patient test results regardless of where the test was performed.

FLOYD PRIMARY CARE
Smith-Jones Lab
35 Sinclair Avenue
Rome, GA 30165
(123) 456-7890
CLIA: 12Do840311

Lab Director: Sandra Marie Smith, MD

Patient ID: 184234
Patient Name: Rice, Charles L.
Date of Birth: 02/20/37
Age: 73 years
Sex: M

Draw Date 05/19/xx
Draw Time: 10:49 AM
Accession #: 71189

Ordering Dr: Smith, Sandra M.

Urinalysis	Result	Reference	Lo	Hi
Color	Yellow	Yellow to amber		
Appearance	Clear	Clear		
Specific Gravity (sp. gr.)	1.010	1.001-1.035		
pH	7.0	4.6 to 8.0		
Protein	Negative	Negative		
Glucose	Negative	Negative		
Ketones	Negative	Negative		
Bilirubin	Negative	Negative		
Blood	Negative	Negative		
Nitrites	Negative	Negative		
Urobilinogen	0.4	0.1 to 1.0		

Action: Patient to be notified of results   **Reviewed by:** SJR   **Date:** 05/19/xx

Medical Record Questions

Place the correct answer in the space provided.

1. What is the normal color of urine? _____

2. Define specific gravity and give the normal sp. gr. of urine. _____

3. This patient's pH was 7.0. Is this higher or lower than the average pH? _____

4. This patient's report indicated a urobilinogen of 0.4. Is this within normal range? _____

5. What would an increased amount of urobilinogen indicate? _____

Medical Terminology • Suffixes • Prefixes • Organization
he Body • Integumentary System • Skelet System • M
ar System • Digestive System • Cardiova ular stem
ood and Lymphatic System • Respiratory System • Ur
stem • **Endocrine System** • Nervous System • Spe

13

LEARNING OUTCOMES

On completion of this chapter, you will be able to:

1. Describe the vital function of the endocrine system.

2. State the description and primary functions of the organs/structures of the endocrine system.

3. Identify the various hormones secreted by the endocrine glands and their hormonal function.

4. Analyze, build, spell, and pronounce medical words.

5. Comprehend the drugs highlighted in this chapter.

6. Describe diagnostic and laboratory tests related to the endocrine system.

7. Identify and define selected abbreviations.

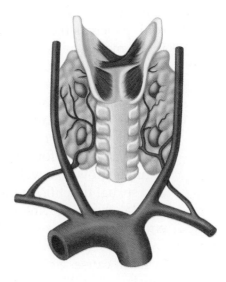

COMBINING FORMS OF THE ENDOCRINE SYSTEM

acid/o	acid	insulin/o	insulin
acr/o	extremity, point	kal/i	potassium (K)
aden/o	gland	myx/o	mucus
adren/	adrenal gland	nephr/o	kidney
andr/o	man	ophthalm/o	eye
cortic/o	cortex	pancreat/o	pancreas
crin/o	to secrete	somat/o	body
estr/o	mad desire	test/o	testicle
galact/o	milk	thym/o	thymus
ger/o	old age	thyr/o	thyroid, shield
gigant/o	giant	toxic/o	poison
gluc/o	sweet, sugar	trop/o	turn
gonad/o	seed	vas/o	vessel
hirsut/o	hairy	viril/o	masculine
insul/o	insulin		

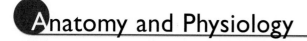natomy and Physiology

The endocrine system is made up of glands, each of which secretes a type of hormone into the bloodstream. The glands of the endocrine system and the hormones they release influence almost every cell, organ, and function of the body. Although the endocrine glands are the body's main hormone producers, some other organs such as the brain, heart, lungs, liver, skin, thymus, and the gastrointestinal mucosa, as well as the placenta during pregnancy, produce and release hormones. The primary glands of the endocrine system are the pituitary, pineal, thyroid, parathyroid, pancreas (islets of Langerhans), adrenals, ovaries in the female, and testes in the male.

The vital function of the endocrine system involves the production and regulation of chemical substances called *hormones*. A hormone is a chemical transmitter that is released in small amounts and transported via the bloodstream to a target organ or other cells. The word *hormone* is derived from the Greek language and means *to excite* or *to urge on*. As the body's chemical messengers, hormones transfer information and instructions from one set of cells to another. They regulate growth, development, mood, tissue function, homeostasis, metabolism, and sexual function in the male and female. Table 13.1 ■ provides an at-a-glance look at the endocrine system. Figure 13.1 ■ shows the primary glands of the endocrine system.

Hyposecretion or hypersecretion of specific hormones of the endocrine system cause or are associated with many pathological conditions. Too much or too little of any hormone can be harmful to the body. Controlling the production of or replacing specific hormones can treat many hormonal disorders and/or conditions.

TABLE 13.1 Endocrine System At-a-Glance

Gland	Primary Functions/Description
Pituitary (hypophysis)	Master gland; has regulatory effects on other endocrine glands
Anterior lobe (adenohypophysis)	Influences growth and sexual development, thyroid function, adrenocortical function; regulates skin pigmentation
Posterior lobe (neurohypophysis)	Stimulates the reabsorption of water and elevates blood pressure; stimulates the uterus to contract during labor, delivery, and parturition; stimulates the release of milk during suckling
Pineal	Helps regulate the release of gonadotropin and controls body pigmentation
Thyroid	Plays vital role in metabolism; regulates the body's metabolic processes; influences bone and calcium metabolism; helps maintain plasma calcium homeostasis
Parathyroid	Maintains normal serum calcium level; plays a role in the metabolism of phosphorus
Pancreas (islets of Langerhans)	Regulates blood glucose levels; plays a vital role in metabolism of carbohydrates, proteins, and fats
Adrenals (suprarenals)	
Adrenal cortex	Regulates carbohydrate metabolism, anti-inflammatory effect; helps body cope during stress; regulates electrolyte and water balance; promotes development of male characteristics
Adrenal medulla	Synthesizes, secretes, and stores catecholamines (dopamine, epinephrine, norepinephrine)
Ovaries	Promote growth, development, and maintenance of female sex organs
Testes	Promote growth, development, and maintenance of male sex organs

The endocrine system and the nervous system work closely together to help maintain homeostasis (a state of equilibrium that is maintained within the body's internal environment). The **hypothalamus**, a collection of specialized cells that are located in the lower central part of the brain, is the primary link between the endocrine and nervous system. Nerve cells in the hypothalamus control the pituitary gland by producing chemicals that either stimulate or suppress hormone secretions from the pituitary. The hypothalamus synthesizes and secretes releasing hormones such as thyrotropin-releasing hormone (TRH) and gonadotropin-releasing hormone (GnRH) and releasing factors such as corticotropin-releasing factor (CRF), growth hormone–releasing factor (GHRF), prolactin-releasing factor (PRF), and melanocyte-stimulating hormone–releasing factor (MRF). The hypothalamus also synthesizes and secretes release-inhibiting hormones such as growth hormone release-inhibiting hormone. It also produces release-inhibiting factors such as prolactin release-inhibiting factor (PIF) and melanocyte–stimulating hormone release-inhibiting factor (MIF). The hypothalamus also exerts direct nervous control over the anterior pituitary and the adrenal medulla and controls the secretion of the hormones epinephrine and norepinephrine. See Table 13.2 ■ for an overview of the endocrine glands, hormones, and hormonal function.

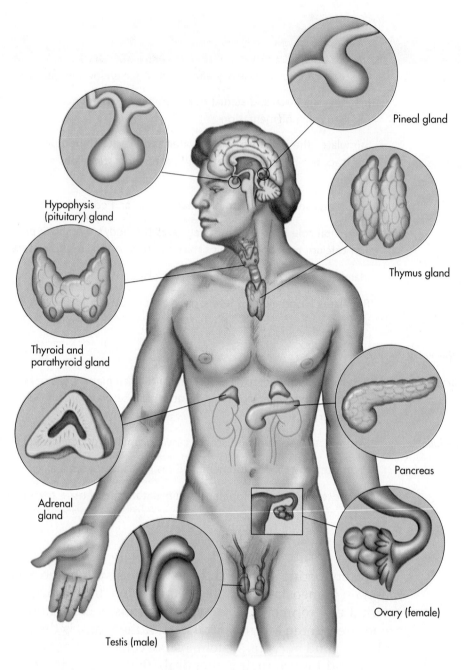

Pineal gland

Thymus gland

Hypophysis
(pituitary) gland

Thyroid and
parathyroid gland

Pancreas

Adrenal
gland

Ovary (female)

Testis (male)

■ **Figure 13.1** Primary glands of the endocrine system.

LIFE SPAN CONSIDERATIONS

Most of the structures and glands of the endocrine system develop during the first 3 months of pregnancy. The endocrine system of the newborn is supplemented by hormones that cross the placental barrier. Both male and female newborns may have swelling of the breast and genitalia from maternal hormones.

TABLE 13.2 Summary of the Endocrine Glands, Hormones, and Hormonal Functions

Endocrine Glands	Hormones	Hormonal Functions
Pituitary gland		
Anterior lobe	Growth hormone (GH) (also called somatotrophin hormone [STH])	Promotes growth and development of bones, muscles, and other organs; enhances protein synthesis, decreases the use of glucose, and promotes fat destruction (lipolysis)
	Adrenocorticotropin hormone (ACTH)	Stimulates growth and development of the adrenal cortex
	Thyroid-stimulating hormone (TSH)	Stimulates growth and development of the thyroid gland
	Follicle-stimulating hormone (FSH)	Stimulates the growth of ovarian follicles in the female and sperm in the male
	Luteinizing hormone (LH)	Stimulates the development of the corpus luteum in the female and the production of testosterone in the male
	Prolactin hormone (PRL) (also called lactogenic hormone [LTH])	Stimulates the development and growth of the mammary glands; important in the initiation and maintenance of milk production during pregnancy. Following childbirth, the act of suckling provides the stimulus for prolactin synthesis and release. When suckling ceases, prolactin secretion slows and milk production decreases and then stops.
	Melanocyte-stimulating hormone (MSH)	Regulates skin pigmentation and promotes the deposit of melanin in the skin after exposure to sunlight
Posterior lobe	Antidiuretic hormone (ADH) (also called vasopressin [VP])	Stimulates the reabsorption of water by the renal tubules and has a pressor effect that elevates the blood pressure
	Oxytocin	Acts on the mammary glands to stimulate the uterus to contract during labor, delivery, and parturition; stimulates the release of milk during suckling
Pineal gland	Melatonin	Helps regulate the release of gonadotropin and influences the body's internal clock
	Serotonin	Stimulates neurotransmitter, vasoconstrictor, and smooth muscle; acts to inhibit gastric secretion

TABLE 13.2 Summary of the Endocrine Glands, Hormones, and Hormonal Functions (continued)

Endocrine Glands	Hormones	Hormonal Functions
Thyroid gland	Thyroxine (T_4)	Maintains and regulates the basal metabolic rate (BMR); influences growth and development, both physical and mental, and the metabolism of fats, proteins, carbohydrates, water, vitamins, and minerals; can be synthetically produced or extracted from animal thyroid glands in crystalline form to be used in the treatment of thyroid dysfunction, especially cretinism, myxedema, and Hashimoto's disease
	Triiodothyronine (T_3)	Influences the basal metabolic rate and is more biologically active than thyroxine
	Calcitonin	Influences bone and calcium metabolism and helps maintain plasma calcium homeostasis; also known as thyrocalcitonin
Parathyroid glands	Parathyroid hormone (PTH) (also called parathormone hormone)	Plays a role in maintenance of a normal serum calcium level and in the metabolism of phosphorus
Islets of Langerhans	Glucagon	Facilitates the breakdown of glycogen to glucose
	Insulin	Plays a role in maintenance of normal blood sugar. It promotes the entry of glucose into the cells, thereby lowering the blood glucose (BG) level.
	Somatostatin	Suppresses the release of glucagon and insulin
Adrenal glands		
Cortex	Cortisol	Regulates carbohydrate, protein, and fat metabolism; needed for gluconeogenesis; increases blood sugar level; provides anti-inflammatory effect; helps body cope during times of stress
	Corticosterone	Essential for normal use of carbohydrates, the absorption of glucose, and gluconeogenesis; also influences potassium (K) and sodium (Na) metabolism
	Aldosterone	Essential in regulating electrolyte and water balance by promoting sodium and chloride reabsorption and potassium excretion
	Testosterone	Influences development of male secondary sex characteristics
	Androsterone	Influences development of male secondary sex characteristics

TABLE 13.2 Summary of the Endocrine Glands, Hormones, and Hormonal Functions (continued)

Endocrine Glands	Hormones	Hormonal Functions
Medulla	Dopamine	Dilates systemic arteries, elevates systolic blood pressure, increases cardiac output, increases urinary output
	Epinephrine (also called adrenaline)	Acts as vasoconstrictor, vasopressor, cardiac stimulant, antispasmodic, and sympathomimetic
	Norepinephrine (also called noradrenaline)	Acts as vasoconstrictor, vasopressor, and neurotransmitter
Ovaries	Estrogens (estradiol, estrone, and estriol)	Essential for the growth, development, and maintenance of female sex organs and secondary sex characteristics; promote the development of the mammary glands; play a vital role in a woman's emotional well-being and sexual drive
	Progesterone	Prepares the uterus for pregnancy
Testes	Testosterone	Essential for normal growth and development of the male accessory sex organs; plays a vital role in the erection process of the penis and thus is necessary for the sexual act, *copulation* (sexual intercourse)
Thymus gland	Thymosin	Promotes the maturation process of T lymphocytes
	Thymopoietin	Influences the production of lymphocyte precursors and aids in their process of becoming T lymphocytes
Gastrointestinal mucosa	Gastrin	Stimulates gastric acid secretion
	Secretin	Stimulates pancreatic juice, bile, and intestinal secretion
	Pancreozymin	Stimulates the pancreas to produce pancreatic juice
	Cholecystokinin	Causes contraction and emptying of the gallbladder, and secretion of pancreatic enzymes
	Enterogastrone	Regulates gastric secretions

PITUITARY GLAND (HYPOPHYSIS)

The **pituitary gland** is a small gray gland located at the base of the brain (Figure 13.1). It lies or rests in a shallow depression of the sphenoid bone known as the *sella turcica*. It is attached by the infundibulum stalk to the hypothalamus. The pituitary is approximately 1 centimeter (cm) in diameter and weighs approximately 0.6 gram (g). It is divided into the anterior lobe (*adenohypophysis*) and the posterior lobe (*neurohypophysis*). The pituitary is also called the **master gland** of the body because of its regulatory effects on the other endocrine glands.

Anterior Lobe

The *adenohypophysis* or **anterior lobe** secretes several hormones that are essential for the growth and development of bones, muscles, other organs, sex glands, the thyroid gland, and the adrenal cortex. The hormones secreted by the anterior lobe and their functions are described in Table 13.2 and shown in Figure 13.2 ■

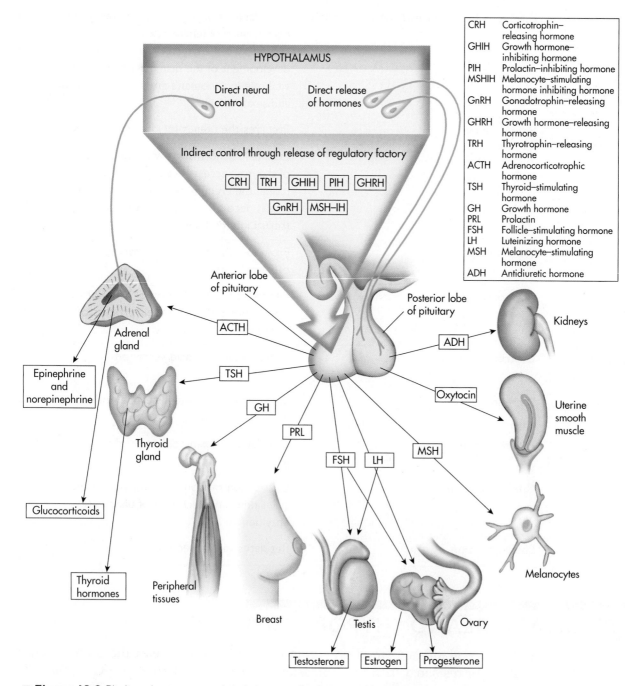

CRH	Corticotrophin–releasing hormone
GHIH	Growth hormone–inhibiting hormone
PIH	Prolactin–inhibiting hormone
MSHIH	Melanocyte–stimulating hormone inhibiting hormone
GnRH	Gonadotrophin–releasing hormone
GHRH	Growth hormone–releasing hormone
TRH	Thyrotrophin–releasing hormone
ACTH	Adrenocorticotrophic hormone
TSH	Thyroid–stimulating hormone
GH	Growth hormone
PRL	Prolactin
FSH	Follicle–stimulating hormone
LH	Luteinizing hormone
MSH	Melanocyte–stimulating hormone
ADH	Antidiuretic hormone

■ **Figure 13.2** Pituitary hormones and their target cells, tissues, and/or organs.

Posterior Lobe

The *neurohypophysis* or **posterior lobe** stores and secretes two important hormones that are synthesized in the hypothalamus. The hormones secreted by the posterior lobe and their functions are described in Table 13.2 and shown in Figure 13.2.

PINEAL GLAND

The **pineal gland** is a small, pine cone–shaped gland located near the posterior end of the corpus callosum. It is less than 1 cm in diameter and weighs approximately 0.1 g (see Figure 13.1). The pineal gland secretes **melatonin** and **serotonin.** Melatonin is a hormone that can be released at night to help regulate the release of gonadotropin. Serotonin is a hormone that is a neurotransmitter, vasoconstrictor, and smooth muscle stimulant and acts to inhibit gastric secretion.

THYROID GLAND

The **thyroid gland** is a large, bilobed gland located in the neck. It is anterior to the trachea and just below the thyroid cartilage. The thyroid is approximately 5 cm long and 3 cm wide and weighs approximately 30 g (see Figure 13.1 and Figure 13.3 ■). It plays a vital role in metabolism and regulates the body's metabolic processes. The hormones secreted by the thyroid gland and their functions are described in Table 13.2.

Hyposecretion of the thyroid hormones T_3 and T_4 results in **cretinism** during infancy (Figure 13.10 on page 454), **myxedema** during adulthood (Figure 13.15 on page 460), and **Hashimoto's disease.** Hypersecretion of the thyroid hormones T_3 and T_4 results in **hyperthyroidism**, which is also called **thyrotoxicosis**, and **Graves' disease, exophthalmic goiter, toxic goiter**, or **Basedow's disease.** Simple or **endemic**

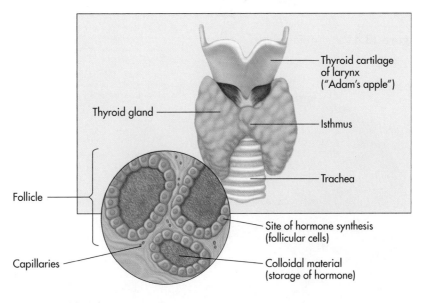

■ Figure 13.3 Thyroid gland.

goiter (Figure 13.14 on page 460) shows an enlargement of the thyroid gland caused by a deficiency of iodine in the diet.

PARATHYROID GLANDS

The **parathyroid glands** are small, yellowish-brown bodies occurring as two pairs located on the dorsal surface and lower aspect of the thyroid gland. Each parathyroid gland is approximately 6 mm in diameter and weighs approximately 0.033 g (see Figure 13.1 and Figure 13.4 ■). The hormone secreted by the parathyroids is *parathyroid (PTH)*, which is also called *parathormone hormone*. This hormone and its functions are described in Table 13.2.

Hyposecretion of PTH can result in **hypoparathyroidism**, which can cause **tetany** (intermittent cramp or tonic muscular contractions). See Figure 13.5 ■ Hypersecretion of PTH can result in **hyperparathyroidism**, which can cause **osteoporosis**, **kidney stones**, and **hypercalcemia.**

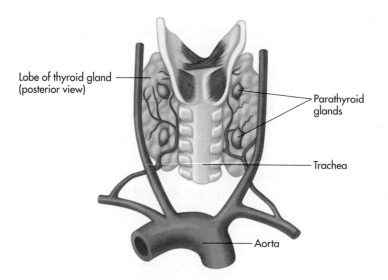

Lobe of thyroid gland
(posterior view)

Parathyroid
glands

Trachea

Aorta

■ **Figure 13.4** Parathyroid glands.

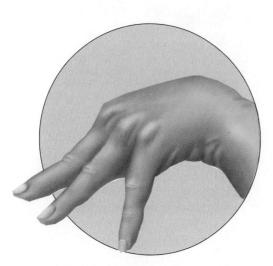

■ **Figure 13.5** Tetany of the hand in hypoparathyroidism.

PANCREAS (ISLETS OF LANGERHANS)

The **islets of Langerhans** are small clusters of cells located within the pancreas (see Figure 13.1 and Figure 13.6 ■). They are composed of three major types of cells: **alpha**, **beta**, and **delta**. The alpha cells secrete the hormone glucagon (see Figure 13.7 ■), which facilitates the breakdown of glycogen to glucose, thereby elevating blood sugar.

The beta cells secrete the hormone insulin (see Figure 13.7), which is essential for the maintenance of normal blood sugar (70–110 mg/100 mL of blood). Insulin is essential to life. It acts to regulate the metabolism of glucose and the process necessary for the intermediary metabolism of carbohydrates, fats, and proteins. It promotes the entry of glucose into the cells, thereby lowering the blood glucose (BG) level. Hyposecretion or inadequate use of insulin may result in **diabetes mellitus (DM).** Hypersecretion of insulin may result in **hyperinsulinism.** The delta cells secrete a hormone, *somatostatin*, which suppresses the release of glucagon and insulin.

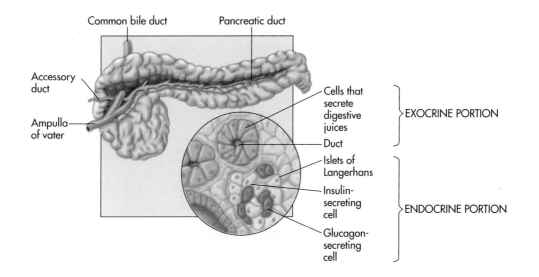

■ **Figure 13.6** Pancreas—an endocrine and exocrine gland.

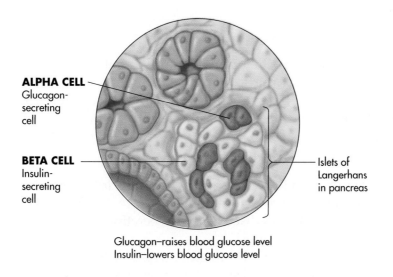

Glucagon–raises blood glucose level
Insulin–lowers blood glucose level

■ **Figure 13.7** Islets of Langerhans.

fyi Untreated diabetes mellitus or complications of diabetes can result in various multisystem effects. Progressive complications include **hyperglycemia** (excessive amount of sugar in the blood) and **hypoglycemia** (deficient amount of sugar in the blood). Hyperglycemia can lead to diabetic **ketoacidosis** (accumulation of ketones and acids in the body due to faulty metabolism of carbohydrates and the improper burning of fats) and the development of a coma when the blood sugar is too high or an insufficient amount of insulin has been received. Hypoglycemia occurs when too much insulin has been taken. Insulin shock is a severe form of hypoglycemia and requires an immediate dose of glucose. Convulsions, coma, and death can occur if the patient is not treated.

LIFE SPAN CONSIDERATIONS

Type 1 diabetes mellitus is usually diagnosed in children and young adults, and was previously known as juvenile diabetes. In Type 1 diabetes, the body does not produce insulin. Insulin is a hormone that is needed to convert sugar (glucose), starches, and other food into energy needed for daily life. The classic symptoms of diabetes mellitus (DM)—**polyuria** (frequent urination), **polydipsia** (excessive thirst), and **polyphagia** (extreme hunger)—appear more rapidly in children. The management of diabetes mellitus during childhood is very difficult because diet, exercise, and medication have to be adjusted and regulated according to the various stages of growth and development of the child.

With aging, the number of tissue receptors decreases, thus diminishing the body's response to hormones. This is especially the case with older adults who develop **Type 2 diabetes mellitus**. In this condition, sufficient insulin is produced, but because the cell receptors are modified and/or reduced, glucose does not enter the cells.

ADRENAL GLANDS (SUPRARENALS)

The **adrenal glands** are two small, triangular-shaped glands located on top of each kidney. Each gland weighs about 5 g and consists of an outer portion or *cortex* and an inner portion called the *medulla* (see Figure 13.1 and Figure 13.8 ■).

Adrenal Cortex

The **cortex** is essential to life due to its secretion of a group of hormones, the glucocorticoids, the mineralocorticoids, and the androgens. The hormones secreted by the adrenal cortex and their functions are described in Table 13.2 and a discussion of these substances and their effects on the body follows.

Glucocorticoids

The two glucocorticoid hormones are *cortisol* and *corticosterone.* Cortisol (hydrocortisone) is the principal steroid hormone secreted by the cortex. Hyposecretion of cortisol can result in **Addison's disease**; hypersecretion can result in **Cushing's disease** (see Figure 13.11 on page 455).

Corticosterone is a steroid hormone secreted by the adrenal cortex. It is essential for the normal use of carbohydrates, the absorption of glucose, and the formation of glycogen in the liver and tissues. It also influences potassium and sodium metabolism.

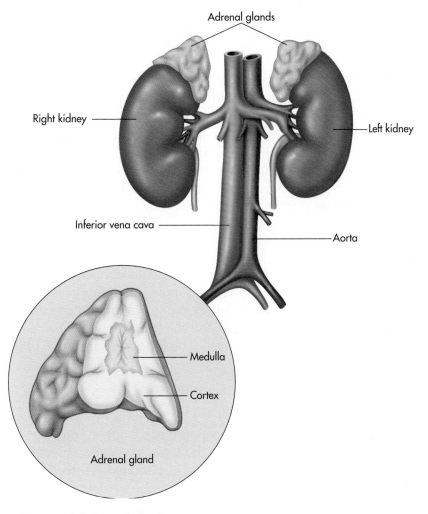

Adrenal glands

Right kidney

Left kidney

Inferior vena cava

Aorta

Medulla

Cortex

Adrenal gland

■ **Figure 13.8** Adrenal glands.

Mineralocorticoids

Aldosterone is the principal **mineralocorticoid** secreted by the adrenal cortex. It is essential in regulating electrolyte and water balance by promoting sodium and chloride reabsorption and potassium excretion. Hyposecretion of this hormone can result in a **reduced plasma volume**, and hypersecretion can result in a condition known as **primary aldosteronism**. In primary aldosteronism, the adrenal glands produce too much aldosterone, causing one to lose potassium and retain sodium. The excess sodium in turn holds onto water, increasing the blood volume and blood pressure. Treatment options for people with primary aldosteronism include medications, lifestyle modifications, and surgery.

Androgens

Androgen refers to a substance or hormone that promotes the development of male characteristics. The two main androgen hormones are *testosterone* and *androsterone.* They are essential for the development of the male secondary sex characteristics.

Adrenal Medulla

The **medulla** synthesizes, secretes, and stores catecholamines, specifically dopamine, epinephrine, and norepinephrine. The hormones secreted by the adrenal medulla and their functions are described in Table 13.2 and a discussion of these substances and their effects on the body follows.

Dopamine

Dopamine is a naturally occurring sympathetic nervous system neurotransmitter that is a precursor of norepinephrine. Dopamine can be supplied as a medication that acts on the sympathetic nervous system. It can be given to increase the amount of dopamine in the brains of patients with Parkinson's disease. Dopamine has varying vasoactive effects depending on the dose at which it is administered. It can act to dilate systemic arteries, elevate systolic blood pressure, increase cardiac output, and increase urinary output.

Epinephrine

Epinephrine (*adrenaline*) acts as a vasoconstrictor, vasopressor, cardiac stimulant, antispasmodic, and sympathomimetic. Its main function is to assist in regulating the sympathetic branch of the autonomic nervous system. It can be synthetically produced and administered *parenterally* (by an injection), *topically* (on a local area of the skin), or by *inhalation* (by nose or mouth). The following are some of the known influences and functions of epinephrine:

- Elevates the systolic blood pressure.
- Increases the heart rate and cardiac output.
- Increases glycogenolysis (conversion of glycogen into glucose), thereby hastening the release of glucose from the liver; this action elevates the blood sugar level and provides the body a spurt of energy; referred to as the *fight-or-flight syndrome*.
- Dilates the bronchial tubes and relaxes air passageways.
- Dilates the pupils to see more clearly.

Norepinephrine

Norepinephrine (*noradrenaline*) acts as a vasoconstrictor, vasopressor, and neurotransmitter. It elevates systolic and diastolic blood pressure, increases the heart rate and cardiac output, and increases glycogenolysis.

OVARIES

The **ovaries** (see Figure 13.1) produce *estrogens* (*estradiol*, *estrone*, and *estriol*) and *progesterone*. Estrogen is the female sex hormone secreted by the graafian follicles of the ovaries. Progesterone is a steroid hormone secreted by the corpus luteum.

TESTES

The **testes** (see Figure 13.1) produce the male sex hormone *testosterone*, which is important for sexual development and sexual behavior and libido, supporting spermatogenesis and erectile function.

PLACENTA

During pregnancy, the **placenta**, containing separate vascular systems of the mother and fetus, serves as an endocrine gland. It produces *chorionic gonadotropin hormone, estrogen,* and *progesterone.*

GASTROINTESTINAL MUCOSA

The **mucosa** of the pyloric area of the stomach secretes the hormone *gastrin,* which stimulates gastric acid secretion. Gastrin also affects the gallbladder, pancreas, and small intestine secretory activities.

The mucosa of the duodenum and jejunum secretes the hormone *secretin,* which stimulates pancreatic juice, bile, and intestinal secretion. The mucosa of the duodenum also secretes *pancreozymin-cholecystokinin,* which stimulates the pancreas. *Enterogastrone,* a hormone that regulates gastric secretions, is also secreted by the duodenal mucosa.

THYMUS

The **thymus** is a bilobed body located in the mediastinal cavity in front of and above the heart (see Figure 13.9 ■). It is composed of lymphoid tissue and is a part of the lymphatic system. It is a ductless glandlike body and secretes the hormones *thymosin* and *thymopoietin.* Thymosin promotes the maturation process of T lymphocytes (thymus dependent), white blood cells that play an important role in cell-mediated immunity. Thymopoietin is a hormone that influences the production of lymphocyte precursors and aids in their process of becoming T lymphocytes.

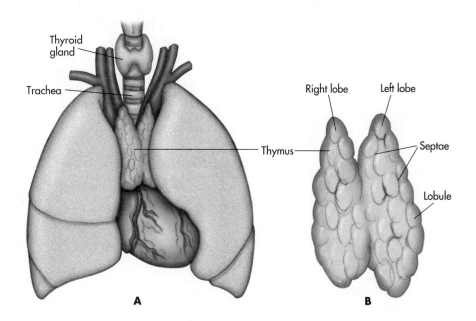

■ **Figure 13.9** Thymus gland. (A) Appearance and position; (B) with anatomic structures.

Anatomy and Physiology Labeling

Identify the structures shown below by filling in the blanks.

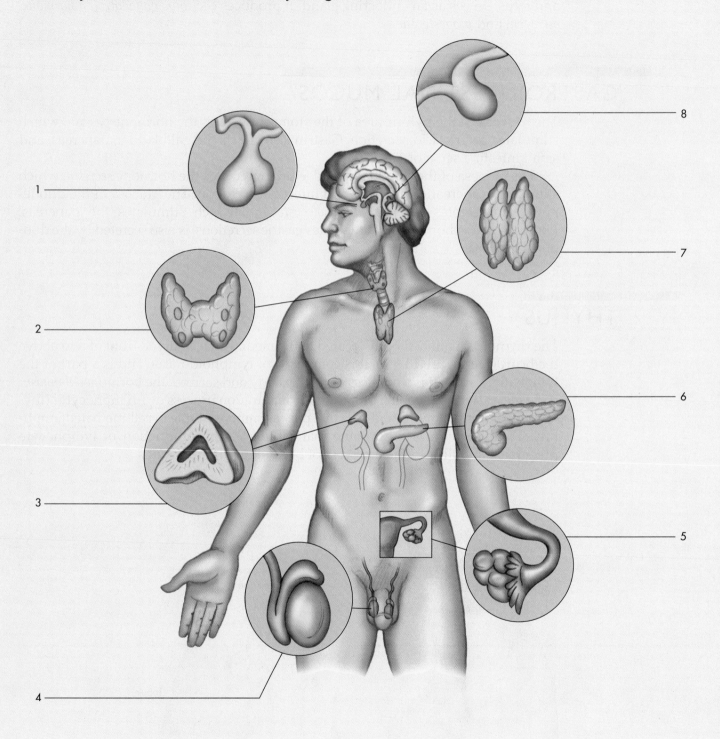

• Building Your Medical Vocabulary •

This section provides the foundation for learning medical terminology. Review the following alphabetized word list. Note how common prefixes and suffixes are repeatedly applied to word roots and combining forms to create different meanings. The word parts are color-coded: prefixes are green, suffixes are blue, **roots/combining forms are red**.

   You will find that some terms have not been divided into word parts. These are common words or specialized terms that are included to enhance your medical vocabulary. See Chapter 1, page 7, to review pronunciation guidelines.

MEDICAL WORD	WORD PARTS		DEFINITION
	Part	**Meaning**	
acidosis (ăs″ ĭ-dō′ sĭs)	acid -osis	acid condition	Condition of excessive acidity of body fluids
acromegaly (ăk″ rō-měg′ ă-lē)	acr/o -megaly	extremity enlargement, large	Characterized (in the adult) by marked enlargement and elongation of the bones of the face, jaw, and extremities. It is caused by an overproduction of growth hormone and is treated by x-ray or surgery.
Addison's disease (ăd′ ĭ-sŭns)			Results from a deficiency in the secretion of adrenocortical hormones; also called *hypoadrenocorticism*. The most common cause of this condition is the result of the body attacking itself (autoimmune disease). For unknown reasons, the immune system views the adrenal cortex as a foreign body, something to attack and destroy. Other causes of Addison's disease include infections of the adrenal glands, spread of cancer to the glands, and hemorrhage into the glands.
adenectomy (ăd″ ĕn-ĕk′ tō-mē)	aden -ectomy	gland surgical excision	Surgical excision of a gland
adenoma (ăd″ ĕ-nō′ mă)	aden -oma	gland tumor	Tumor of a gland
adenosis (ăd″ ĕ-nō′ sĭs)	aden -osis	gland condition	Any disease condition of a gland
adrenal (ăd-rē′ năl)	adren -al	adrenal gland pertaining to	Pertaining to the adrenal glands, triangular bodies that cover the superior surface of the kidneys; also called *suprarenal glands*

454 • CHAPTER THIRTEEN

MEDICAL WORD	WORD PARTS		DEFINITION
	Part	**Meaning**	
adrenalectomy (ăd-rē″ năl-ĕk′ tō-mē)	adren -al -ectomy	adrenal gland pertaining to surgical excision	Surgical excision of an adrenal gland
adrenopathy (ăd″ rĕn-ŏp′ ă-thē)	adren/o -pathy	adrenal gland disease	Any disease of an adrenal gland
androgen (ăn′ drō-jĕn)	andr/o -gen	man formation, produce	Hormones that produce or stimulate the development of male characteristics. The two major androgens are testosterone and androsterone.
catecholamines (kăt″ ĕ-kōl′ ăm-ēns)			Sympathomimetic hormones, epinephrine, norepinephrine, and dopamine
cortisone (kŏr′ tĭ-sōn)	cortis -one	cortex hormone	Glucocorticoid (steroid) hormone secreted by the adrenal cortex; used as an anti-inflammatory agent
cretinism (krē′ tĭn-ĭzm)	cretin -ism	cretin condition	Congenital condition caused by deficiency in secretion of the thyroid hormones and characterized by arrested physical and mental development. Treatment consists of appropriate thyroid replacement therapy. See Figure 13.10 ■

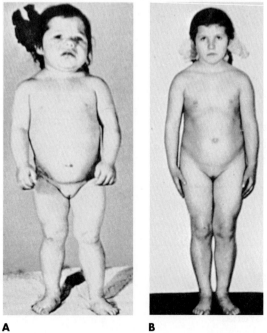

■ **Figure 13.10** (A) A 6-year-old child with congenital hypothyroidism, cretinism, exhibiting marked mental and physical retardation. (B) The same patient after 3 years of thyroxine therapy, which resulted in a spurt of growth and regression of pathological manifestations. Mental retardation is delayed.

A   **B**

MEDICAL WORD	WORD PARTS		DEFINITION
	Part	**Meaning**	
Cushing's disease (koosh´ ĭngs)			Results from hypersecretion of cortisol; symptoms include fatigue, muscular weakness, and changes in body appearance. Prolonged administration of large doses of ACTH can cause Cushing's syndrome. A *buffalo hump* and a *moon face* are characteristic signs of this condition. See Figure 13.11 ▪

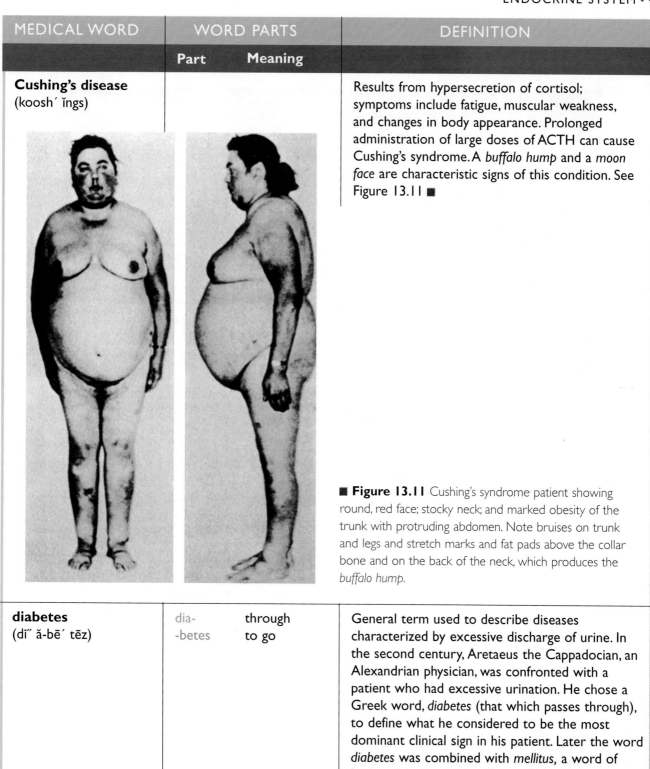

▪ **Figure 13.11** Cushing's syndrome patient showing round, red face; stocky neck; and marked obesity of the trunk with protruding abdomen. Note bruises on trunk and legs and stretch marks and fat pads above the collar bone and on the back of the neck, which produces the *buffalo hump.*

MEDICAL WORD	WORD PARTS		DEFINITION
diabetes (dī˝ ă-bē´ tēz)	dia- -betes	through to go	General term used to describe diseases characterized by excessive discharge of urine. In the second century, Aretaeus the Cappadocian, an Alexandrian physician, was confronted with a patient who had excessive urination. He chose a Greek word, *diabetes* (that which passes through), to define what he considered to be the most dominant clinical sign in his patient. Later the word *diabetes* was combined with *mellitus,* a word of Latin origin that means "honey." In 1670, in those suffering from polyuria, a distinction was made between those patients who had a sweet-tasting urine (diabetes mellitus [DM]) and those patients whose urine had no taste (diabetes insipidus [DI]). There are three major types of diabetes mellitus: Type 1, Type 2, and gestational diabetes. See page 463 for a description of diabetes insipidus.

MEDICAL WORD	WORD PARTS		DEFINITION
	Part	Meaning	

LIFE SPAN CONSIDERATIONS

Once rare, but with the increase in obesity in children doctors are now finding that as many as one out of 20 children who have diabetes has Type 2 diabetes mellitus (DM). It may be possible to prevent the onset of Type 2 DM in both children and adults by making modest lifestyle changes, such as eating a healthy diet, exercising for 30 minutes at least 5 days a week, and maintaining proper body weight for age and body type. Warning signs and symptoms of both Type 1 and Type 2 DM include frequent urination (polyuria), excessive thirst (polydipsia), extreme hunger (polyphagia), unusual weight loss, fatigue, irritability, and blurred vision. In Type 2 DM, tingling or numbness in the feet and frequent vaginal or skin infections can also be symptoms.

MEDICAL WORD	Part	Meaning	DEFINITION
dopamine (dō´ pă-mēn)			Intermediate substance in the synthesis of norepinephrine; used in the treatment of shock because it acts to elevate blood pressure and increase urinary output
dwarfism (dwar´ fizm)	dwarf -ism	small condition	Condition of being abnormally small. It is a medical disorder characterized by an adult height under 4 feet 10 inches (147 cm) and is usually classified as to the underlying condition that is the cause for the short stature. Dwarfism is not necessarily caused by any specific disease or disorder; it can simply be a naturally occurring consequence of a person's genetic makeup.
endocrine (ĕn´ dō-krĭn)	endo- crine	within to secrete	Ductless glands that produce internal secretions (hormones) directly into the bloodstream. See Table 13.2 for examples.
endocrinologist (ĕn″ dō-krĭn-ŏl´ ō-gĭst)	endo- crin/o log -ist	within to secrete study of one who specializes	Physician who specializes in the study of the endocrine system
endocrinology (ĕn″ dō-krĭn-ŏl´ ō-jē)	endo- crin/o -logy	within to secrete study of	Study of the endocrine system
epinephrine (ĕp″ ĭ-nĕf´ rĭn)	epi- nephr -ine	upon kidney substance	Hormone produced by the adrenal medulla; used as a vasoconstrictor and cardiac stimulant to relax bronchospasm and to relieve allergic symptoms; also called *adrenaline*

MEDICAL WORD	WORD PARTS		DEFINITION
	Part	Meaning	
estrogen (ĕs´ trō-jĕn)	estr/o -gen	mad desire formation, produce	Hormones produced by the ovaries, including estradiol, estrone, and estriol; female sex hormones important in the development of secondary sex characteristics and regulation of the menstrual cycle
euthyroid (ū-thī´ royd)	eu- thyr -oid	good, normal thyroid, shield resemble	Normal activity of the thyroid gland
exocrine (ĕks´ ō-krĭn)	exo- crine	out, away from to secrete	Pertains to a type of gland that secretes into ducts (duct glands); examples include sweat glands, salivary glands, mammary glands, stomach, liver, and pancreas
exophthalmic (ĕks˝ ŏf-thăl´ mĭk)	ex- ophthalm -ic	out, away from eye pertaining to	Pertaining to an abnormal condition characterized by a marked protrusion of the eyeballs as often seen in exophthalmic goiter or exophthalmos seen in Graves' disease. People with Graves' ophthalmopathy develop eye problems, including bulging, red or swollen eyes, sensitivity to light, and blurring or double vision. See Figure 13.12 ■

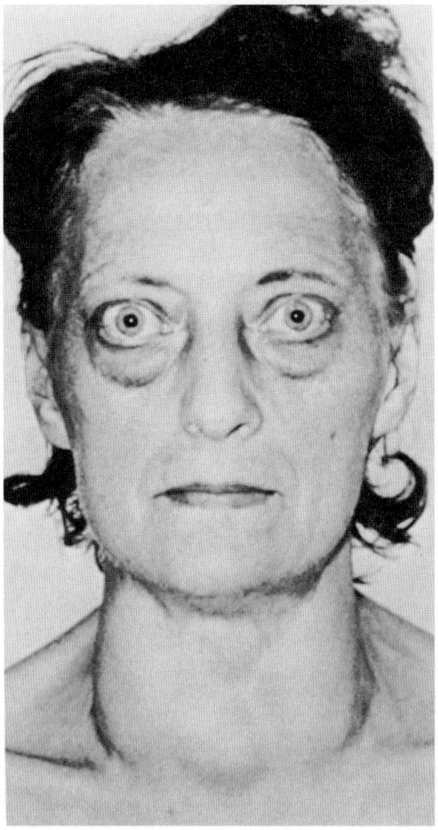

■ **Figure 13.12** Patient with exophthalmos.

| **galactorrhea** (gă-lăk˝ tō-rĭ´ ă) | galact/o -rrhea | milk flow, discharge | Excessive secretion of milk after cessation of nursing |

MEDICAL WORD	WORD PARTS		DEFINITION
	Part	**Meaning**	
gigantism (jī′ găn-tĭzm)	gigant -ism	giant condition	Pathological condition of being abnormally large
glandular (glăn′ dū-lăr)	glandul -ar	little acorn pertaining to	Pertaining to a gland
glucocorticoid (glū″ kō-kŏrt′ ĭ-koyd)	gluc/o cortic -oid	sweet, sugar cortex resemble	General classification of the adrenal cortical hormones, cortisol (hydrocortisone), and corticosterone
hirsutism (hŭr′ sūt-ĭzm)	hirsut -ism	hairy condition	Abnormal condition characterized by excessive growth of hair, especially as occurring in women. See Figure 13.13 ■

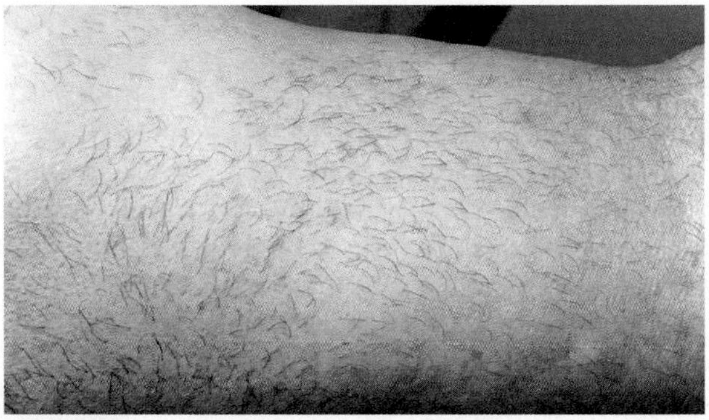

■ **Figure 13.13** Hirsutism.
(Courtesy Jason L. Smith, MD)

MEDICAL WORD	WORD PARTS		DEFINITION
hormone (hor′ mōn)			Class of chemical substance produced by the endocrine glands
hydrocortisone (hī″ drō-kŏr′ tĭ-sōn)	hydro cortis -one	water cortex hormone	Glucocorticoid (steroid) hormone produced by the adrenal cortex; used as an anti-inflammatory agent
hypergonadism (hī″ pĕr-gō′ năd-ĭzm)	hyper- gonad -ism	excessive seed condition	Condition of excessive secretion of the sex glands
hyperinsulinism (hī″ pĕr-ĭn′ sū-lĭn-ĭzm)	hyper- insulin -ism	excessive insulin condition	Condition of excessive amounts of insulin in the blood, causing low blood sugar
hyperkalemia (hī″ pĕr-kă-lē′ mĭ-ă)	hyper- kal -emia	excessive potassium (K) blood condition	Condition of excessive amounts of potassium in the blood

MEDICAL WORD	WORD PARTS		DEFINITION
	Part	**Meaning**	
hyperthyroidism (hī″ pĕr-thī′ royd-ĭzm)	hyper- thyr -oid -ism	excessive thyroid, shield resemble condition	Excessive secretion of thyroid hormone, a condition that can affect many body systems. The most common etiologies of hyperthyroidism are Graves' disease and toxic multinodular goiter. *Graves' disease* is an autoimmnue disease in which antibodies produced by the immune system stimulate the thyroid to produce too much thyroxine. Other forms of hyperthyroidism can be caused by **thyroiditis**, or inflammation of the thyroid gland. Certain benign or malignant tumors can also produce too much thyroid hormone.
hypogonadism (hī″ pō-gō′ năd-ĭzm)	hypo- gonad -ism	deficient seed condition	Condition caused by deficient internal secretion of the gonads
hypoparathyroidism (hī″ pō-păr″ ă-thī′ royd-īzm)	hypo- para- thyr -oid -ism	deficient beside thyroid, shield resemble condition	Deficient internal secretion of the parathyroid glands
hypophysis (hī-pŏf′ ĭ-sĭs)	hypo- -physis	deficient, under growth	Literally means any undergrowth; also called the pituitary gland
hypothyroidism (hī″ pō-thī′ royd-ĭzm)	hypo- thyr -oid -ism	deficient thyroid, shield resemble condition	Pathological condition in which the thyroid gland produces inadequate amounts of thyroid hormone. It can affect many body systems.

LIFE SPAN CONSIDERATIONS

Congenital hypothyroidism (CHT) is a condition that affects infants from birth (congenital) and results from a partial or complete loss of thyroid function (hypothyroidism); it occurs when the thyroid gland fails to develop or function properly. In 80–85% of cases, the thyroid gland is absent, abnormally located, or severely reduced in size. If untreated, it can lead to mental retardation and abnormal growth. In the United States and many other countries, all newborns are tested for congenital hypothyroidism. If treatment begins in the first month after birth, infants usually develop normally.

MEDICAL WORD	WORD PARTS		DEFINITION
	Part	Meaning	

> **fyi** Untreated hypothyroidism can lead to a number of health problems. Constant stimulation of the thyroid to release more hormones can cause the gland to become larger, a condition known as **goiter**. Hashimoto's thyroiditis, an autoimmune disease of the thyroid, is one of the most common causes of goiter. Another type of goiter is an *endemic goiter* that develops in certain geographic regions where the iodine content in food and water is deficient (see Figure 13.14 ■).
>
> ■ **Figure 13.14**
> Endemic goiter.

MEDICAL WORD	Part	Meaning	DEFINITION
insulin (ĭn´ sū-lĭn)	insul -in	insulin chemical	Hormone produced by the beta cells of the islets of Langerhans of the pancreas; acts to regulate the metabolism of glucose and the process necessary for the intermediary metabolism of carbohydrates, fats, and proteins; used in the management of diabetes mellitus
insulinogenic (ĭn˝ sū-lĭn˝ ō-jĕn´ ĭk)	insulin/o -genic	insulin formation, produce	Formation or production of insulin
iodine (ī´ ō-dīn)			Trace mineral that aids in the development and functioning of the thyroid gland
lethargic (lĕ-thar´ jĭk)	letharg -ic	drowsiness pertaining to	Pertaining to drowsiness, sluggish
myxedema (mĭks˝ ĕ-dē´ mă)	myx -edema	mucus swelling	Literally means *condition of mucus swelling*; it is the most severe form of hypothyroidism, characterized by marked edema of the face, a somnolent look, and hair that is stiff and without luster. Without treatment, coma and death can occur. See Figure 13.15 ■

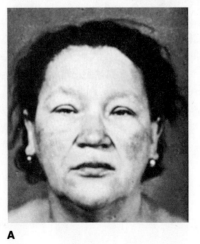
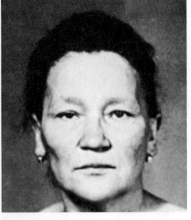

■ **Figure 13.15** (A) A 62-year-old patient with myxedema exhibiting marked edema of the face and a somnolent look. The hair is stiff and without luster. (B) The same patient after 3 months of treatment with thyroxine.

A

B

MEDICAL WORD	WORD PARTS		DEFINITION
	Part	**Meaning**	
norepinephrine (nŏr-ĕp″ĭ-nĕf′rĭn)	nor- epi- nephr -ine	not upon kidney substance	Hormone produced by the adrenal medulla; used as a vasoconstrictor of peripheral blood vessels in acute hypotensive states
oxytocin (ŏk″sĭ-tō′sĭn)			Hormone that stimulates uterine contraction during childbirth and stimulates the release of milk during suckling
pancreatic (păn″krē-ăt′ĭk)	pancreat -ic	pancreas pertaining to	Pertaining to the pancreas
parathyroid glands (păr″ă-thī′royd)	para- thyr -oid	beside thyroid, shield resemble	Endocrine glands located beside the thyroid gland. See Table 13.2.
pineal (pĭn′ē-ăl)	pine -al	pine cone pertaining to	Endocrine gland shaped like a small pine cone
pituitarism (pĭt-ū′ĭ-tă-rĭzm)	pituitar -ism	pituitary gland condition	Any condition of the pituitary gland
pituitary (pĭ-tū′ĭ-tăr″ē)	pituitar -y	pituitary gland pertaining to	Pertaining to the pituitary gland, the hypophysis
progeria (prō-jē′rĭ-ă)	pro- ger -ia	before old age condition	Pathological condition of premature old age occurring in childhood
progesterone (prō-jĕs′tĕr-ōn)	pro- gester -one	before to bear hormone	Hormone produced by the corpus luteum of the ovary, the adrenal cortex, or the placenta; released during the second half of the menstrual cycle
Simmonds' disease (sĭm′mŏnds)			Pathological condition in which complete atrophy of the pituitary gland causes loss of function of the thyroid, adrenals, and gonads; symptoms include premature senility, psychic symptoms, and cachexia; also called *panhypopituitarism*. Treatment involves regular administration of the various hormones whose release is normally dependent on pituitary function.
somatotropin (sō-măt′ō-trō″pĭn)	somat/o trop -in	body turn chemical	Growth-stimulating hormone produced by the anterior lobe of the pituitary gland

MEDICAL WORD	WORD PARTS		DEFINITION
	Part	**Meaning**	
steroids (stĕr´ oydz)	ster -oid	solid resemble	Group of chemical substances that includes hormones, vitamins, sterols, cardiac glycosides, and certain drugs
testosterone (tĕs-tŏs´ tĕr-ōn)	test/o ster -one	testicle solid hormone	Hormone produced by the testes; male sex hormone important in the development of secondary sex characteristics and masculinization
thymectomy (thī-mĕk´ tō-mē)	thym -ectomy	thymus surgical excision	Surgical excision of the thymus gland
thymitis (thī-mī´ tĭs)	thym -itis	thymus inflammation	Inflammation of the thymus gland
thyroid (thī´ royd)	thyr -oid	thyroid, shield resemble	Endocrine gland located in the neck; its shape resembles a shield. See Figure 13.16 ■

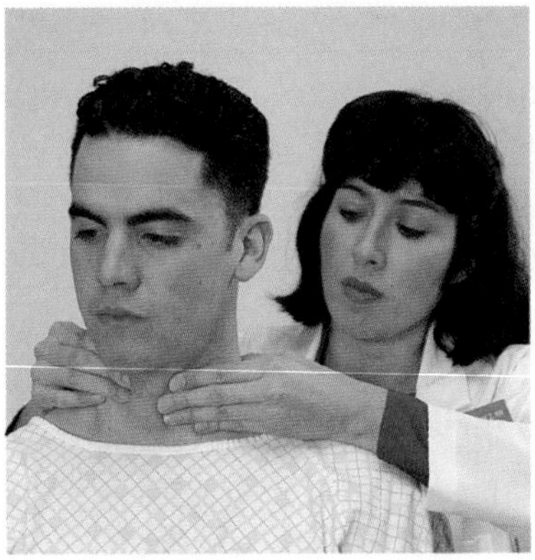

■ **Figure 13.16** Palpating the thyroid gland from behind the patient is a most effective way of assessing the gland for abnormality.

MEDICAL WORD	WORD PARTS		DEFINITION
	Part	Meaning	
thyroidectomy (thī˝ royd-ĕk´ tō-mē)	thyr -oid -ectomy	thyroid, shield resemble surgical excision	Surgical excision of the thyroid gland
thyroiditis (thī˝ royd´ ī´ tĭs)	thyr -oid -itis	thyroid, shield resemble inflammation	Inflammation of the thyroid gland
thyrotoxicosis (thī˝ rō-tŏks˝ ĭ-kō´ sĭs)	thyr/o toxic -osis	thyroid, shield poison condition	Literally means *a poisonous condition of the thyroid gland*; pathological condition caused by an acute oversecretion of thyroid hormones

ENDOCRINE SYSTEM • 463

MEDICAL WORD	WORD PARTS		DEFINITION
	Part	Meaning	
thyroxine (T₄) (thī-rŏks´ ēn)	thyro(x) -ine	thyroid, shield substance	Hormone produced by the thyroid gland; important in growth and development and regulation of the body's metabolic rate and metabolism of carbohydrates, fats, and proteins
vasopressin (VP) (văs˝ ō-prĕs´ ĭn)	vas/o press -in	vessel to press chemical	Hormone produced by the hypothalamus and stored in the posterior lobe of the pituitary gland; also called *antidiuretic hormone (ADH)*. Hyposecretion of this hormone can result in **diabetes insipidus (DI)**, a condition characterized by excessive thirst (*polydipsia*) and excretion of large amounts of diluted urine (*polyuria*). Because of the deficiency of ADH, water is prevented from being reabsorbed into the blood through the renal tubules. *Insipidus* means tasteless, reflecting very dilute and watery urine.
virilism (vĭr´ ĭl-ĭzm)	viril -ism	masculine condition	Pathological condition in which secondary male characteristics, such as growth of hair on face and/or body and deepening of the voice, are produced in a female, usually as the result of adrenal dysfunction or hormonal imbalance or taking medications (androgens)

• Drug Highlights •

TYPE OF DRUG	DESCRIPTION AND EXAMPLES
thyroid hormones	Increase metabolic rate, cardiac output, oxygen consumption, body temperature, respiratory rate, blood volume, and carbohydrate, fat, and protein metabolism; influence growth and development at cellular level. Thyroid hormones are used as supplements or replacement therapy in hypothyroidism, myxedema, and cretinism. EXAMPLES: Levothroid and Synthroid (levothyroxine sodium), Cytomel (liothyronine sodium), and Thyrolar (liotrix)
antithyroid hormones	Inhibit the synthesis of thyroid hormones by decreasing iodine use in manufacture of thyroglobin and iodothyronine; do not inactivate or inhibit thyroxine or triiodothyronine. They are used in the treatment of hyperthyroidism. EXAMPLES: Tapazole (methimazole), potassium iodide solution, and propylthiouracil

TYPE OF DRUG	DESCRIPTION AND EXAMPLES
insulin	Stimulates carbohydrate metabolism by increasing the movement of glucose and other monosaccharides into cells. It also influences fat and carbohydrate metabolism in the liver and adipose cells. It decreases blood sugar, phosphate, and potassium, and increases blood pyruvate and lactate. Insulin is used to treat insulin-dependent diabetes mellitus (IDDM) Type 1, noninsulin-dependent diabetes mellitus (NIDDM) Type 2 when other regimens are not effective, and to treat diabetic ketoacidosis, a complication of diabetes that occurs when the body cannot use sugar (glucose) as a fuel source because the body has no insulin or not enough insulin, and fat is used instead. By-products of fat breakdown, called ketones, build up in the body.
insulin preparations for injection	Insulin is given by subcutaneous injection and is available in various forms such as rapid-acting, intermediate-acting, and long-acting preparations.
rapid acting	EXAMPLES: Novolin R and Humalog Onset of action—$\frac{1}{2}$ hour Appearance—clear
intermediate acting	EXAMPLES: Novolin N and Humulin N Onset of action—1 to 1$\frac{1}{2}$ hours Appearance—cloudy
long acting	EXAMPLE: Levemir Provides up to 24 hours of blood sugar control
oral hypoglycemic agents	Stimulate insulin secretion from pancreatic cells in noninsulin-dependent diabetics with some pancreatic function. They are agents of the sulfonylurea class. EXAMPLES: Diabinese (chlorpropamide), Glucotrol (glipizide), DiaBeta (glyburide), tolazamide, and tolbutamide
hyperglycemic agents	Cause an increase in blood glucose of diabetic patients with severe hypoglycemia (insulin shock). In patients with mild hypoglycemia, the administration of an oral carbohydrate such as orange juice, candy, or a lump of sugar generally corrects the condition. If comatose, the patient is given dextrose solution IV. For management of severe hypoglycemia, the following agents may be used. EXAMPLES: Glucagon (an insulin antagonist), Proglycem (diazoxide), and glucose

• Diagnostic and Lab Tests •

TEST	DESCRIPTION
catecholamines (kăt″ ĕ-kōl′ ă-mēns)	Test performed on urine to determine the amount of epinephrine and nor-epinephrine present. These adrenal hormones increase in times of stress.
corticotropin, corticotropin-releasing factor (kor″ tĭ-kō-trō′ pin)	Test performed on blood plasma to determine the amount of corticotropin present. Increased levels can indicate stress, adrenal cortical hypofunction, and/or pituitary tumors. Decreased **corticotropin-releasing factor (CRF)** levels can indicate adrenal neoplasms and/or Cushing's syndrome.
fasting blood sugar (FBS)	Test performed on blood to determine the level of sugar in the bloodstream. It is done after fasting 8–12 hrs (NPO after midnight) and should be performed the next morning. A FBS of 100–125 mg/dl indicates prediabetes. A FBS of 126 mg/dl indicated diabetes mellitus. Also referred to as *fasting blood glucose (FBG)*.
glucose tolerance test (GTT) (gloo′ kōs)	Blood sugar test performed at specified intervals after the patient has been given a significant amount of glucose. Blood samples are drawn, and the glucose level of each sample is measured. It is more accurate than other blood sugar tests and is used to diagnose diabetes mellitus. A GTT of 140–199 mg/dl indicates prediabetes. A GTT at 200 mg/dl or higher indicates diabetes mellitus.
Hb A1C test	The Hb A1C test is a blood test used to diagnose diabetes, to identify people at risk of developing diabetes, and to monitor how well blood sugar levels are being controlled by the diabetic patient. The Hb A1C test goes by other names, including glycated hemoglobin, glycosylated hemoglobin, hemoglobin A1C, and A1C. In January 2010 the American Diabetes Association (ADA) published revised guidelines with levels of Hb A1C between 5.0 and 5.5% as being within normal range. With each incremental Hb A1C increase, the incidence of diabetes increased; those at a level of 6.5% or greater are considered diabetic, and those between 6.0% and 6.5% are considered at a very high risk for developing diabetes.
17-hydroxycortico-steroids (17-OHCS) (hĭ-drŏk″ sē-kor tĭ-kō)	Test performed on urine to identify adrenocorticosteroid hormones and to determine adrenal cortical function.
17-ketosteroids (17-KS) (kē″ tō-stĕr′ oyds)	Test performed on urine to determine the amount of 17-KS present, the end product of androgens that is secreted from the adrenal glands and testes. It is used to diagnose adrenal tumors.
protein-bound iodine (PBI)	Test performed on serum to indicate the amount of iodine that is attached to serum protein. It can be used to indicate thyroid function.

TEST	DESCRIPTION
radioactive iodine uptake (RAIU) (rā″ dē-ō-ăk′ tĭv ī′ ō-dīn)	Test to measure the ability of the thyroid gland to concentrate ingested iodine. Increased level can indicate hyperthyroidism, cirrhosis, and/or thyroiditis. Decreased level can indicate hypothyroidism.
radioimmunoassay (RIA) (rā″ dē-ō-ĭmŭ″ -nō-ăs′ā)	Standard assay method used to measure minute quantities of specific antibodies and/or antigens. It can be used for clinical laboratory measurements of hormones, therapeutic drug monitoring, and substance abuse screening.
thyroid scan (thī′ royd)	Test to detect tumors of the thyroid gland. The patient is given radioactive iodine 131, which localizes in the thyroid gland, which is then visualized with a scanner device.
thyroxine (T$_4$) (thī-rōks′ ĭn)	Test performed on blood serum to determine the amount of thyroxine present. Increased levels can indicate hyperthyroidism; decreased levels can indicate hypothyroidism.
total calcium	Test performed on blood serum to determine the amount of calcium present. Increased levels can indicate hyperparathyroidism; decreased levels can indicate hypoparathyroidism.
triiodothyronine uptake (T$_3$U) (trī″ ĭ-ō″ dō-thī′ rō-nĭn)	Test performed on blood serum to determine the amount of triiodothyronine present. Increased levels can indicate thyrotoxicosis, toxic adenoma, and/or Hashimoto's struma. Decreased levels can indicate starvation, severe infection, and severe trauma.
ultrasonography (ŭl-tră-sŏn-ŏg′ ră-fē)	Use of high-frequency sound waves as a screening test or as a diagnostic tool to visualize the structure being studied; can be used to visualize the pancreas, thyroid, and any other gland.

• Abbreviations •

ABBREVIATION	MEANING
17-KS	17-ketosteroids
17-OHCS	17-hydroxycorticosteroids
ACTH	adrenocorticotropic hormone
ADA	American Diabetes Association
ADH	antidiuretic hormone
BG	blood glucose
BMR	basal metabolic rate
CHT	congenital hypothyroidism
cm	centimeter
CRF	corticotropin-releasing factor
DI	diabetes insipidus
DM	diabetes mellitus
FBG	fasting blood glucose
FBS	fasting blood sugar
FSH	follicle-stimulating hormone
g	gram
GH	growth hormone
GHRF	growth hormone–releasing factor
GnRF	gonadotropin-releasing factor
GTT	glucose tolerance test
IDDM	insulin-dependent diabetes mellitus
K	potassium
LH	luteinizing hormone
LTH	lactogenic hormone
MIF	melanocyte–stimulating hormone release-inhibiting factor

ABBREVIATION	MEANING
MRF	melanocyte-stimulating hormone–releasing factor
MSH	melanocyte-stimulating hormone
Na	sodium
NIDDM	non-insulin-dependent diabetes mellitus
PBI	protein-bound iodine
PIF	prolactin release-inhibiting factor
PRF	prolactin-releasing factor
PRL	prolactin hormone
PTH	parathyroid (parathormone hormone)
RAIU	radioactive iodine uptake
rDNA	recombinant deoxyribonucleic acid
RIA	radioimmunoassay
STH	somatotropin hormone
T_3	triiodothyronine
T_3U	triiodothyronine uptake
T_4	thyroxine
TFS	thyroid function studies
TH	thyroid hormone
TRH	thyrotropin-releasing hormone
TSH	thyroid-stimulating hormone
VP	vasopressin

• Study and Review • Study and Review • Study and Review
Review • Study and Review • Study and Review • Stu
w • **Study and Review** • Study and Review • Study a

Anatomy and Physiology

Write your answers to the following questions.

1. Name the primary glands of the endocrine system.

a. _____   b. _____

c. _____   d. _____

e. _____   f. _____

g. _____   h. _____

2. State the vital function of the endocrine system. _____

_____

3. Define *hormone*. _____

4. State the vital role of the hypothalamus in regulating endocrine functions. _____

_____

_____

_____

5. Why is the pituitary gland known as the master gland of the body?

_____

6. Name the hormones secreted by the anterior lobe (*adenohypophysis*) of the pituitary gland.

a. _____   b. _____

c. _____   d. _____

e. _____   f. _____

g. _____

7. Name the hormones secreted by the posterior lobe (*neurohypophysis*) of the pituitary gland.

a. _____   b. _____

8. The pineal gland secretes the hormones _____ and _____ .

9. State the vital role of the thyroid gland. _____

10. Name the hormones stored and secreted by the thyroid gland.

    a. _____   **b.** _____

    c. _____

11. Parathyroid (*parathormone hormone*) is essential for the maintenance of a normal level of

    _____ and also plays a role in the metabolism of _____.

12. Insulin is essential for the maintenance of a normal level of _____ .

13. The adrenal cortex secretes a group of hormones known as the _____ , the

    _____ , and the _____ .

14. Name four functions of cortisol.

    a. _____   **b.** _____

    c. _____   **d.** _____

15. Name four functions of corticosterone.

    a. _____   **b.** _____

    c. _____   **d.** _____

16. _____ is the principal mineralocorticoid secreted by the adrenal cortex.

17. Define *androgen*. _____

18. Name the three main catecholamines synthesized, secreted, and stored by the adrenal medulla.

    a. _____   **b.** _____

    c. _____

19. Name three functions of the hormone epinephrine.

    a. _____

    b. _____

    c. _____

20. The ovaries produce the hormones _____ and _____ .

21. The testes produce the hormone _____ .

22. Name the two hormones secreted by the thymus.

    a. _____   **b.** _____

23. Name the four hormones secreted by the gastrointestinal mucosa.

a. _____   b. _____

c. _____   d. _____

Word Parts

PREFIXES

Give the definitions of the following prefixes.

1. dia- _____   **2.** endo- _____

3. eu- _____   **4.** ex- _____

5. exo- _____   **6.** hyper- _____

7. hypo- _____   **8.** para- _____

9. pro- _____   **10.** epi- _____

11. hydro- _____

ROOTS AND COMBINING FORMS

Give the definitions of the following roots and combining forms.

1. acid _____   **2.** acr/o _____

3. aden _____   **4.** aden/o _____

5. cortic _____   **6.** creat _____

7. cretin _____   **8.** andr/o _____

9. crine _____   **10.** crin/o _____

11. dwarf _____   **12.** galact/o _____

13. ger _____   **14.** gigant _____

15. glandul _____   **16.** gluc/o _____

17. gonad _____   **18.** hirsut _____

19. insul _____   **20.** cortis _____

21. insulin/o _____   **22.** kal _____

23. letharg _____   **24.** log _____

25. myx _____   **26.** ophthalm _____

27. pine _____

28. nephr _____

29. pituitar _____

30. ren _____

31. ren/o _____

32. estr/o _____

33. thym _____

34. gester _____

35. thyr _____

36. thyr/o _____

37. toxic _____

38. trop _____

39. viril _____

40. somat/o _____

41. test/o _____

42. ster _____

43. thyrox _____

44. vas/o _____

45. press _____

46. adren _____

47. adren/o _____

48. pancreat _____

SUFFIXES

Give the definitions of the following suffixes.

1. -al _____

2. -gen _____

3. -ar _____

4. -betes _____

5. -ectomy _____

6. -edema _____

7. -emia _____

8. -genic _____

9. -ia _____

10. -ic _____

11. -ism _____

12. -ist _____

13. -itis _____

14. -logy _____

15. -one _____

16. -megaly _____

17. -oid _____

18. -oma _____

19. -osis _____

20. -pathy _____

21. -ine _____

22. -physis _____

23. -in _____

24. -rrhea _____

25. -y _____

Identifying Medical Terms

In the spaces provided, write the medical terms for the following meanings.

1. _____ Any disease condition of a gland

2. _____ Congenital deficiency in secretion of the thyroid hormones characterized by arrested physical and mental development

3. _____ General term used to describe disease characterized by excessive discharge of urine

4. _____ Study of the endocrine system

5. _____ Normal activity of the thyroid gland

6. _____ Pertains to a type of gland that secretes into ducts (duct glands)

7. _____ Pathological condition of being abnormally large

8. _____ General classification of the adrenal cortex hormones

9. _____ Condition of excessive amounts of potassium in the blood

10. _____ Condition caused by deficient internal secretion of the gonads

11. _____ Pertaining to drowsiness; sluggishness

12. _____ Inflammation of the thymus

Spelling

Circle the correct spelling of each medical term.

1. catcholamines / catecholamines
2. cretinism / crtinism
3. exopthalmic / exophthalmic
4. hypothyroidism / hypthyoidism
5. myxedema / myexdema
6. pineal / pinel
7. pituitry / pituitary
8. thyroid / thyoid
9. oxytoin / oxytocin
10. virlism / virilism

Matching

Select the appropriate lettered meaning for each of the following words.

_____ **1.** aldosterone	**a.** Also called *antidiuretic hormone, ADH*
_____ **2.** androgen	**b.** Sympathomimetic hormones, epinephrine, norepinephrine, and dopamine
_____ **3.** catecholamines	**c.** Acts to regulate the metabolism of glucose
_____ **4.** cortisone	**d.** Hormone produced by the thyroid gland
_____ **5.** dopamine	**e.** Essential in regulating electrolyte and water balance by promoting sodium and chloride reabsorption and potassium excretion
_____ **6.** epinephrine	**f.** Hormones that produce or stimulate the development of male characteristics
_____ **7.** insulin	**g.** Glucocorticoid (steroid) hormone used as an anti-inflammatory agent
_____ **8.** iodine	**h.** Intermediate substance in the synthesis of norepinephrine
_____ **9.** thyroxine	**i.** Also called *adrenaline*
_____ **10.** vasopressin	**j.** Trace mineral that aids in the development and functioning of the thyroid gland
	k. Hormone produced by the testes

Abbreviations

Place the correct word, phrase, or abbreviation in the space provided.

1. basal metabolic rate _____

2. diabetes mellitus _____

3. FBS _____

4. GTT _____

5. protein-bound iodine _____

6. PTH _____

7. RIA _____

8. somatotropin hormone _____

9. TFS _____

10. VP _____

Diagnostic and Laboratory Tests

Select the best answer to each multiple-choice question. Circle the letter of your choice.

1. A test performed on urine to determine the amount of epinephrine and norepinephrine present.
   - **a.** catecholamines
   - **b.** corticotropin
   - **c.** protein-bound iodine
   - **d.** total calcium

2. Increased levels can indicate diabetes mellitus, diabetes acidosis, and many other conditions.
   - **a.** protein-bound iodine
   - **b.** total calcium
   - **c.** fasting blood sugar
   - **d.** thyroid scan

3. Test used to detect tumors of the thyroid gland.
   - **a.** thyroxine
   - **b.** total calcium
   - **c.** thyroid scan
   - **d.** protein-bound iodine

4. Blood sugar test performed at specific intervals after the patient has been given a certain amount of glucose.
   - **a.** fasting blood sugar
   - **b.** glucose tolerance test
   - **c.** protein-bound iodine
   - **d.** corticotropin

5. A test used in the diagnosing of adrenal tumors.
   - **a.** 17-HCS
   - **b.** 17-OHCS
   - **c.** 17-KS
   - **d.** 17-HDL

PRACTICAL APPLICATION

CASE STUDY ANALYSIS

This exercise contains information, abbreviations, and medical terminology from an actual medical record or case study that has been adapted for this text. The names and any personal information have been created by the author. Read and study each form or case study and then answer the questions that follow. You may refer to Appendix III, Abbreviations and Symbols, on page A41.

DIABETES CASE STUDY
Meet Matthew J. Marshall

Matthew is a 15 y/o white male c/o being "thirsty, hungry, and urinating a lot." He states, "I am tired and just don't have any energy. I eat like a horse, but I stay hungry. I am afraid that I have 'sugar.' My dad and my grandfather both take insulin."

Signs and Symptoms: Polydipsia, polyphagia, polyuria, and fatigue.
Family history is notable for Type 1 diabetes in father and paternal grandfather; his maternal grandmother has heart disease. **Allergies:** NKDA. Typically, for a patient with this complaint and history, Type 2 diabetes would be considered.

The pertinent findings on physical exam:

Vital Signs: T: 98.4 F; P: 78; R: 18; BP: 132/70

Ht: 5´ 5″

Wt: 160 lb

General Appearance: Overweight for age. BMI: 26.6

Heart: Regular rate and rhythm. No murmurs. Lungs: CTA. Abd: Noted excessive adipose tissue. Soft, nontender, no masses, no liver enlargement. Skin: Warm and dry, no lesions, no discoloration of lower extremities.

The Plan for Diagnosis and Treatment:

1. Send to lab for Hb A1C and schedule FBS, ASAP.

2. Recommend that Matthew attend the next health education seminar. One or both parents are to attend the seminar with him. Explain that individuals who are overweight, have a BMI greater than or equal to 25, and who have immediate family members with diabetes are at a higher risk of developing diabetes. Note: For more information on diabetes, call (800) DIABETES.

3. Patient is to return in one week for test results. If indicated proper medication regimen will be initiated for Matthew.

Case Study Questions

Place the correct answer in the space provided.

1. Why is Matthew concerned that he may have "sugar"?_____

2. To rule out diabetes mellitus, the physician ordered a _____ test and a

_____ ASAP.

3. What are the three classic symptoms of diabetes mellitus that Matthew stated?_____

4. What does the abbreviation FBS mean? _____

5. A BMI over _____ may indicate a higher risk of developing diabetes.

**PEARSON
mymedicalterminologylab**™

MyMedicalTerminologyLab is a premium online homework management system that includes a host of features to help you study. Registered users will find:

- Fun games and activities built within a virtual hospital

- Powerful tools that track and analyze your results—allowing you to create a personalized learning experience

- Videos, flashcards, and audio pronunciations to help enrich your progress

- Streaming lesson presentations and self-paced learning modules

- A space where you and your instructors can view and manage your assignments

Suffixes • Prefixes • Organization of the Body • Integu
ntary System • Skeletal System • Muscular System • Di
ve System • Cardiovascular System • Blood and Lymph
System • Respiratory System • Urinary System • Endo
stem • **Nervous System** • Special Senses: The Ear •

LEARNING OUTCOMES

On completion of this chapter, you will be
able to:

1. Describe the nervous system.

2. State the description and primary functions
   of the organs/structures of the nervous
   system.

3. List the major divisions of the brain and their
   functions.

4. Analyze, build, spell, and pronounce medical
   words.

5. Comprehend the drugs highlighted in this
   chapter.

6. Describe diagnostic and laboratory tests
   related to the nervous system.

7. Identify and define selected abbreviations.

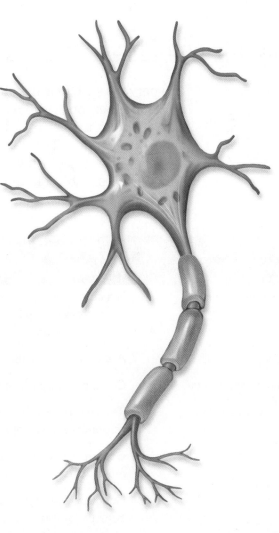

COMBINING FORMS OF THE NERVOUS SYSTEM

cephal/o	head	**lob/o**	lobe
cerebell/o	little brain	**mening/i**	membrane, meninges
cerebr/o	cerebrum	**mening/o**	membrane, meninges
chrom/o	color	**ment/o**	mind
cran/i	skull	**my/o**	muscle
crani/o	skull	**myel/o**	bone marrow, spinal cord
cyt/o	cell	**narc/o**	numbness, sleep, stupor
dendr/o	tree	**neur/i**	nerve
disk/o	a disk	**neur/o**	nerve
dur/o	dura, hard	**pallid/o**	globus pallidus
electr/o	electricity	**papill/o**	papilla
encephal/o	brain	**phe/o**	dusky
esthesi/o	feeling	**poli/o**	gray
fibr/o	fiber	**somn/o**	sleep
gli/o	glue	**spin/o**	a thorn, spine
hypn/o	sleep	**spondyl/o**	vertebra
lamin/o	thin plate	**vag/o**	vagus, wandering
later/o	side	**ventricul/o**	ventricle

Anatomy and Physiology

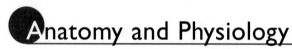

The nervous system is usually described as having two interconnected divisions: the central nervous system (CNS) and the peripheral nervous system (PNS). The CNS includes the brain and spinal cord. It is enclosed by the bones of the skull and spinal column. The PNS consists of the network of nerves and neural tissues branching throughout the body from 12 pairs of cranial nerves and 31 pairs of spinal nerves. Table 14.1 ■ provides an at-a-glance look at the nervous system. See Figure 14.1 ■

TABLE 14.1 Nervous System at-a-Glance

Organ/Structure	Primary Functions/Description
Neurons (nerve cells)	Structural and functional units of the nervous system act as specialized conductors of impulses that enable the body to interact with its internal and external environments
Neuroglia	Act as supporting tissue
Nerve fibers and tracts	Conduct impulses from one location to another
Central nervous system	Receives impulses from throughout the body, processes the information, and responds with an appropriate action
Brain	Governs sensory perception, emotions, consciousness, memory, and voluntary movements
Spinal cord	Conducts sensory impulses to the brain and motor impulses from the brain to body parts; also serves as a reflex center for impulses entering and leaving the spinal cord without involvement of the brain

Organ/Structure	Primary Functions/Description
Peripheral nervous system	Links the central nervous system with other parts of the body
Cranial nerves (12 pairs)	Provide sensory input and motor control, or a combination of these
Spinal nerves (31 pairs)	Carry impulses to the spinal cord and to muscles, organs, and glands
Autonomic nervous system (sympathetic division and parasympathetic division)	Controls involuntary bodily functions such as sweating, secretion of glands, arterial blood pressure, smooth muscle tissue, and the heart. Also stimulates the adrenal gland to release epinephrine (adrenaline), the hormone that causes the familiar adrenaline rush or the "fight-or-flight response."

TABLE 14.1 Nervous System at-a-Glance *(continued)*

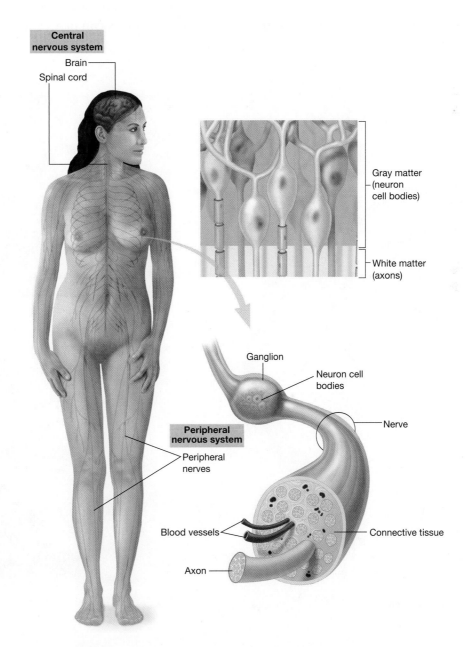

■ **Figure 14.1** The nervous system is described as having two interconnected divisions: the central nervous system (CNS) consisting of the brain and spinal cord and the peripheral nervous system (PNS) consisting of peripheral nerves.

TISSUES OF THE NERVOUS SYSTEM

The nervous system has two principal tissue types. These tissues are made up of **neurons** or nerve cells and their supporting tissues, collectively called **neuroglia**. See Figure 14.2 ■ Neurons are the structural and functional units of the nervous system. These cells are specialized conductors of impulses that enable the body to interact with its internal and external environments. There are several types of neurons, three of which are described in the following sections.

Motor Neurons

Motor neurons cause contractions in muscles and secretions from glands and organs. They also act to inhibit the actions of glands and organs, thereby controlling most of the body's functions. Motor neurons can be described as being *efferent*

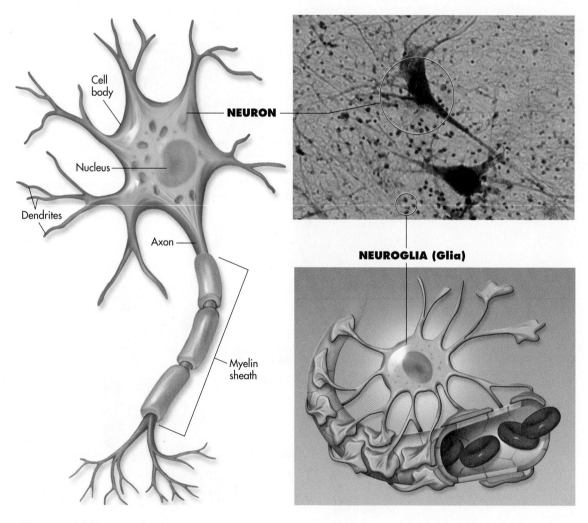

Cell body

Nucleus

Dendrites

Axon

Myelin sheath

NEURON

NEUROGLIA (Glia)

■ **Figure 14.2** Two main types of nerve cells.

processes because they transmit impulses away from the neural cell body to the muscles or organs to be innervated. Motor neurons consist of a nucleated cell body with protoplasmic processes extending away from it in several directions. These processes are known as the **axon** and **dendrites**. Most axons are long and are covered with a fatty substance, the myelin sheath, which acts as an insulator and increases the transmission velocity of the nerve fiber it surrounds. Axons may be as long as several feet and reach from the cell body to the area to be activated. Dendrites resemble the branches of a tree, are short, or unsheathed, and transmit impulses to the cell body. Neurons usually have several dendrites and only one axon.

Sensory Neurons

Sensory neurons differ in structure from motor neurons because they do not have true dendrites. The processes transmitting sensory information to the cell bodies of these neurons are called *peripheral processes,* are sheathed, and resemble axons. They are attached to sensory receptors and transmit impulses to the central nervous system (CNS). After processing the information, the CNS can stimulate motor neurons in response to this sensory information. Sensory neurons are referred to as *afferent nerves* because they carry impulses from the sensory receptors to the synaptic endings in the central nervous system.

Interneurons

Interneurons are called *central* or *associative neurons* and are located entirely within the central nervous system. They function to mediate impulses between sensory and motor neurons.

NERVE FIBERS, NERVES, AND TRACTS

The terms *nerve fiber, nerve,* and *tract* are used to describe neuronal processes conducting impulses from one location to another.

Nerve Fibers

A **nerve fiber** is a single elongated process, the axon of a neuron. Nerve fibers of the peripheral nervous system are wrapped by protective membranes called **sheaths**. The PNS has two types of sheaths: *myelinated* and *unmyelinated*, which are formed by accessory cells. Myelinated fibers have an inner sheath of myelin, a thick, fatty substance, and an outer sheath or **neurilemma** composed of *Schwann cells.* Unmyelinated fibers lack myelin and are sheathed only by the neurilemma. Nerve fibers of the central nervous system do not contain Schwann cells. Therefore, damage to fibers of the CNS is permanent, whereas damage to a peripheral nerve can be reversible.

Nerves

A **nerve** is a collection of nerve fibers, outside the central nervous system. Nerves are usually described as being sensory or **afferent** (*conducting to the CNS*) or motor or **efferent** (*conducting away from the CNS to muscles, organs, and glands*).

Tracts

Groups of nerve fibers within the central nervous system are sometimes referred to as **tracts** when they have the same origin, function, and termination. The spinal cord contains afferent sensory tracts ascending to the brain and efferent motor tracts descending from the brain. The brain itself contains numerous tracts, the largest of which is the *corpus callosum* joining the left and right hemispheres.

TRANSMISSION OF NERVE IMPULSES

Stimulation of a nerve occurs at a *receptor*. There are distinct sensory receptors, ranging from the simplest, which are free nerve endings for pain, to the most complex, as in the retina of the eye for vision. Sensory receptors are specialized to specific types of stimulation such as heat, cold, light, pressure, or pain and react by initiating a chemical change or impulse. The transmission of an impulse by a nerve fiber is based on the **all-or-none principle**. This means that no transmission occurs until the stimulus reaches a set minimum strength, which can vary for different receptors. Once the minimum stimulus or threshold is reached, a maximum impulse is produced. The impulse is then transmitted via a **synapse**, a specialized knoblike branch ending, with the help of certain chemical agents, across a space separating the axon's end knobs from the dendrites of the next neuron or from a motor end plate attached to a muscle. This space is called a **synaptic cleft**, and the chemical agents released are called **neurotransmitters**.

CENTRAL NERVOUS SYSTEM

Consisting of the brain and spinal cord, the **central nervous system (CNS)** receives impulses from throughout the body, processes the information, and responds with an appropriate action. This activity can be at the conscious or unconscious level, depending on the source of the sensory stimulus. Both the brain and spinal cord can be divided into **gray matter** and **white matter**. The gray matter consists of unsheathed cell bodies and true dendrites. The white matter is composed of myelinated nerve fibers. In the spinal cord, the arrangement of white and gray matter results in an H-shaped core of gray cell bodies surrounded by tracts of nerve fibers interconnected to the brain. The reverse is generally true of the brain where the surface layer or cortex is gray matter and most of the internal structures are white matter.

LIFE SPAN CONSIDERATIONS

Neural tube development occurs about the third to fourth week of embryonic life. This development becomes the **central nervous system.** At 6 weeks, a developing fetus's brain waves are measurable. At 28 weeks, the fetal nervous system begins some regulatory functions. By 32 weeks, the developing fetal nervous system is capable of sustaining rhythmic respirations and regulating body temperature. The growth rate of brain and nerve cells is at its most rapid pace up to about 4 years of age.

Brain

The nervous tissue of the **brain** consists of millions of nerve cells and fibers. It is the largest mass of nervous tissue in the body, weighing about 1380 g in the male and 1250 g in the female. The brain is enclosed by three membranes known collectively as the **meninges** (Figure 14.3 ■). From the outside in, these are the *dura mater, arachnoid,* and *pia mater.* The major structures of the brain are the *cerebrum, cerebellum, diencephalon,* and the *brainstem,* which is composed of the *midbrain, pons,* and *medulla oblongata.* See Figure 14.4 ■

LIFE SPAN CONSIDERATIONS

A baby's **brain** has three main structural parts: the **cerebrum**, the **cerebellum**, and the **brainstem.** The cerebrum serves as a control center as it receives, processes, and acts on information. The cerebellum helps coordinate muscle activities and maintains posture and balance. The brainstem maintains vital body functions, such as heartbeat, blood pressure, digestion, and swallowing. While the brain of an infant resembles that of an adult, one area is relatively unrefined. In an infant, the right and left hemispheres of the brain have yet to develop their own specific tasks. However, by the time a child is 3 years old, the two sides of the brain are well on their way to becoming specialized for different tasks.

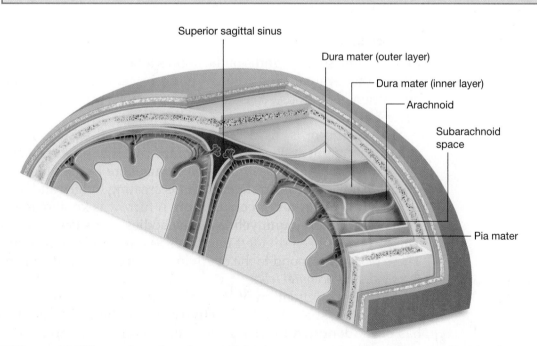

Superior sagittal sinus

Dura mater (outer layer)

Dura mater (inner layer)

Arachnoid

Subarachnoid space

Pia mater

■ **Figure 14.3** The meninges from the outside in: dura mater, arachnoid, and pia mater. Also showing the subarachnoid space and superior sagittal sinus.

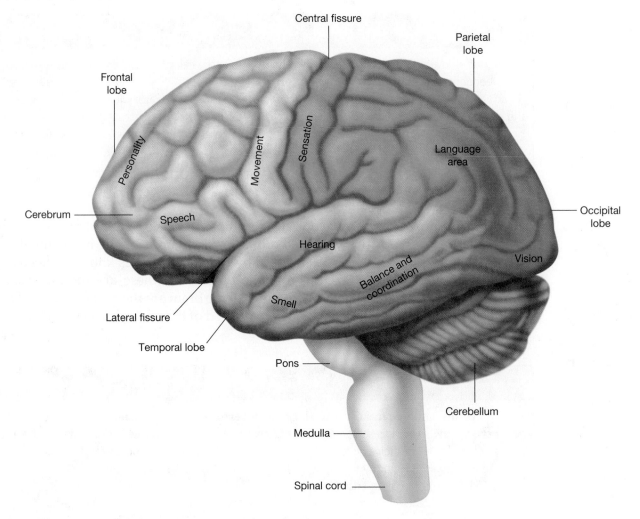

■ **Figure 14.4** Major structures of the brain.

Cerebrum

Representing seven-eighths of the brain's total weight, the **cerebrum** contains nerve centers that evaluate and control all sensory and motor activity, including sensory perception, emotions, consciousness, memory, and voluntary movements. See Table 14.2 ■

The cerebrum is divided by the longitudinal fissure into two cerebral hemispheres, the right and left, that are joined by large fiber tracts (*corpus callosum*) that allow information to pass from one hemisphere to the other. The surface or *cortex* of each hemisphere is arranged in folds creating bulges and shallow furrows. Each bulge is called a **gyrus** or **convolution**. A furrow is known as a **sulcus**. This surface is composed of gray, unmyelinated cell bodies and is known as the **cerebral cortex**. The cortex has been divided into lobes as a means of identifying certain locations. These lobes correspond to the overlying bones of the skull and are the *frontal, parietal, temporal*, and *occipital lobes.*

Electrical stimulation of the various areas of the cortex during neurosurgery has identified specialized cell activity within the different lobes. The **frontal lobe** has been identified as the brain's major motor area and the site for personality and speech. The **parietal lobe** contains centers for sensory input from all parts of the body and is known as the *somesthetic area* and the site for the interpretation

TABLE 14.2 Major Divisions of the Brain and Their Functions

Brain Area	Functions
Cerebrum	Evaluates and controls all sensory and motor activity; sensory perception, emotions, consciousness, memory, and voluntary movements
Cerebellum	Plays an important role in the integration of sensory perception and motor output. Its neural pathways link with the motor cortex, which sends information to the muscles causing them to move, and the spinocerebellar tract, which provides feedback on the position of the body in space (proprioception). The cerebellum integrates these pathways using the constant feedback on body position to fine-tune motor movements. Research shows that the cerebellum also has a broader role in a number of key cognitive functions, including attention and the processing of language, music, and other sensory temporal stimuli.
Diencephalon	
Thalamus	Relay center for all sensory impulses (except olfactory) being transmitted to the sensory areas of the cortex, and relays motor impulses from the cerebellum and the basal ganglia to motor areas of the cortex, thought to be involved with emotions and arousal mechanisms
Hypothalamus	Serves as the principal regulator of autonomic nervous activity that is associated with behavior and expression; also contains hormones that are important for the control of certain metabolic activities such as maintenance of water balance, sugar and fat metabolism, regulation of body temperature, sleep-cycle control, appetite, and sexual arousal.
Brainstem	
Midbrain	Two-way conduction pathway that acts as a relay center for visual and auditory impulses; found in the midbrain are four small masses of gray cells known collectively as the *corpora quadrigemina*. The upper two, called the *superior colliculi*, are associated with visual reflexes. The lower two, or *inferior colliculi*, are involved with the sense of hearing.
Pons	Links the cerebellum and medulla to higher cortical areas; plays a role in somatic and visceral motor control; contains important centers for regulating breathing.
Medulla oblongata	Acts as the cardiac, respiratory, and vasomotor control center; regulates and controls breathing, swallowing, coughing, sneezing, and vomiting as well as heartbeat and arterial blood pressure, thereby exerting control over the circulation of blood

of language. Temperature, pressure, touch, and an awareness of muscle control are some of the sensory activities localized in this area. The **temporal lobe** contains centers for hearing, smell, and language input, and the **occipital lobe** is the primary interpretive processing area for vision. The occipital lobe is directly posterior to the temporal lobe.

Cerebellum

The **cerebellum** is the second largest part of the brain. It occupies a space in the back of the skull, inferior to the cerebrum and dorsal to the pons and medulla oblongata. The cerebellum is oval in shape and divided into lobes by deep fissures. It has a cortex of gray cell bodies, and its interior contains nerve fibers and white matter connecting it to every part of the central nervous system. The cerebellum plays an important part in the coordination of voluntary and involuntary complex patterns of movement and adjusts muscles to maintain posture. See Table 14.2.

Diencephalon

The word **diencephalon** means *second portion of the brain* and refers to the thalamus and hypothalamus.

Thalamus. The **thalamus** is the larger of the two divisions of the diencephalon and is actually two large masses of gray cell bodies joined by a third or intermediate mass. The thalamus serves as a relay center for all sensory impulses (except olfactory) being transmitted to the sensory areas of the cortex. Besides its sensory function, the thalamus also relays motor impulses from the cerebellum and the basal ganglia to motor areas of the cortex. Some impulses related to emotional behavior are also passed from the hypothalamus, through the thalamus, to the cerebral cortex. See Table 14.2.

Hypothalamus. The **hypothalamus** lies beneath the thalamus and is a principal regulator of autonomic nervous activity that is associated with behavior and emotional expression. It also produces neurosecretions for the control of water balance, sugar and fat metabolism, regulation of body temperature, and other metabolic activities. See Table 14.2. The pituitary gland is attached to the hypothalamus by a narrow stalk, the *infundibulum*.

Brainstem

The **brainstem** is the lower part of the brain, adjoining and structurally continuous with the spinal cord. The brainstem provides the main motor and sensory innervation to the face and neck via the cranial nerves. It consists of three structures: the mesencephalon or *midbrain*, the pons, and the medulla oblongata. The brainstem processes visual, auditory, and sensory information and plays an important role in the regulation of cardiac and respiratory function. It also regulates the central nervous system and is pivotal in maintaining consciousness and regulating the sleep cycle.

Midbrain. The **midbrain** is located below the cerebrum and above the pons. The midbrain has four small masses of gray cells known collectively as the **corpora quadrigemina**. The upper two of these masses, called the **superior colliculi**, are associated with visual reflexes such as the tracking movements of the eyes. The lower two, or **inferior colliculi**, are involved with the sense of hearing. See Table 14.2.

Pons. The **pons** is a broad band of white matter located anterior to the cerebellum and between the midbrain and the medulla oblongata. The pons is composed of fiber tracts linking the cerebellum and medulla to higher cortical areas. It also plays a role in somatic and visceral motor control, and contains important centers for regulating breathing. See Table 14.2.

Medulla Oblongata. The **medulla oblongata** connects the pons and the rest of the brain to the spinal cord. All afferent and efferent tracts from the spinal cord either pass through or terminate in the medulla oblongata. It contains nerve centers for regulation and control of breathing, swallowing, coughing, sneezing, vomiting, the heartbeat, and blood pressure. See Table 14.2.

Spinal Cord

The **spinal cord** has an H-shaped gray area of cell bodies encircled by an outer region of white matter. The white matter consists of nerve tracts and fibers providing sensory input to the brain and conducting motor impulses from the brain to spinal neurons. The adult spinal cord is about 44 centimeters (cm) long and extends down the vertebral canal from the medulla to terminate near the junction of the first (L_1) and second (L_2) lumbar vertebrae (Figure 14.5 ■). Between the 12th thoracic (T_{12})

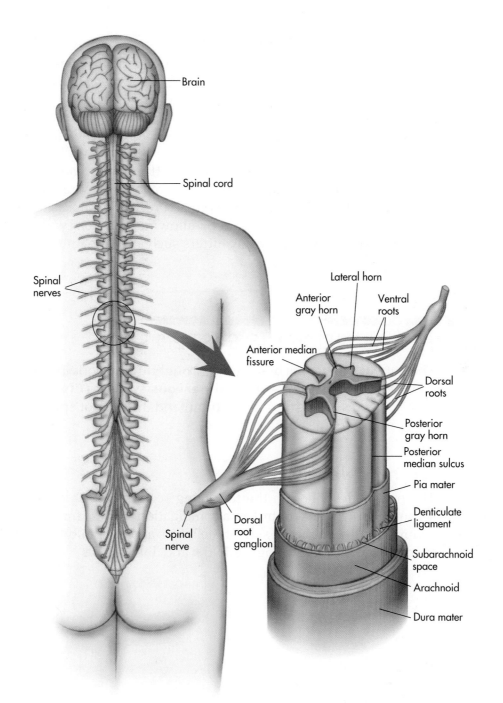

■ **Figure 14.5** Brain, spinal cord, and spinal nerves with an expanded view of a spinal nerve.

and L_1 is a region known as the **conus medullaris**, where the spinal cord becomes conically tapered. The **filum terminale** or terminal thread of fibrous tissue extends from the conus medullaris to the second sacral vertebra. The **cauda equina** (known as the horse's tail) is the terminal portion of the spinal cord that forms the nerve fibers that are the lumbar, sacral, and coccygeal spinal nerves. The functions of the spinal cord are to conduct sensory impulses to the brain, to conduct motor impulses from the brain, and to serve as a reflex center for impulses entering and leaving the spinal cord without direct involvement of the brain.

Cerebrospinal Fluid

The brain and spinal cord are surrounded by **cerebrospinal fluid (CSF)**. This colorless fluid is produced as a filtrate of blood by the *choroid plexuses* within the *ventricles* of the brain. Cerebrospinal fluid circulates through the ventricles, the central canal, and the subarachnoid space. Cerebrospinal fluid is removed from circulation by the **arachnoid villi**, which are small projections of the arachnoid membrane that penetrate the tough outer membrane, the dura mater. The arachnoid villi allow the fluid to drain into the superior sagittal sinus. The normal adult will have between 120 and 150 milliliters (mL) of cerebrospinal fluid in circulation. The fluid serves to cushion the brain and spinal cord from shocks that could cause injury. It also helps to support the brain by allowing it to float within the supporting liquid. It also contains neurotransmitters such as monoamines, acetylcholine (ACh), and neuropeptides.

PERIPHERAL NERVOUS SYSTEM

The network of nerves branching throughout the body from the brain and spinal cord is known as the **peripheral nervous system (PNS)**. There are 12 pairs of cranial nerves that attach to the brain and 31 pairs of spinal nerves connected to the spinal cord.

Cranial Nerves

The nerves described in the following sections attach to the brain and provide sensory input, motor control, or a combination of these functions. They are arranged symmetrically, 12 to each side of the brain, and generally are named for the area or function they serve. See Figure 14.6 ■ and Table 14.3 ■.

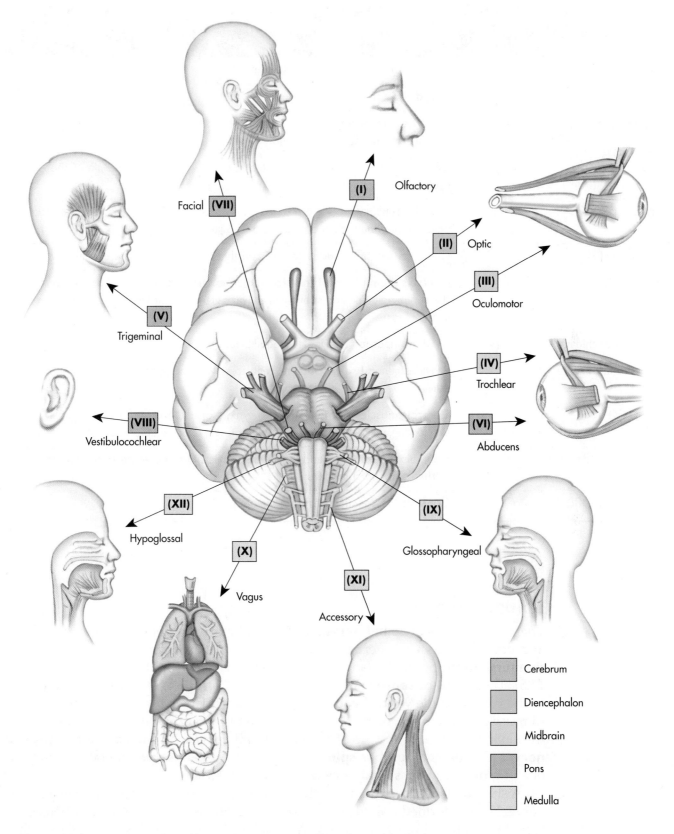

Olfactory
Facial **(VII)**
(I)
(II) Optic
(III) Oculomotor
(V) Trigeminal
(IV) Trochlear
(VIII) Vestibulocochlear
(VI) Abducens
(XII) Hypoglossal
(X) Vagus
(XI) Accessory
(IX) Glossopharyngeal

Cerebrum
Diencephalon
Midbrain
Pons
Medulla

■ **Figure 14.6** Relationship of the 12 cranial nerves to specific regions of the brain.

TABLE 14.3 Cranial Nerves and Functions

Nerve/Number	Function
Olfactory (I)	Detects and provides the sense of smell
Optic (II)	Provides vision
Oculomotor (III)	Conducts motor impulses to four of the six external muscles of the eye and to the muscle that raises the eyelid
Trochlear (IV)	Conducts motor impulses to control the superior oblique muscle of the eyeball
Trigeminal (V)	Provides sensory input from the face, nose, mouth, forehead, and top of the head; motor fibers to the muscles of the jaw (chewing)
Abducens (VI)	Conducts motor impulses to the lateral rectus muscle of the eyeball
Facial (VII)	Controls the muscles of the face and scalp; the lacrimal glands of the eye and the submandibular and sublingual salivary glands; input from the tongue for the sense of taste
Vestibulocochlear (Acoustic) (VIII)	Provides input for hearing and equilibrium
Glossopharyngeal (IX)	Provides general sense of taste; regulates swallowing; controls secretion of saliva
Vagus (X)	Controls muscles of the pharynx, larynx, thoracic, and abdominal organs; swallowing, voice production, slowing of heartbeat, acceleration of peristalsis
Accessory (XI)	Controls the trapezius and sternocleidomastoid muscles, permitting movement of the head and shoulders
Hypoglossal (XII)	Controls the tongue; tongue movements

Spinal Nerves

There are 31 pairs of **spinal nerves** distributed along the length of the spinal cord and emerging from the vertebral canal on either side through the intervertebral foramina. At the point of attachment, each nerve is divided into *two roots* (see Figure 14.5). The **dorsal** or **sensory root** is composed of afferent fibers carrying impulses to the cord, and the **ventral root** contains motor fibers carrying efferent impulses to muscles and organs. Named for the region of the vertebral column from which they exit, there are eight pairs of **cervical spinal nerves**, 12 pairs of **thoracic spinal nerves**, five pairs of **lumbar spinal nerves**, five pairs of **sacral spinal nerves**, and one pair of **coccygeal spinal nerves**. See Figure 14.7 ■

A short distance from the cord, the fibers of the two roots unite to form a spinal nerve. Having formed a single nerve composed of afferent and efferent fibers, each spinal nerve then branches into several smaller nerves. The two primary branches from each spinal nerve are the **dorsal rami** and **ventral rami**. The dorsal rami (*branches*) carry motor and sensory fibers to the muscles and skin of the back and serve an area from the back of the head to the coccyx. The ventral rami, serving a much larger area, carry both motor and sensory fibers to the muscles and organs of the body, including the arms, legs, hands, and feet.

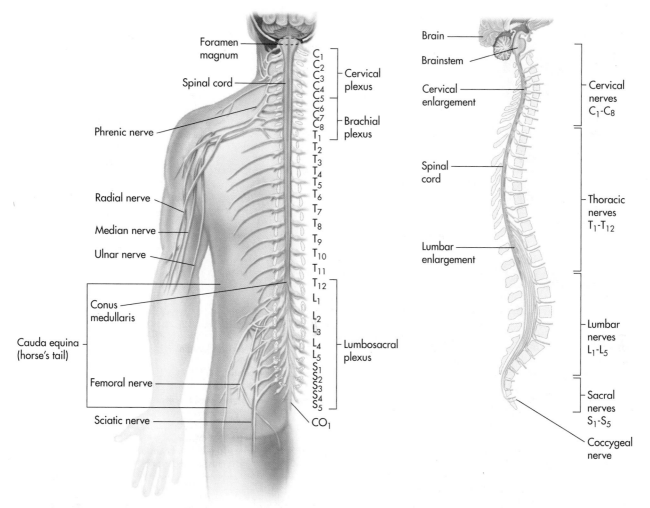

Foramen magnum
Spinal cord
Phrenic nerve
Radial nerve
Median nerve
Ulnar nerve
Conus medullaris
Cauda equina (horse's tail)
Femoral nerve
Sciatic nerve

C1
C2
C3
C4
C5
C6
C7
C8
T1
T2
T3
T4
T5
T6
T7
T8
T9
T10
T11
T12
L1
L2
L3
L4
L5
S1
S2
S3
S4
S5
CO1

Cervical plexus
Brachial plexus
Lumbosacral plexus

Brain
Brainstem
Cervical enlargement
Spinal cord
Lumbar enlargement

Cervical nerves C1-C8
Thoracic nerves T1-T12
Lumbar nerves L1-L5
Sacral nerves S1-S5
Coccygeal nerve

■ **Figure 14.7** The 31 pairs of spinal nerves.

AUTONOMIC NERVOUS SYSTEM

Actually a part of the peripheral nervous system, the **autonomic nervous system (ANS)** controls involuntary bodily functions such as sweating, secretions of glands, arterial blood pressure, smooth muscle tissue, and the heart. The autonomic nervous system is primarily composed of efferent fibers from certain cranial and spinal nerves and can be functionally divided into two divisions, the **sympathetic** and **para-sympathetic**. These two divisions counteract each other's activity to keep the body in a state of homeostasis. See Figure 14.8 ■

Sympathetic Division

Branches from the ventral roots of the 12 thoracic and the first three lumbar spinal nerves form the first part of the **sympathetic division**. The cell bodies of these nerve fibers are located in the *gray matter* of the spinal cord. Just outside the spinal cord, axons of these nerve cells leave the spinal nerves and enter almost immediately into masses of nerve cell bodies, the **sympathetic ganglia**, which form a chain that runs next to the vertebral column. This chain of about 23 ganglia runs from the base of the head to the coccyx and is known as the **sympathetic trunk**. Within the ganglia

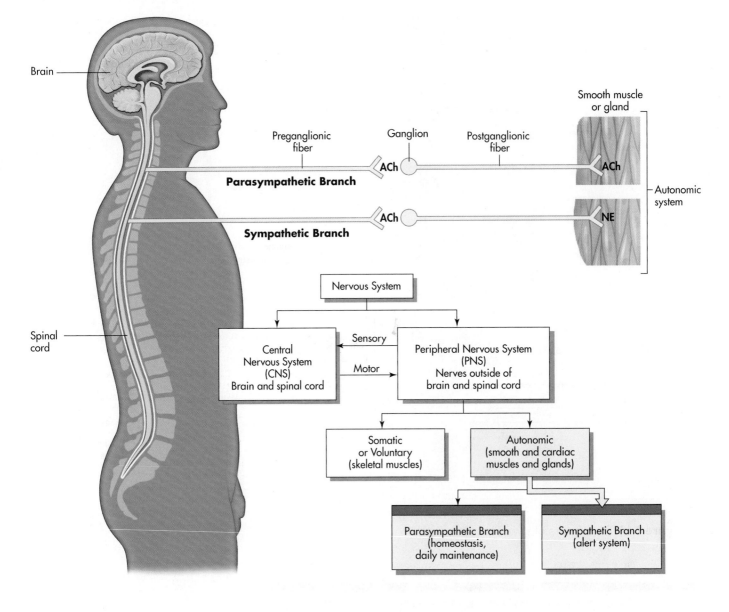

■ **Figure 14.8** General representation of the autonomic nervous system.

of the sympathetic trunk, fibers from the spinal nerves synapse with ganglionic nerve cell bodies. These ganglionic neurons produce long axons that reach to the parts of the body to be innervated. This arrangement, characteristic of autonomic nerves, creates a two-neuron chain as opposed to single-neuron control of regular motor nerves.

Because of the arrangement in which *sympathetic fibers* from spinal nerves synapse with many cell bodies in the sympathetic ganglia, they tend to produce widespread innervation when activated. This condition has been described as preparing the individual for *fight or flight.* During the *fight-or-flight response,* a person experiences increased alertness, increased metabolic rate, decreased digestive and urinary function, an increase in respiration, blood pressure, and heart rate, and a corresponding warming of the body that can activate the sweat glands. The sympathetic system stimulates the adrenal gland to release epinephrine (adrenaline), the hormone that causes the familiar adrenaline rush.

Parasympathetic Division

Very long fibers branching from cranial nerves III, VII, IX, and X, along with long fibers of sacral nerves II, III, and IV, form the first stage of the **parasympathetic division**. Cell bodies for these long fibers are located in the brain and spinal cord. These long fibers extend to ganglia located near the organs to be innervated.

The parasympathetic division works to conserve energy and innervate the digestive system. When activated, it stimulates the salivary and digestive glands, decreases the metabolic rate, slows the heart rate, reduces blood pressure, and promotes the passage of material through the intestines along with absorption of nutrients by the blood.

Anatomy and Physiology Labeling

Identify the structures shown below by filling in the blanks.

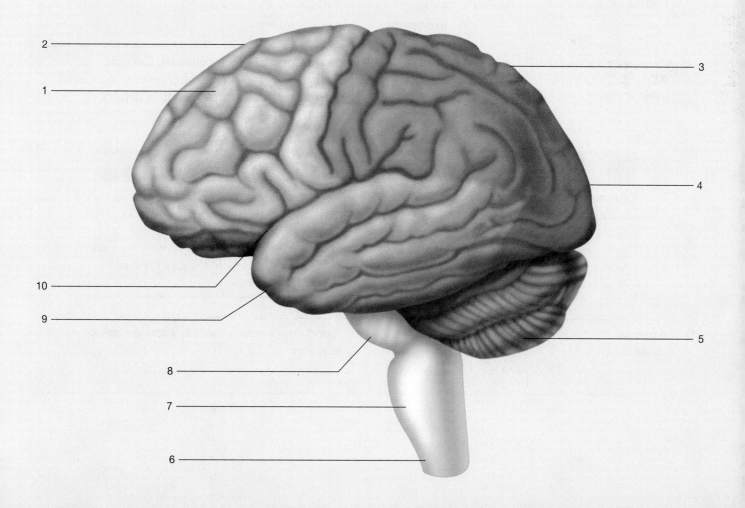

• Building Your Medical Vocabulary •

This section provides the foundation for learning medical terminology. Review the following alphabetized word list. Note how common prefixes and suffixes are repeatedly applied to word roots and combining forms to create different meanings. The word parts are color-coded: prefixes are green, suffixes are blue, roots/combining forms are red.

   You will find that some terms have not been divided into word parts. These are common words or specialized terms that are included to enhance your medical vocabulary. See Chapter 1, page 7, to review pronunciation guidelines.

MEDICAL WORD	WORD PARTS		DEFINITION
	Part	**Meaning**	
acetylcholine (ACh) (ăs″ ĕ-tĭl-kō′ lēn)			Cholinergic neurotransmitter; plays an important role in the transmission of nerve impulses at synapses and myoneural junctions
akathesia (ăk″ ă-thĕ′ zĭă)			Inability to remain still; motor restlessness and anxiety
akinesia (ă″ kĭ-nē′ zĭ-ă)	a- -kinesia	lack of motion, movement	Loss or lack of voluntary motion
Alzheimer's disease (AD) (ahlts′ hĭ-merz)			Severe form of senile dementia. Cortical destruction causes variable degrees of confusion, memory loss, and other cognitive defects.

LIFE SPAN CONSIDERATIONS

Alzheimer's disease (AD) affects a person's ability to carry out activities of daily living (ADL). It is the most common cause of dementia among people age 65 or older. AD involves the parts of the brain that control thought, memory, and language. It usually begins after age 60, and risk goes up with age. It is important to note, however, that AD is not a normal part of aging. Symptoms of Alzhemier's can be described as the 4 A's: anger, aggression, anxiety, and apathy. Eventually, patients need total care.

MEDICAL WORD	WORD PARTS		DEFINITION
amnesia (ăm-nē′ zĭ-ă)	a- mnes -ia	lack of memory condition	Condition in which there is a loss or lack of memory

MEDICAL WORD	WORD PARTS		DEFINITION
	Part	**Meaning**	
amyotrophic lateral sclerosis (ALS) (ă-mī″ ō-trŏf′ ĭk lăt′ ĕr-ăl sklĕ-rō′ sĭs)	a- my/o -troph (y) -ic later -al scler -osis	lack of muscle nourishment pertaining to side pertaining to hardening condition	Muscular weakness, atrophy, with spasticity caused by degeneration of motor neurons of the spinal cord, medulla, and cortex; also called *Lou Gehrig's disease*
analgesia (ăn″ ăl-jē′ zĭ-ă)	an- -algesia	lack of condition of pain	Condition in which there is a lack of the sensation of pain
anencephaly (ăn″ ĕn-sĕf′ ăl-ē)	an- encephal -y	lack of brain condition	Congenital condition in which there is a lack of development of the brain
anesthesia (ăn″ ĕs-thē′ zĭ-ă)	an- -esthesia	lack of feeling	Literally means *loss or lack of the sense of feeling*; a pharmacologically induced reversible state of amnesia, analgesia, loss of responsiveness, loss of skeletal muscle reflexes, and decreased stress response
anesthesiologist (ăn″ ĕs-thē″ zĭ-ŏl′ ō-jĭst)	an- esthesi/o log -ist	lack of feeling study of one who specializes	Physician who specializes in the science of anesthesia
aphagia (ă-fā′ jĭ-ă)	a- -phagia	lack of to eat, swallow	Loss or lack of the ability to eat or swallow
aphasia (ă-fā′ zĭ-ă)	a- -phasia	lack of to speak, speech	Literally means *a lack of the ability to speak*. It is a language disorder in which there is an impairment of producing or comprehending spoken or written language due to brain damage. It can be caused by a stroke, traumatic brain injury, or other brain injury, or it may develop slowly, as in the case of a brain tumor or progressive neurological disease, such as in Alzheimer's or Parkinson's diseases.
apraxia (ă-prăks′ ĭ-ă)	a- -praxia	lack of action	Loss or lack of the ability to use objects properly and to recognize common ones; inability to perform motor tasks or activities of daily living, such as dressing and bathing
asthenia (ăs-thē′ nĭ-ă)	a- -sthenia	lack of strength	Loss or lack of strength

MEDICAL WORD	WORD PARTS		DEFINITION
	Part	**Meaning**	
astrocytoma (ăs″ trō-sī-tō′ mă)	astro- cyt -oma	star-shaped cell tumor	A primary tumor of the brain composed of astrocytes (star-shaped neuroglial cells) characterized by slow growth, cyst formation, metastasis, and malignant glioblastoma within the tumor mass. Surgical intervention is possible in the early developmental stage of the tumor; also called *astrocytic glioma.*
ataxia (ă-tăks′ ĭ-ă)	a- -taxia	lack of order, coordination	Literally means *loss or lack of order;* neurological sign and symptom consisting of lack of coordination of muscle movements. It implies dysfunction of parts of the nervous system that coordinate movement, such as the cerebellum.
bradykinesia (brăd″ ĭ-kĭ-nē′ sĭ-ă)	brady- -kinesia	slow motion, movement	Abnormal slowness of motion
cephalalgia (sĕf″ ă-lăl′ jĭ-ă)	cephal -algia	head pain	Head pain; *headache*
cerebellar (sĕr″ ĕ-bĕl′ ăr)	cerebell -ar	little brain pertaining to	Pertaining to the cerebellum
cerebral palsy (CP) (sĕr″ ĕ-br′ăl pawl′ zē)			Disorder of movement and posture caused by damage to the motor control centers of the developing brain and can occur during pregnancy (about 75%), during childbirth (about 5%), or after birth (about 15%) up to about age 3. Most common permanent disorder of childhood involving four motor dysfunctions: spastic, dyskinetic, ataxic, and mixed. See Figure 14.9 ■

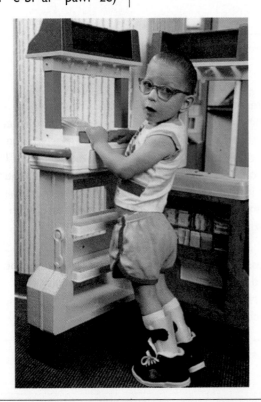

■ **Figure 14.9** Child with cerebral palsy has abnormal muscle tone and lack of physical coordination.

MEDICAL WORD	WORD PARTS		DEFINITION
	Part	Meaning	
cerebrospinal (sĕr″ ĕ-brō-spī´ năl)	cerebr/o spin -al	cerebrum a thorn, spine pertaining to	Pertaining to the cerebrum and the spinal cord
chorea (kō-rē´ ă)			Abnormal involuntary movement disorder, one of a group of neurological disorders called *dyskinesias*; characterized by episodes of rapid, jerky involuntary muscular twitching of the limbs or facial muscles
coma (kō´ ma)			Unconscious state or stupor from which the patient cannot be aroused
concussion (brain) (kōn-kŭsh´ ŭn)	concuss -ion	shaken violently process	Head injury with a transient loss of brain function; may also be called *mild brain injury, mild traumatic brain injury (MTBI), mild head injury (MHI),* and *minor head trauma*
craniectomy (krā″ nĭ-ĕk´ tō-mē)	cran/i -ectomy	skull surgical excision	Surgical excision of a portion of the skull
craniotomy (krā″ nĭ-ŏt´ ō-mē)	crani/o -tomy	skull incision	Literally means *surgical incision into the skull.* It is a surgical operation in which a bone flap is removed from the skull to access the brain. Used to repair defects associated with traumatic head injuries or to repair a cerebral aneurysm. See Figure 14.10 ■

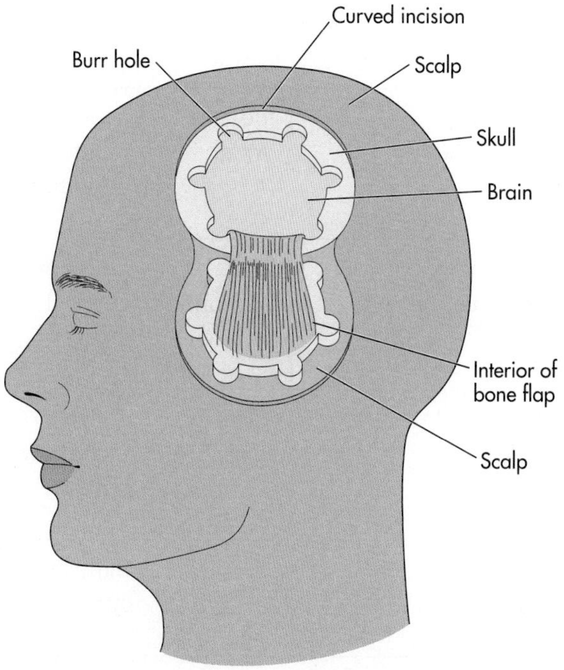

■ **Figure 14.10** In a craniotomy, a portion of the skull and overlying scalp is pulled back to allow access to the brain.

MEDICAL WORD	WORD PARTS		DEFINITION
	Part	Meaning	
deep brain stimulation (DBS)			A surgical procedure used to treat a variety of disabling neurological symptoms—most commonly the debilitating symptoms of Parkinson's disease (PD), such as tremor, rigidity, stiffness, slowed movement, and walking problems; it is also used to treat essential tremor, a common neurological movement disorder. DBS employs a surgically implanted, battery-operated medical device called a *neurostimulator*—similar to a heart pacemaker and approximately the size of a stopwatch—to deliver electrical stimulation to targeted areas in the brain that control movement, blocking the abnormal nerve signals that cause neurological problems. At present, DBS is used only for patients whose symptoms cannot be adequately controlled with medications.

fyi Before the deep brain stimulation (DBS) procedure, a neurosurgeon uses magnetic resonance imaging (MRI), computed tomography (CT) scanning, or microelectrode recording to identify and locate the exact target(s) within the brain (generally, the thalamus, subthalamic nucleus, and globus pallidus) where electrical nerve signals generate the PD or other neurological symptoms. There are three components:

1. The lead (also called an *electrode*)—a thin, insulated wire—is inserted through a small opening in the skull and implanted in the brain. The tip of the electrode is positioned within the targeted brain area.
2. An insulated wire (the *extension*) is passed under the skin of the head, neck, and shoulder, connecting the lead to the neurostimulator.
3. The neurostimulator (the *battery pack*) is usually implanted under the skin near the collarbone, or in some cases, lower in the chest or under the skin over the abdomen.

Once the system is in place, electrical impulses are sent from the neurostimulator up along the extension and the lead and into the brain. These impulses interfere with and block the electrical signals that cause PD symptoms and tremors.

MEDICAL WORD	Part	Meaning	DEFINITION
dementia (dē-měn´ shē-ă)	de- ment -ia	down mind condition	Group of symptoms marked by memory loss and other cognitive functions such as perception, thinking, reasoning, and remembering
diskectomy (dĭs-kěk´ tō-mē)	disk -ectomy	a disk surgical excision	Surgical excision of an intervertebral disk
dyslexia (dĭs-lěks´ ĭ-ă)	dys- -lexia	difficult diction, word, phrase	Condition in which an individual has difficulty in reading and comprehending written language
dysphasia (dĭs-fā´ zĭ-ă)	dys- -phasia	difficult speak, speech	Impairment of speech that may be caused by a brain lesion

MEDICAL WORD	WORD PARTS		DEFINITION
	Part	**Meaning**	
electroencephalo-graph (ē-lĕk″ trō-ĕn-sĕf′ ă-lō-grăf)	electr/o encephal/o -graph	electricity brain instrument for recording	Medical instrument used to record the electrical activity of the brain
electromyography (ē-lĕk″ trō-mī-ŏg′ ră-fē)	electr/o my/o -graphy	electricity muscle recording	Process of recording the contraction of a skeletal muscle as a result of electrical stimulation; used in diagnosing disorders of nerves supplying muscles
encephalitis (ĕn-sĕf′ ă-lī′ tĭs)	encephal -itis	brain inflammation	Inflammation of the brain. There are numerous types of encephalitis, many of which are caused by viral infection. Symptoms include sudden fever, headache, vomiting, photophobia (abnormal visual sensitivity to light), stiff neck and back, confusion, drowsiness, clumsiness, unsteady gait, and irritability.
encephalopathy (ĕn-sĕf′ ă-lōp′ ă-thē)	encephal/o -pathy	brain disease	Any pathological dysfunction of the brain. HIV encephalopathy is called *AIDS-dementia complex*.
endorphins (ĕn-dor′ fĭns)			Chemical substances produced in the brain that act as natural analgesics (*opiates*) and provide feelings of pleasure
epidural (ĕp″ ĭ-dū′ răl)	epi- dur -al	upon dura, hard pertaining to	Literally means *pertaining to situated on the dura mater;* often used to refer to a form of regional anesthesia involving injection of medication via a catheter into the epidural space. This causes both a loss of sensation (anesthesia) and a loss of pain (analgesia), by blocking the transmission of signals through nerves in or near the spinal cord.
epiduroscopy (ep″ ĭ-du-ros′ kō-pē)	epi- dur/o -scopy	upon dura, hard visual examination, to view, examine	Minimally invasive form of surgery that introduces medication via an endoscope into the epidural space; used for back pain relief when all other conservative treatments have failed

MEDICAL WORD	WORD PARTS		DEFINITION
	Part	**Meaning**	
epilepsy (ĕp´ ĭ-lĕp″ sē)	epi- -lepsy	upon seizure	A neurological disorder involving repeated seizures of any type. Seizures are episodes of disturbed brain function that cause changes in attention and/or behavior. The types of seizures experienced by those with epilepsy are classified into four main categories: 1. **Partial seizures** (focal seizures) are those in which electrical disturbances are localized to areas of the brain near the source or focal point of the seizure. 2. **Generalized seizures** (bilateral, symmetrical) are those without local onset that involve both the right and left hemispheres of the brain. 3. **Unilateral seizures** are those in which the electrical discharge is predominantly confined to one of the two hemispheres of the brain. 4. **Unclassified seizures** are those that cannot be placed into one of the other three categories because of incomplete data.

LIFE SPAN CONSIDERATIONS

The majority of epilepsy cases are idiopathic (cause not identified) and symptoms begin during childhood or early adolescence. A child who has a seizure while standing should be gently assisted to the floor and placed in a sidelying position. See Figure 14.11 ■ In adults, epilepsy can occur after severe neurological trauma.

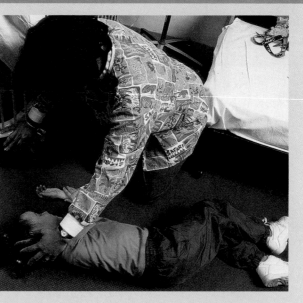

■ **Figure 14.11** A child having a seizure is gently assisted to the floor and placed in a sidelying position.

MEDICAL WORD	WORD PARTS		DEFINITION
ganglionectomy (gang″ lĭ-ō-nĕk´ tō-mē)	ganglion -ectomy	knot surgical excision	Surgical excision of a ganglion (a mass of nerve tissue outside the brain and spinal cord)
glioma (glī-ō´ mă)	gli -oma	glue tumor	Tumor composed of neuroglial tissue

MEDICAL WORD	WORD PARTS		DEFINITION
	Part	**Meaning**	
Guillain-Barré syndrome (gē-yă´ băr-rā)			Pathological condition in which the myelin sheaths covering peripheral nerves are destroyed, resulting in decreased nerve impulses, loss of reflex response, and sudden muscle weakness. Generally an acute viral infection occurs 1–3 weeks before the onset of the syndrome; also called *infectious polyneuritis, acute febrile polyneuritis,* or *acute idiopathic polyneuritis.*
hemiparesis (hĕm˝ ĭ-păr´ ĕ-sĭs)	hemi- -paresis	half weakness	Weakness on one side of the body that can be caused by a stroke, cerebral palsy, brain tumor, multiple sclerosis, and other brain and nervous system diseases
hemiplegia (hĕm˝ ĭ-plē´ jĭ-ă)	hemi- -plegia	half stroke, paralysis	Paralysis of one half of the body when it is divided along the median sagittal plane; total paralysis of the arm, leg, and trunk on the same side of the body. Stroke is the most common cause of this condition. See Figure 14.12B ■

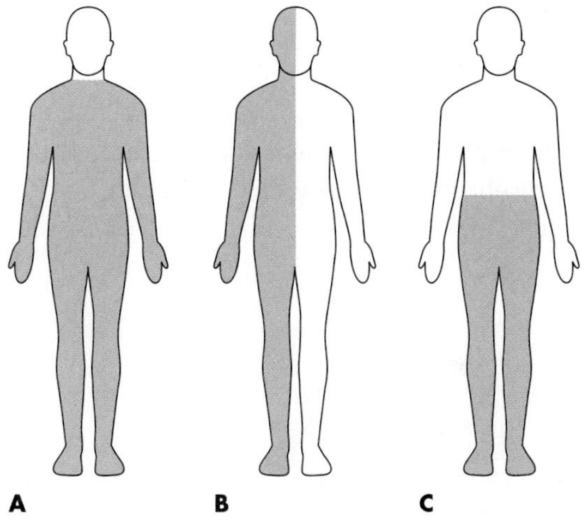

A   **B**   **C**

■ **Figure 14.12** Types of paralysis: (A) Quadriplegia is complete or partial paralysis of the upper extremities and complete paralysis of the lower part of the body. (B) Hemiplegia is paralysis of one half of the body when it is divided along the median sagittal plane. (C) Paraplegia is a paralysis of the lower part of the body.

| **herniated disk syndrome (HDS)** (hĕr-nē-ā´tĕd) | | | Condition in which part or all of the soft, gelatinous central portion of an intervertebral disk (the nucleus pulposus) is forced through a weakened part of the disk. Compression on the nerves can cause *sciatica* or severe lumbar back pain that radiates down one or both legs; also called *herniated intervertebral disk, ruptured disk, herniated nucleus pulposus (HNP),* or *slipped disk.* See Figure 14.13 ■ |

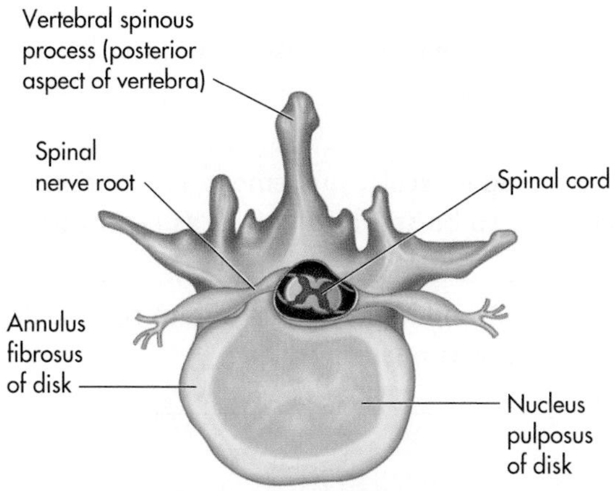

Vertebral spinous process (posterior aspect of vertebra)

Spinal nerve root

Spinal cord

Annulus fibrosus of disk

Nucleus pulposus of disk

■ **Figure 14.13** Herniated intervertebral disk: the herniated nucleus pulposus is applying pressure

MEDICAL WORD	WORD PARTS		DEFINITION
	Part	**Meaning**	
herpes zoster (hĕr' pēz zŏs' tĕr)			Viral disease characterized by painful vesicular eruptions along the segment of the spinal or cranial nerves; also called *shingles*. See Figure 14.14 ■

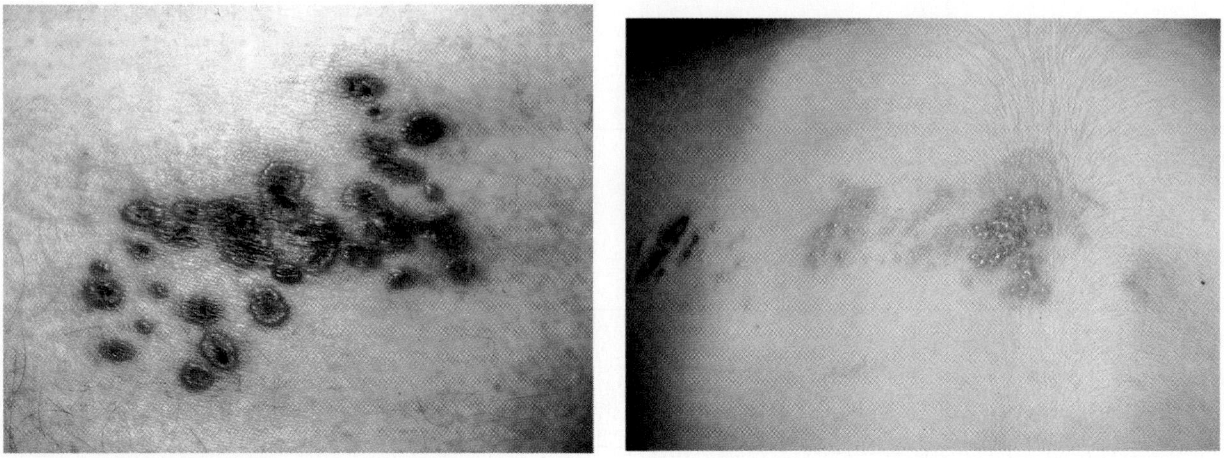

■ **Figure 14.14** Examples of herpes zoster.
(Courtesy of Jason L. Smith, MD)

hydrocephalus (hī″ drō-sĕf′ ă-lŭs)	hydro- cephal -us	water head pertaining to	Condition in which there is an increased amount of cerebrospinal fluid within the brain. See Figure 14.15 ■

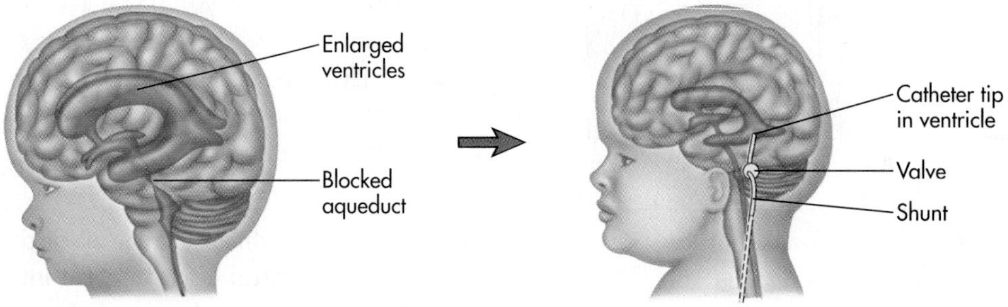

■ **Figure 14.15** Hydrocephalus.

hyperesthesia (hī″ pĕr-ĕs-thē′ zĭ-ă)	hyper- -esthesia	excessive feeling	Increased feelings of sensory stimuli, such as pain, touch, or sound
hyperkinesis (hī″ pĕr-kĭn-ē′ sĭs)	hyper- -kinesis	excessive motion	Increased muscular movement and motion; inability to be still; also known as *hyperactivity*
hypnosis (hĭp-nō′ sĭs)	hypn -osis	sleep condition	Artificially induced trancelike state resembling somnambulism (sleepwalking)

MEDICAL WORD	WORD PARTS		DEFINITION
	Part	**Meaning**	
intracranial (ĭn″ trăh-krā′ nĕ-ăl)	intra- crani -al	within skull pertaining to	Pertaining to within the skull
laminectomy (lăm″ ĭ-nĕk′ tō-mē)	lamin -ectomy	thin plate surgical excision	Surgical excision of a vertebral posterior arch
lobotomy (lō-bŏt′ ō-mē)	lob/o -tomy	lobe incision	Surgical incision into the prefrontal or frontal lobe of the brain
meningioma (mĕn-ĭn″ jĭ-ō′ mă)	mening/i -oma	membrane, meninges tumor	Tumor of the meninges that originates in the arachnoidal tissue
meningitis (mĕn″ ĭn-jĭ′ tĭs)	mening -itis	membrane, meninges inflammation	Inflammation of the meninges of the spinal cord or brain. With early diagnosis and prompt treatment, most patients recover from meningitis. Individuals with bacterial meningitis are usually hospitalized for treatment.

LIFE SPAN CONSIDERATIONS

The child with bacterial meningitis assumes an **opisthotonic** (opisth/o **CF** backward; ton **R** tone/tension; –ic **S** pertaining to) **position**, with the neck and head hyperextended to relieve discomfort. See Figure 14.16 ■

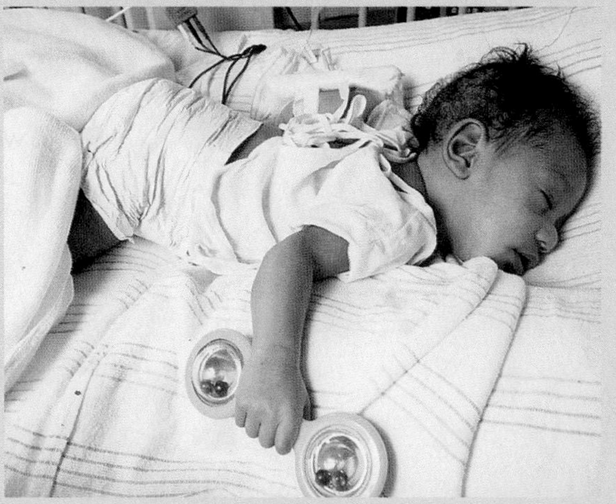

■ **Figure 14.16** Child with bacterial meningitis in an opisthotonic position.

MEDICAL WORD	WORD PARTS		DEFINITION
	Part	**Meaning**	
meningocele (mĕn-ĭn-gō-sēl)	mening/o -cele	membrane, meninges hernia	Congenital hernia (saclike protrusion) in which the meninges protrude through a defect in the skull or spinal column. See Figure 14.17A ■

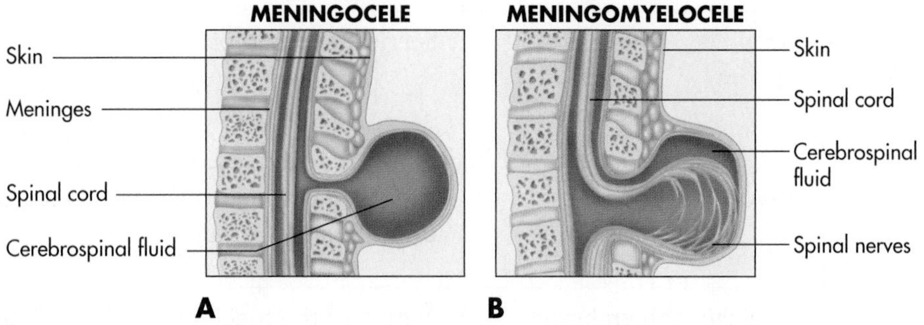

■ **Figure 14.17** Congenital abnormalities of the spine. A. Meningocele. B. Meningomyelocele.

meningomyelocele (mĕn-ĭn″ gō-mī-ĕl′ ō-sēl)	mening/o myel/o -cele	membrane, meninges spinal cord hernia	Congenital herniation of the spinal cord and meninges through a defect in the vertebral column. See Figure 14.17B ■
microcephalus (mī″ krō-sĕf′ ă-lŭs)	micro- cephal -us	small head pertaining to	Abnormally small head; congenital anomaly characterized by an abnormal smallness of the head in relation to the rest of the body
multiple sclerosis (MS) (mŭl′ tĭ-pl sklē′ -rō′ sĭs)	scler -osis	hardening condition	Chronic disease of the central nervous system marked by damage to the myelin sheath. Plaques occur in the brain and spinal cord causing tremor, weakness, incoordination, paresthesia, and disturbances in vision and speech. The multiple effects of MS are shown in Figure 14.18 ■

MEDICAL WORD	WORD PARTS		DEFINITION
	Part	**Meaning**	

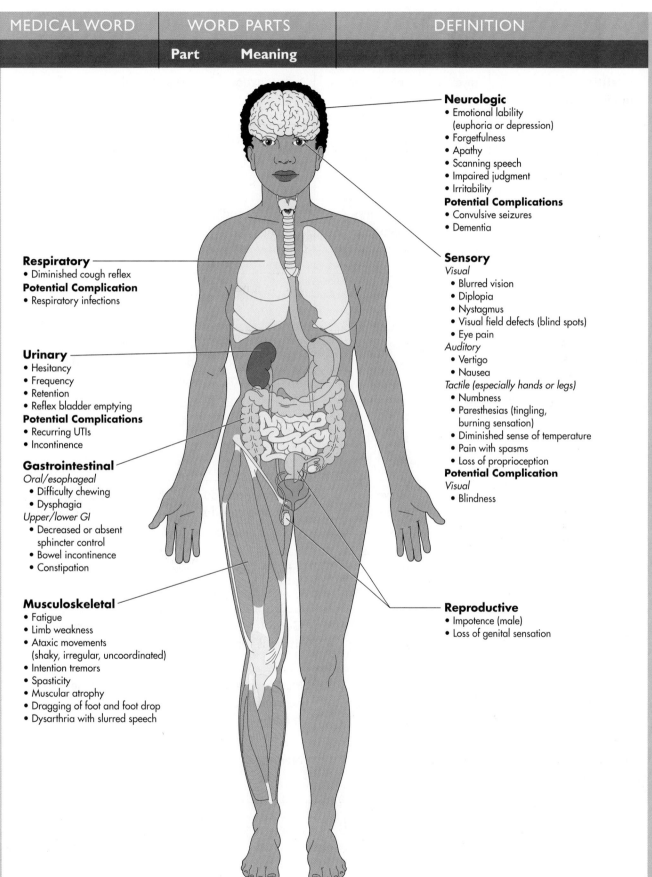

Neurologic
- Emotional lability (euphoria or depression)
- Forgetfulness
- Apathy
- Scanning speech
- Impaired judgment
- Irritability

Potential Complications
- Convulsive seizures
- Dementia

Sensory
Visual
- Blurred vision
- Diplopia
- Nystagmus
- Visual field defects (blind spots)
- Eye pain

Auditory
- Vertigo
- Nausea

Tactile (especially hands or legs)
- Numbness
- Paresthesias (tingling, burning sensation)
- Diminished sense of temperature
- Pain with spasms
- Loss of proprioception

Potential Complication
Visual
- Blindness

Respiratory
- Diminished cough reflex

Potential Complication
- Respiratory infections

Urinary
- Hesitancy
- Frequency
- Retention
- Reflex bladder emptying

Potential Complications
- Recurring UTIs
- Incontinence

Gastrointestinal
Oral/esophageal
- Difficulty chewing
- Dysphagia

Upper/lower GI
- Decreased or absent sphincter control
- Bowel incontinence
- Constipation

Musculoskeletal
- Fatigue
- Limb weakness
- Ataxic movements (shaky, irregular, uncoordinated)
- Intention tremors
- Spasticity
- Muscular atrophy
- Dragging of foot and foot drop
- Dysarthria with slurred speech

Reproductive
- Impotence (male)
- Loss of genital sensation

■ **Figure 14.18** Multisystem effects of multiple sclerosis.

MEDICAL WORD	WORD PARTS		DEFINITION
	Part	Meaning	
myelitis (mī″ ĕ-lī′ tĭs)	myel -itis	spinal cord inflammation	Inflammation of the spinal cord
myelography (mī″ ĕ-lŏg′ ră-fē)	myel/o -graphy	spinal cord recording	X-ray recording of the spinal cord after injection of a radiopaque medium into the spinal canal
narcolepsy (nar′ kō-lĕp″ sē)	narc/o -lepsy	numbness, sleep, stupor seizure	Chronic condition with recurrent attacks of uncontrollable drowsiness and sleep
neuralgia (nū-răl′ jĭ-ă)	neur -algia	nerve pain	Pain in a nerve or nerves
neurasthenia (nū″ răs-thē′ nĭ-ă)	neur -asthenia	nerve weakness	Pathological condition characterized by weakness, exhaustion, and prostration that often accompanies severe depression
neurectomy (nū-rĕk′ tō-mē)	neur -ectomy	nerve surgical excision	Surgical excision of a nerve
neurilemma (nū′ rĭ-lĕm″ mă)	neur/i -lemma	nerve a sheath, husk, rind	Thin membranous sheath that envelops a nerve fiber; also called *sheath of Schwann* or *neurolemma*
neuritis (nū-rī′ tĭs)	neur -itis	nerve inflammation	Inflammation of a nerve
neuroblast (nū′ rō-blăst)	neur/o -blast	nerve germ cell	Germ (embryonic) cell from which nervous tissue is formed
neuroblastoma (nū″ rō-blăs-tō′ mă)	neur/o -blast -oma	nerve germ cell tumor	Malignant tumor composed of cells resembling neuroblasts; occurs mostly in infants and children
neurocyte (nū′ rō-sīt)	neur/o -cyte	nerve cell	Nerve cell, neuron

MEDICAL WORD	WORD PARTS		DEFINITION
	Part	**Meaning**	
neurofibroma (nū″ rō-fǐ-brō′ mǎ)	neur/o fibr -oma	nerve fiber tumor	Fibrous connective tissue tumor of a nerve. See Figure 14.19 ■ ■ **Figure 14.19** Neurofibroma. (Courtesy of Jason L. Smith, MD)
neuroglia (nū-rǒg′ lǐ-ǎ)	neur/o -glia	nerve glue	Supporting or connective tissue cells of the central nervous system (*astrocytes, oligodendroglia, microglia,* and *ependymal cells*)
neurologist (nū-rǒl′ ō-jǐst)	neur/o log -ist	nerve study of one who specializes	Physician who specializes in the study of the nervous system
neurology (Neuro) (nū-rǒl′ ō-jē)	neur/o -logy	nerve study of	The study of the nervous system
neuroma (nū-rō′ mǎ)	neur -oma	nerve tumor	Tumor of nerve cells and nerve fibers
neuropathy (nū-rǒp′ ǎ-thē)	neur/o -pathy	nerve disease	Any pathological nervous tissue disease
neurotransmitter (nū″ rō-trǎns′ mǐt-ěr)			Chemical substances, such as dopamine and acetylcholine, transmitted across a synapse that transmits a signal between two neurons
oligodendroglioma (ǒl″ ǐ-gō-děn″ drō-glǐ-ō′ mǎ)	oligo- dendr/o gli -oma	little tree glue tumor	Malignant tumor derived and composed of oligodendroglia (a type of cell that makes up one component of the tissue of the CNS)
pallidotomy (pǎl″ ǐ-dǒt-ō-mē)	pallid/o -tomy	globus pallidus incision	Surgical destruction of the globus pallidus of the brain done to treat involuntary movements or muscular rigidity in Parkinson's disease

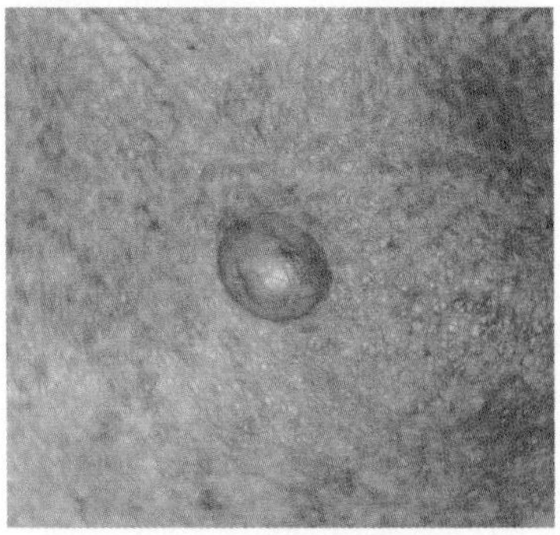

MEDICAL WORD	WORD PARTS		DEFINITION
	Part	**Meaning**	
palsy (pawl´ zē)			Pathological loss of sensation or an impairment of motor function; also called *paralysis*. There are many types of palsy; one example is Bell's palsy, a unilateral paralysis of the facial (VII) nerve. The facial expression is distorted and the patient could be unable to close an eye or control salivation on the affected side.
papilledema (păp˝ ĭl-ĕ-dē´ mă)	papill -edema	papilla swelling	Swelling of the optical disk, usually caused by increased intracranial pressure (ICP); also called *choked disk*
paraplegia (păr˝ ă-plē´ jĭ-ă)	para- -plegia	beside stroke, paralysis	Paralysis of the lower part of the body and of both legs. See Figure 14.12C ■ on page 501.
paresis (păr´ ē-sĭs)			Slight, partial, or incomplete paralysis
paresthesia (păr˝ ĕs-thē´ zĭ-ă)	par- -esthesia	beside feeling	Abnormal sensation, feeling of numbness, prickling, or tingling
Parkinson's disease (păr´ kĭn-sŭnz)			A progressive neurological disorder caused by degeneration of nerve cells in the part of the brain that controls movement. This degeneration creates a shortage of the brain signaling chemical (neurotransmitter) known as *dopamine,* causing the movement impairments that characterize the disease. Often the first symptom of Parkinson's disease is tremor (trembling or shaking) of a limb, especially when the body is at rest. The tremor often begins on one side of the body, frequently in one hand. Other common symptoms include slow movement (*bradykinesia*), an inability to move (*akinesia*), rigid limbs, a shuffling gait, and a stooped posture. Also called *paralysis agitans* or *shaking palsy*. There is no cure for Parkinson's disease. Treatment involves drug therapy to replenish dopamine levels and/or inhibit the effects of the neurotransmitter acetylcholine. Surgical interventions that can be used to stop uncontrollable movements include **pallidotomy** and **deep brain stimulation.**
paroxysm (păr´ ok-sĭzm)			Sudden recurrence of the symptoms of a disease, an exacerbation; also means a *spasm* or *seizure*

MEDICAL WORD	WORD PARTS		DEFINITION
	Part	**Meaning**	
pheochromocytoma (fē-ō-krō″ mō-sĭ-tō′ mă)	phe/o chrom/o cyt -oma	dusky color cell tumor	Chromaffin cell tumor of the adrenal medulla or of the sympathetic nervous system
poliomyelitis (pōl″ ĭ-ō-mī″ ĕl-ī′ tĭs)	poli/o myel -itis	gray spinal cord inflammation	Inflammation of the gray matter of the spinal cord
polyneuritis (pŏl″ ē nū-rī′ tĭs)	poly- neur -itis	many nerve inflammation	Literally means *inflammation involving many nerves*
quadriplegia (kwŏd″ rĭ plē′ jĭ-ă)	quadri- -plegia	four stroke, paralysis	Paralysis of all four extremities and usually the trunk due to injury to the spinal cord in the cervical spine; also called *tetraplegia*. See Figure 14.12A ■ on page 501.
receptor (rē-sĕp′ tōr)			Sensory nerve ending that receives and relays responses to stimuli
Reye's syndrome			Acute disease that causes edema of the brain and increased intracranial pressure, hypoglycemia, and fatty infiltration of the liver and other vital organs; occurs in children and has a relation to aspirin administration; can be viral in origin
sciatica (sī-ăt′ ĭ-kă)			Severe pain along the course of the sciatic nerve
sleep			State of rest for the body and mind; has two distinct types: REM for rapid eye movement, sometimes called *dream sleep,* and NREM for no rapid eye movement
somnambulism (sŏm-năm′ bū-lĭzm)	somn ambul -ism	sleep to walk condition	Condition of sleepwalking
spondylosyndesis (spŏn″ dĭ-lō-sĭn′ dĕ-sĭs)	spondyl/o syn- -desis	vertebra together binding	Surgical procedure to bind vertebra after removal of a herniated disk; also called *spinal fusion*

MEDICAL WORD	WORD PARTS		DEFINITION
	Part	**Meaning**	
stroke			Death of focal brain tissue that occurs when the brain does not get sufficient blood and oxygen; also called *cerebrovascular accident (CVA)* or *brain attack*. If the flow of blood in an artery supplying the brain is interrupted for longer than a few seconds, brain cells can die, causing permanent damage. The interruption can be caused either by bleeding (hemorrhagic stroke) or blood clots in the brain. See Figures 14.20 ■ and 14.21 ■

A *transient ischemic attack (TIA)* is a temporary interference in the blood supply to the brain. It sometimes is referred to as a *ministroke,* and symptoms can last for a few minutes or several hours.

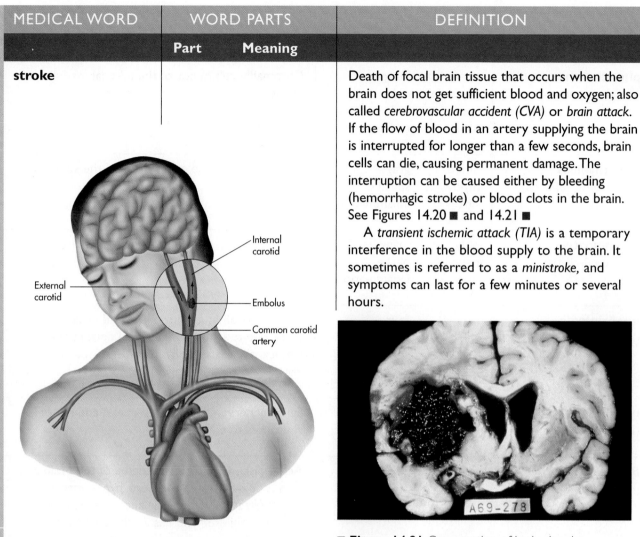

■ **Figure 14.20** Embolus traveling to the brain.

■ **Figure 14.21** Cross-section of brain showing cerebrovascular accident.

LIFE SPAN CONSIDERATIONS

The risk of stroke doubles with each decade after age 35. Stroke occurs in men more often than in women. A very common cause of stroke is atherosclerosis. Fatty deposits and blood platelets collect on the wall of the arteries, forming plaques. Over time, the plaques slowly begin to block the flow of blood. The plaque itself can block the artery enough to cause a stroke.

In some cases, the plaque causes the blood to flow abnormally, which leads to a blood clot. A clot can stay at the site of narrowing and prevent blood flow to all of the smaller arteries it supplies. This type of clot, which does not travel, is called a **thrombus**. In other cases, the clot can travel and wedge into a smaller vessel. A clot that travels is called an **embolism** (see Figure 14.20). Strokes caused by embolisms are commonly associated with cardiovascular pathology, especially heart disorders.

fyi The following sudden symptoms are the warning signs of stroke:
- Numbness or weakness of face, arm, or leg, especially on one side of the body.
- Confusion; trouble speaking or understanding.
- Trouble seeing in one or both eyes.
- Trouble walking, dizziness, loss of balance or coordination.
- Severe headache with no known cause.

MEDICAL WORD	WORD PARTS		DEFINITION
	Part	Meaning	
subdural (sŭb-dū´ răl)	sub- dur -al	below dura, hard pertaining to	Pertaining to below the dura mater
sundowning (sŭn´ dōwnĭng)			Increased agitation or restlessness that occurs in the late afternoon or early evening in patients with cognitive impairment; most common with Alzheimer's-type dementia and Parkinson's disease
sympathectomy (sĭm˝ pă-thĕk´ tō-mē)	sympath -ectomy	sympathy surgical excision	Surgical excision of a portion of the sympathetic nervous system
syncope (sĭn´ kŭ-pē)			Temporary loss of consciousness caused by a lack of blood supply to the brain; also called *fainting*
tactile (tăk´ tĭl)			Pertaining to the sense of touch
Tay–Sachs disease (tā săks´)			Inherited, progressive disease marked by degeneration of brain tissue; predominantly affects Jewish children of Ashkenazi origin
transcutaneous electrical nerve stimulations (TENS) (trăns-kū-tā´ nē-ŭs)			Use of mild electrical stimulation to interfere with the transmission of painful stimuli; has proved useful in relieving pain in some patients
vagotomy (vā-gŏt´ ō-mē)	vag/o -tomy	vagus, wandering incision	Surgical incision of the vagus nerve
ventriculometry (vĕn-trĭk˝ ū-lōm´ ĕtrē)	ventricul/o -metry	ventricle measurement	Measurement of intracranial pressure

• Drug Highlights •

TYPE OF DRUG	DESCRIPTION AND EXAMPLES
analgesics	Inhibit ascending pain pathways in the central nervous system. They increase pain threshold and alter pain perception.
narcotic	EXAMPLES: codeine sulfate, Dilaudid (hydromorphone HCl), Demerol (meperidine HCl), Darvon-N (propoxyphene napsylate), morphine sulfate, and Talwin (pentazocine HCl)
non-narcotic	EXAMPLES: Stadol (butorphanol tartrate) and nalbuphine HCl
analgesics–antipyretics	Act to relieve pain (analgesic effect) and reduce fever (antipyretic effect).
	EXAMPLES: Tylenol (acetaminophen); aspirin; Advil, Motrin, Nuprin (ibuprofen); and Naprosyn, Aleve (naproxen)
sedatives and hypnotics	Depress the central nervous system by interfering with the transmission of nerve impulses. Depending on the dosage, barbiturates, benzodiazepines, and certain other drugs can produce either a sedative or a hypnotic effect. When used as a sedative, the dosage is designed to produce a calming effect without causing sleep. Used as a hypnotic, the dosage is sufficient to cause sleep.
barbiturates	EXAMPLES: pentobarbital and Seconal sodium (secobarbital)
nonbarbiturates	EXAMPLES: chloral hydrate, Dalmane (flurazepam HCl), Restoril (temazepam), and Halcion (triazolam)
antiparkinsonism drugs	Used for palliative relief from such major symptoms as bradykinesia, rigidity, tremor, and disorder of equilibrium and posture. Therapy involves an attempt to replenish dopamine levels and/or inhibit the effects of the neurotransmitter acetylcholine.
	EXAMPLES: Sinemet 25–100 (25 mg of carbidopa and 100 mg of levodopa), Symmetrel (amantadine HCl), levodopa, trihexyphenidyl HCl, Cogentin (benztropine mesylate), Requip (ropinirole), Tasmar (tolcapone), and Stalevo (carbidopa, levodopa, and entacapone)
anticonvulsants	Inhibit the spread of seizure activity in the motor cortex.
	EXAMPLES: Dilantin (phenytoin), Depakene (valproic acid), Tegretol (carbamazepine), Klonopin (clonazepam), and Mysoline (primidone)
cholinesterase inhibitors	Increase the brain's levels of acetylcholine, which helps to restore communication between brain cells. These medications can be used to improve global functioning (including activities of daily living, behavior, and cognition) in some patients with Alzheimer's disease.
	EXAMPLES: Cognex (tacrine), Aricept (donepezil hydrochloride), and Exelon (rivastigmine tartrate)

TYPE OF DRUG	DESCRIPTION AND EXAMPLES
fyi	To date, no treatment can stop Alzheimer's disease (AD). However, for some people in the early and middle stages of the disease, the drugs donepezil (Aricept), rivastigmine (Exelon), galantamine (Razalyne), or memantine (Namenda) can help prevent some symptoms from becoming worse for a limited time. Also, some medicines can help control behavioral symptoms of AD such as sleeplessness, agitation, wandering, anxiety, and depression.

anesthetics	Interfere with the conduction of nerve impulses and are used to produce loss of sensation, loss of pain, muscle relaxation, and/or complete loss of consciousness; block nerve transmission in the area to which they are applied.
local	Block nerve transmission in the area to which they are applied. EXAMPLES: procaine HCl, Xylocaine (lidocaine HCl), and Marcaine (bupivacaine HCl)
general	Affect the central nervous system and produce either partial or complete loss of consciousness. They also produce analgesia, skeletal muscle relaxation, and reduction of reflex activity. EXAMPLES: Suprane (desflurane), isoflurane, Sojurn, Ultane (Sevoflurane)

• Diagnostic and Lab Tests •

TEST	DESCRIPTION
cerebral angiography (sĕr´ ĕ-brăl ăn jī-ŏg´ ră-fē)	Process of making an x-ray record of the cerebral arterial system. A radiopaque substance is injected into an artery of the arm or neck, and x-ray films of the head are taken to visualize cerebral aneurysms, tumors, or ruptured blood vessels.
cerebrospinal fluid (CSF) analysis (sĕr ĕ-brŏ-spī´ năl)	Examination of spinal fluid for color, pressure, pH, and the levels of protein, glucose, and leukocytes. Abnormal results can indicate hemorrhage, tumor, and various disease processes.
computed tomography (CT) (kŏm-pū´ tĕd tō-mŏg˝ ră-fe)	Diagnostic procedure used to study the structure of the brain. Computerized three-dimensional x-ray images allow the radiologist to differentiate among intracranial tumors, cysts, edema, and hemorrhage.
echoencephalography (ĕk ō-ĕn-sĕf´ ă-lŏg´ ră-fē)	Process of using ultrasound to determine the presence of a centrally located mass in the brain.
electroencephalography (EEG) (ē-lĕk-trō-ĕn-sĕf´ ă-lŏg´ ră-fē)	Process of measuring the electrical activity of the brain via an electroencephalograph. Abnormal results can indicate epilepsy, brain tumor, infection, abscess, hemorrhage, and/or coma. Also, brain "death" can be determined by an EEG.

TEST	DESCRIPTION
lumbar puncture (LP) (lŭm´ băr)	Insertion of a needle into the lumbar subarachnoid space for removal of spinal fluid. The fluid is examined for color, pressure, and the level of protein, chloride, glucose, and leukocytes. See Figure 14.22 ■

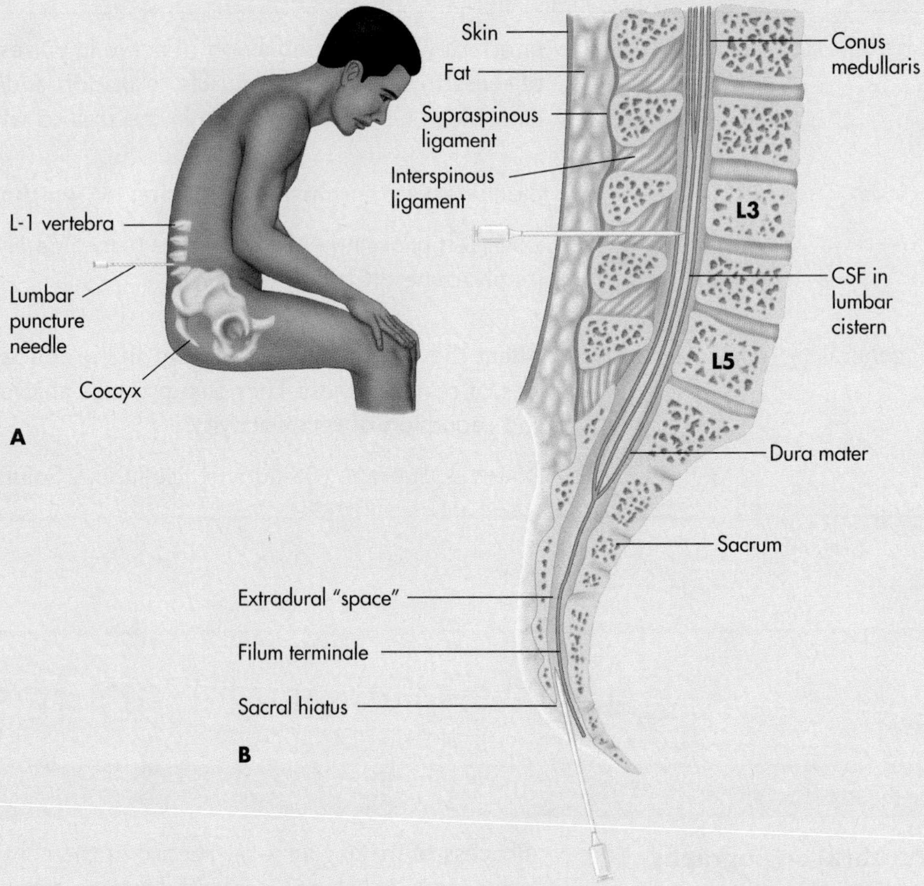

■ **Figure 14.22**
(A) Lumbar puncture, also known as *spinal tap;*
(B) section of the vertebral column showing the spinal cord and membranes with a lumbar puncture needle at L3–4 and in the sacral hiatus.

TEST	DESCRIPTION
myelogram (mī´ ĕ-lō-grăm)	X-ray of the spinal canal after the injection of a radiopaque dye. Useful in diagnosing spinal lesions, cysts, herniated disks, tumors, and nerve root damage.
neurological examination (nū˝ -rō-lōj´ ĭk)	Assessment of a patient's vision; hearing; sense of taste, smell, touch, and pain; position; temperature; gait; and muscle strength, coordination, and reflex action to determine neurological status.
positron emission tomography (PET) (pŏz´ ĭ-trŏn ē-mĭsh´ ŭn tō-mŏg´ ră-fē)	Computer-based nuclear imaging procedure that can produce three-dimensional pictures of actual organ functioning. Useful in locating brain lesion, identifying blood flow and oxygen metabolism in stroke patients, showing metabolic changes in Alzheimer's disease, and studying biochemical changes associated with mental illness.
ultrasonography, brain (ŭl-tră-sŏn-ŏg´ ră-fē)	Use of high-frequency sound waves to record echoes on an oscilloscope and film. Used as a screening test or diagnostic tool.

• Abbreviations •

ABBREVIATION	MEANING	ABBREVIATION	MEANING
ACh	acetylcholine	ICP	intracranial pressure
AD	Alzheimer's disease	LP	lumbar puncture
ADL	activities of daily living	mL	milliliter
ALS	amyotrophic lateral sclerosis	MHT	minor head trauma
ANS	autonomic nervous system	MS	multiple sclerosis
cm	centimeter	MTBI	mild traumatic brain injury
CNS	central nervous system	Neuro	neurology
CP	cerebral palsy	NREM	no rapid eye movement (sleep)
CSF	cerebrospinal fluid	PET	positron emission tomography
CT	computerized tomography	PNS	peripheral nervous system
CVA	cerebrovascular accident	REM	rapid eye movement (sleep)
DBS	deep brain stimulation	TENS	transcutaneous electrical
EEG	electroencephalogram		nerve stimulation
HDS	herniated disk syndrome	TIA	transient ischemic attack
HNP	herniated nucleus pulposus		

and Review • Study and Review • Study and Review
Review • Study and Review • Study and Review • Stu
w • **Study and Review** • Study and Review • Study a

Anatomy and Physiology

Write your answers to the following questions.

1. Name the two interconnected divisions of the nervous system.

a. _____   **b.** _____

2. _____ are the structural and functional units of the nervous system.

3. Describe an *axon.* _____

4. Describe a *dendrite.* _____

5. State an action of sensory neurons. _____

6. Define the following terms:

a. *Nerve fiber* _____

b. *Nerve* _____

c. *Tracts* _____

7. The central nervous system consists of the _____ and the _____

_____.

8. Name the three meninges enclosing the brain.

a. _____   **b.** _____

c. _____

9. Name the seven major divisions of the brain.

a. _____   **b.** _____

c. _____   **d.** _____

e. _____   **f.** _____

g. _____

10. The _____ has been identified as the brain's major motor area.

11. The parietal lobe is also known as the _____ _____

12. The temporal lobe contains centers for _____ and

_____ input.

13. The occipital lobe is the primary area for _____.

14. State the functions of the thalamus.

a. _____   **b.** _____

15. State three functions of the hypothalamus.

a. _____   **b.** _____

c. _____

16. The cerebellum plays an important role in the integration of _____ and

_____.

17. State five functions of the medulla oblongata.

a. _____   **b.** _____

c. _____   **d.** _____

e. _____

18. State the three functions of the spinal cord.

a. _____   **b.** _____

c. _____

19. The normal adult has between _____ and _____

mL of cerebrospinal fluid in circulation.

20. State four functions of the autonomic nervous system.

a. _____   **b.** _____

c. _____   **d.** _____

21. Name the two divisions of the autonomic nervous system.

a. _____   **b.** _____

Word Parts

PREFIXES

Give the definitions of the following prefixes.

1. a- _____
2. an- _____

3. astro- _____
4. brady- _____

5. de- _____
6. dys- _____

7. epi- _____
8. hemi- _____

9. hydro- _____
10. hyper- _____

11. intra- _____
12. micro- _____

13. oligo- _____
14. par- _____

15. para- _____
16. poly- _____

17. quadri- _____
18. sub- _____

ROOTS AND COMBINING FORMS

Give the definitions of the following roots and combining forms.

1. ambul _____
2. dur/o _____

3. cephal _____
4. later _____

5. cerebell _____
6. cerebr/o _____

7. chrom/o _____
8. concuss _____

9. cran/l _____
10. crani/o _____

11. cyt _____
12. dendr/o _____

13. disk _____
14. dur _____

15. electr/o _____
16. encephal _____

17. encephal/o _____
18. esthesi/o _____

19. narc/o _____
20. ganglion _____

21. gli _____
22. hypn _____

23. pallid/o _____
24. lamin _____

25. lob/o _____

26. log _____

27. mening _____

28. mening/i _____

29. mening/o _____

30. ment _____

31. mnes _____

32. myel _____

33. myel/o _____

34. my/o _____

35. neur _____

36. neur/i _____

37. neur/o _____

38. papill _____

39. phe/o _____

40. poli/o _____

41. scler _____

42. spin _____

43. spondyl/o _____

44. somn _____

45. sympath _____

46. vag/o _____

47. ventricul/o _____

SUFFIXES

Give the definitions of the following suffixes.

1. -al _____

2. -algesia _____

3. -algia _____

4. -ar _____

5. -asthenia _____

6. -blast _____

7. -cele _____

8. -cyte _____

9. -desis _____

10. -ectomy _____

11. -edema _____

12. -esthesia _____

13. -glia _____

14. -gram _____

15. -graph _____

16. -graphy _____

17. -ia _____

18. -ic _____

19. -ion _____

20. -ism _____

21. -ist _____

22. -itis _____

23. -kinesia _____

24. -kinesis _____

25. -lepsy _____

26. -lemma _____

27. -lexia _____

29. -troph(y) _____

31. -scopy _____

33. -osis _____

35. -pathy _____

37. -phasia _____

39. -sthenia _____

41. -tomy _____

43. -y _____

28. -logy _____

30. -metry _____

32. -oma _____

34. -paresis _____

36. -phagia _____

38. -praxia _____

40. -taxia _____

42. -us _____

Identifying Medical Terms

In the spaces provided, write the medical terms for the following meanings.

1. _____ Condition in which there is a loss or lack of memory

2. _____ Condition in which there is a lack of the sensation of pain

3. _____ Loss or lack of the ability to eat or swallow

4. _____ Neurological sign and symptom consisting of lack of coordination of muscle movements

5. _____ Head pain; headache

6. _____ Pertaining to the cerebellum

7. _____ Surgical excision of a portion of the skull

8. _____ Condition in which an individual has difficulty in reading and comprehending written language

9. _____ Inflammation of the brain

10. _____ Literally means pertaining to, situated on the dura mater

11. _____ Slight paralysis that affects one side of the body

12. _____ Inflammation of the meninges of the spinal cord or brain

13. _____ Pain in a nerve or nerves

14. _____ Inflammation of a nerve

15. _____ Nerve cell, neuron

16. _____ The study of the nervous system

17. _____ Tumor of nerve cells and nerve fibers

18. _____ Pathological loss of sensation or an impairment of motor function

19. _____ Literally means inflammation involving many nerves

20. _____ Condition of sleepwalking

21. _____ Surgical incision of the vagus nerve

22. _____ Measurement of intracranial pressure

Spelling

Circle the correct spelling of each medical term.

1. anesthesia / anesthsia

2. bradkinesia / bradykinesia

3. cerebrospinal / cerebospinal

4. craniotomy / cranitomy

5. epilepsy / epilepisy

6. meningioma / meningoma

7. meningmyelcele / meningomyelocele

8. neuropathy / neurpathy

9. poliomyelitis / poiliomyelitis

10. ventriulmetry / ventriculometry

Matching

Select the appropriate lettered meaning for each of the following words.

_____ 1. acetylcholine

_____ 2. Alzheimer's disease

_____ 3. stroke

_____ 4. endorphins

_____ 5. epilepsy

_____ 6. palsy

_____ 7. diskectomy

_____ 8. epiduroscopy

_____ 9. dementia

_____ 10. sciatica

a. Group of symptoms marked by memory loss and other cognitive functions

b. Chemical substances produced in the brain that act as natural analgesics (*opiates*) and provide feelings of pleasure

c. Cerebrovascular accident

d. Severe form of senile dementia

e. A neurological disorder involving repeated seizures of any type

f. Used for back pain relief when all other conservative treatments have failed

g. Cholinergic neurotransmitter

h. Pathological loss of sensation or an impairment of motor function

i. Severe pain along the course of the sciatic nerve

j. Surgical excision of an intervertebral disk

k. Anxiety syndrome and panic disorder

Abbreviations

Place the correct word, phrase, or abbreviation in the space provided.

1. Alzheimer's disease _____

2. amyotrophic lateral sclerosis _____

3. CNS _____

4. CP _____

5. computerized tomography _____

6. herniated disk syndrome _____

7. ICP _____

8. LP _____

9. MS _____

10. positron emission tomography _____

Diagnostic and Laboratory Tests

Select the best answer to each multiple-choice question. Circle the letter of your choice.

1. Diagnostic procedure used to study the structure of the brain.
   a. computed tomography
   b. echoencephalography
   c. electroencephalography
   d. myelogram

2. Process of using ultrasound to determine the presence of a centrally located mass in the brain.
   a. computed tomography
   b. echoencephalography
   c. electroencephalography
   d. myelogram

3. X-ray of the spinal canal after the injection of a radiopaque dye.
   a. cerebral angiography
   b. computed tomography
   c. myelogram
   d. ultrasonography

4. Computer-based nuclear imaging procedure that can produce three-dimensional pictures of actual organ functioning.
   a. electroencephalography
   b. myelogram
   c. ultrasonography
   d. positron emission tomography

5. Use of high-frequency sound waves to record echoes on an oscilloscope and film.
   a. electroencephalography
   b. myelogram
   c. ultrasonography
   d. positron emission tomography

PRACTICAL APPLICATION

MEDICAL RECORD ANALYSIS

This exercise contains information, abbreviations, and medical terminology from an actual medical record or case study that has been adapted for this text. The names and any personal information have been created by the author. Read and study each form or case study and then answer the questions that follow. You may refer to Appendix III, Abbreviations and Symbols, on page A41.

OXFORD NEUROLOGICAL CENTER
7894 Hazelbrook Drive
Centreville, VA 30120
(123) 456-7890

Marcus James Madison, MD Charles Robert Jones, MD Nagoya T. Yung, MD

Summary Report

Patient: Brown, James E. **Age:** 78 **Sex:** Male **Date:** 05/19/xx

---

James E. Brown, age 78, has rather advanced Parkinson's disease, present for 7 years. It is affecting his activities of daily living (ADL). He has difficulty bathing, dressing, and has frequent falls. He has marked hesitancy on changing directions and unsteadiness with fatigue. He can brush his teeth and wash his face.

On neurological examination he did have mild to moderate impairment in cognition and short-term memory, although he is oriented to time, place, and person. He has a mild tremor, worse in the left arm than the right. He has rigidity in the upper extremities. He has marked difficulty in movement, with long delays in initiating movement and frequent freezing in place. He has postural instability. He has mild dysarthria (difficult articulation of speech). His gait is characterized by shuffling strides. He can arise from a chair with difficulty only after multiple attempts. Deep tendon reflexes are symmetrical, and toes are downgoing. Cranial nerves are unremarkable.

He has been on Sinemet 25–100 mg tid for the last 6 years. I have asked him to increase his Sinemet dose to qid. Mr. Brown is to return to our office in 3 months.

Marcus James Madison, MD

Medical Record Questions

Place the correct answer in the space provided.

1. On neurological examination Mr. Brown did have mild to moderate impairment in

_____ and short-term memory.

2. Mr. Brown has a mild _____, worse in the left arm than the right.

3. What does *dysarthria* mean? _____

4. Sinemet 25–100 mg is classified as a/an _____ drug.

5. Why is this drug prescribed for Mr. Brown? _____

anization of the Body • Integumentary System • Skeleta
ystem • Muscular System • Digestive System • Cardiov
ar System • Blood and Lymphatic System • Respiratory
stem • Urinary System • Endocrine System • Nervous
stem • **Special Senses: The Ear** • Special Senses: The

15

LEARNING OUTCOMES

On completion of this chapter, you will be able to:

1. State the description and primary functions of the ear.

2. Analyze, build, spell, and pronounce medical words.

3. Comprehend the drugs highlighted in this chapter.

4. Describe diagnostic and laboratory tests related to the ear.

5. Identify and define selected abbreviations.

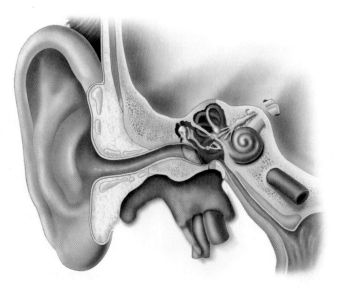

COMBINING FORMS OF THE EAR

audi/o	to hear	**neur/o**	nerve
aur/i	ear	**ot/o**	ear
chol/e	gall or bile	**pharyng/e**	pharynx
cochle/o	land snail	**presby/o**	old
electr/o	electricity	**py/o**	pus
labyrinth/o	maze, inner ear	**scler/o**	hardening
laryng/o	larynx, voice box	**staped/o**	stapes, stirrup
mast/o	mastoid process, breast-shaped	**steat/o**	fat
myring/o	eardrum, tympanic membrane	**tympan/o**	eardrum, tympanic membrane

Anatomy and Physiology

The **ear** is generally described as having three distinct divisions: the external ear, the middle ear, and the inner ear, each with distinct functions. The ear contains structures for both the sense of hearing and the sense of balance. The eighth cranial nerve, also called the acoustic or auditory nerve, carries nerve impulses for both hearing and balance from the ear to the brain. Table 15.1 ■ provides an at-a-glance look at the ear. The ear and its anatomic structures are shown in Figure 15.1 ■

TABLE 15.1 Special Senses: The Ear at-a-Glance

Organ/Structure	Primary Functions/Description
External ear	
Auricle (pinna)	Collects and directs sound waves into the auditory canal and then into the tympanic membrane
External acoustic meatus (auditory canal)	Numerous glands line the canal and secrete cerumen (earwax) to lubricate and protect the ear
Tympanic membrane (eardrum)	Separates the external ear from the middle ear and is not actually part of the external ear
Middle ear	
Contains the ossicles: malleus, incus, and stapes; has several openings; is lined with mucous membrane	Transmits sound vibrations from the tympanic membrane to the cochlea Equalizes external/internal air pressure on the tympanic membrane
Inner ear	
Cochlea	Located on the basilar membrane is the **organ of Corti** containing hair cell sensory receptors for the sense of hearing

TABLE 15.1 Special Senses: The Ear at-a-Glance *(continued)*

Organ/Structure	Primary Functions/Description
Vestibule	Contains the utricle and saccule, membranous pouches containing perilymph. The utricle communicates with the semicircular canals and contains hair cell sensory receptors connected to fibers from the eighth cranial nerve. These hair cells react to the force of gravity and movement of **otoliths**, and are a part of the sense of equilibrium.
Semicircular canals	Contain nerve endings in the form of hair cells that note changes in the position of the head and reports such movement to the brain through fibers leading to the eighth cranial nerve

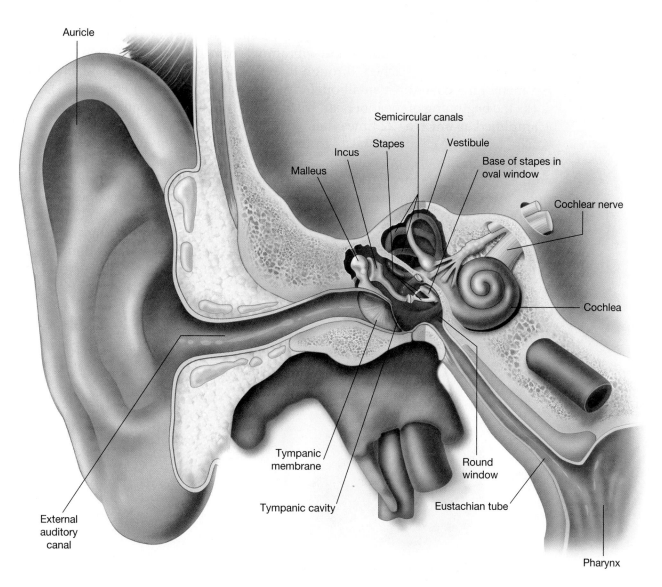

■ **Figure 15.1** The ear and its anatomic structures.

EXTERNAL EAR

The **external ear** is the appendage on the side of the head consisting of the **auricle** or **pinna** and the *external acoustic meatus*. The auricle (pinna) is the external portion of the ear that serves to protect the **tympanic membrane** (eardrum), as well as to collect and direct sound waves through the **ear canal** to the eardrum. About 1¼ inches long, the canal contains modified sweat glands that secrete **cerumen**, or **earwax**. Too much cerumen can block sound transmission.

MIDDLE EAR

The **middle ear**, separated from the external ear by the eardrum, is an air-filled cavity (**tympanic cavity**) carved out of the temporal bone. This cavity contains three specialized small bones or **ossicles** instrumental to the hearing process. These ossicles are the **malleus (hammer), incus (anvil)**, and **stapes (stirrup)**. See Figure 15.2 ■ These bones mechanically transmit sound vibrations from the tympanic membrane, to which the malleus is attached, through the incus to the stapes, which attaches to a thin membrane covering a small opening, the oval window (see Figure 15.1), that marks the beginning of the inner ear. During transmission, tympanic vibrations can be amplified as much as 22 times their original force.

The tympanic cavity connects to the throat/nasopharynx via the **eustachian tube**. This ear–throat connection makes the ear susceptible to infection. The spread of infection from the throat along this membrane to the middle ear is called **otitis media (OM).** The continued spread of infection to one of the mastoid bones is called **mastoiditis.** The eustachian tube functions to equalize air pressure on both sides of the eardrum. Normally the walls of the tube are collapsed. Swallowing and chewing actions open the tube to allow air in or out, as needed for equalization. Equalizing air pressure ensures that the eardrum vibrates maximally when struck by sound waves.

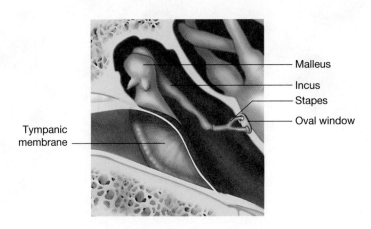

Malleus
Incus
Stapes
Oval window

Tympanic membrane

■ **Figure 15.2** The ossicles of the middle ear along with the oval window and tympanic membrane.

LIFE SPAN CONSIDERATIONS

At 36 weeks, the **earlobes** of the fetus are soft and around 40 weeks they become firm. In newborns, the wall of the ear canal is pliable because of underdeveloped cartilage and bone. The eustachian tube in infants is shorter and straighter than in older children and adults. Because of this, an infant or young child is more predisposed to developing an ear infection. When this occurs, the child's ears should be examined very carefully. See Figure 15.3 ■

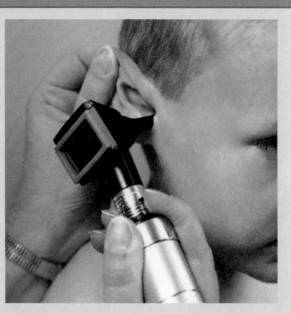

■ **Figure 15.3** To examine a child's ear, the pinna should be pulled back and up for children over 3 years; the pinna should be pulled down and back for children under 3 years of age.

INNER EAR

The **inner ear** consists of a membranous labyrinth or mazelike network of canals located within a bony labyrinth. These structures are called **labyrinths** because of their complicated shapes. The bony labyrinth, located in the temporal bone, consists of the *cochlea, vestibule,* and three *semicircular canals.* Within the bony labyrinth but separated from it by a pale fluid called **perilymph**, is the membranous labyrinth, filled with a fluid called **endolymph.** This membranous labyrinth contains the actual hearing cells, the *hair cells of the organ of Corti.*

Cochlea

The **cochlea** is a spiral-shaped bony structure containing the cochlear duct; it is so named because it resembles a snail shell. The spiral cavity of the bony cochlea is partitioned into three tubelike channels that run the entire length of the spiral. Two membranes form these tubelike areas. The *basilar membrane* forms the lower channel or *scala tympani,* and the *vestibular membrane (Reissner's membrane)* forms the upper channel, which is called the *scala vestibuli.* Between the two scala is a space, the *cochlear duct,* formed by the vestibular membrane on top and the basilar membrane as a floor. Located on the basilar membrane is the **organ of Corti** containing hair cell sensory receptors for the sense of hearing. The fluid perilymph fills the scala vestibuli and scala tympani. A different fluid, endolymph, fills the cochlear duct (see Figure 15.4 ■).

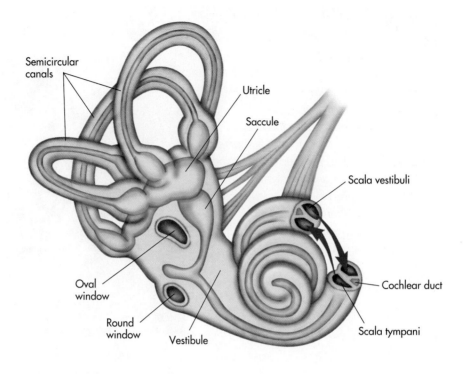

Semicircular
canals

Utricle

Saccule

Scala vestibuli

Cochlear duct

Oval
window

Scala tympani

Round
window

Vestibule

■ **Figure 15.4** The cochlea.

The Process of Hearing

In the process of hearing, sound waves are collected by the auricle (pinna) and directed through the external auditory canal to the tympanic membrane (eardrum), causing it to vibrate. These vibrations move the three small bones of the middle ear (malleus, incus, and stapes). The movement of the stapes at the oval window sets up pressure waves in the auditory fluids (perilymph and endolymph). The waves distort the basilar membrane and cause the vibration of the hair cells of the organ of Corti. These vibrations are picked up by auditory nerve fibers that transmit an electric nerve signal to the cerebral cortex of the brain, where it is interpreted as sound. The path of sound vibrations is shown in Figure 15.5 ■

Vestibule

The **vestibule** is a bony structure located between the cochlea and the three semicircular canals. The bony vestibule contains the **utricle** and **saccule**, membranous pouches containing perilymph. The utricle communicates with the semicircular canals and contains hair cell sensory receptors connected to fibers from the eighth cranial nerve. These hair cells bend to the forces of gravity and movement of otoliths and are a part of the sense of *equilibrium.*

Semicircular Canals

Located at right angles to each other are the superior, posterior, and inferior **semicircular canals.** Within the bony canals are the membranous semicircular ducts containing endolymph. At the base of each canal is an enlargement called an **ampulla** containing nerve endings in the form of hair cells. Changes in the position of the head cause the fluid in the canals to flow against these sensory receptors, which, in

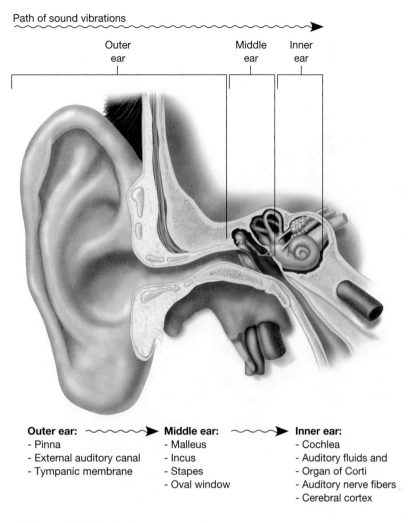

Path of sound vibrations

Outer ear | Middle ear | Inner ear

Outer ear:
- Pinna
- External auditory canal
- Tympanic membrane

Middle ear:
- Malleus
- Incus
- Stapes
- Oval window

Inner ear:
- Cochlea
- Auditory fluids and
- Organ of Corti
- Auditory nerve fibers
- Cerebral cortex

■ **Figure 15.5** Path of sound vibrations.

turn, report such movement to the brain through fibers leading to the eighth cranial nerve. Dizziness and motion sickness are associated with the continued movement of the fluid in the semicircular canals due to gravitational influences and the resulting sensory sensation in these areas.

LIFE SPAN CONSIDERATIONS

With aging, changes occur in the external, middle, and inner ear. The skin of the auricle can become dry and wrinkled. Production of cerumen declines and is drier. There is also dryness of the external canal, which causes itching. Hairs in the external canal become coarser and longer, especially in males. The eardrum thickens, and the bony joints in the middle ear degenerate.

Changes in the inner ear affect sensitivity to sound, understanding of speech, and balance. Degenerative changes include atrophy of the cochlea, the cochlear nerve cells, and the organ of Corti. These changes lead to the hearing loss, **presbycusis**, which is common in the older adult. Noisy surroundings make it difficult for older adults to discriminate between sounds, thereby impairing communication and socialization. The hearing distance (HD) of older adults can also be impaired.

Anatomy and Physiology Labeling

Identify the structures shown below by filling in the blanks.

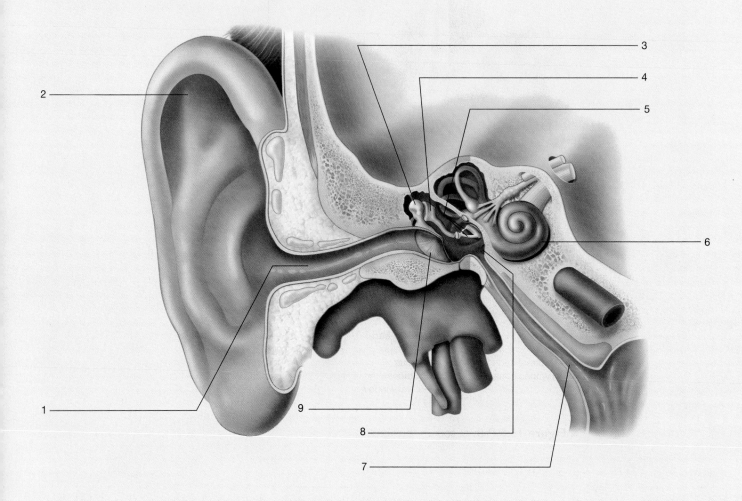

• Building Your Medical Vocabulary •

This section provides the foundation for learning medical terminology. Review the following alphabetized word list. Note how common prefixes and suffixes are repeatedly applied to word roots and combining forms to create different meanings. The word parts are color-coded: prefixes are green, suffixes are blue, roots/combining forms are red.

    You will find that some terms have not been divided into word parts. These are common words or specialized terms that are included to enhance your medical vocabulary. See Chapter 1, page 7, to review pronunciation guidelines.

MEDICAL WORD	WORD PARTS		DEFINITION
	Part	Meaning	
acoustic (ă-koos´ tĭk)	acoust -ic	hearing pertaining to	Pertaining to the sense of hearing
audiogram (ŏ´ dĭ-ō-grăm˝)	audi/o -gram	to hear a mark, record	Record of hearing by audiometry
audiologist (ŏ˝ dĭ-ŏl´ ō-jĭst)	audi/o log -ist	to hear study of one who specializes	One who specializes in diagnosing disorders of hearing
audiology (ŏ˝ dĭ-ŏl´ ō-jĭ)	audi/o -logy	to hear study of	Study of hearing disorders
audiometer (ŏ dĭ-ŏm´ ĕ-tĕr)	audi/o -meter	to hear instrument to measure	Medical instrument used to measure hearing
audiometry (ŏ˝ dĭ-ŏm´ ĕ-trē)	audi/o -metry	to hear measurement	Measurement of the hearing sense
audiphone (ŏ´ dĭ-fōn)	aud/i phone	to hear voice	Medical instrument that conveys sound to the auditory nerve through teeth or bone
auditory (ŏ´ dĭ-tō˝ rē)	auditor -y	hearing pertaining to	Pertaining to the sense of hearing
aural (ŏ´ răl)	aur -al	the ear pertaining to	Pertaining to the ear

MEDICAL WORD	WORD PARTS		DEFINITION
	Part	**Meaning**	
auricle (ŏ´ rĭ-kl)	aur/i -cle	ear small	External portion of the ear, known as the *pinna* (pin' na)
binaural (bĭn-aw´ răl)	bin aur -al	twice ear pertaining to	Pertaining to both ears
cerumen (sē-roo´ měn)			Earwax, the yellowish substance secreted by the glands in the auditory canal of the external ear
cholesteatoma (kō″ lē-stē″ ă-tō´ mă)	chol/e steat -oma	gall or bile fat tumor	Tumorlike mass filled with epithelial cells and cholesterol
cochlea (kŏk´ lē-ă)			Portion of the inner ear shaped like a snail shell; contains the *organ of Corti*
deafness			Complete or partial loss of the ability to hear. *Hearing impairment* is often used to describe a minimal loss of hearing as compared to the use of the word *deafness* when there is complete or extensive loss of hearing. See Figure 15.6 ■

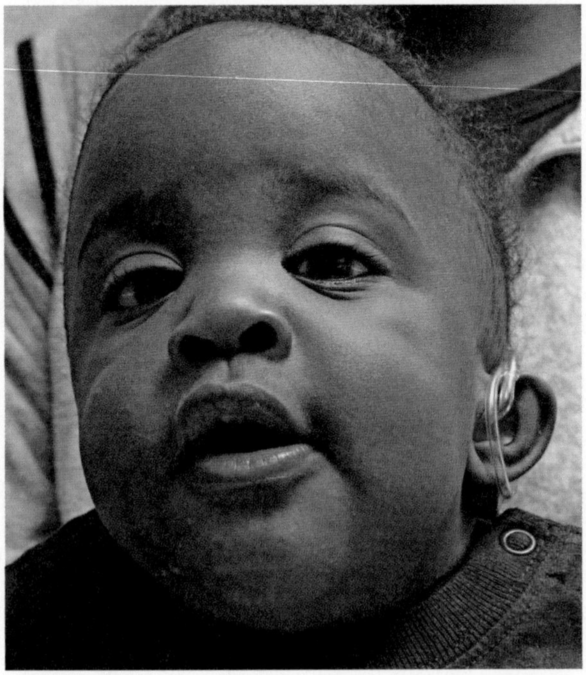

■ **Figure 15.6** A child with a hearing impairment wears a hearing aid (as noted in his left ear).

MEDICAL WORD	WORD PARTS		DEFINITION
	Part	**Meaning**	

LIFE SPAN CONSIDERATIONS

Sustained noise over 85 decibels (db, dB) can cause permanent **hearing loss**. Risk doubles with each 5-decibel increase. About two in every 10 teens have lost some of their hearing ability from exposure to noise and are not aware of it, according to a study conducted at the University of Florida. See Figure 15.7 ■ Standard hearing tests given to middle and high school students identified some hearing loss in 17% of the students. High-pitched sounds are the first to be affected by noise exposure. As hearing loss progresses, a person can start to have difficulty hearing, particularly when there is noise in the background. Excessive noise can permanently damage the hair cell sensory receptors of the organ of Corti. These receptors are instrumental in transmitting sound to the brain.

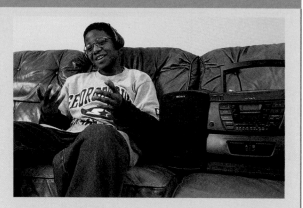

■ **Figure 15.7** Listening to loud music with headphones or at rock concerts is a frequent cause of hearing loss among teenagers and young adults.

MEDICAL WORD	WORD PARTS		DEFINITION
	Part	**Meaning**	
ear			Contains structures for both the sense of hearing and the sense of balance
electrocochleography (ē-lĕk″ trō-kŏk″ lē-ŏg′ ră-fē)	electr/o cochle/o -graphy	electricity land snail recording	Recording of the electrical activity produced when the cochlea is stimulated
endaural (ĕn′ dŏ″ răl)	end- aur -al	within ear pertaining to	Pertaining to within the ear
endolymph (ĕn′ dō-lĭmf)	endo- -lymph	within serum, clear fluid	Clear fluid contained within the labyrinth of the ear
equilibrium (ē″ kwĭ-lĭb′ rē-ŭm)			State of balance
eustachian tube (ū-stā′ kē-ăn)			Narrow tube between the middle ear and the throat that serves to equalize pressure on both sides of the eardrum

MEDICAL WORD	WORD PARTS		DEFINITION
	Part	**Meaning**	
fenestration (fĕn″ ĕs-trā′ shŭn)	fenestrat -ion	window process	Surgical operation in which a new opening is made in the labyrinth of the inner ear to restore hearing
incus (ing′ kŭs)			Middle of the three ossicles; also called the *anvil*
labyrinth (lăb′ ĭ-rĭnth)			The inner ear; made up of the *vestibule, cochlea,* and *semicircular canals*
labyrinthectomy (lăb″ ĭ-rĭn-thĕk′ tō-mē)	labyrinth -ectomy	maze, inner ear surgical excision	Surgical excision of the labyrinth
labyrinthitis (lăb″ ĭ-rĭn-thī′ tĭs)	labyrinth -itis	maze, inner ear inflammation	Inflammation of the labyrinth
labyrinthotomy (lăb″ ĭ-rĭn-thŏt′ ō-mē)	labyrinth/o -tomy	maze, inner ear incision	Incision of the labyrinth
malleus (măl′ ē-ŭs)			Largest of the three ossicles; also called the *hammer*
mastoidalgia (măs″ toyd-ăl′ jĭ-ă)	mast -oid -algia	mastoid process, breast-shaped resemble pain	Pain in the mastoid process (a bony protuberance of the skull near the ear)
mastoiditis (măs″ toyd-ī′ tĭs)	mast -oid -itis	mastoid process, breast-shaped resemble inflammation	Inflammation of one of the mastoid bones; characterized by fever, headache, and malaise

MEDICAL WORD	WORD PARTS		DEFINITION
	Part	Meaning	
Ménière's disease (mān″ ē-ārz)			An abnormality of the inner ear causing a host of symptoms, including vertigo (severe dizziness), tinnitus (a roaring sound in the ears), fluctuating hearing loss, and the sensation of pressure or pain in the affected ear. Symptoms are associated with a change in fluid volume within the labyrinth and can occur suddenly and arise daily or as infrequently as once a year.
monaural (mŏn-aw´ răl)	mon(o)- aur -al	one ear pertaining to	Pertaining to one ear
myringectomy (mĭr-ĭn-jĕk´ tō-mē)	myring -ectomy	eardrum, tympanic membrane surgical excision	Surgical excision of the tympanic membrane
myringoplasty (mĭr-ĭn´ gō-plăst″ ē)	myring/o -plasty	eardrum, tympanic membrane surgical repair	Surgical repair of the tympanic membrane
myringoscope (mĭr-ĭn´ gō-skōp)	myring/o -scope	eardrum, tympanic membrane instrument for examining	Medical instrument used to examine the eardrum
myringotome (mĭ-rĭn´ gō-tōm)	myring/o -tome	eardrum, tympanic membrane instrument to cut	Surgical instrument used for cutting the eardrum
myringotomy (mĭr-ĭn-gŏt´ ō-mē)	myring/o -tomy	eardrum, tympanic membrane incision	Surgical incision of the tympanic membrane to remove unwanted fluids from the ear

MEDICAL WORD	WORD PARTS		DEFINITION
	Part	Meaning	
ossicle (ŏs´ ĭ-kl)			Small bone; any one of the three bones of the middle ear: the *malleus,* the *incus,* or the *stapes*
otic (ō´ tĭk)	ot -ic	ear pertaining to	Pertaining to the ear
otitis (ō-tī´ tĭs)	ot -itis	ear inflammation	Inflammation of the ear
otitis media (ō-tī´ tĭs mē´ dē-ă)	ot -itis med -ia	ear inflammation middle condition	Inflammation of the middle ear

LIFE SPAN CONSIDERATIONS

Otitis media is often difficult to detect in children because most children affected by this disorder do not yet have sufficient speech and language skills to tell others what is bothering them. Common signs of otitis media include:

- Unusual irritability; fussiness
- Difficulty sleeping; night awakening
- Tugging or pulling at one or both ears (see Figure 15.8 ■)
- Fever
- Fluid draining from the ear
- Loss of balance
- Unresponsiveness to quiet sounds or other signs of hearing difficulty such as sitting too close to the television or being inattentive

Note: Children age 2 and younger who attend day care centers are 36 times more likely to contract ear infections, pneumonia, and meningitis than stay-at-home children. Most middle ear infections are a result of an upper respiratory infection (URI) that has spread through the eustachian tube.

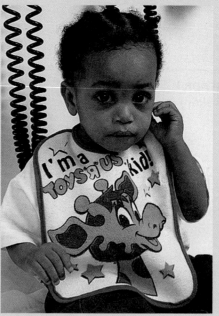

■ **Figure 15.8** This young child is pulling at the ear and acting fussy, two important signs of otitis media.

| **otodynia** (ō˝ tō-dĭn´ ĭ-ă) | ot/o -dynia | ear pain | Pain in the ear, earache; also referred to as *otalgia* |

MEDICAL WORD	WORD PARTS		DEFINITION
	Part	**Meaning**	
otolaryngologist (ō″tō-lar″ĭn-gŏl″ō-jĭst)	ot/o laryng/o log -ist	ear larynx, voice box study of one who specializes	Physician who specializes in the study of the ear and larynx (*voice box*)
otolaryngology (ō″tō-lar″ĭn-gŏl′ō-jē)	ot/o laryng/o -logy	ear larynx, voice box study of	Study of the ear and larynx (*voice box*)
otolith (ō′tō-lĭth)	ot/o -lith	ear stone	Ear stone
otomycosis (ō″tō-mĭ-kō′sĭs)	ot/o myc -osis	ear fungus condition	Fungal infection of the ear
otoneurology (ō″tō-nū-rŏl′ō-jē)	ot/o neur/o -logy	ear nerve study of	Specialized diagnosis and treatment of the ear and its neurological association
otopharyngeal (ō″tō-far-ĭn′jē-āl)	ot/o pharyng/e -al	ear pharynx pertaining to	Pertaining to the ear and pharynx
otoplasty (ō′tō-plăs″tē)	ot/o -plasty	ear surgical repair	Plastic surgical repair of the ear
otopyorrhea (ō″tō-pī″ō-rē′ă)	ot/o py/o -rrhea	ear pus flow	Pus in the ear
otorhinolaryngology (ENT) (ō″tō-rī″nō-lăr″ĭn-gŏl′ō-jē)	ot/o rhin/o laryng/o -logy	ear nose larynx study of	Study of the ear, nose, and larynx (*voice box*). The medical specialty is often referred to as *ENT* (*ear, nose, throat*); in this case, *throat* is used in a broad sense instead of *larynx*.
otosclerosis (ō″tō-sklē-rō′sĭs)	ot/o scler -osis	ear hardening condition	Hardening (stiffening) condition of the ear structures characterized by progressive deafness

MEDICAL WORD	WORD PARTS		DEFINITION
	Part	**Meaning**	
otoscope (ō´ tō-skōp)	ot/o -scope	ear instrument for examining	Medical instrument used to examine the ear. See Figure 15.9 ■ An inspection of the walls of the auditory canal should find no sign of irritation, discharge, or a foreign object. The walls are normally pink and some cerumen is present. The tympanic membrane is usually pearly gray and translucent. It reflects light and the ossicles are visible.
			■ **Figure 15.9** The otoscope is positioned in the ear prior to examination of the auditory canal.
oval window			Membrane in the middle ear into which the footplate of the stapes fits
perilymph (pĕr´ ĭ-lĭmf)	peri- -lymph	around serum, pale fluid	Serum fluid of the inner ear
presbycusis (prĕz˝ bĭ-kū´ sĭs)	presby -cusis	old hearing	Impairment of hearing that occurs with aging
stapedectomy (stā˝ pē-dĕk´ tō-mē)	staped -ectomy	stapes, stirrup surgical excision	Surgical excision of the stapes in the middle ear to improve hearing, especially in cases of otosclerosis. The stapes is replaced by a prosthesis.
stapes (stā´ pēz)			Innermost of the ossicles in the middle ear; also called the *stirrup*

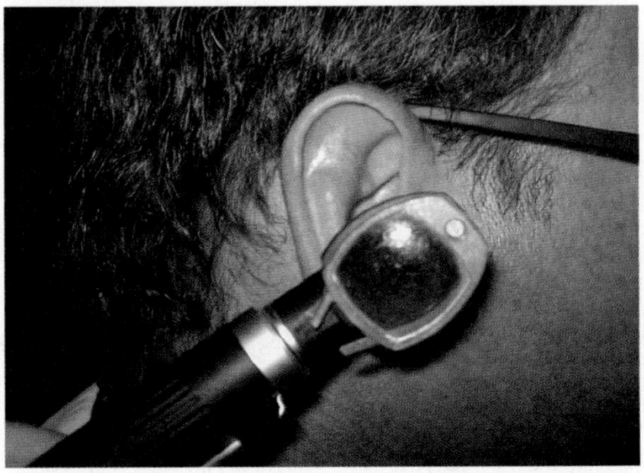

MEDICAL WORD	WORD PARTS		DEFINITION
	Part	**Meaning**	
tinnitus (tĭn-ī´ tŭs)			The sensation of ringing or roaring sounds in one or both ears is a symptom associated with damage to the auditory cells in the inner ear. It can also be a symptom of other health problems.

fyi According to estimates by the American Tinnitus Association, at least 12 million Americans have tinnitus. Of these, at least 1 million experience it so severely that it interferes with their daily activities, such as hearing, working, and sleeping. There are several possible causes of tinnitus:

- **Hearing loss.** Doctors and scientists have discovered that people with different kinds of hearing loss, primarily from presbycusis or trauma-related damage to the inner ear, also have tinnitus.
- **Loud noise.** Too much exposure to loud noise can cause noise-induced hearing loss and tinnitus.
- **Medicine.** More than 200 medicines can cause tinnitus.
- **Other health problems.** Allergies, tumors, and problems in the heart and blood vessels, jaws, and neck can cause tinnitus.

A patient can be referred to an *otolaryngologist* for diagnosis and/or an *audiologist*, who performs hearing tests. Although there is no cure for tinnitus, scientists and doctors have discovered several treatments that can provide some relief such as hearing aids, medications, and maskers, which are small electronic devices that use sound to make tinnitus less noticeable.

MEDICAL WORD	WORD PARTS		DEFINITION
tuning fork			Instrument used medically in a hearing test, which, when struck at the forked end, vibrates and thus can be heard and felt
tympanectomy (tĭm″ păn-ĕk tō-mē)	tympan -ectomy	eardrum, tympanic membrane surgical excision	Surgical excision of the tympanic membrane (eardrum)
tympanic (tĭm-păn´ ĭk)	tympan -ic	eardrum, tympanic membrane pertaining to	Pertaining to the eardrum (tympanic membrane)

MEDICAL WORD	WORD PARTS		DEFINITION
	Part	Meaning	
tympanic thermometer			Electronic thermometer used to determine internal body temperature by measuring it from the tympanic membrane and its surrounding tissues. See Figure 15.10 ■ and Figure 15.11 ■

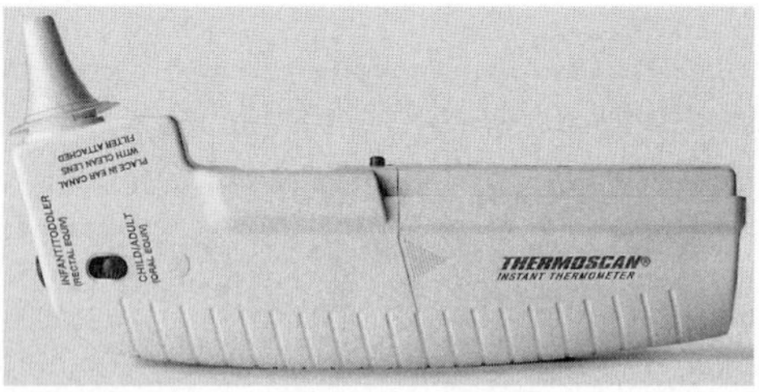

■ **Figure 15.10** Thermoscan instant thermometer (Courtesy of Thermoscan, Inc., San Diego, CA)

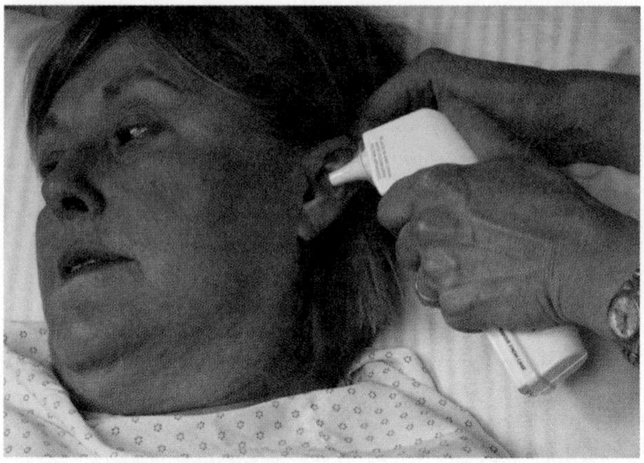

■ **Figure 15.11** Use of the tympanic thermometer to measure body temperature.

MEDICAL WORD	WORD PARTS		DEFINITION
	Part	Meaning	
tympanitis (tĭm-păn-ĭ´ tĭs)	tympan -itis	eardrum, tympanic membrane inflammation	Inflammation of the eardrum (tympanic membrane)
tympanoplasty (tĭm˝ păn-ō-plăs´ tē)	tympan/o -plasty	eardrum, tympanic membrane surgical repair	Surgical repair of the tympanic membrane (eardrum)
utricle (ū´ trĭk-l)			Small, saclike structure of the labyrinth of the inner ear
vertigo (ver´ tĭ-gō)			Sensation of instability and loss of equilibrium; patients feel like they are spinning in space or objects around them are spinning. Caused by a disturbance in the semicircular canal of the inner ear or the vestibular nuclei of the brainstem.

• Drug Highlights •

TYPE OF DRUG	DESCRIPTION AND EXAMPLES
analgesic	Used to relieve pain without causing loss of consciousness. EXAMPLES: Tylenol (acetaminophen); Advil, Motrin (ibuprofen); aspirin
antipyretic	Agent that reduces fever. EXAMPLES: Tylenol (acetaminophen), aspirin NOTE: In children, aspirin should not be used as an analgesic or antipyretic because of the risk of Reye's syndrome.
antibiotics	Used to treat infectious diseases; can be natural or synthetic substances that inhibit the growth of or destroy microorganisms, especially bacteria.
penicillins	Act by interfering with bacterial cell wall synthesis among newly formed bacterial cells. Penicillins are contraindicated in patients who are known to be allergic or hypersensitive to any of its varieties or to any of the cephalosporins. EXAMPLES: penicillin G, ampicillin, penicillin V, piperacillin, and amoxicillin
cephalosporins	Chemically and pharmacologically related to the penicillins, they act by inhibiting bacterial cell wall synthesis, thereby promoting the death of the developing microorganisms. Hypersensitivity to cephalosporins and/or penicillins can result in an allergic reaction. EXAMPLES: cefazolin sodium, cefaclor, Keflex (cephalexin), and Suprax (cefixime)
tetracyclines	Primarily bacteriostatic and active against a wide range of gram-negative and gram-positive microorganisms, they inhibit protein synthesis in the bacterial cell. NOTE: Contraindicated in children 8 years of age and younger; they cause permanent discoloration of tooth enamel. EXAMPLES: Sumycin, tetracycline hydrochloride; Declomycin DMCT (demeclocycline HCl); and Doryx, Vibramycin (doxycycline)
erythromycin	Works by inhibiting protein synthesis in susceptible bacteria. These drugs can be used for patients who are allergic to penicillin. EXAMPLES: ERY-TAB, EES, EryPed, and Erythrocin
drugs used to treat vertigo	Vertigo is a sensation of movement, when the person is not moving, that can be caused by a lesion or other process affecting the brain, the eighth cranial nerve, or the labyrinthine system of the ear. Drugs used for vertigo include anticholinergics, antihistamines, and antidopamines. EXAMPLES: dimenhydrinate, Benadryl (diphenhydramine HCl), Antivert (meclizine HCl), promethazine HCl, Transderm-scop (scopolamine)

• Diagnostic and Lab Tests •

TEST	DESCRIPTION
auditory-evoked response (aw′dĭ-tō rē-ĕ-vōkd′)	Response to auditory stimuli (sound) that can be measured independently of the patient's subjective response. Use of an electroencephalograph can determine the intensity of sound and presence of response. This test is useful to test the hearing of children who are too young for standard tests, autistic, hyperkinetic, and/or retarded.
electronystagmography (ENG) (ē-lĕk″ trō-nĭs tăg-mŏg′ ră-fē)	Recording eye movement in response to specific stimuli, such as sound; used to determine the presence and location of a lesion in the vestibule of the ear, to help diagnose unilateral hearing loss of unknown origin, and to help identify the cause of vertigo, tinnitus, and dizziness.
pure tone audiometry	Method of testing pure tones by providing calibrated tones to a person via earphones, allowing that person to increase the sound level until it can just be heard. Various strategies are used, but pure tone audiometry with tones starting at about 125 Hz (cycles/second) and increasing by octaves, half-octaves, or third-octaves to about 8000 Hz is typical. Hearing tests of right and left ears are generally done independently. The results of such tests are summarized in audiograms. Audiograms compare hearing to the normal threshold of hearing, which varies with frequency, as illustrated by the hearing curves. The audiogram is normalized to the hearing curve so that a straight horizontal line at 0 represents normal hearing.
otoscopy (ō-tŏs′ kō-pē)	Visual examination of the external auditory canal and the tympanic membrane via an otoscope. Pneumatic otoscopy uses a special attachment on the otoscope. This allows the examiner to direct a light stream of air toward the eardrum. The directed air current should then cause the tympanic membrane to vibrate. With dysfunction there is little or no vibration noted.

TEST	DESCRIPTION

fyi When examining the tympanic membrane with an otoscope, the position, mobility, color, and degree of translucency are evaluated and described. The normal tympanic membrane is in the neutral position (neither retracted nor bulging), pearly gray, translucent, and responds briskly to positive and negative pressure, indicating an air-filled space. An abnormal tympanic membrane can be retracted or bulging and immobile or poorly mobile in pneumatic **otoscopy**. The position of the tympanic membrane is a key for differentiating acute otitis media and otitis media with effusion. In acute otitis media, the tympanic membrane is usually bulging and purulent fluid is present in the middle ear (Figure 15.12 ■).

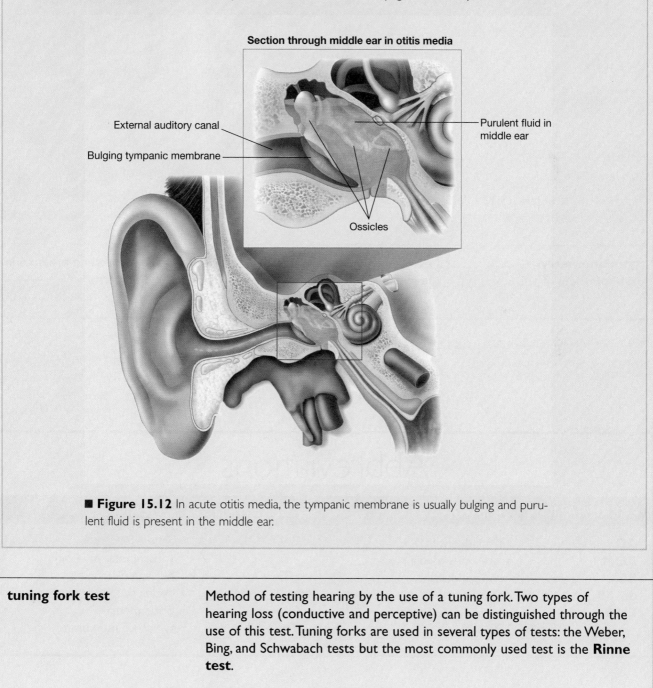

Section through middle ear in otitis media

External auditory canal

Bulging tympanic membrane

Purulent fluid in middle ear

Ossicles

■ **Figure 15.12** In acute otitis media, the tympanic membrane is usually bulging and purulent fluid is present in the middle ear.

tuning fork test	Method of testing hearing by the use of a tuning fork. Two types of hearing loss (conductive and perceptive) can be distinguished through the use of this test. Tuning forks are used in several types of tests: the Weber, Bing, and Schwabach tests but the most commonly used test is the **Rinne test**.

TEST	DESCRIPTION
Rinne test (rĭn´ nē)	The Rinne test utilizes a tuning fork to compare bone conduction (BC) hearing with air conduction (AC). After being struck, the vibrating tuning fork is held on the mastoid process until sound is no longer heard. The fork is then immediately placed just outside the ear. Normally, the sound is audible at the ear. See Figure 15.13 ■

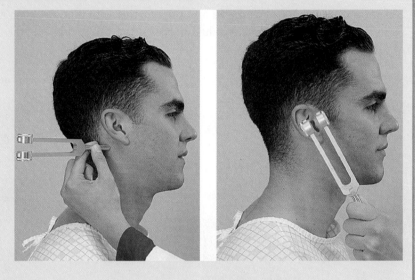

■ **Figure 15.13** Administration of the Rinne test.

tympanometry (tĭm″ păn-nŏm´ ĕ-trē)	Measurement of the movement of the tympanic membrane and pressure in the middle ear. It is used for detecting middle ear disorders.

• Abbreviations •

ABBREVIATION	MEANING	ABBREVIATION	MEANING
AC	air conduction	ENT	ear, nose, throat (otorhinolaryngology)
AOM	acute otitis media		
BC	bone conduction	HD	hearing distance
db, dB	decibel	Hz	cycles/second
ENG	electronystagmography	OM	otitis media
		TM	tympanic membrane

Anatomy and Physiology

Write your answers to the following questions.

1. The ears contain structures for both the sense of _____ and the sense of
   _____ .

2. Name the three divisions of the ear.

   a. _____   **b.** _____

   c. _____

3. The external ear consists of the _____ and the _____ .

4. Which structure of the external ear collects sound waves? _____

5. State the two functions of cerumen.

   a. _____   **b.** _____

6. Name the three ossicles of the middle ear.

   a. _____   **b.** _____

   c. _____

7. State the function of the ossicles.

   _____

8. State two functions of the middle ear.

   a. _____   **b.** _____

9. The bony labyrinth of the inner ear consists of the _____ , _____ ,
   and the _____ .

10. Name the three divisions of the membranous labyrinth.

    a. _____   **b.** _____

    c. _____

11. Located on the basilar membrane is the _____ , containing hair cell sensory receptors for
    the sense of hearing.

12. The _____ is a bony structure located between the cochlea and the three
    semicircular canals.

13. The auditory nerve is also known as the _____ .

14. Dizziness and _____ are associated with the continued movement of the fluid in the semicircular canals due to gravitational influences.

15. Name the two types of fluid found in the ear.

    a. _____   **b.** _____

Word Parts

PREFIXES

Give the definitions of the following prefixes.

1. end- _____   **2.** endo- _____

3. peri- _____   **4.** bin- _____

5. mon(o)- _____

ROOTS AND COMBINING FORMS

Give the definitions of the following roots and combining forms.

1. acoust _____ **2.** aud/i _____

3. audi/o _____ **4.** auditor _____

5. aur _____ **6.** chol/e _____

7. cochle/o _____ **8.** electr/o _____

9. labyrinth _____ **10.** labyrinth/o _____

11. laryng/o _____ **12.** log _____

13. mast _____ **14.** myc _____

15. myring _____ **16.** myring/o _____

17. neur/o _____ **18.** ot _____

19. ot/o _____ **20.** pharyng/e _____

21. phone _____ **22.** presby _____

23. py/o _____ **24.** rhin/o _____

25. scler _____ **26.** staped _____

27. steat _____ **28.** tympan _____

29. aur/i _____

30. fenestrat _____

31. med _____

32. tympan/o _____

SUFFIXES

Give the definitions of the following suffixes.

1. -al _____

2. -algia _____

3. -cusis _____

4. -dynia _____

5. -ectomy _____

6. -gram _____

7. -graphy _____

8. -ic _____

9. -ist _____

10. -itis _____

11. -lith _____

12. -logy _____

13. -lymph _____

14. -meter _____

15. -metry _____

16. -oid _____

17. -oma _____

18. -osis _____

19. -plasty _____

20. -rrhea _____

21. -scope _____

22. -tome _____

23. -tomy _____

24. -y _____

25. -cle _____

26. -ion _____

27. -ia _____

Identifying Medical Terms

In the spaces provided, write the medical terms for the following meanings.

1. _____ One who specializes in diagnosing disorders of hearing

2. _____ Measurement of the hearing sense

3. _____ Pertaining to the sense of hearing

4. _____ Pertaining to within the ear

5. _____ Inflammation of the labyrinth

6. _____ Surgical repair of the tympanic membrane

7. _____ Surgical instrument used for cutting the eardrum

8. _____ Pain in the ear, earache

9. _____ Study of the ear and larynx

10. _____ Pertaining to the ear and pharynx

11. _____ Medical instrument used to examine the ear

12. _____ Serum fluid of the inner ear

13. _____ Surgical excision of the stapes of the ear

14. _____ Surgical excision of the tympanic membrane

15. _____ The sensation of ringing or roaring sounds in one or both ears

Spelling

Circle the correct spelling of each medical term.

1. acostic / acoustic

2. audilogy / audiology

3. cholestoma / cholesteatoma

4. electrocochleography / electrochleography

5. labyrinthitis / labrinthitis

6. myringplasty / myringoplasty

7. otomycosis / otomcosis

8. otoscerosis / otosclerosis

9. typanic / tympanic

10. typanitis / tympanitis

Matching

Select the appropriate lettered meaning for each of the following words.

_____ 1. auricle

_____ 2. binaural

_____ 3. cerumen

_____ 4. equilibrium

_____ 5. fenestration

_____ 6. labyrinth

_____ 7. myringotomy

_____ 8. ossicle

_____ 9. tympanoplasty

_____ 10. vertigo

a. State of balance

b. Inner ear

c. Small bone

d. Surgical repair of the tympanic membrane

e. Pertaining to both ears

f. Sensation of instability, loss of equilibrium

g. Surgical operation in which a new opening is made in the labyrinth

h. External portion of the ear

i. Earwax

j. Surgical incision of the tympanic membrane

k. Organ of hearing

Abbreviations

Place the correct word, phrase, or abbreviation in the space provided.

1. air conduction _____

2. bone conduction _____

3. db, dB _____

4. electronystagmography _____

5. ENT _____

6. hearing distance _____

7. otitis media _____

Diagnostic and Laboratory Tests

Select the best answer to each multiple-choice question. Circle the letter of your choice.

1. The response to auditory stimuli that can be measured independent of the patient's subjective response.
   a. auditory-evoked response   **c.** tuning fork test
   b. electronystagmography   **d.** otoscopy

2. Recording of eye movement in response to specific stimuli.
   a. auditory-evoked response   **c.** tympanometry
   b. electronystagmography   **d.** otoscopy

3. Visual examination of the external auditory canal and the tympanic membrane.
   a. tuning fork test   **c.** electronystagmography
   b. tympanometry   **d.** otoscopy

4. Measurement of the movement of the tympanic membrane.
   a. tuning fork tests   **c.** otoscopy
   b. tympanometry   **d.** electronystagmography

5. This test utilizes a tuning fork to compare bone conduction (BC) hearing with air conduction (AC).
   a. Rinne test   **c.** otoscopy
   b. tympanometry   **d.** electronystagmography

PRACTICAL APPLICATION

MEDICAL RECORD ANALYSIS

This exercise contains information, abbreviations, and medical terminology from an actual medical record or case study that has been adapted for this text. The names and any personal information have been created by the author. Read and study each form or case study and then answer the questions that follow. You may refer to Appendix III, Abbreviations and Symbols, on page A41.

HOLLY HILL OTOLARYNGOLOGY CLINIC
112 Dogwood Blvd.
Kingwood, Texas 77339
(123) 456-7890
William R. Patel, MD, King Louis Lataif,
MD, Brittany Nicole Benz, MD

May 10, 20xx
Starr J. Bentley, MD
235 Maple Lane
Kingwood, Texas 77339
Re: Takeshia Chamberlain

Dear Doctor Bentley,
Thank you for your referral of Takeshia Chamberlain, age 2, seen in my office on April 25, 20xx. When seen, Takeshia had a fever of 102.2° F, with noted dark circles under both eyes and appeared to be in moderate pain. Child was pulling on her left ear and upon examination left TM red, dull, and bulging, diffuse light reflex with loss of landmark. Pneumatic otoscopy revealed immobile left TM. Right TM pearly gray, landmarks intact. Nasal mucosa dark red and swollen, with moderate amount of discharge. Oral mucosa erythematous with yellow-white exudates, no lesions. Uvula rises in midline with phonation. Gag reflex present. No lymphadenopathy. Neck supple. Lungs CTA and heart normal rate and rhythm. No murmurs. Skin: no rashes or lesions, warm to the touch.

A diagnosis of acute otitis media (AOM) left ear was confirmed.

I ordered acetaminophen (Tylenol) liquid, 1.6 mL (1 teaspoon) PO every 4 hours prn for pain and fever. Amoxicillin (Amoxil) suspension 40mg per kg per day, in three divided doses, every 8 hours for 10 days for infection. Instructed the mother on the adverse reactions to penicillin and explained that she should not give the antibiotic with soft drinks or fruit juices because the acid in these products could destroy the effectiveness of the drug. Stressed the importance of the baby taking the antibiotic as ordered for the entire 10 days and around the clock, every 8 hours. Instructed the mother to bring the baby back to the clinic if symptoms do not improve in 48–72 hours. Scheduled a follow-up visit for 3 weeks.

Best regards,
William R. Patel, MD

Medical Record Questions

Place the correct answer in the space provided.

1. In Takeshia the signs and symptoms of acute otitis media included a fever of _____ and

   the child _____ on her left ear.

2. The diagnosis was determined by a visual examination of the ear called pneumatic _____ ,
   a physical examination of the child, and the signs and symptoms presented.

3. Acetaminophen (Tylenol) is classified as a (n) _____ and is given to relieve

   _____ and reduce _____ .

4. Amoxicillin (Amoxil) is a(n) _____ and is given for _____ .

5. The _____ in soft drinks and fruit juices can destroy the effectiveness of the

   _____ drug.

PEARSON
mymedicalterminologylab

**MyMedicalTerminologyLab is a premium online homework management system that includes
a host of features to help you study. Registered users will find:**

• Fun games and activities built within a virtual hospital

• Powerful tools that track and analyze your results—allowing you to create a personalized learning experience

• Videos, flashcards, and audio pronunciations to help enrich your progress

• Streaming lesson presentations and self-paced learning modules

• A space where you and your instructors can view and manage your assignments

gumentary System • Skeletal System • Muscular System
Digestive System • Cardiovascular System • Blood and
mphatic System • Respiratory System • Urinary System
ndocrine System • Nervous System • Special Senses: T
ar • **Special Senses: The Eye** • Female Reproductive

16

LEARNING OUTCOMES

On completion of this chapter, you will be able to:

1. State the description and primary functions of the eye.

2. Analyze, build, spell, and pronounce medical words.

3. Comprehend the drugs highlighted in this chapter.

4. Describe diagnostic and laboratory tests related to the eye.

5. Identify and define selected abbreviations.

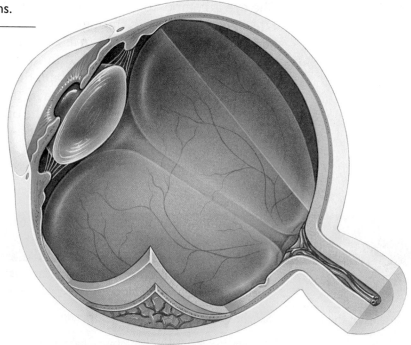

COMBINING FORMS OF THE EYE

ambly/o	dull	my/o	muscle
anis/o	unequal	ocul/o	eye
blephar/o	eyelid	ophthalm/o	eye
choroid/o	choroid	opt/o	eye
conjunctiv/o	to join together, conjunctiva	orth/o	straight
cor/o	pupil	phac/o	lens
corne/o	cornea	phak/o	lentil, lens
cry/o	cold	phot/o	light
cycl/o	ciliary body	presby/o	old
dacry/o	tear, lacrimal duct, tear duct	pupill/o	pupil
dipl/o	double	rad/i	radiating out from a center
electr/o	electricity	retin/o	retina
fibr/o	fiber	scler/o	sclera, hardening
foc/o	focus	stigmat/o	point
goni/o	angle	ton/o	tone, tension
irid/o	iris	trich/o	hair
kerat/o	cornea	trop/o	turn
lacrim/o	tear, lacrimal duct, tear duct	uve/o	uvea
lent/o	lens	xen/o	foreign material
metr/o	measure	xer/o	dry
mi/o	less, small		

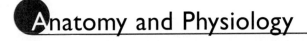natomy and Physiology

The **eye** is composed of special anatomical structures that work together to facilitate sight. Light passes through the cornea, pupil, lens, and the vitreous body to stimulate sensory receptors (*rods* and *cones*) in the **retina** or innermost layer of the eye. **Vision** is made possible through the coordinated actions of nerves that control the movement of the eyeball, the amount of light admitted by the pupil, the focusing of that light on the retina by the lens, and the transmission of the resulting sensory impulses to the brain by the optic nerve. The brain permits the perception of vision. Table 16.1 ■ provides an at-a-glance look at the eye. Figure 16.1 ■ shows the internal structures of the eye.

TABLE 16.1 Special Senses: The Eye at-a-Glance

Organ/Structure	Primary Functions/Description
Orbit	Contains the eyeball; cavity is lined with fatty tissue that cushions the eyeball and has several openings through which blood vessels and nerves pass
Muscles of the eye	Six short muscles provide support and rotary movement of the eyeball
Eyelids	Protect the eyeballs from intense light, foreign particles, and impact; permits the eye to remain moist

TABLE 16.1 Special Senses: The Eye at-a-Glance (continued)

Organ/Structure	Primary Functions/Description
Conjunctiva	Acts as a protective covering for the exposed surface of the eyeball and helps keep the eyelid and eyeball moist
Lacrimal apparatus	Produces, stores, and removes tears that cleanse and lubricate the eye
Eyeball	Organ of vision
Sclera	Outer layer of the eyeball composed of fibrous connective tissue; at the front of the eye, it is visible as the white of the eye and ends at the cornea
Cornea	Transparent anterior portion of the eyeball, which bends light rays and helps to focus them on the surface of the retina
Choroid	Pigmented vascular membrane that prevents internal reflection of light
Ciliary body	Smooth muscle that forms a part of the ciliary body that governs the convexity of the lens; secretes nutrient fluids that nourish the cornea, the lens, and surrounding tissues
Iris	Colored membrane attached to the ciliary body (can appear as blue, brown, green, hazel, or gray) with a circular opening in its center, the pupil, and two muscles that contract; regulates the amount of light admitted by the pupil
Retina	Innermost layer with photoreceptive cells; translates light waves focused on its surface into nerve impulses
Lens	Sharpens the focus of light on the retina (accommodation [Acc])

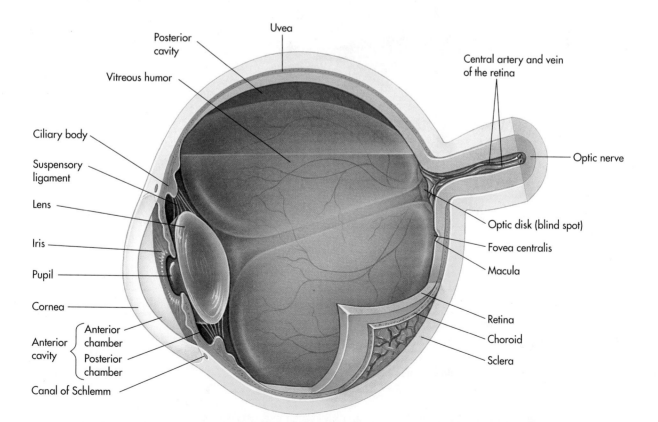

■ **Figure 16.1** Internal structure of the eye.

EXTERNAL STRUCTURES OF THE EYE

The orbit, the muscles of the eye, the eyelids, the conjunctiva, and the lacrimal apparatus make up the external structures of the eye.

Orbit

The **orbit** is a cone-shaped cavity in the front of the skull that contains the *eyeball.* Formed by the combination of several bones, this cavity is lined with fatty tissue that cushions the eyeball and has several **foramina** (openings) through which blood vessels and nerves pass. The **optic foramen** is the short canal through the lesser wing of the sphenoid bone at the apex of the orbit that gives passage to the optic nerve and the ophthalmic artery.

Muscles of the Eye

Six eye muscles control movement of the eye, allowing it to follow a moving object and move precisely. Of the six, four are rectus muscles and two are oblique muscles. *Rectus muscles* allow a person to see up, down, right, and left. *Oblique muscles* allow the eyes to turn to see upper left and upper right, lower left and lower right. See Figure 16.2 ■ The eye muscles also help maintain the shape of the eyeball.

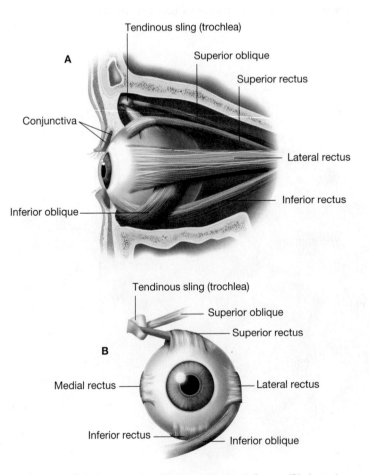

■ **Figure 16.2** Eye muscles. (A) Lateral view, left eye. (B) Anterior view, left eye.

Eyelids

Each eye has a pair of **eyelids** that are continuous with the skin, cover the eyeball, and protect it from intense light, foreign particles, and impact. Through their blinking motion, eyelids keep the eyeball's surface lubricated and free from dust and debris. Known as the *superior* and *inferior palpebrae,* those movable "curtains" join to form a **canthus** or angle at either corner of the eye. The slit between the eyelids is called the **palpebral fissure** through which light reaches the inner eye.

The edges of the eyelids contain eyelashes that help protect the eyeball by preventing foreign matter, such as insects, smoke, dust, or dirt particles, from coming into contact with the eyeball. Along the inner margin of the thin skin of the lid, *meibomian glands* secrete sebum, an oily substance that helps keep the eyelids from sticking together. These glands are embedded in the tarsal plate of each eyelid and are called *tarsal glands* and *palpebral glands.*

Conjunctiva

Lining the underside of each eyelid and reflected onto the anterior portion of the eyeball is a mucous membrane known as the **conjunctiva**. This membrane acts as a protective covering for the exposed surface of the eyeball.

Lacrimal Apparatus

Included in the **lacrimal apparatus** are those structures that produce, store, and remove the tears that cleanse and lubricate the eye. These structures are the lacrimal gland, located in the outer corner of each eyelid, lacrimal canaliculi (ducts), the lacrimal sac, and the nasolacrimal duct, which empties into the nasal cavity (see Figure 16.3 ■).

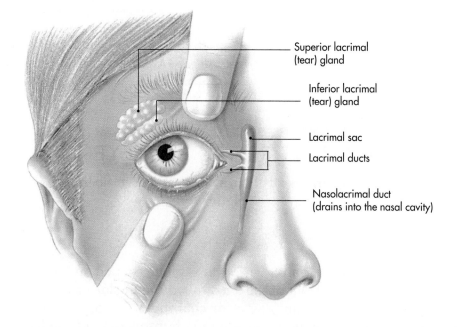

Superior lacrimal
(tear) gland

Inferior lacrimal
(tear) gland

Lacrimal sac

Lacrimal ducts

Nasolacrimal duct
(drains into the nasal cavity)

■ **Figure 16.3** Lacrimal glands and lacrimal canaliculi (ducts).

Lacrimal Gland

Located above the outer corner of the eye, the **lacrimal gland** secretes tears through approximately 12 ducts onto the surface of the conjunctiva of the upper lid. This fluid washes across the anterior surface of the eye and is collected by the *lacrimal canaliculi* (ducts).

Lacrimal Canaliculi

The **lacrimal canaliculi** are the two ducts at the inner corner of the eye that collect tears and drain into the lacrimal sac.

Lacrimal Sac

The enlargement of the upper portion of the lacrimal duct is known as the **lacrimal sac.** Tears secreted by the lacrimal glands are pulled into this sac and subsequently forced into the nasolacrimal duct by the blinking action of the eyelids. The sac is dilated and pulls in fluid as the muscles associated with blinking close the lids. The sac constricts, forcing the fluid down the nasolacrimal duct as the lids are opened.

Nasolacrimal Duct

The passageway draining lacrimal fluid into the nose is known as the **nasolacrimal duct.** The lacrimal sac is the enlarged upper portion of this duct.

LIFE SPAN CONSIDERATIONS

The eyes begin to develop as an outgrowth of the forebrain in the 4-week-old embryo. At 24 weeks, the eyes are structurally complete. At 28 weeks, eyebrows and eyelashes are present, and the eyelids open. The newborn can see, and **visual acuity** is estimated to be around 20/400. Most newborns appear to have crossed eyes because their eye muscles are not fully developed. At first, the eyes appear to be blue or gray. Permanent coloring becomes fixed between 6 and 12 months of age. Tears do not appear until approximately 1 to 3 months because the lacrimal gland ducts are immature. Depth perception begins to develop around 9 months of age. Visual acuity improves with age and by the age of 2 or 3 years, it is around 20/30 or 20/20. Children are farsighted until about 5 years of age.

INTERNAL STRUCTURES OF THE EYE

The eyeball, its various structures, and the nerve fibers connecting it to the brain make up the internal eye (see Figure 16.1).

Eyeball

The **eyeball** is the organ of vision. It is globe shaped and is divided into two cavities. The space in front of the lens, called the **ocular cavity**, is further divided by the iris into **anterior** and **posterior chambers.** The anterior chamber is filled with a watery fluid known as the **aqueous humor.** Behind the lens is a much larger cavity filled with a jellylike material, the **vitreous humor**, which maintains the eyeball's spherical shape. The three layers forming the outer, middle, and inner surfaces of the eyeball as well as the lens and its functions are discussed here.

Outer Layer

The eyeball's outer layer is composed of the **sclera** or white of the eye and the **cornea** or transparent anterior portion of the eye's fibrous outer surface. The curved surface of the cornea is important because it bends light rays and helps to focus them on the surface of the retina.

Middle Layer

Known as the **uvea**, the middle layer of the eyeball, lying just below the sclera, consists of the iris, the ciliary body, and the choroid.

The **iris** is a colored membrane attached to the ciliary body and suspended between the lens and the cornea in the aqueous humor. It has a circular opening in its center—the **pupil**—and two muscles that contract or dilate to regulate the amount of light admitted by the pupil.

The **ciliary body** is a thickened portion of the vascular membrane to which the iris is attached. Smooth muscle forming a part of the ciliary body governs the convexity of the lens. The ciliary body secretes nutrient fluids (the *aqueous humor*) that nourish the cornea, the lens, and the surrounding tissues.

The **choroid** is a pigmented vascular membrane that prevents internal reflection of light.

Inner Layer

The innermost layer of the eye, or **retina**, is richly supplied with blood vessels and contains photoreceptive cells that translate light waves focused on its surface into nerve impulses. See Figure 16.4 ■

The photoreceptor cells of the retina are the **rods** and **cones.** Rods are sensitive to dim light and used for night vision. Cones are sensitive to bright light and color vision. Most of the approximately 6 million cone cells are grouped into a small area

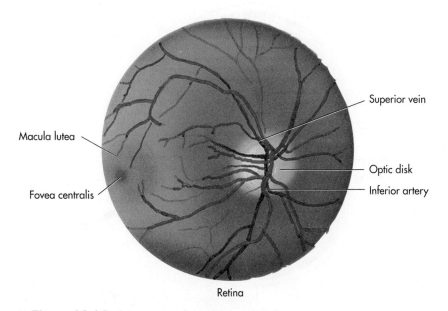

Macula lutea

Superior vein

Fovea centralis

Optic disk

Inferior artery

Retina

■ **Figure 16.4** Retina as seen through an ophthalmoscope.

called the **macula lutea.** In the center of the macula lutea is a small depression, the **fovea centralis**, which is the central focusing point within the eye; it contains only cone cells. The eye contains approximately 120 million rods that are sensitive to dim light. They contain **rhodopsin**, a pigment necessary for night vision.

The point at which nerve fibers from the retina converge to form the optic nerve is known as the **optic disk.** At the optic disk, fibers of the optic nerve extend to the thalamus and on to the visual cortical areas of the brain. The absence of rods and cones in the area of the optic disk creates a *blind spot* on the surface of the retina, located about 3 millimeters to the nasal side of the macula. It is the only part of the retina that is insensitive to light.

Lens

A colorless crystalline body biconvex in shape and enclosed in a transparent capsule, the **lens** is suspended by ligaments just behind the iris. Contraction and relaxation of the ciliary muscle control the tension of the suspensory ligaments to change the shape of the lens. The function of the lens is to sharpen the focus of light on the retina. This process, called **accommodation (Acc)**, is reflexive in nature and combines changes in the size of the pupil, the curvature of the lens, and the convergence of the optic axes to keep the image in the same place on both retinae. Accommodation occurs for both near and distant vision.

HOW SIGHT OCCURS

When a person views external objects, the light rays strike the eye and then pass through the cornea, pupil, aqueous humor, lens, and vitreous humor. They then reach the retina and stimulate the rods and cones. An upside-down image is relayed along nerve impulses to the optic nerve. The images are transferred to the brain, which turns the images into a right-side-up image. This image is the one that the person sees. See Figures 16.5 ■ and 16.6 ■

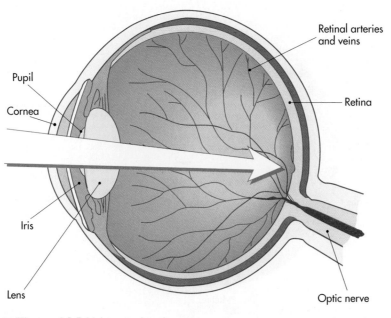

■ **Figure 16.5** Light entering the eye.

EYE

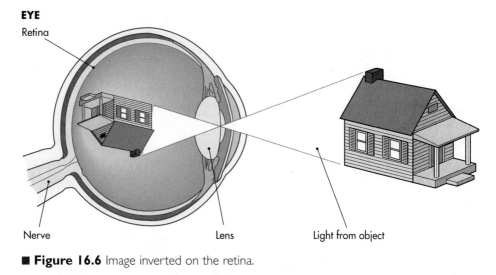

■ **Figure 16.6** Image inverted on the retina.

Anatomy and Physiology Labeling

Identify the structures shown below by filling in the blanks.

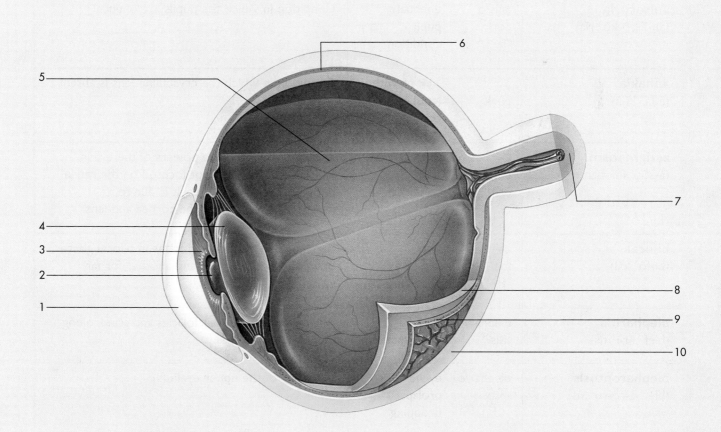

• Building Your Medical Vocabulary •

This section provides the foundation for learning medical terminology. Review the following alphabetized word list. Note how common prefixes and suffixes are repeatedly applied to word roots and combining forms to create different meanings. The word parts are color-coded: prefixes are green, suffixes are blue, **roots/combining forms are red**.

   You will find that some terms have not been divided into word parts. These are common words or specialized terms that are included to enhance your medical vocabulary. See Chapter 1, page 7, to review pronunciation guidelines.

MEDICAL WORD	WORD PARTS		DEFINITION
	Part	**Meaning**	
accommodation (Acc) (ă-kŏm″ ō-dā′ shn)			Process by which the eyes make adjustments to see objects at various distances
amblyopia (ăm″ blĭ-ō′ pĭ-ă)	ambly -opia	dull vision	Dullness of vision; reduced or dimness of vision; also called *lazy eye*
anisocoria (ăn-ī″ sō-kŏ′ rĭă)	anis/o cor -ia	unequal pupil condition	Condition in which the pupils are unequal
aphakia (ă-fā′ kĭ-ă)	a- phak -ia	lack of, without lentil, lens condition	Condition in which the crystalline lens is absent
astigmatism (ă-stĭg′ mă-tĭzm)	a- stigmat -ism	lack of, without point condition	Defect in the refractive powers of the eye in which a ray of light is not focused on the retina but is spread over an area. It is due to a misshapen curvature of the cornea and lens.
bifocal (bī-fō′ kăl)	bi- foc -al	two focus pertaining to	Pertaining to having two foci, as in bifocal glasses; one foci for near vision and another for far vision
blepharitis (blĕf″ ăr-ī′ tĭs)	blephar -itis	eyelid inflammation	Inflammation of the hair follicles and glands along the edges of the eyelids
blepharoptosis (blĕf″ ă-rō-tō′ sĭs)	blephar/o -ptosis	eyelid prolapse, drooping	Drooping of the upper eyelid(s)

MEDICAL WORD	WORD PARTS		DEFINITION
	Part	Meaning	
cataract (kăt″ ə răkt′)			Opacity of the crystalline lens or its capsule; most often occurs in older adults. See Figure 16.7 ▪ The most common symptoms of a cataract are cloudy or blurry vision; problems with light, including headlights that seem too bright at night, glare from lamps or very bright sunlight, and seeing a halo around lights; colors that seem faded; poor night vision; double or multiple vision; and frequent need for changes in eyeglass or contact lens prescription. Surgery is the only effective treatment for a cataract. See *phacoemulsification* on page 575.

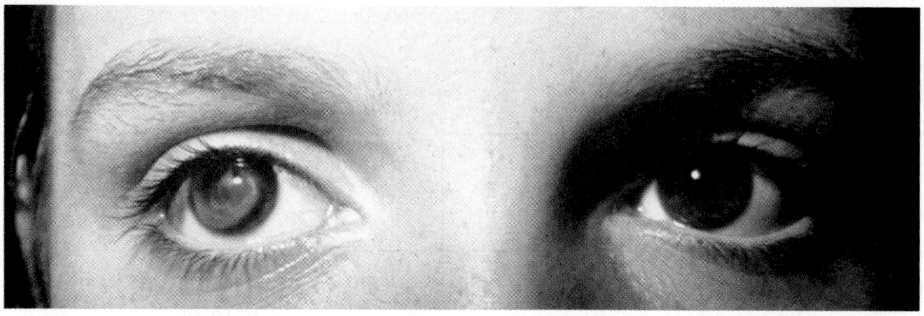

▪ **Figure 16.7** Cataract of the right eye.

MEDICAL WORD	WORD PARTS		DEFINITION
chalazion (kă-lā′ zĭ-ŏn)			Small, hard, painless cyst of a sebaceous gland of the eyelids
choroiditis (kō″ royd-ī′ tĭs)	choroid -itis	choroid inflammation	Inflammation of the vascular coat of the eye
conjunctivitis (kŏn-junk″ tĭ-vi tĭs)	conjunctiv -itis	to join together, conjunctiva inflammation	Inflammation of the conjunctiva that can be caused by allergens, irritating substances (shampoo, dirt, smoke, pool chlorine), bacteria, viruses, or sexually transmitted diseases (STDs). The type called *pinkeye* is usually infectious and contagious.

MEDICAL WORD	WORD PARTS		DEFINITION
	Part	**Meaning**	

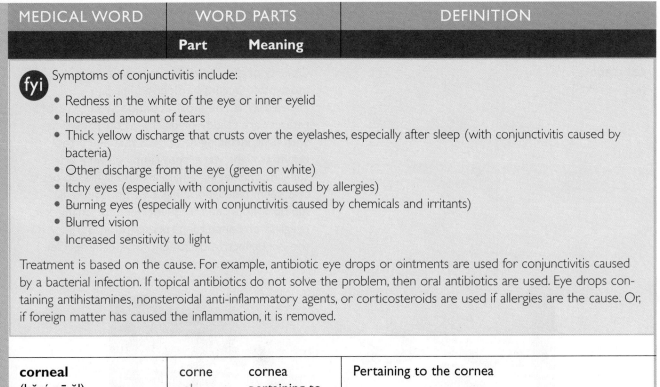

(fyi) Symptoms of conjunctivitis include:

- Redness in the white of the eye or inner eyelid
- Increased amount of tears
- Thick yellow discharge that crusts over the eyelashes, especially after sleep (with conjunctivitis caused by bacteria)
- Other discharge from the eye (green or white)
- Itchy eyes (especially with conjunctivitis caused by allergies)
- Burning eyes (especially with conjunctivitis caused by chemicals and irritants)
- Blurred vision
- Increased sensitivity to light

Treatment is based on the cause. For example, antibiotic eye drops or ointments are used for conjunctivitis caused by a bacterial infection. If topical antibiotics do not solve the problem, then oral antibiotics are used. Eye drops containing antihistamines, nonsteroidal anti-inflammatory agents, or corticosteroids are used if allergies are the cause. Or, if foreign matter has caused the inflammation, it is removed.

MEDICAL WORD	Part	Meaning	DEFINITION
corneal (kŏr´ nē-ăl)	corne -al	cornea pertaining to	Pertaining to the cornea
corneal transplant (kŏr´ nē-ăl)			Surgical process of transferring the cornea from a donor to a patient
cryosurgery (krī´´ ō-sur´ jur-ē)	cry/o surgery	cold surgery	Type of surgery that uses extreme cold to destroy tissue or to produce well-demarcated areas of cell injury; can be used in the removal of cataracts and in the repair of retinal detachment
cycloplegia (sī´´ klō-plē´ jĭ-ă)	cycl/o -plegia	ciliary body stroke, paralysis	Paralysis of the ciliary muscle
dacryoma (dăk´´ rĭ-ŏ´ mă)	dacry -oma	tear, lacrimal duct, tear duct tumor	Tumorlike swelling caused by obstruction of the tear duct(s)
diplopia (dĭp-lō´ pĭ-ă)	dipl/o -opia	double sight, vision	Double vision. Note that the suffix begins with a vowel, so the "o" on the combining form *dipl/o* is dropped.
electroretinogram (ē-lěk´´ trō-rět´ ĭ-nō-grăm)	electr/o retin/o -gram	electricity retina mark, record	Record of the electrical response of the retina to light stimulation

MEDICAL WORD	WORD PARTS		DEFINITION
	Part	Meaning	
emmetropia (EM) (ĕm″ ĕ-trō′ pĭ-ă)	em-	in	Normal or perfect vision. See Figure 16.8A ■
	metr	measure	
	-opia	sight, vision	

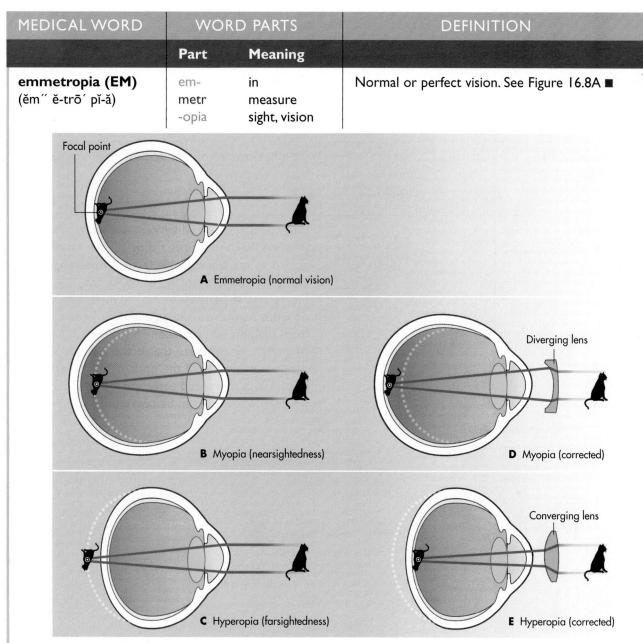

■ **Figure 16.8** Normal vision and visual abnormalities. (A) In normal vision, the lens focuses the visual image on the retina. Common problems with the accommodation mechanism involve (B) myopia, the inability to lengthen the focal distance enough to focus the image of a distant object on the retina and (C) hyperopia, the inability to shorten the focal distance adequately for nearby objects. These conditions can be corrected by placing appropriately shaped lenses in front of the eyes. (D) Diverging lens is used to correct myopia and (E) converging lens is used to correct hyperopia.

entropion (ĕn-trō-pē-ŏn)	en-	in	Turning inward of the margin of the lower eyelid
	trop	turn	
	-ion	process	
enucleation (ē-nū″ klē-ā′ shŭn)	enucleat	to remove the kernel of	Process of removing an entire part or mass without rupture, as the eyeball from its orbit
	-ion	process	

MEDICAL WORD	WORD PARTS		DEFINITION
	Part	Meaning	
esotropia (ST) (ĕs″ ō-trō′ pĭ-ă)	eso- trop -ia	inward turn condition	Condition in which the eye or eyes turn inward; *crossed* eyes
exotropia (XT) (ĕks″ ō-trō′ pē-ă)	ex(o)- trop -ia	out turn condition	Turning outward of one or both eyes
glaucoma (glaw-kō′ mă)			Disease characterized by *increased intraocular pressure (IOP)*. The three major categories of glaucoma are closed-angle (acute), open-angle (chronic), and congenital glaucoma. See Figure 16.9 ■ Glaucoma occurs when the aqueous humor is blocked and drains too slowly from the anterior chamber. This causes a buildup of intraocular pressure that is too high for the proper functioning of the optic nerve. When glaucoma is diagnosed early and managed properly, blindness can be prevented.

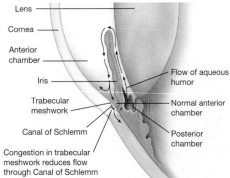

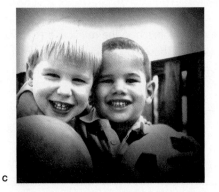

■ **Figure 16.9** In glaucoma, the accumulation of aqueous humor in the anterior chamber of the eye causes pressure to build, resulting in eventual loss of vision. (A) and (B) show two forms of glaucoma; (C) shows the narrowing of the optic field that is a typical symptom of untreated glaucoma.

MEDICAL WORD	WORD PARTS		DEFINITION
	Part	**Meaning**	

MEDICAL WORD	WORD PARTS		DEFINITION
gonioscope (gō´ nĭ-ō-skōp)	goni/o -scope	angle instrument for examining	Instrument used to examine the angle of the anterior chamber of the eye
hemianopia (hĕm´´ ē-ă-nŏ´ pē-ă)	hemi- an- -opia	half lack of sight, vision	Inability (blindness) to see half of the field of vision
hyperopia (HT) (hī´´ pĕr-ō´ pĭ-ă)	hyper- -opia	beyond sight, vision	Vision defect in which parallel rays come to a focus beyond the retina; *farsightedness*. See Figure 16.8C ■ and E ■
intraocular (ĭn´´ trăh-ŏk´ ū-lăr)	intra- ocul -ar	within eye pertaining to	Pertaining to within the eye
iridectomy (ĭr´´ ĭ-dĕk´ tō-mē)	irid -ectomy	iris surgical excision	Surgical excision of a portion of the iris
iridocyclitis (ĭr´´ ĭd-ō-sī-klī´ tĭs)	irid/o cycl -itis	iris ciliary body inflammation	Inflammation of the iris and ciliary body
keratitis (kĕr´´ ă-tī´ tĭs)	kerat -itis	cornea inflammation	Inflammation of the cornea
keratoconjunctivitis (kĕr´´ ă-tō-kŏn-jŭnk´´ tĭ-vī´ tĭs)	kerat/o conjunctiv -itis	cornea to join together, conjunctiva inflammation	Inflammation of the cornea and the conjunctiva

MEDICAL WORD	WORD PARTS		DEFINITION
	Part	**Meaning**	
keratoplasty (kĕr´ ă-tō-plăs˝ tē)	kerat/o -plasty	cornea surgical repair	Surgical repair of the cornea
lacrimal (lăk´ rĭm-ăl)	lacrim -al	tear, lacrimal duct, tear duct pertaining to	Pertaining to the tears
laser (lā´ zĕr)			Acronym for *light amplification by stimulated emission of radiation*

fyi Laser surgery can be used to treat glaucoma, including the following types:

1. Laser peripheral iridotomy (LPI) in which a small hole is made in the iris to allow it to fall back from the fluid channel and help the fluid drain.
2. Argon laser trabeculoplasty (ALT) in which a laser beam opens the fluid channels of the eye, helping the drainage system to work better.
3. Selective laser trabeculoplasty (SLT), a type of laser surgery that uses a combination of frequencies allowing the laser to work at very low levels. It treats specific cells selectively and leaves untreated portions of the trabecular meshwork (the meshlike drainage canals surrounding the iris) intact.
4. When medication and/or laser surgery does not lower the intraocular pressure of the eye, the doctor could recommend a procedure called *filtering microsurgery*. This procedure makes a tiny drainage hole in the sclera (*sclerostomy*). The new drainage hole allows fluid to flow out of the eye and thereby helps lower eye pressure. This prevents or reduces damage to the optic nerve.

macular degeneration (măk´ ū-lăr dē´ gĕn-ēr˝ă -shŭn)			Degeneration of the macular area of the retina, an area important in the visualization of fine details. The two basic types of macular degeneration are dry and wet. In the dry type, the deterioration of the retina is associated with the formation of small yellow deposits (*drusen*), under the macula. This leads to a thinning and drying out of the macula. The amount of central vision loss is directly related to the location and amount of retinal thinning caused by the drusen. There is no known treatment or cure for the dry type of macular degeneration. Approximately 10% of the cases of macular degeneration are the wet (exudative) type. In this type of macular degeneration, abnormal blood vessels (known as *subretinal neovascularization*) grow under the retina and macula. These new blood vessels can then bleed and leak fluid, thereby causing the macula to bulge or lift up, thus distorting or destroying central vision. This can cause rapid and severe vision loss. If vision is to be saved, immediate laser surgery should be done in the early stages of wet macular degeneration.

MEDICAL WORD	WORD PARTS		DEFINITION
	Part	**Meaning**	

LIFE SPAN CONSIDERATIONS

Macular degeneration is an incurable, age-related, progressive eye disease that affects more than 10 million Americans. It is the leading cause of blindness for those ages 55 and older. For the first time, researchers have linked gene defects to macular degeneration, which could lead to the ability to identify people at high risk for the disorder and perhaps ways to treat or prevent vision loss.

LIFE SPAN CONSIDERATIONS

Stargardt's disease, also known as *juvenile macular degeneration*, is an inherited disease that usually manifests itself between the ages of 7 and 12. Scientists' current theory is that Stargardt's disease causes the eye's central vision to deteriorate because the rod cells just outside the macula erode, which eventually harms the retinal pigment epithelium (RPE). As the RPE fails, the disease can spread to the macula's cone cells, causing macular degeneration's characteristic loss of central vision. Vision loss is usually slow until the 20/40 level and then rapidly progresses to the 20/200 level. Unfortunately, in some cases, vision can degenerate to 10/200 in a period of months. Peripheral vision generally remains.

Presently there is no cure for Stargardt's disease, nor has any treatment been proven to improve visual loss or to retard the progression of the disease.

MEDICAL WORD	WORD PARTS Part	Meaning	DEFINITION
microlens (mǐ′ krō-lĕns)			Small, thin corneal contact lens
miotic (mǐ-ŏt′ ǐk)	mi/o -tic	less, small pertaining to	Pertaining to an agent that causes the pupil to contract
mydriatic (mǐd″ rǐ-ăt′ ǐk)	mydriat -ic	dilation, widen pertaining to	Pertaining to an agent that causes the pupil to dilate
myopia (MY) (mǐ-ŏ′ pǐ-ă)			Vision defect in which parallel rays come to a focus in front of the retina; *nearsightedness*. See Figure 16.8B ■ and D ■
nyctalopia (nǐk″ tă-lō′ pǐ-ă)	nyctal -opia	night sight, vision	Condition in which the individual has difficulty seeing at night; *night blindness*
nystagmus (nǐs-tăg′ mŭs)			Involuntary, constant, rhythmic movement of the eyeball
ocular (ŏk′ ū-lar)	ocul -ar	eye pertaining to	Pertaining to the eye

MEDICAL WORD	WORD PARTS		DEFINITION
	Part	**Meaning**	
ocular fundus (ŏk´ ū-lar fŭn-dŭs)			Posterior inner part of the eye as seen with an ophthalmoscope
ophthalmologist (ŏf″ thăl-mŏl´ ō-jĭst)	ophthalm/o log -ist	eye study of one who specializes	Physician who specializes in the study of the eye
ophthalmology (ŏf″ thăl-mŏl´ ō-jē)	ophthalm/o -logy	eye study of	Study of the eye
ophthalmoscope (ŏf″ thăl´ mō-skōp)	ophthalm/o -scope	eye instrument for examining	Medical instrument used to examine the interior of the eye. See Figure 16.10 ■

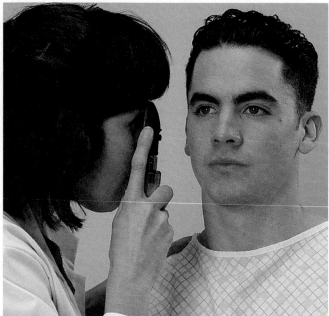

■ **Figure 16.10** Use of an ophthalmoscope to examine the interior of the eye.

optic (op´ tĭk)	opt -ic	eye pertaining to	Pertaining to the eye
optician (ŏp-tĭsh´ ăn)	opt -ician	eye specialist	One who specializes in making optical products and accessories, such as eyeglasses. This person is not a physician.
optometrist (ŏp-tŏm´ ĕ-trĭst)	opt/o metr -ist	eye measure one who specializes	One who specializes in examining the eyes for refractive errors and providing appropriate corrective lenses. This person is not a physician but is trained and licensed as a doctor of optometry (OD).

MEDICAL WORD	WORD PARTS		DEFINITION
	Part	Meaning	
optomyometer (ŏp″ tō-mī-ŏm´ ĕt-ĕr)	opt/o my/o -meter	eye muscle instrument to measure	Instrument used to measure the strength of the muscles of the eye
orthoptics (or-thŏp´ tĭks)	orth opt -ic (s)	straight eye pertaining to	Study and treatment of defective binocular vision resulting from defects in ocular musculature; also a technique of eye exercises for correcting defective binocular vision
phacoemulsification (făk″ ō-ē´ mŭl´ sĭ-fĭ-kā″ shŭn)	phac/o emulsificat -ion	lens disintegrate process	Process of using ultrasound to disintegrate a cataract by inserting a needle through a small incision and aspirating the disintegrated cataract. See Figure 16.11 ■

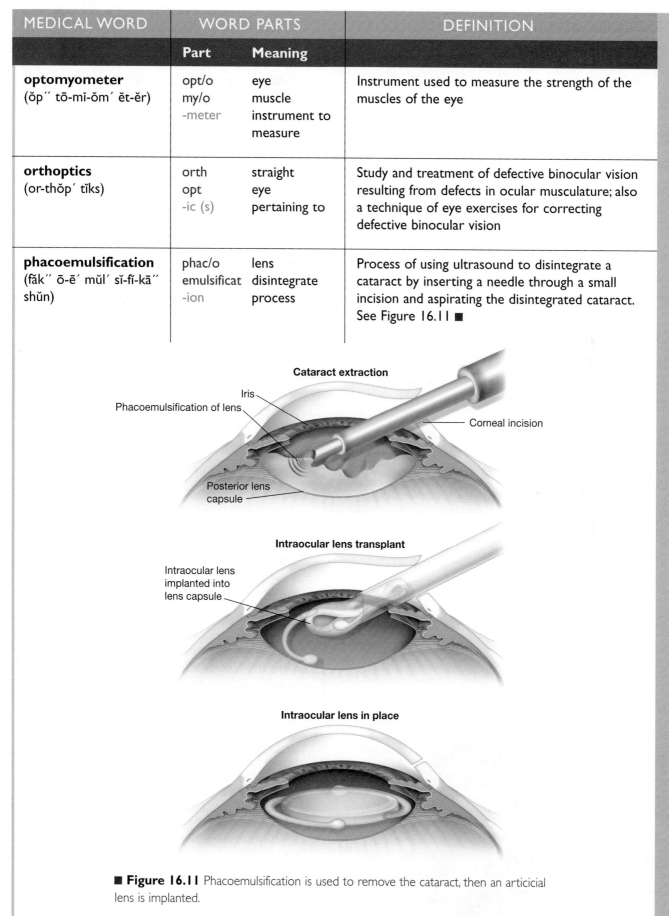

Cataract extraction

Iris

Phacoemulsification of lens

Corneal incision

Posterior lens capsule

Intraocular lens transplant

Intraocular lens implanted into lens capsule

Intraocular lens in place

■ **Figure 16.11** Phacoemulsification is used to remove the cataract, then an articicial lens is implanted.

MEDICAL WORD	WORD PARTS		DEFINITION
	Part	**Meaning**	
phacolysis (făk-ŏl″ ĭ-sĭs)	phac/o -lysis	lens destruction, to separate	Surgical destruction and removal of the crystalline lens in the treatment of a cataract
phacosclerosis (făk″ ō-sklĕr-ō′ sĭs)	phac/o scler -osis	lens hardening, sclera condition	Condition of hardening of the crystalline lens
photocoagulation (fō″ tō-kō-ăg″ ū-lā′ shŭn)	phot/o coagulat -ion	light to clot process	Process of altering proteins in tissue by the use of light energy such as the laser beam; used to treat retinal detachment, retinal bleeding, intraocular tumors, and/or macular degeneration (wet)
photophobia (fō″ tō-fō′ bĭ-ă)	phot/o -phobia	light fear	Unusual intolerance to light
presbyopia (prĕz″ bĭ-ō′ pĭ-ă)	presby -opia	old sight, vision	Vision defect in which parallel rays come to a focus beyond the retina; occurs normally with aging; also called *hyperopia* (farsightedness). See Figure 16.8C.
pupillary (pū′ pĭ-lĕr-ē)	pupill -ary	pupil pertaining to	Pertaining to the pupil
radial keratotomy (rā′ dē-ăl kĕr-ă′ tŏt′ ō-mē)	rad/i -al kerat/o -tomy	radiating out from a center pertaining to cornea incision	Surgical procedure that can be performed to correct nearsightedness (*myopia*). Delicate spoke-like incisions are made in the cornea to flatten it, thereby shortening the eyeball so that light reaches the retina. Vision is not improved for all patients, and complications could lead to blindness.
retinal detachment (rĕt′ ĭ-năl dē-tăch′mĕnt)			Separation of the retina from the choroid layer of the eye that can be caused by trauma or can occur spontaneously. See Figure 16.12 ■

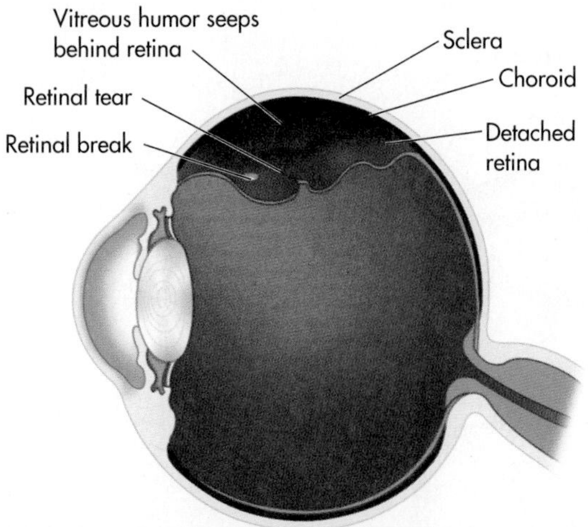

Vitreous humor seeps behind retina
Retinal tear
Retinal break
Sclera
Choroid
Detached retina

■ **Figure 16.12** Retinal detachment.

MEDICAL WORD	WORD PARTS		DEFINITION
	Part	Meaning	
retinitis (rĕt″ ĭ-nī′ tĭs)	retin -itis	retina inflammation	Inflammation of the retina
retinitis pigmentosa (rĕt″ ĭ-nī′ tĭs pĭg″ mēnt′ ŏsă)			Chronic progressive disease marked by bilateral primary degeneration of the retina beginning in childhood and leading to blindness by middle age. Night blindness and a reduced field of vision are early clinical signs of this disease.
retinoblastoma (rĕt″ ĭ-nō-blăs-tō′ mă)	retin/o -blast -oma	retina germ cell tumor	Malignant tumor arising from the germ cell of the retina
retinopathy (rĕt″ ĭn-ŏp′ ă-thē)	retin/o -pathy	retina disease	Any disease of the retina. In the United States, *diabetic retinopathy* is the leading cause of new blindness in people ages 20–74. See Figure 16.13 ■

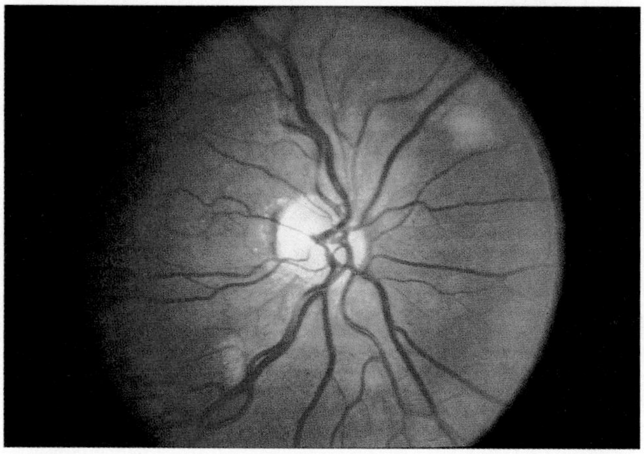

■ **Figure 16.13** Appearance of the ocular fundus in diabetic retinopathy. (Courtesy of the National Eye Institute, National Institutes of Health)

retrolental fibroplasia (RLF) (rĕt″ rō-lĕn-tăl fĭ-brō-plā-sē-ă)	retro- lent -al fibr/o -plasia	behind lens pertaining to fiber formation	Disease of the retinal vessels present in premature infants; can be caused by excessive use of oxygen in the incubator; can cause retinal detachment and blindness
scleritis (sklē-rī′ tĭs)	scler -itis	hardening, sclera inflammation	Inflammation of the sclera (white of the eye)
strabismus (stră-bĭz′ mŭs)	strabism -us	a squinting structure	Disorder of the eye in which the optic axes cannot be directed to the same object; *squinting*
sty(e) (stī)			Inflammation of one or more of the sebaceous glands of the eyelid; also called a *hordeolum*

MEDICAL WORD	WORD PARTS		DEFINITION
	Part	**Meaning**	
tonography (tō-nŏg´ ră-fē)	ton/o -graphy	tone recording	Recording of intraocular pressure used in detecting glaucoma
tonometer (tŏn-ŏm´ ĕ-tĕr)	ton/o -meter	tone instrument to measure	Medical instrument used to measure intraocular pressure. See Figure 16.14 ■

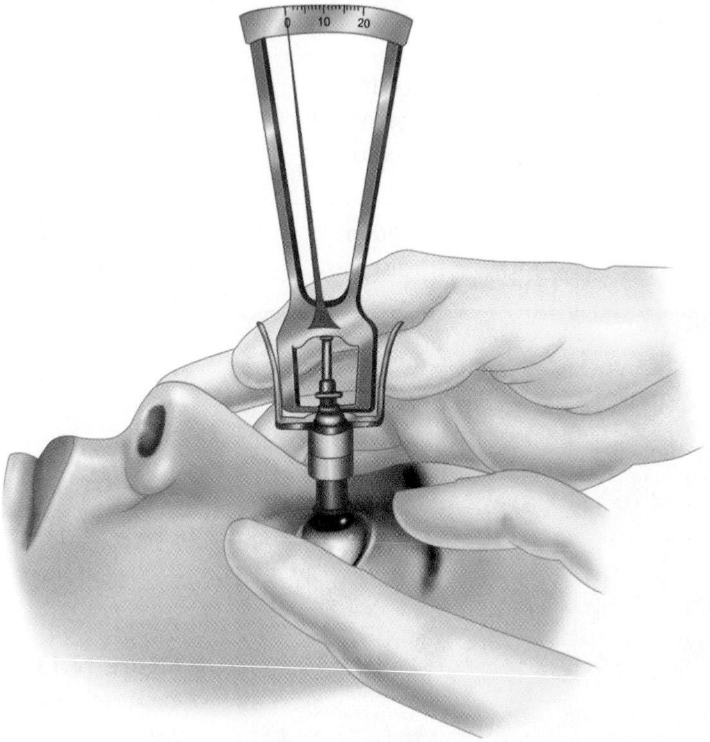

■ **Figure 16.14** Schiötz tonometer for measuring intraocular pressure.

MEDICAL WORD	WORD PARTS		DEFINITION
trichiasis (trĭk-ī´ ăs-ĭs)	trich -iasis	hair condition	Condition of ingrowing eyelashes that rub against the cornea, causing a constant irritation to the eyeball
trifocal (trĭ-fō´ căl)	tri- foc -al	three focus pertaining to	Pertaining to having three foci
uveal (ū´ vē-ăl)	uve -al	uvea pertaining to	Pertaining to the second or vascular coat of the eye
uveitis (ū-vē-ī´ tĭs)	uve -itis	uvea inflammation	Inflammation of the uvea (consists of the iris, ciliary body, and choroid, and forms the pigmented layer)

MEDICAL WORD	WORD PARTS		DEFINITION
	Part	Meaning	
xenophthalmia (zĕn″ ŏf-thăl′ mē-ă)	xen	foreign material	Inflamed eye condition caused by foreign material
	ophthalm	eye	
	-ia	condition	
xerophthalmia (zē-rŏf-thăl′ mē-ă)	xer	dry	Eye condition in which the conjunctiva is dry
	ophthalm	eye	
	-ia	condition	

• Drug Highlights •

TYPE OF DRUG	DESCRIPTION AND EXAMPLES
drugs used to treat glaucoma	Either increase the outflow of aqueous humor, decrease its production, or produce both of these actions.
prostaglandin analogues	Work by increasing the drainage of intraocular fluid, thereby decreasing intraocular pressure.
	EXAMPLES: Travatan (travoprost ophthalmic solution 0.004%), Lumigan (bimatoprost ophthalmic solution 0.03%), and Xalatan (latanoprost)
adrenergic drugs	Increase drainage of intraocular fluid.
	EXAMPLES: Propine ophthalmic solution and USP 0.1% (epinephrine)
alpha antagonist	Works both to decrease production of fluid and increase drainage.
	EXAMPLE: Alphagan P (brimonide tartrate ophthalmic solution 0.1%)
beta blockers	Decrease production of intraocular fluid.
	EXAMPLES: Akbeta (levobunolol HCl ophthalmic solution, USP), carteolol HCl ophthalmic solution, Timolol Maleate, Betoptic S (betaxolol HCl 0.25%), Betagan Liquifilm Sterile Ophthalmic Solution (levobunolol), OptiPranolol (metipranolol), Timoptic-XE (timolol maleate ophthalmic gel forming solution), Betimol (timolol hemihydrate), and Ocupress (carteolol HCl)
carbonic anhydrase inhibitors	Decrease production of intraocular fluid.
	EXAMPLES: Azopt (brinzolamide ophthalmic suspension 1%), Diamox Sequels Sustained Release Capsules (acetazolomide), and Trusopt (dorzolamide)
cholinergic (miotic)	Increases drainage of intraocular fluid.
	EXAMPLE: Pilocarpine HCl Ophthalmic Solution

TYPE OF DRUG	DESCRIPTION AND EXAMPLES
cholinesterase	Increases drainage of intraocular fluid.
	EXAMPLE: Phospholine Iodide (echothiophate)
combination of beta blocker and carbonic anhydrase inhibitor	Decreases production of intraocular fluid.
	EXAMPLE: Cosopt (dorzolomide HCl timolol maleate ophthalmic solution)
mydriatics	Agents used to dilate the pupil (mydriasis); can be anticholinergics or sympathomimetics.
anticholinergics	Dilate the pupil and interfere with the ability of the eye to focus properly (cycloplegia). They are used primarily as an aid in refraction, during internal examination of the eye, in intraocular surgery, and in the treatment of anterior uveitis and secondary glaucomas.
	EXAMPLES: atropine sulfate, Mydriacyl (tropicamide)
sympathomimetics	Produce mydriasis without cycloplegia. Pupil dilation is obtained as the drug causes contraction of the dilator muscle of the iris. They also affect intraocular pressure by decreasing production of aqueous humor while increasing its outflow from the eye.
	EXAMPLES: Propine (dipivefrin HCl), Albalon (naphazoline HCl), epinephrine HCl, and neosynephrine (phenylephrine HCl)
antibiotics	Used to treat infectious diseases, especially those caused by bacteria. Those used for the eye can be in the form of an ointment, cream, or solution.
	EXAMPLES: chloramphenicol, polymyxin B sulfate, moxifloxacin (Vigamox), and gatifloxacin (Zymar)
antifungal agent	Natacyn (natamycin) is used to treat fungal infections of the eye, such as blepharitis, conjunctivitis, and keratitis.
antiviral agents	Stoxil and Herplex (idoxuridine) are potent antiviral agents used to treat keratitis caused by the herpes simplex virus. Vira-A (vidarabine) and Viroptic (trifluridine) are also used to treat viral infections of the eye and are effective in the treatment of herpes simplex infections.

• Diagnostic and Lab Tests •

TEST	DESCRIPTION
color vision tests	Use of polychromatic (multicolored) charts or an *anomaloscope* (a device for detecting color blindness) to assess an individual's ability to recognize differences in color. A person who is color blind will not see the number 27 in the circle in Figure 16.15 ■

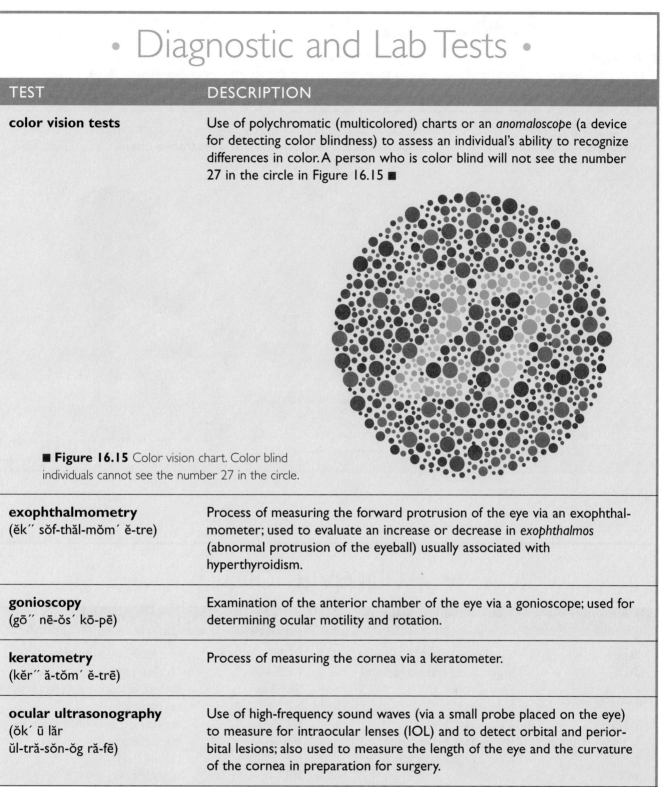

■ **Figure 16.15** Color vision chart. Color blind individuals cannot see the number 27 in the circle.

exophthalmometry (ĕk″ sŏf-thăl-mŏm′ ĕ-tre)	Process of measuring the forward protrusion of the eye via an exophthalmometer; used to evaluate an increase or decrease in *exophthalmos* (abnormal protrusion of the eyeball) usually associated with hyperthyroidism.
gonioscopy (gō″ nē-ŏs′ kō-pē)	Examination of the anterior chamber of the eye via a gonioscope; used for determining ocular motility and rotation.
keratometry (kĕr″ ă-tŏm′ ĕ-trē)	Process of measuring the cornea via a keratometer.
ocular ultrasonography (ŏk′ ū lăr ŭl-tră-sŏn-ŏg ră-fē)	Use of high-frequency sound waves (via a small probe placed on the eye) to measure for intraocular lenses (IOL) and to detect orbital and periorbital lesions; also used to measure the length of the eye and the curvature of the cornea in preparation for surgery.
ophthalmoscopy (ŏf-thăl-mŏs′ kō-pē)	Examination of the interior of the eyes via an ophthalmoscope; used to view the retina and identify changes in the blood vessels and to diagnose systemic diseases.

TEST	DESCRIPTION
tonometry (tŏn-ŏm´ ĕ-trē)	Measurement of the intraocular pressure (IOP) of the eye via a tonometer; used to screen for and detect glaucoma. See Figure 16.14.
visual acuity (VA) (vĭzh´ ū-ăl ă-kū´ ĭ-tē)	Acuteness or sharpness of vision. A Snellen eye chart can be used to test it; the patient reads letters of various sizes from a distance of 20 feet. Normal vision is 20/20. See Figure 16.16 ■

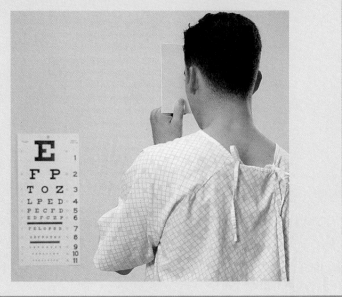

■ **Figure 16.16** Test of distance vision using the Snellen eye chart.

• Abbreviations •

ABBREVIATION	MEANING	ABBREVIATION	MEANING
Acc	accommodation	**RLF**	retrolental fibroplasias
ALT	argon laser trabeculoplasty	**RPE**	retinal pigment epithelium
EM	emmetropia	**SLT**	selective laser trabeculoplasty
HT	hyperopia	**ST**	esotropia
IOL	intraocular lens	**STDs**	sexually transmitted diseases
IOP	intraocular pressure	**VA**	visual acuity
LPI	laser peripheral iridotomy	**VF**	visual field
MY	myopia	**XT**	exotropia

y and Review • Study and Review • Study and Revie
Review • Study and Review • Study and Review • St
ew • **Study and Review** • Study and Review • Study

Anatomy and Physiology

Write your answers to the following questions.

1. The external structures of the eye are the _____ , _____ ,

   _____ , _____ , and the _____

   _____ .

2. The orbit is lined with _____ _____ , which cushions the eyeball.

3. The optic foramen is an opening for the _____ _____ and

   _____ _____ .

4. State the functions of the muscles of the eye.

   a. _____

   b. _____

5. Each eye has a pair of eyelids that function to protect the eyeball from _____ ,

   _____ _____ , and _____ .

6. Describe the conjunctiva and state its function. _____

   _____

7. Define *lacrimal apparatus.* _____

   _____

8. The internal structures of the eye are the _____ , _____ , and

   the _____ _____ .

9. The eyeball is the organ of _____ .

10. The point at which nerve fibers from the retina converge to form the optic nerve is known as the

    _____ _____ .

11. Define *accommodation.* _____

    _____

12. Match the following terms and definitions by placing the correct letter on the line provided.

_____ **1.** aqueous humor

_____ **2.** vitreous humor

_____ **3.** iris

_____ **4.** sclera

_____ **5.** uvea

_____ **6.** pupil

_____ **7.** retina

_____ **8.** rods and cones

_____ **9.** lens

_____ **10.** cornea

a. White of the eye

b. Colored membrane attached to the ciliary body

c. Watery fluid

d. Opening in the center of the iris

e. Jellylike material

f. Middle layer of the eyeball

g. Transparent anterior portion of the eyeball

h. Innermost layer of the eyeball

i. Photoreceptor cells

j. Colorless crystalline body

Word Parts

PREFIXES

Give the definitions of the following prefixes.

1. a- _____

2. bi- _____

3. en- _____

4. em- _____

5. eso- _____

6. hyper- _____

7. intra- _____

8. tri- _____

9. ex(o)- _____

10. hemi- _____

11. an- _____

12. retro- _____

ROOTS AND COMBINING FORMS

Give the definitions of the following roots and combining forms.

1. ambly _____

2. conjunctiv _____

3. anis/o _____

4. blephar _____

5. blephar/o _____

6. choroid _____

7. cry/o _____

8. cor _____

9. corne _____

10. cycl _____

11. cycl/o _____

12. enucleat _____

13. dacry _____

14. mi/o _____

15. electr/o _____

16. foc _____

17. goni/o _____

18. irid _____

19. irid/o _____

20. kerat _____

21. kerat/o _____

22. lacrim _____

23. log _____

24. metr _____

25. my _____

26. my/o _____

27. nyctal _____

28. ocul _____

29. ophthalm _____

30. ophthalm/o _____

31. opt _____

32. opt/o _____

33. phac/o _____

34. phak _____

35. phot/o _____

36. presby _____

37. pupill _____

38. retin _____

39. retin/o _____

40. scler _____

41. stigmat _____

42. ton/o _____

43. trop _____

44. uve _____

45. xen _____

46. xer _____

47. mydriat _____

48. orth _____

49. emulsificat _____

50. coagulat _____

51. rad/i _____

52. lent _____

53. fibr/o _____

54. strabism _____

55. trich _____

SUFFIXES

Give the definitions of the following suffixes.

1. -al _____

2. -ar _____

3. -ary _____

4. -blast _____

5. -iasis _____

6. -ectomy _____

7. -gram _____

8. -graphy _____

9. -ia _____

10. -ic _____

11. -ician _____

12. -ion _____

13. -ism _____

14. -ist _____

15. -itis _____

16. -logy _____

17. -lysis _____

18. -plasia _____

19. -meter _____

20. -oma _____

21. -opia _____

22. -osis _____

23. -pathy _____

24. -phobia _____

25. -plasty _____

26. -plegia _____

27. -ptosis _____

28. -scope _____

29. -tic _____

30. -tomy _____

31. -us _____

Identifying Medical Terms

In the spaces provided, write the medical terms for the following meanings.

1. _____ Dullness of vision

2. _____ Pertaining to having two foci

3. _____ Drooping of the upper eyelid(s)

4. _____ Pertaining to the cornea

5. _____ Tumorlike swelling caused by obstruction of the tear duct(s)

6. _____ Double vision

7. _____ Normal or perfect vision

8. _____ Pertaining to within the eye

9. _____ Inflammation of the cornea

10. _____ Surgical repair of the cornea

11. _____ Pertaining to tears

12. _____ Pertaining to the eye

13. _____ Unusual intolerance to light

Spelling

Circle the correct spelling of each medical term.

1. astigmatism / astigmatims
2. cyloplegia / cycloplegia
3. irdectomy / iridectomy
4. ophthalmologist / opthalmologist
5. pacosclerosis / phacosclerosis
6. pupilary / pupillary
7. retinoblastoma / retinblastoma
8. scleritis / sleritis
9. tonmeter / tonometer
10. ueal / uveal

Matching

Select the appropriate lettered meaning for each of the following words.

_____ 1. anomaloscope

_____ 2. entropion

_____ 3. cataract

_____ 4. hemianopia

_____ 5. phacoemulsification

_____ 6. photocoagulation

_____ 7. radial keratotomy

_____ 8. retrolental fibroplasia

_____ 9. strabismus

_____10. sty(e)

a. Disorder of the eye in which the optic axes cannot be directed to the same object

b. Disease of the retinal vessels present in premature infants

c. Process of using ultrasound to disintegrate a cataract

d. Use of a laser to treat retinal detachment and/or retinal bleeding

e. Device used to detect color blindness

f. Turning inward of the margin of the lower eyelid

g. Surgical procedure performed to correct myopia

h. Inability to see half of the field of vision

i. _Hordeolum_

j. Opacity of the crystalline lens or its capsule

k. Disease characterized by increased intraocular pressure

Abbreviations

Place the correct word, phrase, or abbreviation in the space provided.

1. accommodation _____

2. EM _____

3. HT _____

4. intraocular lens _____

5. esotropia _____

6. MY _____

7. VA _____

8. IOP _____

9. visual field _____

10. XT _____

Diagnostic and Laboratory Tests

Select the best answer to each multiple-choice question. Circle the letter of your choice.

1. Process of measuring the forward protrusion of the eye.
   a. gonioscopy
   b. keratometry
   c. exophthalmometry
   d. tonometry

2. Process of measuring the cornea.
   a. gonioscopy
   b. keratometry
   c. exophthalmometry
   d. tonometry

3. Used to identify changes in the blood vessels in the eye and to diagnose systemic diseases.
   a. exophthalmometry
   b. gonioscopy
   c. ophthalmoscopy
   d. tonometry

4. Process of measuring the intraocular pressure of the eye.
   a. exophthalmometry
   b. gonioscopy
   c. ophthalmoscopy
   d. tonometry

5. Process used to measure the acuteness or sharpness of vision.
   a. color vision tests
   b. ultrasonography
   c. tonometry
   d. visual acuity

PRACTICAL APPLICATION

MEDICAL RECORD ANALYSIS

This exercise contains information, abbreviations, and medical terminology from an actual medical record or case study that has been adapted for this text. The names and any personal information have been created by the author. Read and study each form or case study and then answer the questions that follow. You may refer to Appendix III, Abbreviations and Symbols, on page A41.

Instructions for Outpatient Cataract Surgery

Before Surgery

1. Your surgery has been scheduled for Tuesday, August 2, 20xx, as an outpatient at: Dewdrop Surgery Center.

2. Report to the center the day of surgery at 7:10 A.M.

3. The afternoon before surgery and the morning of surgery, use the antibiotics Vigamox and Zymar drops in the right eye to help prevent a bacterial infection. Afternoon and evening before surgery, 1 drop at 3:00, 5:00, 7:00, and 9:00 P.M.

4. Do not eat or drink anything the morning of surgery, except a sip of water to take your medications.

5. Do not wear makeup, fingernail polish, or jewelry to the center.

6. If you are normally taking any medications in the morning, especially heart or blood pressure medications, be sure to take them before you come to the center for surgery. However, if you take insulin or diabetes medication, do not take it until you get home from surgery.

7. Go by the outpatient surgery department at Dewdrop Center to pre-admit any time before the day of surgery.

After Surgery

1. You may go home shortly after surgery. Be sure to bring someone to drive you home. You may resume normal activities but do not engage in vigorous exercise on the day of surgery. Be careful not to have a fall.

2. The shield may be removed 6 hours after surgery. **DO NOT PUT ANY PRESSURE ON YOUR EYE AND DO NOT RUB YOUR EYE.** Put the Vigamox/Zymar drops in 3 times before you go to bed.

3. Return to Dr. Cedric Emmanuel's office on Wednesday, August 3, 20xx, at 10:25 A.M. and further instructions will be given. Bring all your eye drops to the office with you.

4. Continue any medications that you are taking unless otherwise instructed. Resume your usual diet.

5. If you have mild pain, take Tylenol Regular-strength (325 mg) acetaminophen: Two tablets every 4–6 as needed, not to exceed 12 tablets in 24 hours. If the pain is severe call Dr. Cedric Emmanuel: Office & Beeper (123) 456-7890.

Medical Record Questions

Place the correct answer in the space provided.

1. What type of medication is Vigamox and why is it ordered for this patient? _____

2. What type of medication is Zymar and why is it ordered for this patient? _____

3. Should the patient take his or her heart and blood pressure medicine the morning of surgery?

_____

4. When should the patient go by the Dewdrop Surgery Center to pre-admit?

_____

5. If the patient has mild pain what should he or she take? _____

---

igestive System • Cardiovascular System • Blood and L
natic System • Respiratory System • Urinary System •
ndocrine System • Nervous System • Special Senses: Th

• Female Reproductive System • Special Senses: T
with an Overview of Obstetrics • Male Reprod

17

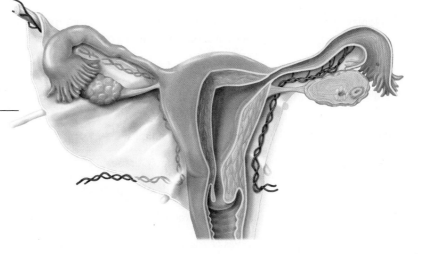

LEARNING OUTCOMES

On completion of this chapter, you will be able to:

1. State the description and primary functions of the organs/structures of the female reproductive system.

2. Define obstetrics and summarize the process of fertilization.

3. State the definition of pregnancy and describe its four stages.

4. Describe the three stages of labor.

5. Analyze, build, spell, and pronounce medical words.

6. Comprehend the drugs highlighted in this chapter.

7. Describe diagnostic and laboratory tests related to this chapter.

8. Identify and define selected abbreviations.

COMBINING FORMS OF THE FEMALE REPRODUCTIVE SYSTEM

abort/o	to miscarry	metr/i	womb, uterus
cervic/o	cervix, neck	metr/o	womb, uterus
coit/o	a coming together	my/o	muscle
colp/o	vagina	o/o	ovum, egg
culd/o	cul-de-sac	oophor/o	ovary
cyst/o	bladder	pareun/o	lying beside, sexual intercourse
fibr/o	fibrous tissue		
gynec/o	female	rect/o	rectum
hyster/o	womb, uterus	salping/o	fallopian tube
mamm/o	breast	uter/o	uterus
mast/o	breast	vagin/o	vagina
men/o	month, menses, menstruation	venere/o	sexual intercourse
		vers/o	turning

Anatomy and Physiology

The female reproductive system consists of a left and a right ovary, which are the female's primary sex organs, and the following accessory sex organs: two fallopian tubes, the uterus, the vagina, the vulva, and two breasts. The vital function of the female reproductive system is to perpetuate the species through sexual or germ cell reproduction. Table 17.1 ■ provides an at-a-glance look at the female reproductive system. See Figures 17.1 ■ and 17.2 ■

TABLE 17.1 Female Reproductive System at-a-Glance

Organ/Structure	Primary Functions/Description
Uterus	Provides a place for the nourishment and development of the fetus during pregnancy; contracts rhythmically and powerfully to help push out the fetus during the process of birthing
Fallopian tubes	Serve as ducts to convey the ovum from the ovary to the uterus and to convey spermatozoa from the uterus toward each ovary
Ovaries	Produce ova and hormones
Vagina	Female organ of copulation (sexual intercourse), serves as a passageway for the discharge of menstruation and a passageway for the birth of a fetus
Vulva	External female genitalia
Mons pubis	Provides pad of fatty tissue
Labia majora	Provides two folds of adipose tissue
Labia minora	Lying within the labia majora, encloses the vestibule
Vestibule	Serves as the entrance to the urethra, the vagina, and two excretory ducts of Bartholin's glands
Clitoris	Erectile tissue that is homologous to the penis of the male; produces pleasurable sensations during the sexual act
Breasts	Following childbirth, mammary glands produce milk

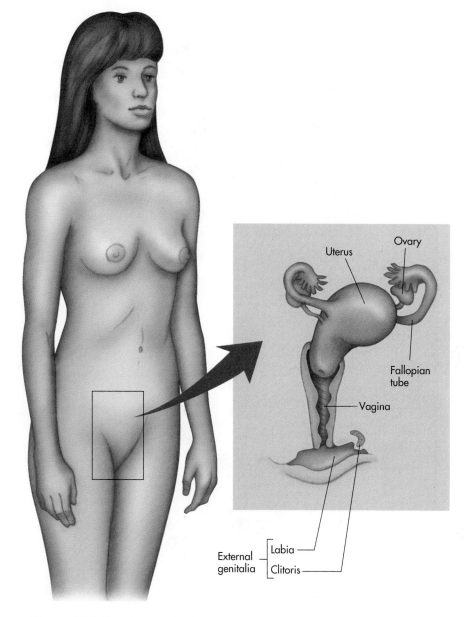

External genitalia { Labia, Clitoris

■ **Figure 17.1** Female reproductive system.

UTERUS

The **uterus** is a muscular, hollow, pear-shaped organ that is about 8 centimeters (cm) long, 5 cm wide, and 2.5 cm thick. The normal position of the uterus, known as **anteflexion**, is with the cervix pointing toward the lower end of the sacrum and the fundus toward the suprapubic region. See Figure 17.3 ■ An average uterus weighs between 30 and 40 grams (g), which is 1–1.4 ounces (oz).

The uterus can be divided into two anatomical regions: the body and the cervix. The *uterine body* or *corpus* is the larger (upper) portion. The *fundus* is the rounded portion of the uterine body above the openings of the fallopian tubes. The uterine body ends at a constricted central area known as the *isthmus*. The cervix is the lowermost cylindrical portion of the uterus that extends from the isthmus to the vagina.

The uterus is suspended in the anterior part of the pelvic cavity, halfway between the sacrum and the symphysis pubis, above the bladder, and in front of the rectum.

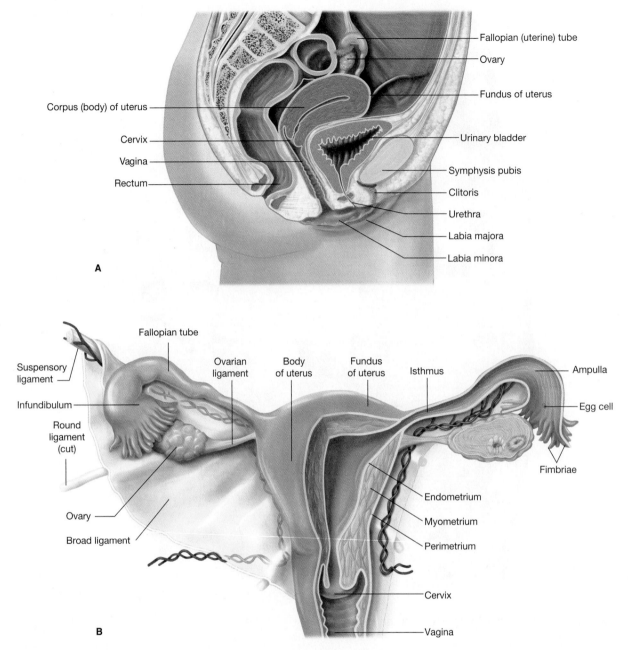

Fallopian (uterine) tube

Ovary

Fundus of uterus

Corpus (body) of uterus

Cervix

Vagina

Rectum

Urinary bladder

Symphysis pubis

Clitoris

Urethra

Labia majora

Labia minora

A

Suspensory ligament

Fallopian tube

Ovarian ligament

Body of uterus

Fundus of uterus

Isthmus

Ampulla

Infundibulum

Round ligament (cut)

Egg cell

Fimbriae

Ovary

Broad ligament

Endometrium

Myometrium

Perimetrium

Cervix

Vagina

B

■ **Figure 17.2** Female organs of reproduction and associated structures.

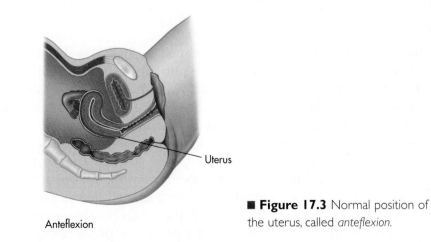

Uterus

Anteflexion

■ **Figure 17.3** Normal position of the uterus, called *anteflexion*.

A number of ligaments support the uterus and hold it in position: two broad ligaments, two round ligaments, two uterosacral ligaments, and the ligaments that are attached to the bladder.

Uterine Wall

The wall of the uterus consists of three layers: the **perimetrium** or outer layer, the **myometrium** or muscular middle layer, and the **endometrium**, which is the mucous membrane lining the inner surface of the uterus. See Figure 17.2. The endometrium is composed of columnar epithelium and connective tissue and is supplied with blood by both straight and spiral arteries. It undergoes marked changes in response to hormonal stimulation during the menstrual cycle.

Abnormal Positions of the Uterus

The uterus can become malpositioned because of weakness of any of its supporting ligaments. Trauma, disease processes of the uterus, or multiple pregnancies can contribute to the weakening of the supporting ligaments. The following terms describe some of the abnormal positions (see Figure 17.4 ■) of the uterus:

Retroversion. Turned backward with the cervix pointing forward toward the symphysis pubis.

Retroflexion. Bent backward at an angle with the cervix usually unchanged from its normal position.

Anteversion. Fundus turned forward toward the pubis with the cervix tilted up toward the sacrum.

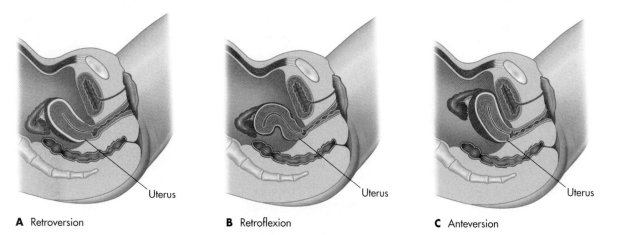

A Retroversion   **B** Retroflexion   **C** Anteversion

■ **Figure 17.4** Displacement of the uterus within the uterine cavity. (A) Retroversion is a backward tilting. (B) Retroflexion is a backward bending. (C) Anteversion is a forward titling.

FALLOPIAN TUBES

Also called the **uterine tubes** or **oviducts**, the **fallopian tubes** extend laterally from either side of the uterus and end near each ovary. An average, normal fallopian tube is about 11.5 cm long and 6 mm wide. Its wall is composed of three layers: the **serosa** or outermost layer, composed of connective tissue; the **muscular layer**, containing inner circular and outer longitudinal layers of smooth muscle; and the **mucosa** or inner layer, consisting of simple columnar epithelium.

Anatomical Features of the Fallopian Tubes

The **isthmus** is the constricted portion of the fallopian tube nearest the uterus. From the isthmus, the tube continues laterally and widens to form a section called the **ampulla**. Beyond the ampulla, the tube continues to expand and ends as a funnel-shaped opening. This end of the tube is called the **infundibulum**, and its opening is the **ostium**. Surrounding each ostium are **fimbriae** or *fingerlike structures* (see Figure 17.2) that work to propel the discharged ovum into the tube, where ciliary action aids in moving it toward the uterus. Should the ovum become impregnated by a spermatozoon while in the tube, the process of **fertilization** occurs.

FERTILIZATION

Fertilization is the process in which a sperm penetrates an ovum and unites with it. See Figure 17.5 ■ At this time, the 23 chromosomes from the male combine with the 23 chromosomes from the female to make a new life. Fertilization generally occurs within 24 hours following ovulation and usually takes place in the fallopian tube. A single sperm penetrates the ovum, and the resulting cell is called a **zygote.**

By this event, called **conception**, the gender and other biological traits of the new individual are determined. The fertilized ovum or zygote is genetically complete and

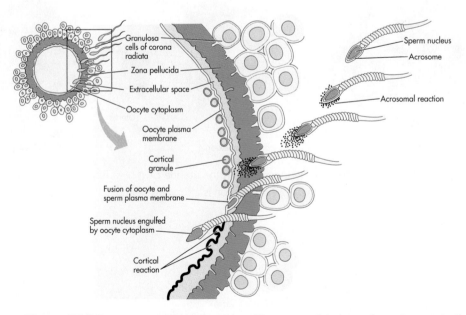

■ **Figure 17.5** Sperm penetration of an ovum. The sequential steps of oocyte penetration by a sperm are depicted moving from top to bottom.

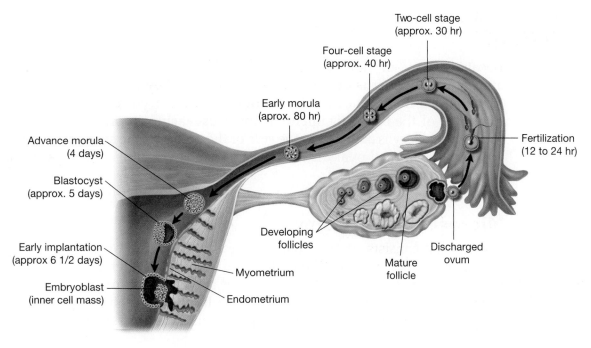

■ **Figure 17.6** During ovulation, the ovum leaves the ovary and enters the fallopian tube. Subsequent changes in the fertilized ovum from conception to implantation are depicted.

immediately begins to divide, forming a solid mass of cells called a **morula.** See Figure 17.6 ■ The cells of the morula continue to divide, and by the time the developing **embryo** (the term for the stage of development between weeks 2 and 8) reaches the uterus, it is a hollow ball of cells known as a **blastocyst,** which consists of an outer layer of cells and an inner cell mass. As the blastocyst develops, it forms a structure with two cavities, the **yolk sac** and **amniotic cavity.** In humans, the yolk sac is the site of formation of the first red blood cells and the cells that will become ovum and sperm.

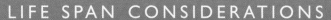

LIFE SPAN CONSIDERATIONS

The sex of a child is determined at the time of fertilization. When a spermatozoon carrying the X sex chromosome fertilizes the X-bearing ovum, the result is a female child (X + X = female). When the X-bearing ovum is fertilized by the Y-bearing spermatozoon, a male child is produced (X + Y = male). Sex differentiation occurs early in the embryo. At 16 weeks, the external **genitals** of the fetus are recognizably male or female. This difference can be seen during ultrasonography. See Figure 17.7 ■

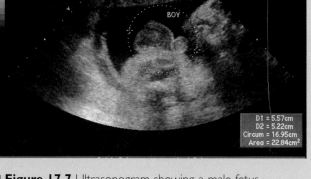

■ **Figure 17.7** Ultrasonogram showing a male fetus.
(Courtesy of Nancy West)

OVARIES

Located on either side of the uterus, the **ovaries** are almond-shaped organs attached to the uterus by the ovarian ligament. They lie close to the fimbriae of the fallopian tubes. The anterior border of each ovary is connected to the posterior layer of the broad ligament by the **mesovarium** (portion of the peritoneal fold). Each ovary is attached to the side of the pelvis by the **suspensory ligaments**. An average, normal ovary is about 4 cm long, 2 cm wide, and 1.5 cm thick. See Figure 17.8 ■

Microscopic Anatomy

Each ovary consists of two distinct areas: the **cortex** or outer layer and the **medulla** or inner portion. The cortex contains small secretory sacs or follicles in three stages of development. These stages are known as **primary**, **growing**, and **graafian** or mature stage. The ovarian medulla contains connective tissue, nerves, blood and lymphatic vessels, and some smooth muscle tissue in the region of the hilus.

Function of the Ovaries

The anterior lobe of the pituitary gland, which produces the *gonadotropic hormones* FSH and LH, primarily control the functional activity of the ovaries. These abbreviations are for *follicle-stimulating hormone*, which is instrumental in the development of the ovarian follicles, and *luteinizing hormone*, which stimulates the development of the **corpus luteum**, a small yellow mass of cells that develops within a ruptured ovarian follicle.

Two functions have been identified for the ovary: the production of ova, female reproductive cells, and the production of hormones.

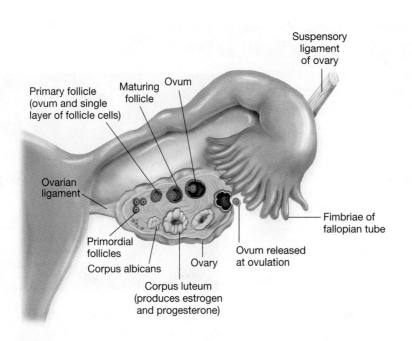

■ **Figure 17.8** Ovary.

Production of Ova

Each month a *graafian follicle* ruptures on the ovarian cortex, and an **ovum** (singular of ova) discharges into the pelvic cavity, where it enters the fallopian tube. This process is known as **ovulation.** In an average, normal woman more than 400 ova may be produced during her reproductive years (see Figure 17.8).

Production of Hormones

The ovaries are also endocrine glands, producing **estrogen**, the female sex hormone secreted by the ovarian follicles, and **progesterone**, a steroid hormone secreted by the corpus luteum that is important in the maintenance of pregnancy. These hormones are essential in promoting growth and development and maintaining the female secondary sex organs and characteristics. These hormones also prepare the uterus for pregnancy, promote development of the mammary glands, and play a vital role in a woman's emotional well-being and sexual drive.

VAGINA

The **vagina** is a musculomembranous tube extending from the vestibule to the uterus (see Figures 17.2 and 17.9 ■). It is 10–15 cm in length and situated between the bladder and the rectum. It is lined by mucous membrane made up of *squamous epithelium*. A fold of mucous membrane, the **hymen**, partially covers the external opening of the vagina.

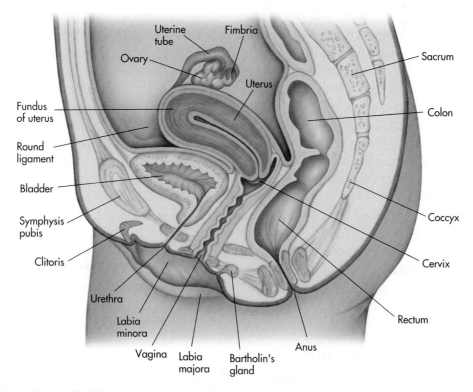

■ **Figure 17.9** Sagittal section of the female pelvis showing organs of the reproductive system.

VULVA

The **vulva** consists of the following five organs that comprise the external female genitalia (see Figure 17.9):

Mons pubis. A pad of fatty tissue of triangular shape and, after puberty, covered with pubic hair. It may be referred to as the *mons veneris* or *mound of Venus* and is the rounded area over the *symphysis pubis.*

Labia majora. The two folds of adipose tissue, which are large liplike structures, lying on either side of the vaginal opening.

Labia minora. Two thin folds of skin that lie within the labia majora and enclose the vestibule.

Vestibule. The cleft between the labia minora. It is approximately 4–5 cm long and 2 cm wide. Four major structures open into it: the urethra, the vagina, and two excretory ducts of the Bartholin glands.

Clitoris. A small organ consisting of sensitive erectile tissue that is homologous to the penis of the male. It is located between the anterior labial commissure and partially hidden by the anterior portion of the labia minora.

The **perineum** is the region bounded by the inferior edges of the pelvis. In the female, it is located between the vulva and the anus. It is a muscular sheet that forms the pelvic floor and during childbirth it can be torn and cause injury to the anal sphincter. To avoid such an injury, an *episiotomy*, a surgical procedure to prevent tearing of the perineum and facilitate delivery of the infant, may be performed.

BREASTS

The **breasts** or mammary glands are compound alveolar structures consisting of 15–20 glandular tissue lobes separated by septa of connective tissue. Most women have two breasts that lie anterior to the pectoral muscles and curve outward from the lateral margins of the sternum to the anterior border of the axilla (Figure 17.10 ■). The size of the breast can vary greatly according to age, heredity, and adipose (fatty) tissue present.

The **areola** is the dark, pigmented area found in the skin over each breast, and the *nipple* is the elevated area in the center of the areola. During pregnancy, the areola changes from its pinkish color to a dark brown or reddish color. The areola is supplied with a row of small sebaceous glands that secrete an oily substance to keep it resilient. The *lactiferous glands* consist of 20–24 glands in the areola of the nipple and, during **lactation** (the process of milk secretion), conveys it to a suckling infant. See Figure 17.10.

The hormone **prolactin**, which is produced by the anterior lobe of the pituitary, stimulates the mammary glands to produce milk after childbirth. Other hormones playing a role in milk production are insulin and glucocorticoids. **Colostrum**, a thin yellowish secretion, is the *first milk* and contains mainly serum and white blood cells.

Breastfeeding

Breastfeeding is the act of providing milk to a baby from the mother's breasts. Mature mother's milk and its precursor, colostrum, are considered to be the most balanced foods available for normal infants. Breast milk is sterile, easily digested, nonallergenic,

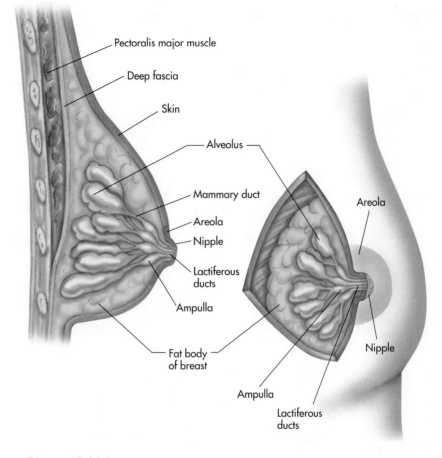

■ Figure 17.10 Breast.

and transmits maternal antibodies that protect against various infections and illnesses. In addition, the baby's suckling causes the release of **oxytocin** in the mother, which stimulates uterine contractions and promotes the return of the uterus to its normal nonpregnant size and state.

LIFE SPAN CONSIDERATIONS

The American Academy of Pediatrics currently recommends the following:

Pediatricians and parents should be aware that exclusive breastfeeding is sufficient to support optimal growth and development for approximately the first 6 months of life and provides continuing protection against diarrhea and respiratory tract infection. Breastfeeding should be continued for at least the first year of life.

MENSTRUAL CYCLE

The menstrual cycle is a periodic recurrent series of changes occurring in the uterus, ovaries, vagina, and breasts. It is regulated by the complex interaction of hormones: luteinizing hormone (LH) and follicle-stimulating hormone (FSH), which are produced by the pituitary gland, and the female sex hormones estrogen and progesterone, which are produced by the ovaries. The onset of the **menstrual cycle**, *menarche*, occurs at

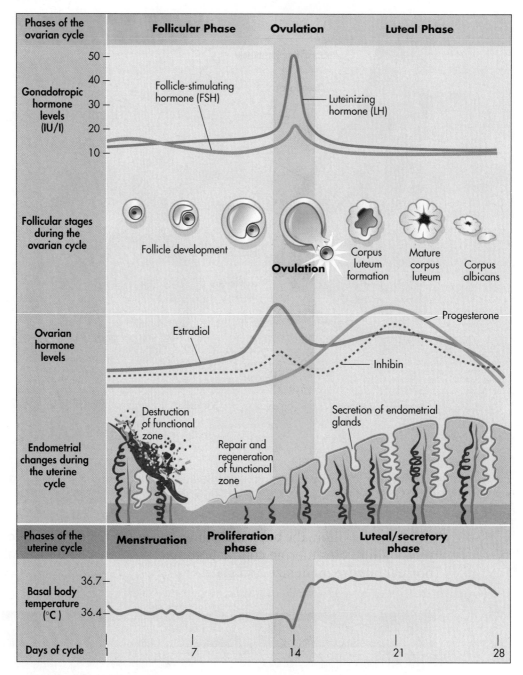

Figure 17.11 Hormonal regulation of the female reproductive cycle.

the age of **puberty** and ceases at **menopause.** The menstrual cycle occurs during a woman's reproductive years, except during **pregnancy.** The first day of bleeding is counted as the beginning of each menstrual cycle (day 1). The cycle ends just before the next menstrual period. The menstrual cycle occurs every 21–40 days and has three phases: follicular phase, ovulation, and the luteal phase. See Figure 17.11 ■

Follicular Phase

Menstruation, which marks the first day of the follicular phase, is characterized by the discharge of a bloody fluid from the uterus accompanied by a shedding of the endometrium. This phase averages 4–5 days and is considered to be the first to the fifth days of the cycle.

Ovulatory Phase

The **ovulatory phase** is characterized by the stimulation of estrogen, the thickening and vascularization of the endometrium, along with the maturing of the ovarian follicle. This phase begins about the fifth day and ends at the time of rupture of the graafian follicle (release of the egg), usually 36 hours after the surge in luteinizing hormone begins. About 12–24 hours after the egg is released, this surge can be detected by measuring the luteinizing hormone level in the urine. If the egg is not fertilized within 12–48 hours of being released, it disintegrates. The ovulatory phase occurs about 14 days before the onset of menstruation.

Luteal or Secretory Phase

The **luteal phase** follows ovulation. It last about 14 days, unless fertilization occurs, and ends just before a menstrual period. During this phase, the corpus luteum in the ovary is developing and secreting progesterone. Progesterone causes the mucus in the cervix to thicken, making the entry of sperm or bacteria into the uterus less likely. It also causes the body temperature to increase slightly during the luteal phase and remain elevated until a menstrual period begins. This increase in temperature can be used to estimate whether ovulation has occurred. In the second part of the luteal phase, the estrogen level increases, also stimulating the endometrium to thicken. In response to the increase in estrogen and progesterone levels, the breasts may swell and become tender. If the egg is not fertilized, the corpus luteum degenerates after 14 days, and a new menstrual cycle begins.

Premenstrual or Ischemic Time Period

During the **premenstrual** time period, the coiled uterine arteries become constricted, the endometrium becomes anemic and begins to shrink, and the corpus luteum decreases in functional activity. This time period lasts about 2 days and ends with the occurrence of menstruation.

OVERVIEW OF OBSTETRICS

Obstetrics (OB) is the branch of medicine that pertains to the care of women during pregnancy, childbirth, and the postpartum period, which is also called the **puerperium.** A physician specializing in this medical field is known as an **obstetrician.**

PREGNANCY

Pregnancy can be defined as a temporary condition that occurs within a woman's body from the time of conception through the embryonic and fetal periods to birth. The normal term of pregnancy is approximately 40 weeks (280 days); this equals

10 lunar months or 9⅓ calendar months. The length of pregnancy is called the **gestation period** and is divided into three segments of 3 months, each called **trimesters.**

Human development follows three stages: the *preembryonic stage* is the first 14 days of development after the ovum is fertilized; the *embryonic stage* begins in the third week after fertilization; and the *fetal stage* begins in the ninth week. See Figure 17.12 ■

During the fifth week of development, the embryo has a marked C-shaped body and a rudimentary tail. At 7 weeks, the head of the embryo is rounded and nearly erect. The eyes have shifted forward and are closer together, and the eyelids begin to form. At 9 weeks, every organ system and external structure is present, and the developing embryo is now called a **fetus**. See Figure 17.13 ■

At 14 weeks, the skin of the fetus is so transparent that blood vessels are visible beneath it. More muscle tissue and body skeleton have developed and holds the fetus more erect. At 20 weeks, the fetus weighs approximately 435–465 g and measures about 19 cm. The skin is less transparent due to subcutaneous deposits of brown fat. Fingernails and toenails have developed and "woolly" hair covers the head. See Figure 17.14 ■

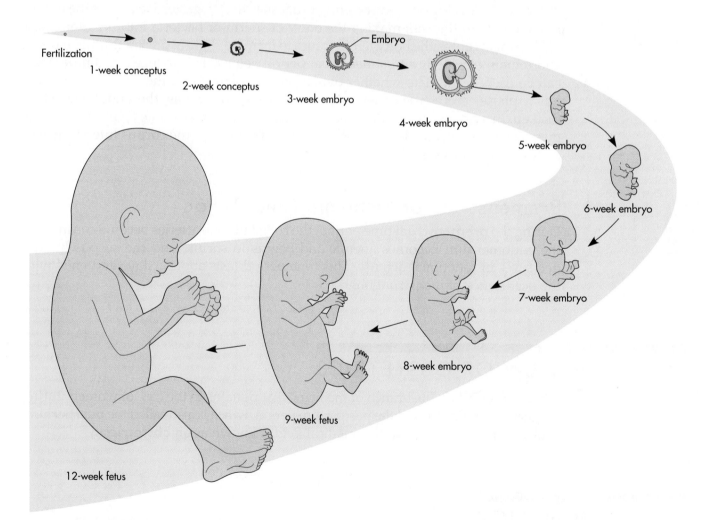

Fertilization

1-week conceptus

2-week conceptus

3-week embryo

4-week embryo

Embryo

5-week embryo

6-week embryo

7-week embryo

8-week embryo

9-week fetus

12-week fetus

■ **Figure 17.12** Actual size of a human conceptus from fertilization to the early fetal stage. The embryonic stage begins in the 3rd week after fertilization; the fetal stage begins in the 9th week.

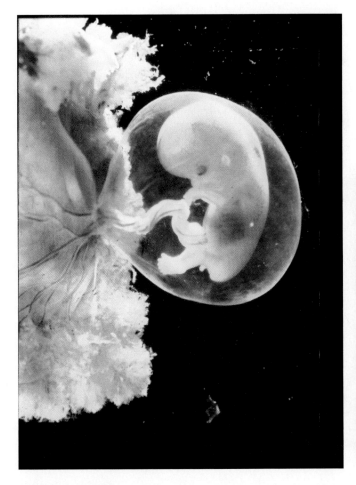

■ **Figure 17.13** Fetus at 9 weeks.
Every organ system and external structure is present.
(Source: Lennart Nilsson/Albert Bonniers Förlag AB, *A Child Is Born*, New York: Dell
Publishing)

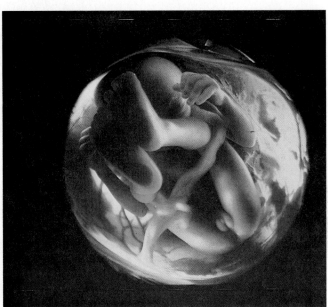

■ **Figure 17.14** Fetus at 20 weeks.
The fetus weighs approximately 435–465 g and measures
about 19 cm. Subcutaneous deposits of brown fat make the
skin less transparent. "Woolly" hair covers the head, and nails
have developed on the fingers and toes.
(Source: Lennart Nilsson/Albert Bonniers Förlag AB, *A Child Is Born*, New York:
Dell Publishing)

Pregnancy is divided into four stages:

1. **Prenatal stage.** Time period between conception and onset of labor; refers to both the care of the woman during pregnancy and the growth and development of the fetus. Figure 17.15 ■ shows the position of the fetus in a full-term pregnancy.

2. **Labor.** Time period during which forceful contractions move the fetus down the birth canal and expel it from the uterus during childbirth.

3. **Parturition.** Time period of actively giving birth; also known as **childbirth** or **delivery.**

4. **Postpartum period** or **puerperium.** Six-week time period following childbirth and expulsion of the placenta. The female reproductive organs usually return to an essentially prepregnant condition in which *involution of the uterus* (return of the uterus to normal size after childbirth) occurs.

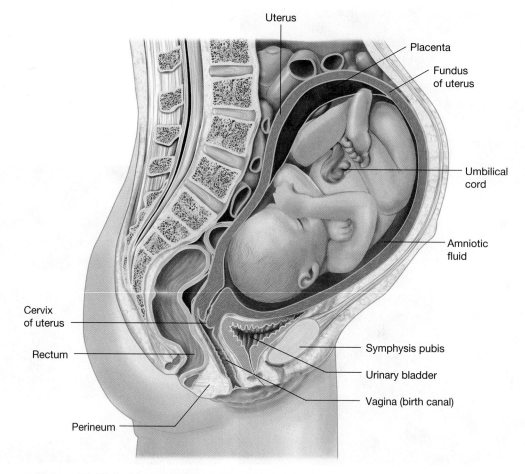

■ **Figure 17.15** Position of fetus in full-term pregnancy.

LABOR AND DELIVERY

Labor is the process by which forceful contractions move the fetus down the birth canal and expel it from the uterus during childbirth. The signs and symptoms that labor is about to start can occur from hours to weeks before the actual onset of labor. Signs of impending labor include:

- **Braxton Hicks contractions.** Irregular contractions that begin in the second trimester and intensify as full term approaches.

- **Increased vaginal discharge.** Normally clear and nonirritating discharge caused by fetal pressure.

- **Lightening.** The descent of the baby into the pelvis. The expectant mother will notice that she can breathe easier and often states, "The baby has dropped." This may occur 2–3 weeks before the first stage of labor begins.

- **Bloody show.** Thick mucus mixed with pink or dark-brown blood. As the cervix softens, effaces, and dilates, the mucous plug that has sealed the uterus during pregnancy is dislodged from the cervix and small capillaries are torn, producing the bloody show.

- **Rupture of the membranes.** Occurs when the amniotic sac (bag of waters) ruptures.

Note: When the membranes do not rupture on their own, they will be ruptured by the attending physician or midwife. This is known as **AROM**: **a**rtificial **r**upture **of m**embranes.

- **Energy spurt or nesting.** Occurs in many women shortly before the onset of labor. They may suddenly have the energy to clean their houses and do things that they have not had the energy to do previously.

- **Weight loss.** Loss of 1–3 pounds shortly before labor can occur as hormone changes cause excretion of extra body water.

Stages of Labor

True labor is characterized by rhythmic contractions that develop a regular pattern and are more frequent, more intense, and last longer. A general feeling of discomfort is felt in the lower back and lower abdomen. A bloody show is often present, and progressive effacement and dilation of the cervix occur. Labor is divided into three stages: dilation, expulsion, and placental (see Figure 17.16 ■):

- **First stage: Dilation.** Begins with the onset of true labor and lasts until the cervix is fully dilated to 10 cm.

- **Second stage: Expulsion.** Continues after the cervix is dilated to 10 cm until the delivery of the baby. During this stage an **episiotomy**, a surgical procedure performed to prevent tearing of the perineum and to facilitate delivery of the fetus, may be performed.

LIFE SPAN CONSIDERATIONS

The newborn baby usually has a cone-shaped or molded head due to its journey down the birth canal. It is covered with **vernix caseosa**, a protective cheesy substance that covers the fetus during intrauterine life. The baby will present with **lanugo**, fine downy hair that covers the body, especially the shoulders, back, forehead, and temple. The external **genitalia**, the male or female reproductive organs, are usually enlarged.

- **Third stage: Placental.** Delivery of the placenta.

  The **placenta** is a highly vascular organ that anchors the developing fetus to the uterus and provides the means by which the fetus receives its nourishment and oxygen. It also functions as an excretory, respiratory, and endocrine organ, which produces human chorionic gonadotropin (hCG). The placenta consists of a fetal portion and a maternal portion. The fetal portion has a shiny, slightly grayish appearance and is formed by a coming together of chorionic villi in which the umbilical vein and arteries intertwine to form the **umbilical cord**. The maternal portion develops from the decidual basalis of the uterus. It has a red, beefy-looking appearance. The mature placenta is 15–18 centimeters (cm) (6–7 inches) in diameter and weighs approximately 450 grams (about 1 pound). When expelled following parturition, it is known as the **afterbirth**.

  The time it takes to deliver the placenta is anywhere from 5 to 30 minutes. The placenta is expelled in one or two ways: the **Schultze mechanism**, with the fetal surface presenting, or the **Duncan mechanism** presenting the maternal surface. The placenta is examined to be certain that all of it has been expelled. Any small portion of the placenta that remains in the uterus could interfere with uterine contractions

A

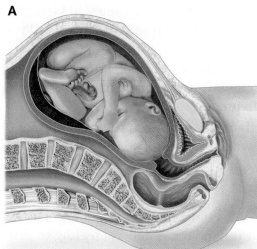

DILATION STAGE:
Uterine contractions dilate cervix

B

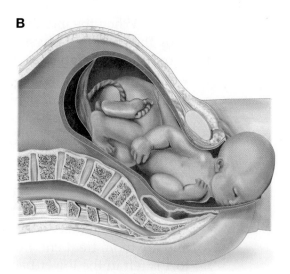

EXPULSION STAGE:
Birth of baby or expulsion

C

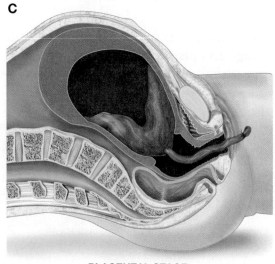

PLACENTAL STAGE:
Delivery of placenta

■ **Figure 17.16** Three stages of labor and delivery.

after the birth of the baby and contribute to infection. To control bleeding from the vessels that supplied the placenta during pregnancy, the uterus must contract and remain contracted after placental expulsion.

Newborn Assessment

The first assessment of the newborn involves using the Apgar score. It is performed immediately following the birth of the baby. This method was developed by Virginia Apgar (U.S. anesthesiologist, 1909–1974) as the first objective evaluation of newborns in 1952 and since then, the Apgar score has become the standard tool for assessing newborn babies. The five assessments of the Apgar score are a mnemonic based on Virginia's last name. Ratings are based on **A**ppearance (color), **P**ulse (heartbeat), **G**rimace (reflex), **A**ctivity (muscle tone), and **R**espiration (breathing). The score is taken at 1 and 5 minutes after birth, the high score being 10 and the low score being 1. See Table 17.2 ■

TABLE 17.2 The Apgar Score

Sign	0	1	2
Heart rate	Absent	Less than 100/min	More than 100/min
Respiratory effort	Absent	Slow, irregular	Regular or crying
Reflex irritability	No response	Grimace, frown	Cry, cough
Muscle tone	Limp	Some motion, some flexion of extremities, some resistance to extension of extremities	Active, spontaneous flexion, good tone
Color	Cyanotic or pale	Body pink, extremities cyanotic	Completely pink

Anatomy and Physiology Labeling

Identify the structures shown below by filling in the blanks.

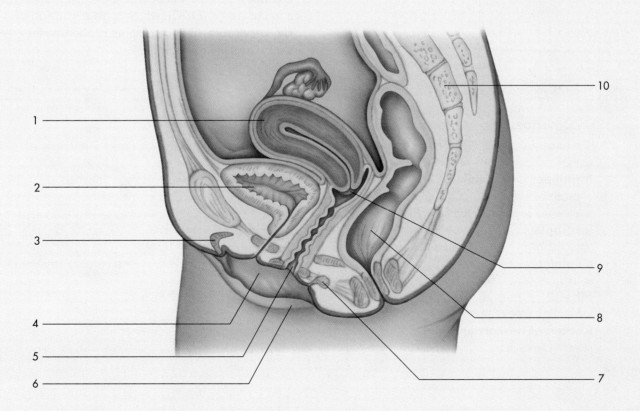

• Building Your Medical Vocabulary •

This section provides the foundation for learning medical terminology. Review the following alphabetized word list. Note how common prefixes and suffixes are repeatedly applied to word roots and combining forms to create different meanings. The word parts are color-coded: prefixes are green, suffixes are blue, roots/combining forms are red.

You will find that some terms have not been divided into word parts. These are common words or specialized terms that are included to enhance your medical vocabulary. See Chapter 1, page 7, to review pronunciation guidelines.

MEDICAL WORD	WORD PARTS		DEFINITION
	Part	Meaning	
abortion (AB) (a-bōr´ shŭn)	abort -ion	to miscarry process	Process of miscarrying (either spontaneous or induced); termination of the pregnancy before the fetus is viable (capable of living outside of the uterus). Treatment during or after a miscarriage includes measures to prevent hemorrhage and infection. With any type of miscarriage, the patient should see her health care provider as soon as possible. If the abortion is incomplete and not all tissue has been expelled, a dilation and curettage (D&C), which is an expansion of the cervical canal and scraping of the uterine wall, is usually performed.

fyi The risk for spontaneous abortion is higher in women over age 35, in women with systemic diseases such as diabetes mellitus or thyroid conditions, and women with a history of three or more prior spontaneous abortions. The types of spontaneous abortions or miscarriages include the following.

Threatened. Uterine bleeding or spotting is accompanied by cramping or low-back pain. The cervix is not dilated. See Figure 17.17A ■

Imminent or inevitable. Uterine bleeding or spotting is accompanied by cramping or low back pain. The cervix is dilated. Miscarriage is inevitable when there is dilation or effacement of the cervix or rupture of the membranes. See Figure 17.17B ■

Incomplete. Some products of conception have been expelled, but some remain in the uterus. Bleeding and cramps may persist when the miscarriage is not complete. See Figure 17.17C ■

Complete. All of the products of conception are expelled. A completed miscarriage can be confirmed by an ultrasound.

Missed. A pregnancy demise in which nothing is expelled. It is not known why this occurs. Signs of this would be a loss of pregnancy symptoms and the absence of fetal heart tones.

Recurrent miscarriage (RM). Defined as three or more consecutive first-trimester miscarriages. Also referred to as habitual abortion.

MEDICAL WORD	WORD PARTS		DEFINITION
	Part	**Meaning**	

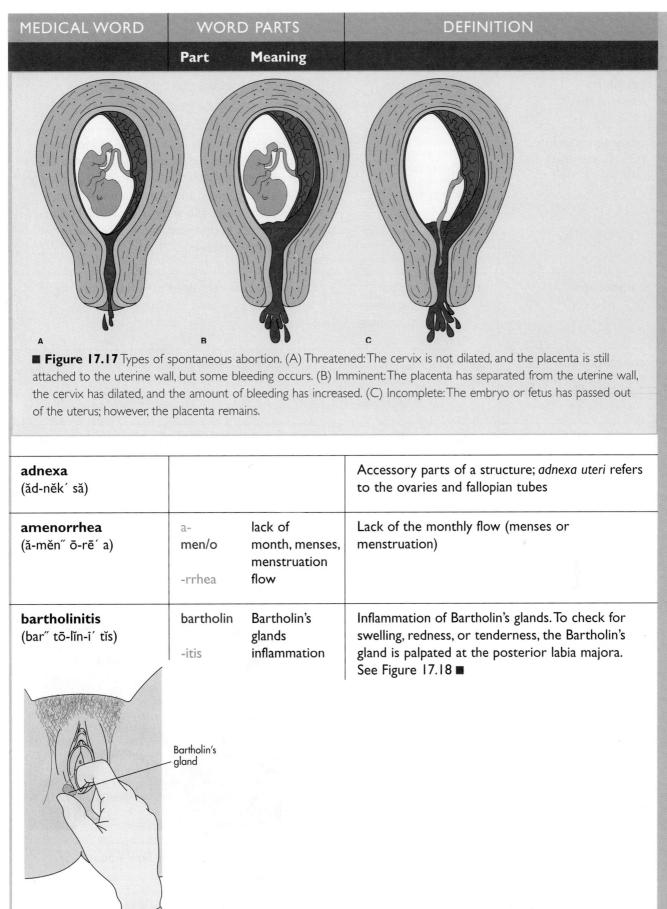

■ **Figure 17.17** Types of spontaneous abortion. (A) Threatened: The cervix is not dilated, and the placenta is still attached to the uterine wall, but some bleeding occurs. (B) Imminent: The placenta has separated from the uterine wall, the cervix has dilated, and the amount of bleeding has increased. (C) Incomplete: The embryo or fetus has passed out of the uterus; however, the placenta remains.

MEDICAL WORD	Part	Meaning	DEFINITION
adnexa (ăd-něk′ să)			Accessory parts of a structure; *adnexa uteri* refers to the ovaries and fallopian tubes
amenorrhea (ă-měn″ ō-rē′ a)	a- men/o -rrhea	lack of month, menses, menstruation flow	Lack of the monthly flow (menses or menstruation)
bartholinitis (bar″ tō-lĭn-ī′ tĭs)	bartholin -itis	Bartholin's glands inflammation	Inflammation of Bartholin's glands. To check for swelling, redness, or tenderness, the Bartholin's gland is palpated at the posterior labia majora. See Figure 17.18 ■

Bartholin's gland

■ **Figure 17.18** Palpating Bartholin's glands.

MEDICAL WORD	WORD PARTS		DEFINITION
	Part	**Meaning**	
cervicitis (sĕr-vĭ-sī´ tĭs)	cervic -itis	cervix inflammation	Inflammation of the uterine cervix
cesarean section **(CS, C-section)**			Delivery of the fetus by means of an incision through the abdominal cavity and then into the uterus. Elective C-section is indicated for known cephalopelvic (head to pelvis) disproportion, malpresentations, and active herpes infection. Fetal distress is the most common cause for an emergency C-section.
colposcope (kŏl´ pō-skōp)	colp/o -scope	vagina instrument for examining	Medical instrument used to examine the vagina and cervix by means of a magnifying lens
contraception (kŏn˝ tră-sĕp´ shŭn)	contra- cept -ion	against receive process	Process of preventing conception
culdocentesis (kŭl˝ dō-sĕn-tē´ sĭs)	culd/o -centesis	cul-de-sac surgical puncture	Surgical puncture of the cul-de-sac for removal of fluid
cystocele (sĭs´ tō-sēl)	cyst/o -cele	bladder hernia	Hernia of the bladder that protrudes into the vagina
Doppler ultrasound (dăp´ lr ŭl´ trăh-sŏund)			Procedure using an audio transformation of high-frequency sounds to monitor the fetal heartbeat (FHB). See Figure 17.19 ■
dysmenorrhea (dĭs˝ mĕn-ō-rē´ ă)	dys- men/o -rrhea	difficult, painful month, menses, menstruation flow	Difficult or painful monthly flow (menses or menstruation)

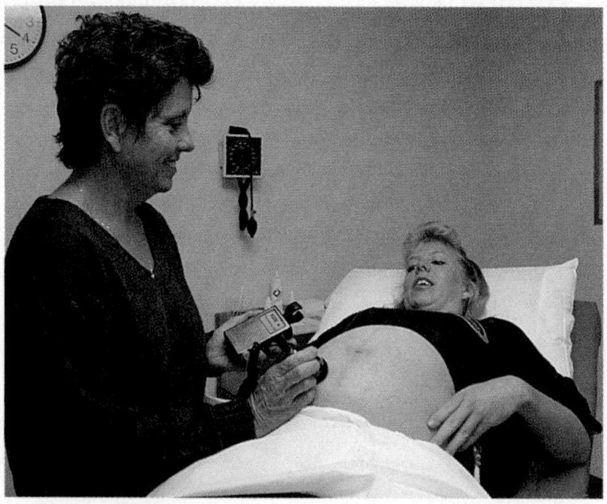

■ **Figure 17.19** Listening to the fetal heartbeat (FHB) with a Doppler device.

MEDICAL WORD	WORD PARTS		DEFINITION
	Part	**Meaning**	
dyspareunia (dĭs´ pă-rū´ nĭ-ă)	dys- pareun -ia	difficult, painful lying beside, sexual intercourse condition	Difficult or painful sexual intercourse (copulation)
eclampsia (ĕ-klămp´ sē-ă)	ec- lamp(s) -ia	out to shine condition	Complication of severe preeclampsia that involves seizures; also known as *toxemia* or *pregnancy-induced hypertension (PIH)*
ectopic pregnancy (ĕk-tŏp´ĭk prĕg´năn-sē)			A pregnancy that occurs when the fertilized egg is implanted in one of various sites, the most common being a fallopian tube; also referred to as a *tubal pregnancy*. See Figure 17.20 ■ This type of pregnancy is life threatening to the mother and almost always fatal to her fetus. It is the leading cause of pregnancy-related death in African American women.

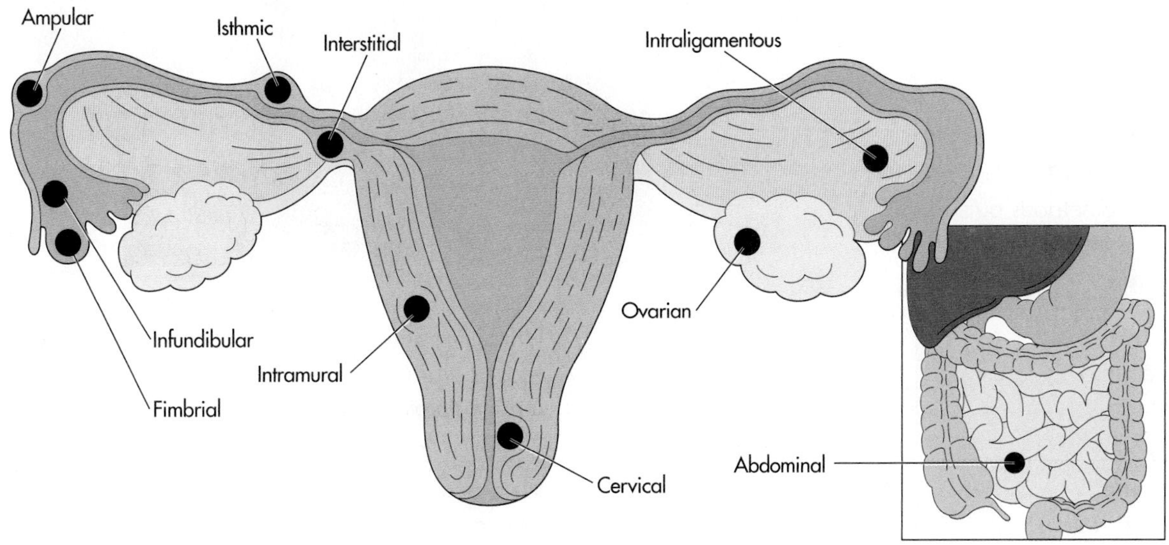

■ **Figure 17.20** Various implantation sites in ectopic pregnancy. The most common site is within the fallopian tube, hence the term *tubal pregnancy*.

MEDICAL WORD	WORD PARTS		DEFINITION
	Part	**Meaning**	
endometriosis (ĕn″ dō-mē″ trĭ-ō′ sĭs)	endo- metr/i -osis	within uterus condition	Pathological condition in which endometrial tissue has been displaced to various sites in the abdominal or pelvic cavity. This tissue responds to cyclic hormonal signals. Because it is outside the uterus and cannot be cast off each month, the tissue causes bleeding, with the formation of scars and adhesions. This is generally what causes daily or monthly cyclic pain. See Figure 17.21 ■

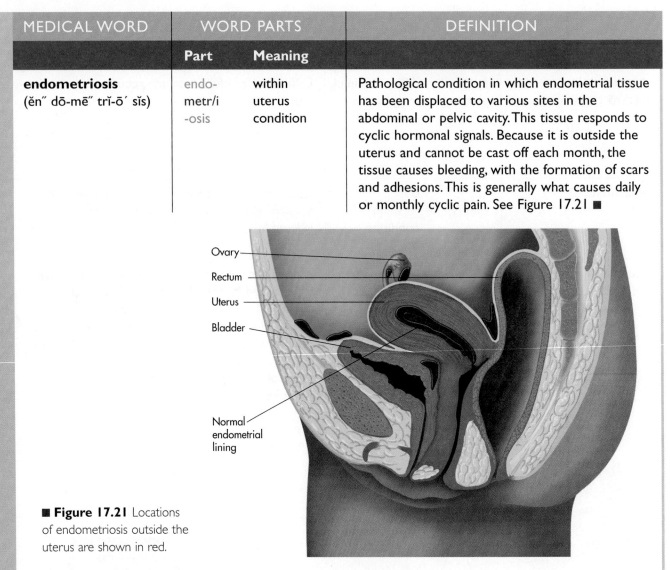

Ovary
Rectum
Uterus
Bladder
Normal endometrial lining

■ **Figure 17.21** Locations of endometriosis outside the uterus are shown in red.

| **fibroma**
(fĭ-brō′ mă) | fibr
-oma | fibrous tissue
tumor | Fibrous tissue tumor; also called *fibroid tumor,* the most common benign tumor found in women. See *uterine fibroid.* |
| **genitalia**
(jĕn-ĭ-tăl′ ĭ-ă) | genital
-ia | belonging to birth
condition | Male or female reproductive organs. See Figure 17.22 ■ |

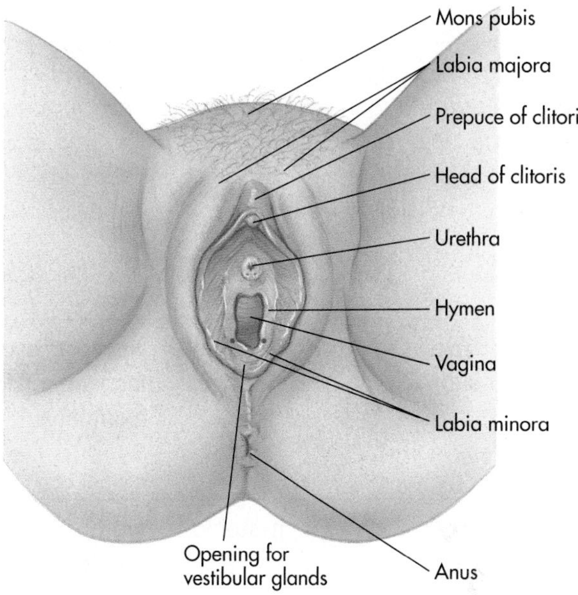

MEDICAL WORD	WORD PARTS		DEFINITION
	Part	Meaning	

■ **Figure 17.22** External female genitalia (vulva).

MEDICAL WORD	WORD PARTS		DEFINITION
	Part	Meaning	
gravida (grăv´ ĭ-dă)			Refers to any pregnancy, regardless of duration, including the present one; when used in the recording of an obstetrical history, indicates the number of pregnancies, for example, **nulligravida** refers to a woman who has never been pregnant and is written as Gravida 0, **primigravida** refers to a woman who is pregnant for the first time and is written as Gravida 1, **multigravida** refers to a woman who has been pregnant more than once and is written as Gravida 2 (3, 4, 5, etc.).
group B streptococcus (GBS) (strĕp´´ tō-kŏk´ ŭs)			Type of bacterium commonly found in the vagina and intestinal tract; found in 10–25% of all pregnant women; it can cause life-threatening infections in the newborn
gynecologist (gī´´ nĕ-kōl´ ō-jĭst)	gynec/o log -ist	female study of one who specializes	Physician who specializes in the study of the female, especially the diseases of the female reproductive organs and the breasts
gynecology (GYN) (gī´´ nĕ-kōl´ ō-jē)	gynec/o -logy	female study of	Study of the female, especially the diseases of the female reproductive organs and the breasts
hymenectomy (hī´´ mĕn-ĕk´ tō-mē)	hymen -ectomy	hymen surgical excision	Surgical excision of the membranous fold of tissue (the hymen) that partially or completely covers the vaginal opening

MEDICAL WORD	WORD PARTS		DEFINITION
	Part	**Meaning**	
hysterectomy (hĭs″ tĕr-ĕk′ tō-mē)	hyster -ectomy	womb, uterus surgical excision	Surgical excision of the uterus.

fyi When the entire uterus, including the cervix, fallopian tubes, and ovaries, is removed during a hysterectomy, it is referred to as a *panhysterosalpingo-oophorectomy*. If a woman has not yet reached menopause, a hysterectomy stops menstruation (monthly periods), as well as ending her ability to become pregnant.

Often one or both ovaries and fallopian tubes are removed at the same time a hysterectomy is done. When both ovaries and both tubes are removed, it is called a *bilateral salpingo-oophorectomy*. This procedure causes *surgical menopause* in women who are premenopausal.

MEDICAL WORD	WORD PARTS		DEFINITION
hysteroscope (hĭs′ tĕr-ō-skōp)	hyster/o -scope	womb, uterus instrument for examining	Instrument used in the biopsy of uterine tissue before 12 weeks of gestation. This tissue is then analyzed for chromosome arrangement, DNA sequence, and genetic defects.
hysterotomy (hĭs″ tĕr-ŏt′ ō-mē)	hyster/o -tomy	womb, uterus incision	Incision into the uterus, commonly combined with a laparotomy (surgical incision into the abdomen) during a cesarean section. Hysterotomies are also performed during fetal surgery.
intrauterine (ĭn′ tră-ū′ tĕr-ĭn)	intra- uter -ine	within uterus pertaining to	Pertaining to within the uterus
laser ablation (lā′ zĕr ăb-lā′ shŭn)			Procedure that uses a laser to destroy the uterine lining. A biopsy is performed before the procedure to make sure no cancer is present. This procedure can be used for disabling menstrual bleeding. It causes sterility.
linea nigra (lĭn′ē-ă nĭ′gră)			Dark line on the abdomen that runs from above the umbilicus to the pubis during pregnancy. See Figure 17.23 ■

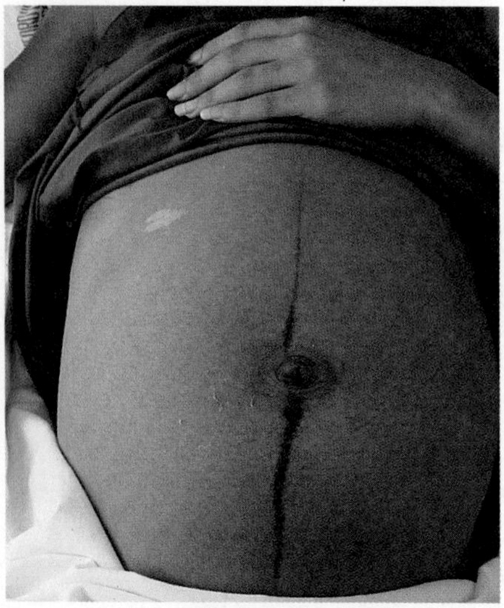

■ **Figure 17.23**
Linea nigra.

MEDICAL WORD	WORD PARTS		DEFINITION
	Part	Meaning	
lochia (lō´ kē-ă)			Vaginal discharge occurring after childbirth. At first it is blood-tinged (*rubra*); then, after 3 or 4 days, it becomes pink and brown-tinged (*serosa*); after that, it becomes yellow and then turns to white (*alba*). Lochia typically last 2–4 weeks.
lumpectomy (lŭm-pěk´ tō-mē)	lump -ectomy	lump surgical excision	Surgical removal of a tumor from the breast. This procedure removes only the tumor and some surrounding tissue but no lymph nodes; usually not considered for large tumors, although the latest strategy involves shrinking large tumors with chemotherapy so that they become small enough to be removed by this method. See Figure 17.24 ▪

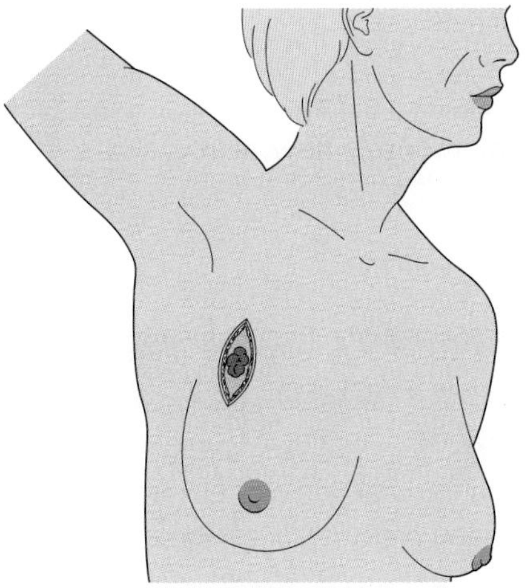

Lumpectomy

▪ **Figure 17.24** A lumpectomy removes only the tumor and a small margin of surrounding tissue.

mammoplasty (măm´ ō-plăs˝ tē)	mamm/o -plasty	breast surgical repair	Surgical repair of the breast
mastectomy (măs-těk´ tō-mē)	mast -ectomy	breast surgical excision	Surgical excision of the breast. See Figure 17.25 ▪

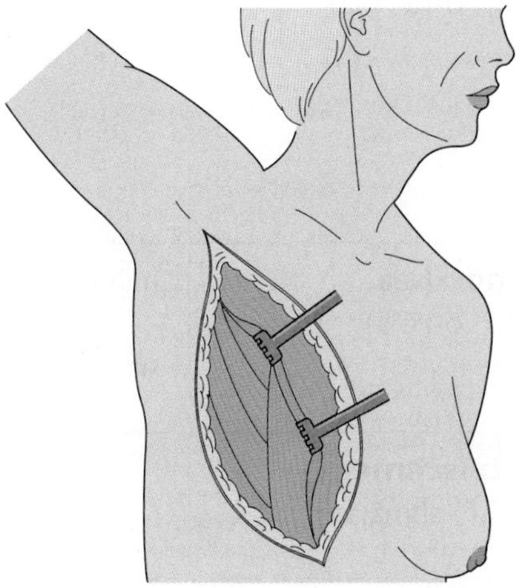

▪ **Figure 17.25** A modified radical mastectomy removes all breast tissue and the underarm lymph nodes but leaves the underlying muscles.

Modified radical mastectomy

MEDICAL WORD	WORD PARTS		DEFINITION
	Part	**Meaning**	
mastitis (măs-tī´ tis)	mast -itis	breast inflammation	Inflammation of the breast that occurs most commonly in women who are breastfeeding. It is caused by bacteria that enter through a crack or abrasion of the nipple. Generalized symptoms include fever, chills, and headache. Localized symptoms include breast pain, redness, tenderness, and swelling.
menarche (mĕn-ar´ kē)	men -arche	month, menses, menstruation beginning	Beginning of the monthly flow (menses, menstruation)
menopause (mĕn´ ō-pawz)	men/o pause	month, menses, menstruation cessation	Cessation of the monthly flow; also called *climacteric*

LIFE SPAN CONSIDERATIONS

At about 50 years of age, men and women begin experiencing bodily changes that are directly related to **hormonal** production. In women, the ovaries cease to produce estrogen and progesterone. With decreased production of the female hormones, estrogen and progesterone, women enter the phase of life known as **menopause**.

The symptoms of menopause vary from being hardly noticeable to being severe. Symptoms can include irregular periods, hot flashes, vaginal dryness, insomnia, joint pain, headache, emotional instability, irritability, and depression. Breast tissue can lose its firmness, and pubic and axillary hair becomes sparse. Without estrogen, the uterus becomes smaller, the vagina shortens, and vaginal tissues become drier. There can be loss of bone mass leading to **osteoporosis**.

menorrhagia (mĕn˝ ō-rā´ jĭ-ă)	men/o -rrhagia	month, menses, menstruation to burst forth	Excessive uterine bleeding at the time of a menstrual period, either in number of days or amount of blood or both. Can be caused by such conditions as uterine fibroid tumors, pelvic inflammatory disease, or by an endocrine imbalance.
menorrhea (mĕn˝ ō-rē´ă)	men/o -rrhea	month, menses, menstruation flow	Normal monthly flow (menses, menstruation)
mittelschmerz (mĭt´ ĕl-shmārts)			Abdominal pain that occurs midway between the menstrual periods at ovulation
myometritis (mī˝ ō-mē-trī´ tĭs)	my/o metr -itis	muscle womb, uterus inflammation	Inflammation of the muscular wall of the uterus

MEDICAL WORD	WORD PARTS		DEFINITION
	Part	**Meaning**	
oligomenorrhea (ŏl″ ĭ-gō-měn″ ō-rē´ă)	oligo- men/o -rrhea	scanty month, menses, menstruation flow	Scanty monthly flow (menses, menstruation)
oogenesis (ō″ ō-jěn´ ě-sĭs)	o/o -genesis	ovum, egg formation, produce	Formation of the ovum
oophorectomy (ō″ ŏf-ō-rěk´ tō-mê)	oophor -ectomy	ovary surgical excision	Surgical excision of an ovary
ovulation (ŏv″ ū-lā´ shŭn)	ovulat -ion	little egg process	Process in which an ovum is discharged from the cortex of the ovary; periodic ripening and rupture of a mature graafian follicle and the discharge of an ovum from the cortex of the ovary. Occurs approximately 14 days before the onset of the next menstrual period. See Figure 17.26 ■

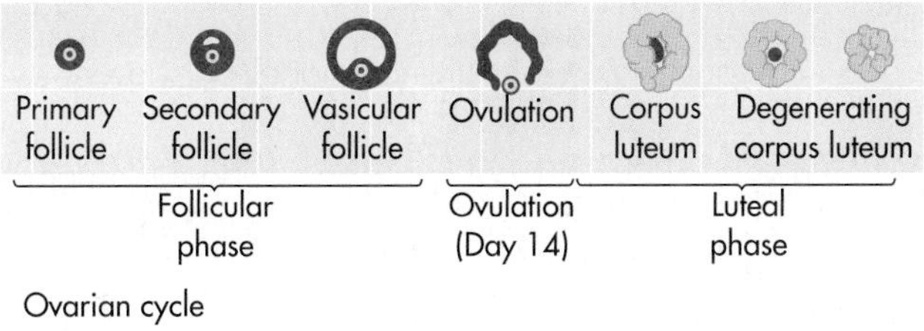

Ovarian cycle

■ **Figure 17.26** Changes in the ovarian follicles during the 28-day ovarian cycle.

para			Means to bear or bring forth; refers to a woman who has given birth after 20 weeks gestation, regardless of whether the infant is born alive or dead. When used in the recording of an obstetrical history, *para* or *Para* is used to indicate the number of births. For example, **multipara** refers to a woman who has given birth to two or more children and is written as Para 2 (3, 4, 5, etc.); **nullipara** refers to a woman who has not given birth after more than 20 weeks of gestation and is written as Para O; and **primipara** refers to a woman who has had one birth at more than 20 weeks gestation, regardless of whether the infant was born alive or dead, and is written as Para 1.
pelvic inflammatory disease (PID) (pěl´ vĭk ĭn-flăm´ ă-tŏr´ ē)			Infection of the upper genital area; can affect the uterus, ovaries, and fallopian tubes.

MEDICAL WORD	WORD PARTS		DEFINITION
	Part	Meaning	

fyi Pelvic inflammatory disease (PID) is the most common and serious complication of sexually transmitted diseases (STDs) among women. This infection of the upper genital area occurs when disease-causing organisms migrate upward from the vagina and cervix into the upper genital area. If untreated, it can cause scarring, which can lead to infertility, tubal pregnancy, chronic pelvic pain, and other serious consequences. Infertility occurs in approximately 20% of women who have had PID.

perimenopause (pĕr-ĭ-mĕn´ ō-pawz)	peri-	around	Period of gradual changes that lead into menopause, affecting a woman's hormones, body, and feelings. It can be a stop–start process that can take months or years. Hormone levels fluctuate, thereby causing changes in the menstrual cycle, which becomes irregular.
	men/o	month, menses, menstruation	
	pause	cessation	

fyi A nonprescription regimen for perimenopause includes:

Exercise. Aerobic, weight-bearing, and/or stretching exercises at least 30 minutes to an hour, four to five times a week.

Diet. High in fruits and vegetables and low in saturated fat. Reduce intake of caffeine, alcohol, hot beverages, and spicy foods.

The National Institutes of Health (NIH) reports some evidence for the efficacy of including soy preparations in one's diet for perimenopausal symptoms, while not making a definitive statement about its use. Study data indicate no serious safety concerns using soy products short term.

Note: Soy contains phytoestrogens that are similar to estrogen and isoflavones. Blueberries and cherries also contain bioflavonoids, which are a source of phytoestrogens. Flaxseeds and flaxseed oil are lignans—also phytoestrogens—and can help relieve hot flashes and vaginal dryness. These lignans also can have a stabilizing effect on hormone-related mood swings.

| **placenta previa** (plă-sen´tă prē´vē-ă) | | | In this condition, the placenta is improperly implanted in the lower uterine segment. The fetus receives less oxygen and the expectant mother has an increased risk of hemorrhage and infection. Placenta previa is classified as one of four degrees (Figure 17.27 ■): 1. **Total placenta previa.** The placenta completely covers the internal os. 2. **Partial placenta previa.** The placenta partially covers the internal os. 3. **Marginal placenta previa.** The edge of the placenta is at the margin of the internal os. 4. **Low-lying placenta.** The placenta is implanted in the lower segment but does not reach the internal os, although it is in close proximity to it. The most common symptom of placenta previa is painless uterine bleeding during the second half of pregnancy. Bleeding can be scanty or profuse (hemorrhage). When this occurs, the expectant mother is advised to go to the hospital. |

MEDICAL WORD	WORD PARTS		DEFINITION
	Part	**Meaning**	
			To determine a diagnosis, a transabdominal ultrasound examination is performed to pinpoint the placenta's location. A vaginal examination usually is avoided because it could trigger heavy bleeding. A woman who has been diagnosed with placenta previa may need to stay in the hospital until delivery. If the bleeding stops, as it often does, her physician continues to monitor the expectant mother and her baby.

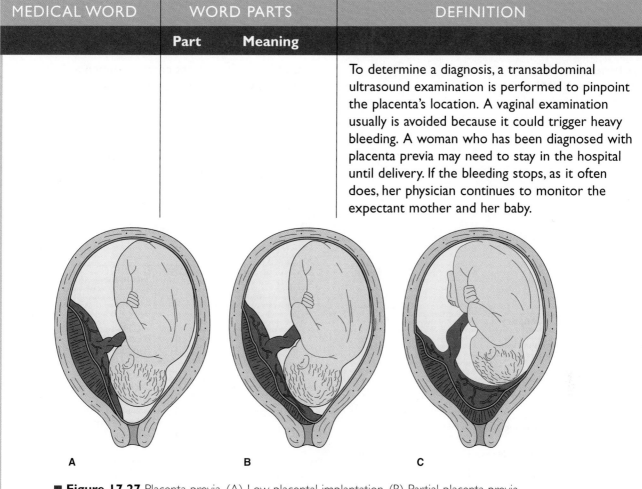

A   B   C

■ **Figure 17.27** Placenta previa. (A) Low placental implantation. (B) Partial placenta previa. (C) Total placenta previa.

MEDICAL WORD	WORD PARTS		DEFINITION
	Part	Meaning	
postcoital (pōst-kō´ ĭt-ăl)	post- coit -al	after a coming together pertaining to	Pertaining to after sexual intercourse
preeclampsia (prē˝ ē-klămp´ sē-ă)	pre- ec- lamp(s) -ia	before out to shine condition	Serious complication of pregnancy characterized by increasing hypertension, proteinuria (abnormal concentrations of urinary protein), and edema, also known as *toxemia* or *pregnancy-induced hypertension (PIH)*

MEDICAL WORD	WORD PARTS		DEFINITION
	Part	**Meaning**	
premenstrual syndrome (PMS) (prē-měn-stroo-ăl)			Condition that affects certain women and can cause distressful symptoms that begin 2 weeks before the onset of menstruation. The cause is unknown but may be due to the amount of prostaglandin produced, a deficient or excessive amount of estrogen or progesterone, or an interrelationship between these factors. The multisystem effects of premenstrual syndrome are presented in Figure 17.28 ■

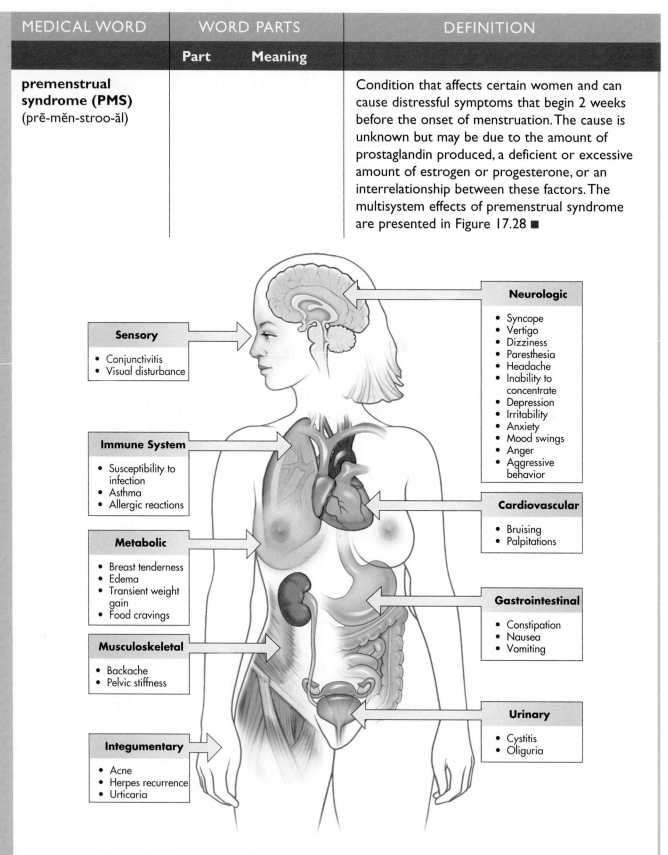

Sensory
- Conjunctivitis
- Visual disturbance

Immune System
- Susceptibility to infection
- Asthma
- Allergic reactions

Metabolic
- Breast tenderness
- Edema
- Transient weight gain
- Food cravings

Musculoskeletal
- Backache
- Pelvic stiffness

Integumentary
- Acne
- Herpes recurrence
- Urticaria

Neurologic
- Syncope
- Vertigo
- Dizziness
- Paresthesia
- Headache
- Inability to concentrate
- Depression
- Irritability
- Anxiety
- Mood swings
- Anger
- Aggressive behavior

Cardiovascular
- Bruising
- Palpitations

Gastrointestinal
- Constipation
- Nausea
- Vomiting

Urinary
- Cystitis
- Oliguria

■ **Figure 17.28** Multisystem effects of premenstrual syndrome.

MEDICAL WORD	WORD PARTS		DEFINITION
	Part	**Meaning**	
rectovaginal (rĕk″ tō-văj′ ĭ-năl)	rect/o vagin -al	rectum vagina pertaining to	Pertaining to the rectum and vagina
retroversion (rĕt″ rō-vur′ shŭn)	retro- vers -ion	backward turning process	Process of being turned backward, such as the displacement of the uterus with the cervix pointed forward. See Figure 17.4A on page 596.
salpingectomy (săl″ pĭn-jĕk′ tō-mē)	salping -ectomy	fallopian tube surgical excision	Surgical excision of a fallopian tube
salpingitis (săl″ pĭn-jī′ tĭs)	salping -itis	fallopian tube inflammation	Inflammation of a fallopian tube
salpingo-oophorectomy (săl′ pĭng″ gō-ō″ ŏf-ō- rĕk′ tō-mē)	salping/o oophor -ectomy	fallopian tube ovary surgical excision	Surgical excision of an ovary and a fallopian tube
toxic shock syndrome (TSS)			A serious bacterial infection caused by *Staphylococcus aureus* bacteria. Symptoms of TSS start suddenly with vomiting, high fever (temperature at least 102° F [38.8° C]), a rapid drop in blood pressure (with lightheadedness or fainting), watery diarrhea, headache, sore throat, and muscle aches. A type of related infection, streptococcal toxic shock syndrome (STSS), is caused by streptococcus bacteria. Within 48 hours of infection, blood pressure drops dangerously low, and the person may have fever, dizziness, confusion, difficulty breathing, and a weak and rapid pulse. The skin may be pale, cool, and moist, with a rash that sometimes peels later. The area around an infected wound can become swollen, red, and have areas of severely damaged or dying flesh. The liver and kidneys may begin to fail, and bleeding problems may develop.

fyi Toxic shock syndrome (TSS) was originally linked to the use of tampons, but is now also known to be associated with use of the contraceptive sponge and diaphragm birth control methods. Streptococcal toxic shock syndrome (STSS) most often appears after streptococcus bacteria have invaded areas of injured skin, such as cuts and scrapes, surgical wounds, and even chickenpox blisters.

MEDICAL WORD	WORD PARTS		DEFINITION
	Part	Meaning	
uterine fibroid (ū´ tĕr-ĭn fī-broyd)	uter -ine fibr -oid	uterus pertaining to fibrous tissue resemble	Benign fibrous tumor of the uterus made up of muscle cells and other tissues that grow within the wall of the uterus; the most common benign tumors in women of childbearing age; also called *uterine leiomyoma*. Fibroids are classified into three groups based on where they grow, such as just underneath the lining of the uterus, between the muscles of the uterus, or on the outside of the uterus. Most fibroids grow within the wall of the uterus, and some grow on stalks (called *peduncles*) that grow out from the surface of the uterus or into the cavity of the uterus. See Figure 17.29 ■

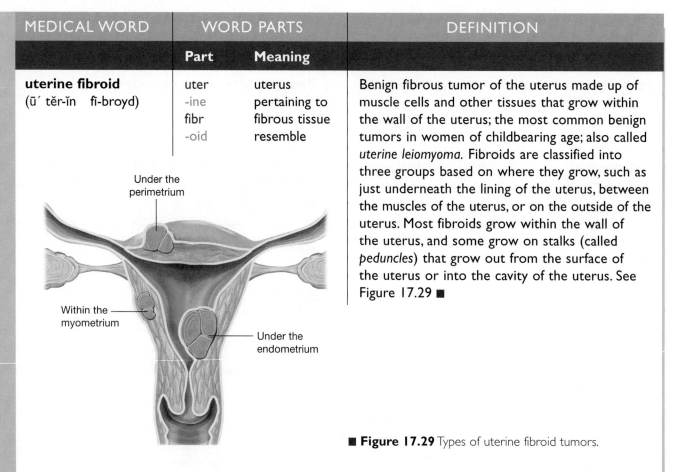

Under the perimetrium

Within the myometrium

Under the endometrium

■ **Figure 17.29** Types of uterine fibroid tumors.

fyi Types of surgery used to treat uterine fibroids include:

- *Dilation and curettage* (D&C) is a procedure that involves enlarging the cervix (dilation) and then scraping (curettage) out portions of the lining of the uterus. It is considered to be minor surgery performed in a hospital, ambulatory surgery center, or clinic.
- *Myomectomy* is a surgery to remove fibroids without taking out the healthy tissue of the uterus. It can be major surgery (with an abdominal incision) or minor surgery. The type, size, and location of the fibroids determine what type of procedure is done.
- *Hysterectomy* is a surgery to remove the uterus and is the only sure way to cure uterine fibroids. This surgery is used when a woman's fibroids are large or if she has heavy bleeding and is either near or past menopause and/or does not want to become pregnant in the future.

| **vaginitis**
(văj″ ĭn-i´ tĭs) | vagin
-itis | vagina
inflammation | Inflammation of the vagina |
| **venereal**
(vē-nē´ rē-ăl) | venere

-al | sexual intercourse
pertaining to | Pertaining to or resulting from sexual intercourse. See Sexually Transmitted Diseases in Chapter 18, "Male Reproductive System," on pages 660–663. |

• Drug Highlights •

TYPE OF DRUG	DESCRIPTION AND EXAMPLES
female hormones	
estrogens	Natural female sex hormone secreted by the ovarian follicles. Used for a variety of conditions including amenorrhea, dysfunctional uterine bleeding (DUB), and hirsutism as well as in palliative therapy for breast cancer in women and prostatic cancer in men. They are also used as hormone therapy (HT) in the treatment of uncomfortable symptoms that are related to menopause. EXAMPLES: Premarin (conjugated estrogens, USP), Estrace (estradiol), Estraderm (estradiol) transdermal system, Ogen (estropipate), and Menest (esterified estrogens)
progestogens/progestins	Natural female steroid hormone secreted by the corpus luteum. When produced synthetically, progesterones can be used to prevent uterine bleeding; combined with estrogen they can be used for treatment of amenorrhea. They may be used in cases of infertility and threatened or habitual miscarriage. Progesterone is responsible for changes in the uterine endometrium during the second half of the menstrual cycle, development of maternal placenta after implantation, and development of mammary glands. EXAMPLES: Provera (medroxyprogesterone acetate), norethindrone acetate, and Prometrium (natural progesterone)
contraceptives	
birth control pills (BCP)	Oral contraceptives (OC) containing mixtures of estrogen and progestin in various levels of strength that are nearly 100% effective when used as directed. The estrogen in the pill inhibits ovulation, and the progestin inhibits pituitary secretion of luteinizing hormone (LH), causes changes in the cervical mucus that renders it unfavorable to penetration by sperm, and alters the nature of the endometrium. EXAMPLES: Micronor, Brevicon, Lo/Ovral, and Nor-QD
birth control patch	Ortho Evra is the first transdermal birth control patch that continuously delivers two synthetic hormones, progestin (norelgestromin) and estrogen (ethinyl estradiol). The patch impedes pregnancy by preventing the ovaries from releasing eggs (ovulation) and thickening the cervical mucus. The patch is applied directly to the skin (buttocks, abdomen, upper torso, or upper outer arm) and has an effectiveness rate of 95%.

TYPE OF DRUG	DESCRIPTION AND EXAMPLES
injectable	Depo-Provera is an injectable contraceptive that is given four times a year. It contains medroxyprogesterone acetate, a synthetic drug that is similar to progesterone. Depo-Provera prevents pregnancy by stopping the ovaries from releasing eggs (ovulation) and thickens the cervical mucus. When used correctly, it can prevent pregnancy over 99% of the time.
intrauterine device (IUD)	Small device that is placed within the uterus to prevent pregnancy. It is usually made of soft, flexible, ultralight plastic and is 99.2% to 99.9% effective as birth control. Two types are available: ParaGard and Mirena. ParaGard uses copper around the plastic. Anyone allergic to copper should not use it. Mirena releases small amounts of a synthetic progesterone over time and can be left in place for up to 5 years. IUDs do not protect against sexually transmitted diseases (STDs) or the human immunodeficiency virus (HIV). See Figure 17.30 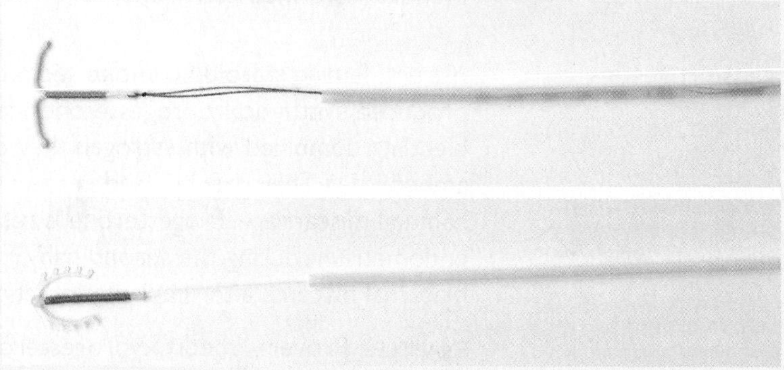 ■

■ **Figure 17.30** Examples of intrauterine devices (IUDs).

• Diagnostic and Lab Tests •

TEST	DESCRIPTION
amniocentesis (ăm″ nĭ-ō -sĕn-tĕ′ sĭs)	Surgical puncture of the amniotic sac to obtain a sample of amniotic fluid containing fetal cells that are examined. It can be determined whether the fetus has Down syndrome, neural tube defects, Tay–Sachs disease, or other genetic defects. Determines chromosomal abnormalities and biochemical disorders. See Figure 17.31 ■

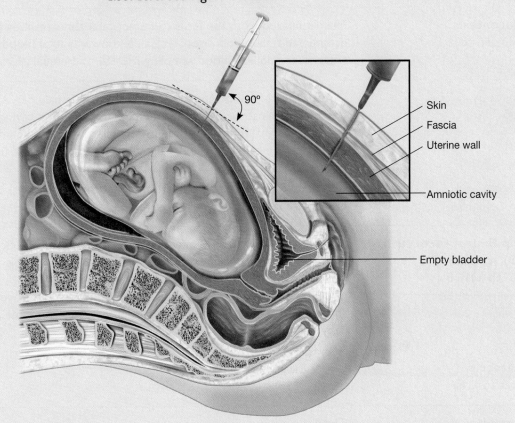

■ **Figure 17.31** Amniocentesis. The woman is usually scanned by ultrasound to determine the placental site and to locate a pocket of fluid. As the needle is inserted, three levels of resistance are felt when the needle penetrates the skin, fascia, and uterine wall. When the needle is placed within the amniotic cavity, amniotic fluid is withdrawn.

TEST	DESCRIPTION
blood grouping (A, B, AB, and O)	Determines blood type.
breast examination	Visual inspection and manual examination of the breast for changes in contour, symmetry, dimpling of skin, retraction of the nipple(s), and the presence of lumps.

TEST	DESCRIPTION
chorionic villus sampling (CVS) (kō″ rē-ŏn-ĭk vĭl′ŭs)	Determine chromosomal abnormalities and biochemical disorders (Down syndrome, Tay–Sachs disease, and cystic fibrosis).
colposcopy (kŏl-pŏs′ kō-pē)	Visual examination of the vagina and cervix via a colposcope. Abnormal results can indicate cervical or vaginal erosion, tumors, and dysplasia.
complete blood count	Check for anemia, infection, or cell abnormalities.
cordocentesis (kor-dō-sēn-tē′sĭs)	Examine blood from the fetus to detect fetal abnormalities (Down syndrome and fetal blood disorders); also known as fetal blood sampling, percutaneous umbilical blood sampling [PUBS], and umbilical vein sampling.
culdoscopy (kŭl-dŏs′ kō-pē)	Direct visual examination of the viscera of the female pelvis through a culdoscope. The instrument is introduced into the pelvic cavity through the posterior vaginal fornix. Can be used to diagnose ectopic pregnancy and to determine the cause of pelvic pain and to check for pelvic masses.
estrogen (es′ trō-jĕns)	Test done on urine or blood serum to determine the level of estrone, estradiol, and estriol.
Group B streptococcus (GBS) screening (strĕp″ tō-kŏk′ ŭs)	Screen for vaginal strep B infection. It is to be performed between the 35th and 37th week of pregnancy. Any time other than this will not be significant to show if the expectant mother is carrying GBS during her time of delivery. Note: When the expectant mother tests positive, intravenous antibiotics are recommended during delivery, to reduce the chance of the baby becoming infected with GBS.
hematocrit (hē-măt′ ō-krĭt)	Check for anemia during pregnancy.
hemoglobin (hē m″ ō-glō′ bĭn)	Check for anemia during pregnancy.
hepatitis B screen (hĕp″ ă-tī′ tĭs)	Identify carriers of hepatitis.
human chorionic gonadotropin (hCG) (kō″ rē-ŏn-ĭk gŏn″ ă-dō-trō′ĭn)	Determine the presence of hCG, which is secreted by the placenta. A positive result usually indicates pregnancy.
human immunodeficiency virus (HIV) screen (ĭm″ ū-nō-dĕ-fĭsh′ ĕn-sē)	Identify HIV infection.

TEST	DESCRIPTION
hysterosalpingography (HSG) (hĭs″ tĕr-ō -săl″ pĭn-gŏg′ ră-fē)	X-ray of the uterus and fallopian tubes after the injection of a radiopaque substance. Size and structure of the uterus and fallopian tubes can be evaluated. Uterine tumors, fibroids, tubal pregnancy, and tubal occlusion can be observed. Also used for treatment of an occluded fallopian tube.
laparoscopy (lăp-ăr-ŏs′ kō-pē)	Visual examination of the abdominal cavity. A flexible, lighted instrument (laparoscope) is inserted through a periumbilical incision to examine the ovaries and fallopian tubes.
mammography (măm-ŏg′ ră-fē)	Specific type of imaging that uses a low-dose x-ray system for examination of the breasts. A mammography exam is called a *mammogram*. The two types of mammograms are *screening,* which is generally used to detect breast cancer or other changes in the breast tissue in women who do not have symptoms, and *diagnostic,* which can be ordered when a screening mammogram shows something abnormal in the breast. It is the most effective means of detecting early breast cancers.
maternal blood glucose	Screen for gestational diabetes. If the level of glucose is moderately elevated, a more conclusive glucose tolerance test (GTT) may be ordered.
nonstress test (NST)	Identify fetal compromise in conditions with poor placenta function, such as hypertension, diabetes mellitus, or post-term gestation (pregnancy lasting beyond 42 weeks).
Papanicolaou (Pap) smear (păp′ ăh-nĭk″ ō-lă′ oo)	Screening technique to aid in the detection of cervical cancer. Both false-positive and false-negative results have been experienced with Pap smears. It is a screening procedure. Pap smear results are generally reported as within normal limits (WNL), abnormal squamous cells of undetermined significance (Ascus), mild dysplasia (CIN [cervical intraepithelial neoplasia] I), moderate dysplasia (CIN II), and severe dysplasia and/or carcinoma in-situ (CIN III).
pregnanediol (prĕg″ nān-dī-ŏl)	Urine test to determine menstrual disorders or possible abortion.
quad marker screen (AFP, hCG, UE, and inhibin-A)	Measure high and low levels of alpha-fetoprotein (AFP) (a protein produced by the baby's liver) and abnormal levels of human chorionic gonadotropin (hCG) (a hormone produced by the placenta), unconjugated estriol (UE) (a hormone produced in the placenta and in the baby's liver), and inhibin-A (a hormone produced by the placenta). To assess probabilities of potential genetic disorders.
Rh factor (positive or negative)	Determine risk for maternal–fetal blood incompatibility.

TEST	DESCRIPTION
rubella (German measles) titer (roo-běl′ lă tǐ′ tēr)	Determine immunity to rubella.
TORCH panel (tōrch)	Screen for toxoplasmosis, rubella, cytomegalovirus (CMV), and herpes simplex virus (HSV).
toxoplasmosis screen (tŏks-ō-plăs-mō′sǐs)	Determine toxoplasmosis infection.
ultrasound (ŭl′ tră-sŏund)	**Uses during pregnancy include:** • Confirm viable pregnancy. • Confirm fetal heartbeat (FHB). • Measure the crown-rump length or gestational age. • Confirm ectopic pregnancy. • Confirm molar pregnancy (hydatidiform mole or hydatid mole). • Assess abnormal gestation. • Diagnose fetal malformation and structural abnormalities. • Confirm multiple pregnancies. • Determine gender of the baby. • Identify placenta location. • Confirm intrauterine death. • Observe fetal presentation and movements. • Identify uterine and pelvic abnormalities of the mother during pregnancy.
urinalysis (ū′ rǐ-năl′ i-sǐs)	Check for infection, renal disease, or diabetes.
wet mat or wet-prep	Examination of vaginal discharge for the presence of bacteria and yeast. Vaginal smear placed on a microscopic slide, wet with normal saline, and then viewed under a microscope by the physician.

• Abbreviations •

ABBREVIATION	MEANING	ABBREVIATION	MEANING
AB	abortion	**HSG**	hysterosalpingography
AH	abdominal hysterectomy	**IUD**	intrauterine device
AROM	artificial rupture of membranes	**HIV**	human immunodeficiency virus
Ascus	atypical squamous cells of undetermined significance	**LH**	luteinizing hormone
BCP	birth control pill	**NST**	nonstress test
CIN	cervical intraepithelial neoplasia	**OB**	obstetrics
cm	centimeter	**OC**	oral contraceptive
CS, C-section	cesarean section	**OTC**	over-the-counter
CVS	chorionic villus sampling	**Pap**	Papanicolaou (smear)
D&C	dilation and curettage	**PID**	pelvic inflammatory disease
DES	diethylstilbestrol	**PIH**	pregnancy-induced hypertension
DUB	dysfunctional uterine bleeding		
FHB	fetal heartbeat	**PMS**	premenstrual syndrome
g	gram	**STDs**	sexually transmitted diseases
GBS	Group B streptococcus	**STSS**	streptococcal toxic shock syndrome
hCG	human chorionic gonadotropin		
HT	hormone therapy	**TSS**	toxic shock syndrome

• Study and Review • Study and Review • Study a

Anatomy and Physiology

Write your answers to the following questions.

1. List the primary and accessory sex organs of the female reproductive system.

a. _____   b. _____

c. _____   d. _____

e. _____   f. _____

2. The normal position of the uterus is known as _____

3. Define *fundus.* _____

4. Name the three layers of the uterine wall.

a. _____   b. _____

c. _____

5. State two primary functions associated with the uterus.

a. _____

b. _____

6. Define the following terms.

a. *Retroflexion* _____

_____

b. *Anteversion* _____

_____

c. *Retroversion* _____

_____

7. The fallopian tubes are also called the _____ _____ or

_____ .

8. Should the ovum become impregnated by a spermatozoon while in the fallopian tube, the process of

_____ occurs.

632

9. State the two functions of the ovary.

a. _____   b. _____

10. State the three functions of the vagina.

a. _____   b. _____

c. _____

11. The breasts or _____ _____ are compound alveolar structures.

12. The _____ is the dark pigmented area found in the skin over each breast, and the

_____ is the elevated area in its center.

13. Define *colostrum*. _____

_____

14. Name the three phases of the menstrual cycle.

a. _____   b. _____

c. _____

Overview of Obstetrics

Write your answers to the following questions.

1. _____ is the branch of medicine that pertains to the care of women during pregnancy, childbirth, and the postpartum period.

2. _____ is the process in which a sperm penetrates an ovum.

3. The fertilized ovum is also known as a _____

4. As the blastocyst develops, it forms a structure with two cavities, the _____ and

_____ .

5. Pregnancy is divided into four stages. Describe each of these stages.

a. Prenatal stage _____

b. Labor _____

c. Parturition _____

d. Postpartum period_____

6. Labor is divided into three stages. Describe each of these stages.

a. First stage _____

b. Second stage _____

c. Third stage _____

Word Parts

PREFIXES

Give the definitions of the following prefixes.

1. a- _____
2. contra- _____
3. dys- _____
4. ec- _____
5. endo- _____
6. intra- _____
7. oligo- _____
8. peri- _____
9. post- _____
10. retro- _____
11. pre- _____

ROOTS AND COMBINING FORMS

Give the definition of the following roots and combining forms.

1. abort _____
2. bartholin _____
3. cept _____
4. cervic _____
5. coit _____
6. colp/o _____
7. culd/o _____
8. cyst/o _____
9. fibr _____
10. genital _____
11. gynec/o _____
12. hymen _____
13. hyster _____
14. hyster/o _____
15. lamp(s) _____
16. log _____
17. mamm/o _____
18. mast _____
19. men _____
20. men/o _____
21. metr _____
22. metr/i _____
23. my/o _____
24. o/o _____
25. oophor _____
26. ovulat _____
27. par _____
28. pause _____
29. rect/o _____
30. salping _____
31. salping/o _____
32. uter _____
33. vagin _____
34. venere _____

35. vers _____   **36.** lump _____

37. pareun _____

SUFFIXES
Give the definitions of the following suffixes.

1. -al _____   **2.** -arche _____

3. -cele _____   **4.** -centesis _____

5. -ectomy _____   **6.** -genesis _____

7. -ia _____   **8.** -ine _____

9. -ion _____   **10.** -ist _____

11. -itis _____   **12.** -oma _____

13. -osis _____   **14.** -plasty _____

15. -rrhagia _____   **16.** -rrhea _____

17. -scope _____   **18.** -oid _____

Identifying Medical Terms

In the spaces provided, write the medical terms for the following meanings.

1. _____ Inflammation of the uterine cervix

2. _____ Difficult or painful monthly flow

3. _____ Fibrous tissue tumor

4. _____ Study of the female

5. _____ Surgical excision of the hymen

6. _____ Surgical repair of the breast

7. _____ Normal monthly flow

8. _____ Formation of the ovum

9. _____ Difficult or painful sexual intercourse

10. _____ Male or female reproductive organs

Spelling

Circle the correct spelling of each medical term.

1. bartholinitis / bartolinitis

2. hysterotomy / hystrotomy

3. menorhagia / menorrhagia

4. oophorectomy / oophorectmy

5. salpingitis / salpinitis

6. vajinitis / vaginitis

7. veneral / venereal

8. menarche / menache

9. oligomenorrhea / oligomenorhea

10. postcotal / postcoital

Matching

Select the appropriate lettered meaning for each of the following words.

_____ 1. laser ablation

_____ 2. lumpectomy

_____ 3. menarche

_____ 4. mittelschmerz

_____ 5. ovulation

_____ 6. gynecologist

_____ 7. contraception

_____ 8. perimenopause

_____ 9. hysterotomy

_____ 10. rectovaginal

a. Beginning of the monthly flow (menses, menstruation)

b. Surgical removal of a tumor from the breast

c. Abdominal pain that occurs midway between the menstrual periods at ovulation

d. Process in which an ovum is discharged from the cortex of the ovary

e. Procedure that uses a laser to destroy the uterine lining

f. Pertaining to the rectum and vagina

g. Period of gradual changes that lead into menopause

h. Physician who specializes in the study of the female

i. Incision into the uterus

j. Process of preventing conception

k. Lack of monthly flow (menses, menstruation)

Abbreviations

Place the correct word, phrase, or abbreviation in the space provided.

1. AH _____

2. DES _____

3. birth control pill _____

4. intrauterine device _____

5. pelvic inflammatory disease _____

6. cervical intraepithelial neoplasia_____

7. DUB _____

8. PMS _____

9. dilation and curettage _____

10. toxic shock syndrome _____

Diagnostic and Laboratory Tests

Select the best answer to each multiple-choice question. Circle the letter of your choice.

1. X-ray of the uterus and fallopian tubes after the injection of a radiopaque substance.
  a. hysterosalpingography   **c.** culdoscopy
  b. laparoscopy   **d.** mammography

2. Used to examine the ovaries and fallopian tubes.
  a. colposcopy   **c.** laparoscopy
  b. culdoscopy   **d.** mammography

3. Process of obtaining pictures of the breast by use of x-rays.
  a. colposcopy   **c.** laparoscopy
  b. culdoscopy   **d.** mammography

4. Screening technique to aid in the detection of cervical/uterine cancer and cancer precursors.
  a. colposcopy   **c.** estrogens
  b. Papanicolaou (Pap smear)   **d.** mammography

5. Urine test that determines menstrual disorders or possible abortion.
  a. wet mat or wet-prep   **c.** Pap smear
  b. culdoscopy   **d.** pregnanediol

PRACTICAL APPLICATION

SOAP: CHART NOTE ANALYSIS

This exercise will make you aware of information, abbreviations, and medical terminology typically found in a gynecology patient's chart note. The names and any personal information have been created by the author. Read and study each form or case study and then answer the questions that follow. You may refer to Appendix III, Abbreviations and Symbols, on page A41.

Patient: Smith, Ann M.   **Date:** 2/21/XX

Dob: 01/24/1957   **Age:** 54   **Sex:** Female

Insurance: Best Care Insurance

Allergies: Penicillin

Subjective: 54 y/o white female presents with complaints of irregular periods, hot flashes, and trouble sleeping. She states, "Sex with my husband has become uncomfortable and I am very moody. I am really having trouble with hot flashes. I wake up in the middle of the night soaked—especially my hair and neck." When asked about her children, she indicates that she has two children, one daughter who is an English teacher and one son who is a pharmacist. She also states that she has never had an abortion. Her LMP was 11/21/XX.

Objective:

Vital Signs: T: 98.8 F; **P:** 70; **R:** 16; **BP:** 120/78

Ht: 5′ 3″

Wt: 135 lb

General Appearance: Attractive, well-groomed, and pleasant. Noted a slight nervousness and concern during initial interview.

GYN:

Breasts: Symmetrical, no palpable masses or tenderness, no dimpling or skin changes

External genitalia: No lesions or inflammation, normal hair distribution with thinning

Cervix: Pink, smooth, no cervical motion tenderness; Pap smear performed

Adnexa uteri: Nontender, no masses

Uterus: NSSC, noted retroversion position, firm, slightly enlarged, with possible uterine fibroid tumor

Rectal exam: No fissures, hemorrhoids, or skin lesions in perianal area. Sphincter tone good, no prolapse. No masses or tenderness.

Pregnancies: Gravida 2 Para 2 Abortions 0

Assessment: Perimenopause

P

Plan: Patient elected the nonprescription treatment for 6 months. To be reevaluated August 20XX.

1. Schedule mammogram ASAP. If WNL, then annually.

2. Advised to use over-the-counter water-soluble vaginal lubricant for intercourse and moisturizer for vaginal dryness.

3. Advised to go to the laboratory for CBC, cholesterol, triglycerides, and glucose. Check TSH, FSH, and estradiol levels to R/O thyroid disorder and obtain hormone baseline levels.

4. Recommended she take a multivitamin and mineral complex that contains 400 mcg of folic acid. Also, take 1500 mg of calcium with Vitamin D daily and an antioxidant.

5. Schedule a pelvic ultrasound to R/O uterine fibroid tumor, ASAP.

6. Recommend a bone density study before reevaluation in August.

Chart Note Questions

Place the correct answer in the space provided.

1. What is the abbreviation for gynecology? _____

2. What does the statement, "I wake up in the middle of the night soaked—especially my hair and neck," indicate?

_____

3. What is the medical word for difficult or painful sexual intercourse? _____

4. What does Gravida 2 indicate? _____

5. Why is a pelvic ultrasound recommended? _____

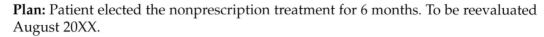

MyMedicalTerminologyLab is a premium online homework management system that includes a host of features to help you study. Registered users will find:

- Fun games and activities built within a virtual hospital

- Powerful tools that track and analyze your results—allowing you to create a personalized learning experience

- Videos, flashcards, and audio pronunciations to help enrich your progress

- Streaming lesson presentations and self-paced learning modules

- A space where you and your instructors can view and manage your assignments

18

LEARNING OUTCOMES

On completion of this chapter, you will be able to:

1. State the description and primary functions of the organs/structures of the male reproductive system.

2. Analyze, build, spell, and pronounce medical words.

3. Explain the causes, symptoms, and treatments of selected sexually transmitted diseases.

4. Comprehend the drugs highlighted in this chapter.

5. Provide the description of diagnostic and laboratory tests related to the male reproductive system.

6. Identify and define selected abbreviations.

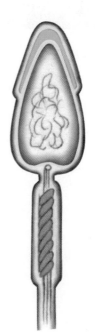

COMBINING FORMS OF THE MALE REPRODUCTIVE SYSTEM

artific/i	not natural	**orchid/o**	testicle
balan/o	glans penis	**prostat/o**	prostate
cis/o	to cut	**sperm/o**	seed, sperm
crypt/o	hidden	**sperm/i**	seed, sperm
didym/o	testis	**spermat/o**	seed, sperm
ejaculat/o	to throw out	**testicul/o**	testicle
gon/o	genitals	**varic/o**	twisted vein
gynec/o	female	**vas/o**	vessel
mast/o	breast	**vesicul/o**	seminal vesicle
mit/o	thread	**zo/o**	animal
orch/o	testicle		

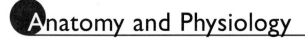natomy and Physiology

The male reproductive system consists of the testes, various ducts, the urethra, and the following accessory glands: bulbourethral, prostate, and the seminal vesicles. The supporting structures and accessory sex organs are the scrotum and the penis. The vital function of the male reproductive system is to provide the sperm cells necessary to fertilize the ovum, thereby perpetuating the species. Table 18.1 ■ provides an at-a-glance look at the male reproductive system. See Figure 18.1 ■

TABLE 18.1 Male Reproductive System at-a-Glance

Organ/Structure	Primary Functions/Description
Scrotum	Acts as a natural climate control center for the testicles in order to maintain viability of sperm. The temperature in the scrotum is a degree or two lower than the usual body temperature of 98.6°F, which would kill sperm.
Penis	Acts as male organ of copulation and urination; site of the orifice for the elimination of urine and semen from the body
Testes	Provide the male sex hormone, testosterone, provided by cells within them; contain seminiferous tubules that are the site of sperm formation and development
Epididymis	Acts as site for the maturation of sperm
Vas deferens	Acts as excretory duct of the testis
Seminal vesicles	Produce a slightly alkaline fluid that becomes a part of the seminal fluid or semen
Prostate gland	Secretes an alkaline fluid that aids in maintaining the viability of spermatozoa
Bulbourethral or Cowper's glands	Produce a mucous secretion before ejaculation, which becomes a part of the semen
Urethra	Transmits urine and semen out of the body

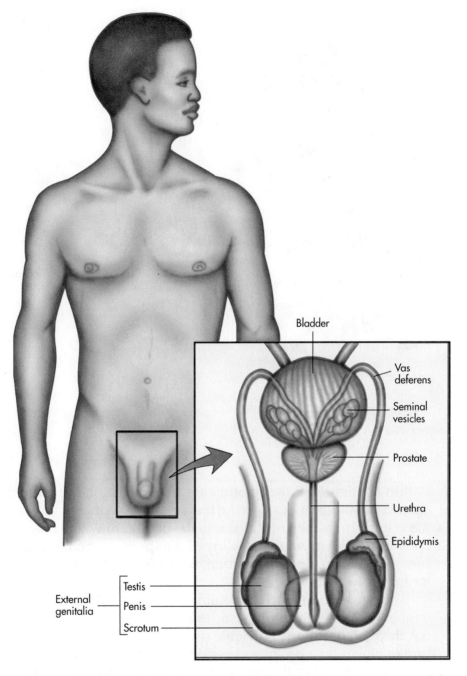

■ **Figure 18.1** Male reproductive system: seminal vesicles, prostate, urethra, vas deferens, epididymis, and external genitalia.

EXTERNAL ORGANS

In the male, the scrotum, the testes, and the penis are the external organs of reproduction. See Figures 18.1 and 18.2 ■

Scrotum

The **scrotum** is a pouchlike structure located behind and below the penis. It is suspended from the perineal region and is divided by a septum into two sacs, each containing one of the testes along with its connecting tube called the **epididymis**.

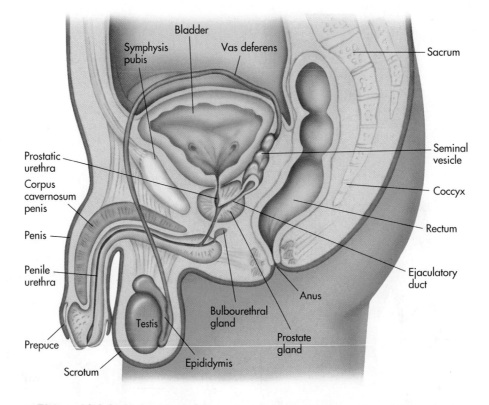

■ **Figure 18.2** Sagittal section of the male pelvis, showing the organs of the reproductive system.

Within the tissues of the scrotum are fibers of smooth muscle that contract in the absence of sufficient heat, giving the scrotum a wrinkled appearance. This contractile action brings the testes closer to the perineum where they can absorb sufficient body heat to maintain the viability of the **spermatozoa**. These changes in the scrotum illustrate its primary function, which is to act as a natural climate control center for the testicles.

The temperature in the scrotum is a degree or two lower than the usual body temperature of 98.6° F. The testicles need this lower temperature in order to carry out their job of producing viable sperm. If the testicles are kept at body temperature or higher for a prolonged period, infertility or sterility can result. The scrotum continually monitors the environment for temperature changes and responds automatically in the way that is best for the production of healthy sperm.

Under normal conditions, the walls of the scrotum are generally free of wrinkles, and it hangs loosely between the thighs (Figure 18.1).

Testes

The male has two ovoid-shaped organs, the **testes**, located within the scrotum. See Figure 18.3 ■ Each testis is about 4 cm long and 2.5 cm wide. The interior of each testis is divided into about 250 wedge-shaped lobes by fibrous tissues. Coiled within each lobe are one to three small tubes called the **seminiferous tubules**, which are the site of the development of male reproductive cells, the **spermatozoa**. Cells within the testes also produce the male sex hormone, **testosterone**, which is responsible for the development of secondary male characteristics during puberty and maintaining them through adulthood.

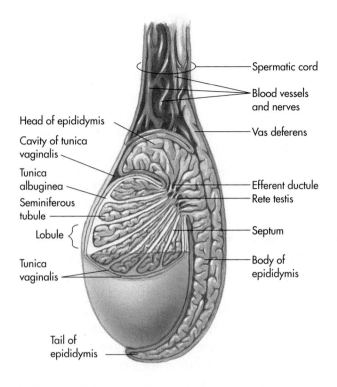

Figure 18.3 Sagittal view of the testis showing interior anatomy.

LIFE SPAN CONSIDERATIONS

Puberty is defined as a period of rapid change in the lives of boys and girls during which time the reproductive organs mature and become functionally capable of reproduction. In the male, puberty generally begins around 12 years of age when the genitals start to increase in size and the shoulders broaden and become muscular. As testosterone is released, secondary sexual characteristics develop, such as pubic and axillary hair, increase in size of the penis and testes, voice changes (deepening), facial hair, erections, and nocturnal emissions.

Testosterone is essential for normal growth and development of the male accessory sex organs. It plays a vital role in the erection process of the penis and thus is necessary for the reproductive act, copulation. Additionally, testosterone affects the growth of hair on the face, muscular development, and vocal timbre. The *seminiferous tubules* form a plexus or network called the *rete testis* from which 15–20 small ducts, the efferent ductules, leave the testis and open into the epididymis (see Figures 18.1 and 18.2).

Penis

The **penis** is the external male sex organ and is composed of erectile tissue covered with skin. The size and shape of the penis varies, with an average erect penis being 15–20 cm in length. The penis has three longitudinal columns of erectile tissue that are capable of significant enlargement when engorged with blood, as is the case during sexual stimulation. Two of these columns, located side by side, form the greater part of the penis. These columns are known as the *corpora cavernosa penis.* The third longitudinal column, the *corpus spongiosum,* has the same function as the first two columns but contains the penile portion of the urethra and tends to be more elastic when in an erectile state. The *corpus spongiosum,* at its distal end, expands to form the *glans penis,* the cone-shaped head of the penis, and is the site of the urethral orifice. It is covered with loose skin folds called the **foreskin** or prepuce. See Figure 18.2. The foreskin contains glands that secrete a lubricating fluid called *smegma.* The foreskin can be removed by a surgical procedure known as **circumcision.** See Figure 18.7 on page 652.

The erectile state in the penis results when sexual stimulation causes large quantities of blood from dilated arteries supplying the penis to fill the cavernous spaces in the erectile tissue. When the arteries constrict, the pressure on the veins in the area is reduced, thus allowing more blood to leave the penis than enters, and the penis returns to its normal state. The functions of the penis are to serve as the male organ of **copulation** (sexual intercourse) and as the site of the orifice for the elimination of urine and semen from the body.

LIFE SPAN CONSIDERATIONS

In the newborn, the scrotum can appear large at birth. One or both testes can fail to descend into the scrotum, causing a condition called **cryptorchidism.** The foreskin of the penis can be tight at birth, causing **phimosis**, a condition of narrowing of the opening of the prepuce wherein the foreskin cannot be drawn back over the glans penis. Congenital defects such as **epispadias** (urethra opens on the dorsum of the penis) and **hypospadias** (urethra opens on the underside of the penis) can be present. See Figure 18.10 on page 654.

INTERNAL ORGANS

In the male, the epididymis, the vas deferens, the seminal vesicles, the prostate gland, the bulbourethral glands, and the urethra are the internal organs of reproduction.

Epididymis

Each testis is connected by efferent ductules to an **epididymis**, which is a coiled tube laying on the posterior aspect of the testis. The epididymis is between 13 and 20 feet in length but is coiled into a space less than 2 inches (5 cm) long and ends in the ductus deferens. Each epididymis functions as a site for the maturation of **sperm** (Figure 18.4 ■) and as the first part of the duct system through which sperm pass on their journey to the urethra (Figures 18.1 and 18.2).

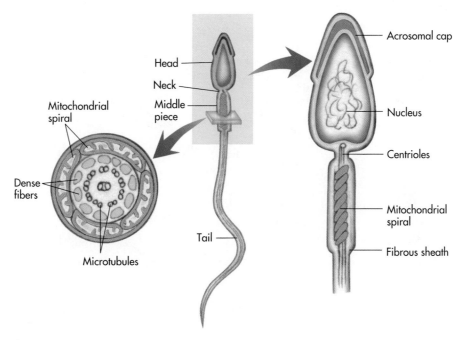

■ **Figure 18.4** Basic structure of a spermatozoon (sperm).

Vas Deferens

The **vas deferens**, also called the **ductus deferens**, is a slim muscular tube, about 30–45 cm in length, and is a continuation of the epididymis (Figures 18.1 and 18.2). It conveys sperm from the epididymis to the ejaculatory duct. It has been described as the *excretory duct* of the testis and extends from a point adjacent to the testis to enter the abdomen through the inguinal canal. Between the testis and the part of the abdomen known as the *internal inguinal ring*, the vas deferens is contained within a structure known as the **spermatic cord** that also contains arteries, veins, lymphatic vessels, and nerves.

Seminal Vesicles

There are two **seminal vesicles**, each connected by a narrow duct to a vas deferens, which then forms a short tube, the **ejaculatory duct**, which penetrates the base of the prostate gland and opens into the prostatic portion of the urethra (Figures 18.1 and 18.5 ■). The seminal vesicles produce a slightly alkaline fluid that becomes a part of the seminal fluid or semen.

Prostate Gland

The **prostate gland** is about 4 cm wide and weighs about 20 g. It is composed of glandular, connective, and muscular tissue and lies behind the urinary bladder (Figure 18.1 and 18.5). It surrounds the first 2.5 cm of the urethra and secretes an alkaline fluid that aids in maintaining the viability of spermatozoa. Enlargement of the prostate, called **benign prostatic hyperplasia (BPH),** is a condition that can occur in older men. In this condition, the prostate obstructs the urethra and interferes with the normal passage of urine. When this occurs, a **prostatectomy** can be performed to remove a part of the gland. The prostate gland can also be a site for cancer in older men.

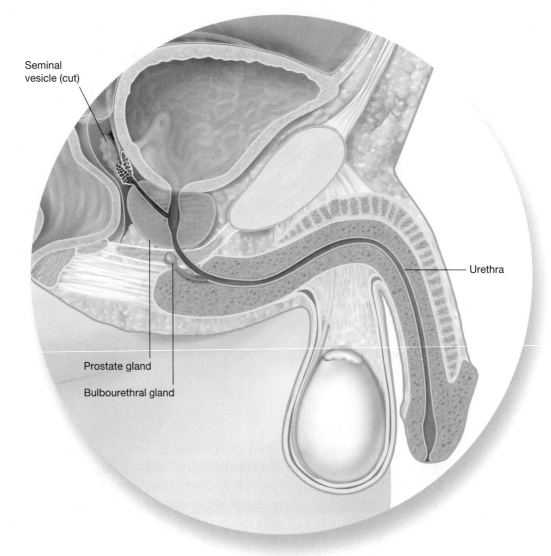

Seminal
vesicle (cut)

Urethra

Prostate gland

Bulbourethral gland

■ **Figure 18.5** Sagittal view of the male pelvis showing the seminal vesicle, ejaculatory duct, prostate gland, bulbourethral glands, and urethra.

LIFE SPAN CONSIDERATIONS

With aging, the prostate gland enlarges and its glandular secretions decrease, the testes become smaller and firmer, the production of testosterone gradually decreases, and pubic hair becomes sparser and stiffer.

In a healthy, normal male, **spermatogenesis** and the ability to have erections last a lifetime. However, sexual arousal can be slowed with a longer refractory period between erections. In men, a normal *refractory period* is the time span between orgasms during which time they are not physically able to have another orgasm. In older men the refractory time lengthens.

Bulbourethral Glands

The **bulbourethral glands**, or *Cowper's glands*, are two small pea-sized glands located below the prostate and on either side of the urethra. A duct about 2.5 cm long connects them with the wall of the urethra. The bulbourethral glands produce a mucous secretion before ejaculation, which becomes a component of semen.

Urethra

The male **urethra** is approximately 20 cm long and is divided into three sections: prostatic, membranous, and penile. It extends from the urinary bladder to the external urethral orifice at the head of the penis. It serves the duel function of transmitting urine and semen out of the body.

Anatomy and Physiology Labeling

Identify the structures shown below by filling in the blanks.

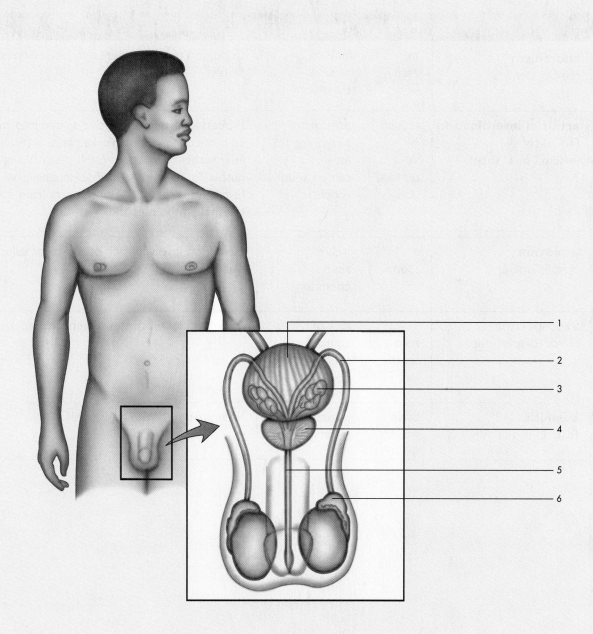

1
2
3
4
5
6

• Building Your Medical Vocabulary •

This section provides the foundation for learning medical terminology. Review the following alphabetized word list. Note how common prefixes and suffixes are repeatedly applied to word roots and combining forms to create different meanings. The word parts are color-coded: prefixes are green, suffixes are blue, roots/combining forms are red.

You will find that some terms have not been divided into word parts. These are common words or specialized terms that are included to enhance your medical vocabulary. See Chapter 1, page 7, to review pronunciation guidelines.

MEDICAL WORD	Part	Meaning	DEFINITION
anorchism (ăn-ōr′ kĭzm)	an- orch -ism	lack of testicle condition	Condition in which there is a lack of one or both testes
artificial insemination (ăr″ tĭ-fĭsh′ ăl ĭn-sĕm″ ĭn-ā′ shŭn)	artific/i -al in- seminat -ion	not natural pertaining to into semen, seed process	Process of artificially placing semen into the vagina so that conception can take place. *Artificial insemination homologous (AIH)* means using the husband's semen and *artificial insemination heterologous* refers to using sperm from a donor other than the husband.
aspermia (ă-spĕr′ mē-ă)	a- sperm -ia	lack of seed condition	Condition involving lack of sperm or failure to ejaculate sperm
azoospermia (ă-zō″ ō-spĕr′ mē-ă)	a- zo/o sperm -ia	lack of animal seed condition	Condition in which the semen lacks spermatozoa
balanitis (băl″ ă-nī′ tĭs)	balan -itis	glans inflammation	Inflammation of the glans penis

MEDICAL WORD	WORD PARTS		DEFINITION
	Part	**Meaning**	
benign prostatic hyperplasia (BPH) (bē-nīn´ prŏs-tăt´-ĭk hī´´ pĕr-plā´zē-a)			Enlargement of the prostate gland. As the prostate enlarges, it compresses the urethra, thereby restricting the normal flow of urine. See Figure 18.6 ■ This restriction generally causes a number of symptoms and can be referred to as *prostatism*. **Prostatism** is any condition of the prostate gland that interferes with the flow of urine from the bladder. Symptoms usually include weak or difficult-to-start urine stream; feeling that the bladder is not empty; need to urinate often, especially at night; feeling of urgency (a sudden need to urinate); abdominal straining; decrease in size and force of the urinary stream; and interruption of the stream.

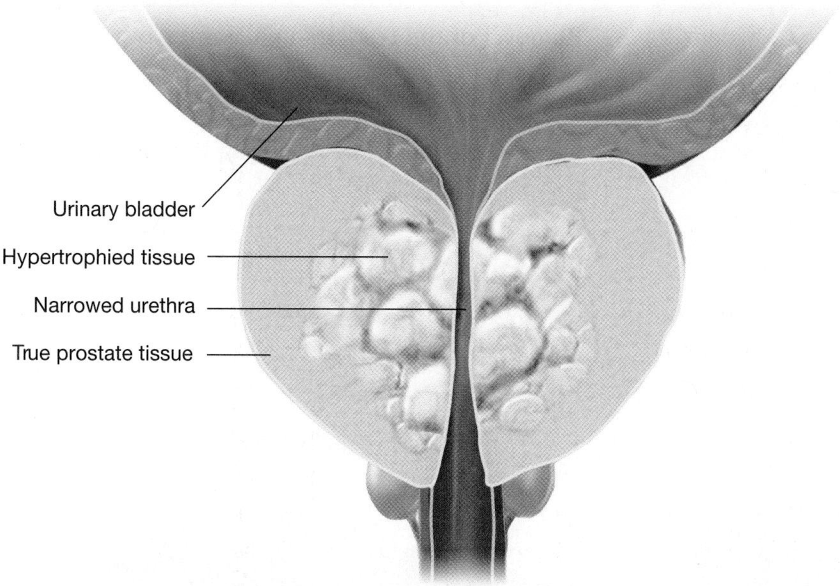

Urinary bladder
Hypertrophied tissue
Narrowed urethra
True prostate tissue

■ **Figure 18.6** Benign prostatic hyperplasia (BPH) showing an enlarged prostate compressing the urethra.

LIFE SPAN CONSIDERATIONS

By age 60, four out of five men have an enlarged prostate. Treatment for benign prostatic hyperplasia includes drug therapy (see Drug Highlights, page 664), nonsurgical procedures, and/or surgery.

Nonsurgical treatments include:

1. **Transurethral microwave thermotherapy (TUMT)**. A device called a Prostatron employs microwaves to heat and destroy excess prostate tissue, sending computer-regulated microwaves through a catheter to heat-selected portions of the prostate to at least 111°F. A cooling system protects the urinary tract during the procedure.
2. **Transurethral needle ablation (TUNA)**. A minimally invasive treatment that delivers low-level radiofrequency energy through twin needles to burn away a well-defined region of the enlarged prostate. Shields protect the urethra from heat damage. Improves urine flow and relieves symptoms with fewer side effects when compared with transurethral resection of the prostate (TURP).

MEDICAL WORD	WORD PARTS		DEFINITION
	Part	Meaning	

Types of surgery used for benign prostatic hyperplasia include:

1. **Transurethral resection of the prostate (TURP or TUR)**. During this procedure, the most common form of surgery used for this condition, an endoscopic instrument that has ocular and surgical capabilities is introduced directly through the urethra to the prostate and small pieces of the prostate gland are removed by using an electrical cutting loop.
2. **Transurethral incision of the prostate (TUIP)**. Used to widen the urethra by making a few small cuts in the bladder neck where the urethra joins the bladder and in the prostate gland itself.
3. **Open surgery**. Used when a transurethral procedure cannot be done: when the gland is greatly enlarged, when there are complicating factors, or when the bladder has been damaged and needs to be repaired.
4. **Laser surgery**. Employs side-firing laser fibers and ND:YAG (Neodimium Doped Yttrium Aluminum Garnet) lasers to vaporize obstructing prostate tissue.

MEDICAL WORD	WORD PARTS		DEFINITION
castrate (kăs′ trāt)	castr -ate	to prune use	Removal of the testicles in a man or ovaries in a woman; *to geld; to spay*
circumcision (sĕr″ kŭm-sĭ′ shŭn)	circum- cis -ion	around to cut process	Surgical procedure of removing the foreskin of the penis. See Figure 18.7 ■

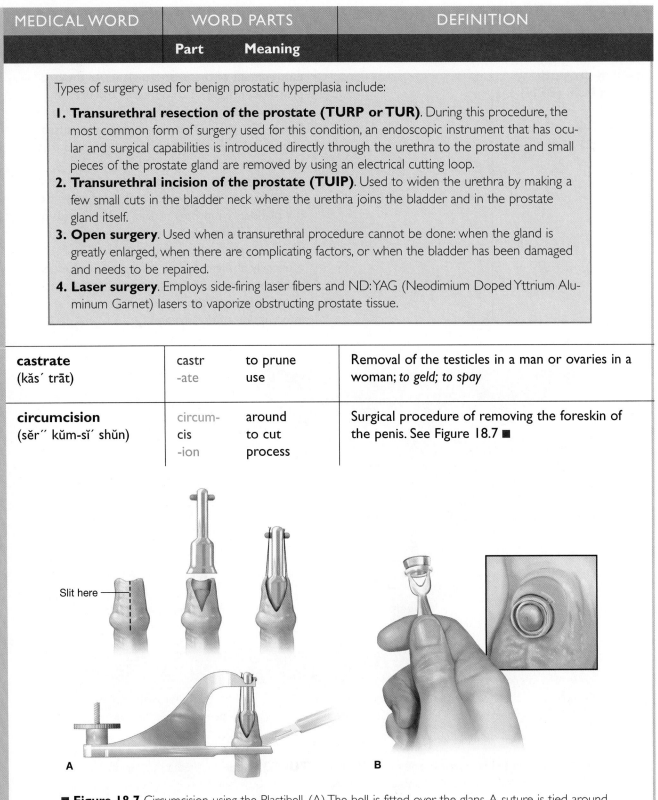

■ **Figure 18.7** Circumcision using the Plastibell. (A) The bell is fitted over the glans. A suture is tied around the bell's rim, and then the excess prepuce is cut away. (B) The plastic rim remains in place for 3–4 days until healing occurs. The bell may be allowed to fall off; it is removed if still in place after 8 days.

MEDICAL WORD	WORD PARTS	DEFINITION
cloning (klōn′ ing)		Process of creating a genetic identical of an individual organism through asexual reproduction

MEDICAL WORD	WORD PARTS		DEFINITION
	Part	Meaning	
coitus (kō´ ĭ-tŭs)			Sexual intercourse between a man and a woman; *copulation*
condom (kŏn´ dŭm)			Thin, flexible protective sheath, usually rubber (latex), worn over the penis during copulation to help prevent impregnation (block the passage of sperm) or venereal disease (VD)
condyloma (kŏn´´ dĭ-lō´ mă)			Wartlike growth on the skin, most often seen on the external genitalia; either viral or syphilitic in origin. See Figure 18.8 ■

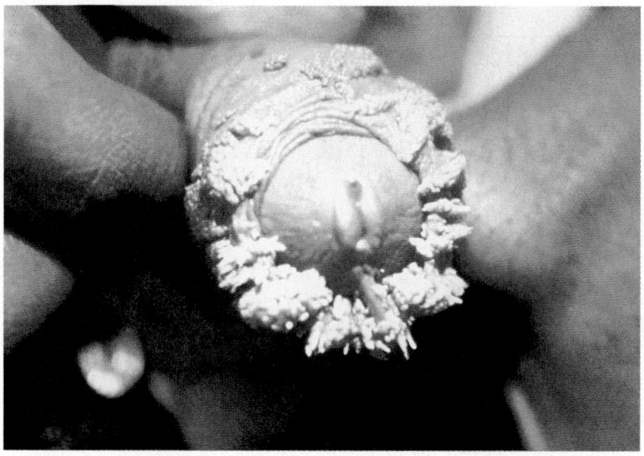

■ **Figure 18.8** Genital warts.

(Courtesy of the Centers for Disease Control and Prevention)

cryptorchidism (krĭpt-ōr´ kĭzm)	crypt orchid -ism	hidden testicle condition	Condition in which one or both testes fail to descend into the scrotum. See Figure 18.9 ■

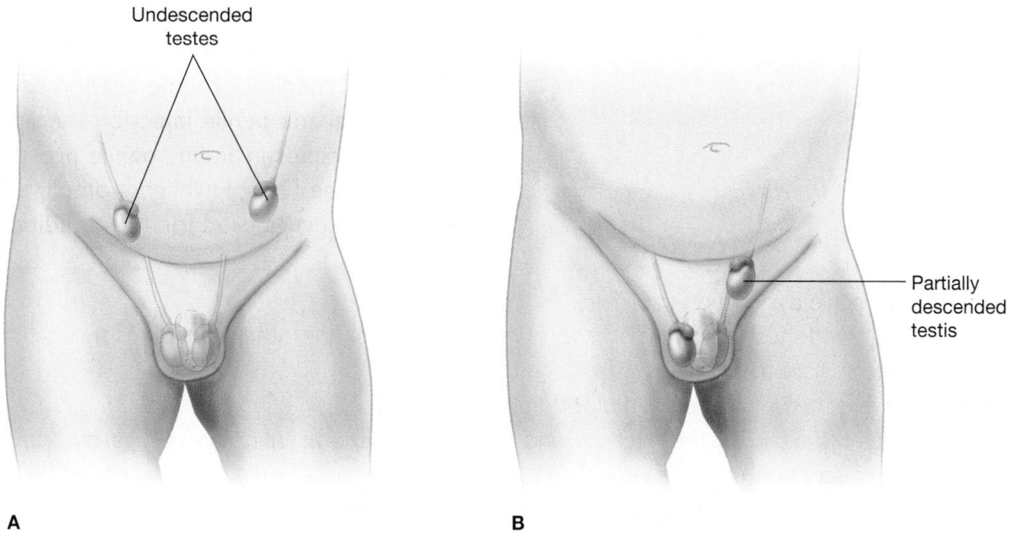

■ **Figure 18.9** Cryptochordism showing (A) undescended testes and (B) a partially descended testis.

ejaculation (ē-jăk´´ ū-lā´ shŭn)	ejaculat -ion	to throw out process	Process of expulsion of seminal fluid and sperm from the male urethra

MEDICAL WORD	WORD PARTS		DEFINITION
	Part	**Meaning**	
epididymitis (ĕp″ ĭ-dĭd″ ĭ-mī′ tĭs)	epi- didym -itis	upon testis inflammation	Inflammation of the epididymis
epispadias (ĕp″ ĭ-spā′ dĭ-ăs)	epi- spadias	upon a rent, an opening	Congenital defect in which the urethra opens on the dorsum of the penis. See Figure 18.10A ▪

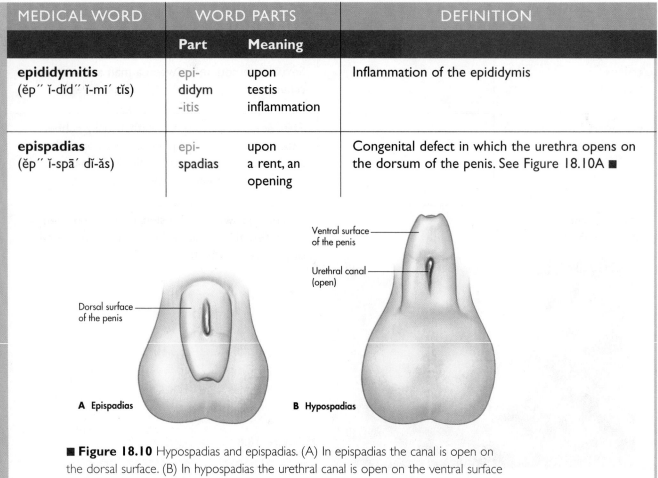

Ventral surface of the penis

Urethral canal (open)

Dorsal surface of the penis

A Epispadias

B Hypospadias

▪ **Figure 18.10** Hypospadias and epispadias. (A) In epispadias the canal is open on the dorsal surface. (B) In hypospadias the urethral canal is open on the ventral surface of the penis.

erectile dysfunction (ED) (ĕ-rĕk′ tĭl dĭs-fŭnk′ shŭn)			Inability to achieve and maintain penile erection sufficient to complete satisfactory intercourse. Many treatment options for ED are available today. These include the vacuum constriction device (VCD); oral medications; medication patches and gels; urethral and penile injection therapies; and surgical therapies including penile prostheses (implants). See Drug Highlights on page 665 for examples of drugs used for this condition.

fyi Physical causes of erectile dysfunction include:

• Vascular diseases.   Arteriosclerosis, hypertension, high cholesterol, and other conditions that can cause obstruction of blood flow to the penis
• Diabetes.   Can alter nerve function and blood flow to the penis
• Prescription drugs.   Certain antihypertensive and cardiac medications, antihistamines, psychiatric medications, and other prescription drugs
• Substance abuse.   Excessive smoking, alcohol, and illegal drugs constrict blood vessels
• Neurological diseases.   Multiple sclerosis, Parkinson's disease, and other diseases can interrupt nerve impulses to the penis
• Surgery.   Prostate, colon, bladder, and other types of pelvic surgery may damage nerves and blood vessels
• Spinal injury.   Interruptions of nerve impulses from the spinal cord to the penis
• Other.   Hormonal imbalance, kidney failure, dialysis, and reduced testosterone levels

MEDICAL WORD	WORD PARTS		DEFINITION
	Part	**Meaning**	
eugenics (ū-jĕn´ ĭks)	eu- -genic(s)	good formation, produce	Study and control of the bringing forth of offspring as a means of improving genetic characteristics of future generations
gamete (găm´ ēt)			Mature reproductive cell of the male or female; *a spermatozoon or ovum*
gonorrhea (GC) (gŏn˝ ŏ-rē´ă)	gon/o -rrhea	genitals flow	Highly contagious venereal disease of the genital mucous membrane of either sex; the infection is transmitted by the gonococcus *Neisseria gonorrhoeae.*
gynecomastia (ji˝ nĕ-kō-măs´ tĭ-ă)	gynec/o mast -ia	female breast condition	Pathological condition of excessive development of the mammary glands in the male
herpes genitalis (hĕr´ pēz jĕn-ĭ-tăl´ ĭs)			Highly contagious venereal disease of the genitalia of either sex; caused by herpes simplex virus–2 (HSV-2).
heterosexual (hĕt˝ ĕr-ō-sĕk´ shū-ăl)	hetero- sexu -al	different sex pertaining to	Pertaining to the opposite sex; refers to an individual who has a sexual preference and relationship with the opposite sex
homosexual (hō˝ mō-sĕks´ ū-ăl)	homo- sexu -al	similar, same sex pertaining to	Pertaining to the same sex; refers to an individual who has a sexual preference and relationship with the same sex
hydrocele (hī´ drō-sēl)	hydro- -cele	water hernia, swelling, tumor	Accumulation of fluid in a saclike cavity. One that occurs during prenatal development is caused by a failure of the closure of the canal between the peritoneal cavity and the scrotum. See Figure 18.11A ■

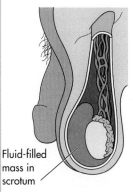

Fluid-filled mass in scrotum

A. Hydrocele

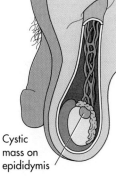

Cystic mass on epididymis

B. Spermatocele

Dilation of pampiniform venous complex

C. Varicocele

■ **Figure 18.11** Common disorders of the scrotum. (A) and (B) Hydroceles and spermatoceles do not usually require treatment unless they become large and cause pain. (C) Varicoceles are usually treated to prevent infertility.

MEDICAL WORD	WORD PARTS		DEFINITION
	Part	**Meaning**	
hypospadias (hī″ pō-spă′ dĭ-ăs)	hypo- spadias	under a rent, an opening	Congenital defect in which the urethra opens on the underside of the penis. See Figure 18.10B.
infertility (ĭn″ fĕr-tĭl′ ĭ-tē)			Inability of a heterosexual couple to produce a viable offspring
mitosis (mī-tō′ sĭs)	mit -osis	thread condition	Ordinary condition of cell division
oligospermia (ŏl″ ĭ-gō-spĕr′ -mĭ-ă)	oligo- sperm -ia	scanty seed condition	Condition in which there is insufficient (scanty) amount of spermatozoa in the semen
orchidectomy (or″ kĭ-dĕk′ tō-mē)	orchid -ectomy	testicle surgical excision	Surgical excision of a testicle
orchidotomy (or″ kĭd-ŏt′ ō-mē)	orchid/o -tomy	testicle incision	Incision into a testicle
orchiditis (or-kī′ tĭs)	orchid -itis	testicle inflammation	Inflammation of a testicle
parenchyma (păr-ĕn′ kĭ-mă)	par- enchyma	beside to pour	Essential cells of a gland or organ that are concerned with its function
phimosis (fĭ-mō′ sĭs)	phim -osis	a muzzle condition	A condition that can be present at birth in which there is narrowing of the opening of the prepuce and the foreskin cannot be drawn back over the glans penis. *When this condition occurs later in life, it can be an emergency if blood flow is blocked to the penis.*
prepuce (prē′ pūs)			Foreskin over the glans penis in the male

MEDICAL WORD	WORD PARTS		DEFINITION
	Part	**Meaning**	
prostate cancer (prŏs´ tāt)			Malignant tumor of the prostate gland. See Figure 18.12 ■ Diagnosis of prostate cancer can be confirmed with a medical history; physical examination, including a digital rectal exam (DRE) (Figure 18.13 ■); and results of a PSA blood test. The physician performs a digital rectal exam to assess the size and condition (firm, soft, hard) of the prostate gland.

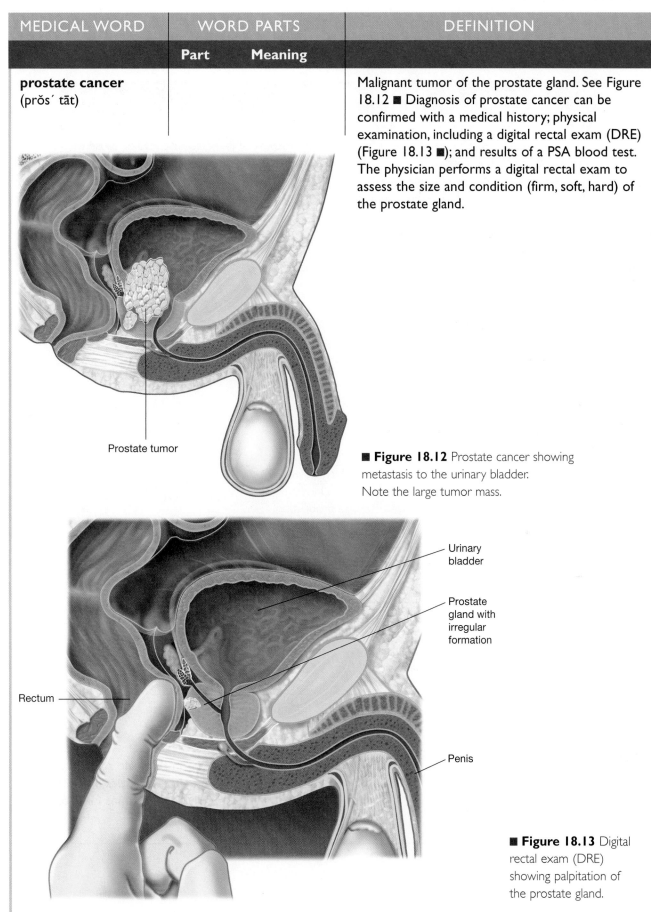

Prostate tumor

■ **Figure 18.12** Prostate cancer showing metastasis to the urinary bladder. Note the large tumor mass.

Urinary bladder

Prostate gland with irregular formation

Rectum

Penis

■ **Figure 18.13** Digital rectal exam (DRE) showing palpitation of the prostate gland.

MEDICAL WORD	WORD PARTS		DEFINITION
	Part	**Meaning**	

LIFE SPAN CONSIDERATIONS

Prostate cancer is the most common type of cancer found in American men and by age 50, up to one in four men have some cancerous cells in the prostate gland. It is the second leading cause of cancer death in men, exceeded only by lung cancer. While one man in six will have prostate cancer during his lifetime, only one man in 32 will die of this disease. A man is more likely to die *with* prostate cancer than to die *from* prostate cancer.

fyi Prostate cancer is graded and staged for aggressiveness based on how far it has spread throughout the body. CT scans and bone scans help in staging, but sometimes it becomes clear only at the time of surgery. Following are the stages of prostate cancer:

- Stages A and B are confined to the prostate gland.
- Stage C has spread to other tissues near the prostate gland.
- Stage D has spread to lymph nodes or sites in the body a distance away from the prostate.

The proper management of the many stages of prostate cancer is controversial. Depending on the grade and stage of the cancer, some options are as follows:

- Chemotherapy
- Cryosurgery to freeze cancer cells
- External radiation to the prostate and pelvis
- Hormone therapy
- Radioactive implants put directly into the prostate, which slowly kill cancer cells
- Surgery to remove part or all of the prostate and surrounding tissue
- Surgical removal of the testicles to block testosterone production
- Watchful waiting and monitoring only

A significant number of prostate cancer patients use complementary and alternative medicine (CAM) as part of their treatment according to a new study, but do not tell their doctors about these therapies, which could have a negative effect on their care.

MEDICAL WORD	WORD PARTS		DEFINITION
prostatectomy (prŏs″ tă-tĕk´ tō-mē)	prostat -ectomy	prostate surgical excision	Surgical excision of the prostate
prostatitis (prŏs″ tă-tī´ tĭs)	prostat -itis	prostate inflammation	Inflammation of the prostate
puberty (pū´ ber-tē)			Stage of development in the male and female when secondary sex characteristics begin to develop and the individual becomes functionally capable of reproduction

MEDICAL WORD	WORD PARTS		DEFINITION
	Part	Meaning	
semen (sē´ měn)			Fluid-transporting medium for spermatozoa discharged during ejaculation
spermatoblast (spĕr-măt´ ō-blăst)	spermat/o -blast	seed, sperm immature cell, germ cell	Sperm germ cell
spermatocele (spĕr-măt´ ō-sēl)	spermat/o -cele	seed, sperm hernia, swelling, tumor	Cystic swelling of the epididymis that contains spermatozoa; is mobile, usually painless, and requires no treatment. See Figure 18.11B ■
spermatogenesis (spĕr˝ măt-ō-jĕn´ ĕ-sĭs)	spermat/o -genesis	seed, sperm formation, produce	Formation of spermatozoa
spermatozoon (spĕr˝ măt-ō-zō´ ŏn)	spermat/o zoon	seed, sperm life	Male sex cell; plural form is spermatozoa
spermicide (spĕr´ mĭ-sīd)	sperm/i -cide	seed, sperm to kill	Agent that kills sperm
syphilis (sĭf´ ĭ-lĭs)			Infectious venereal disease caused by Treponema pallidum, which is transmitted sexually.
testicular (tĕs-tĭk´ ū-lar)	testicul -ar	testicle pertaining to	Pertaining to a testicle
varicocele (văr´ ĭ-kō-sēl)	varic/o -cele	twisted vein hernia, swelling, tumor	Enlargement and twisting of the veins of the spermatic cord. See Figure 18.11C ■

MEDICAL WORD	WORD PARTS		DEFINITION
	Part	**Meaning**	
vasectomy (văs-ĕk´ tō-mē)	vas -ectomy	vessel surgical excision	Surgical procedure in which the vas deferens are tied off and cut apart, providing sterility by preventing transport of sperm out of the testes. See Figure 18.14 ■

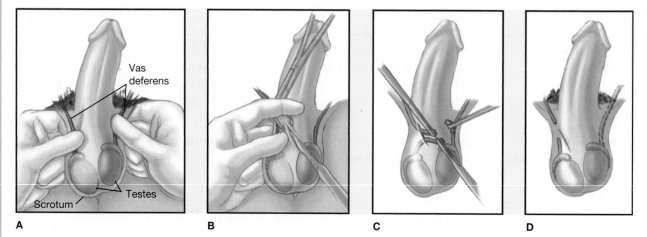

A   B   C   D

■ **Figure 18.14** Vasectomy. (A) The spermatic cords are located as they ascend from the scrotum. (B) The vas deferens are severed. (C) A 1 cm section is removed. (D) The cut ends cannot reconnect thereby preventing the passage of sperm cells and providing surgical sterilization.

fyi A vasectomy does not affect a man's ability to achieve orgasm, ejaculate, or achieve erections. After 4–6 weeks, sperm are no longer present in the semen. A semen specimen must be examined and found to be totally free of sperm a month or more after vasectomy before the patient can rely on the vasectomy for birth control.

vesiculitis (vĕ-sĭk″ ū-lĭ´ tĭs)	vesicul -itis	seminal vesicle inflammation	Inflammation of a seminal vesicle

SEXUALLY TRANSMITTED DISEASES

Sexually transmitted diseases (STDs) can occur in men, women, and children. They are passed from person to person through sexual contact or from mother to child. Table 18.2 ■ is a summary of the most common sexually transmitted diseases.

TABLE 18.2 Sexually Transmitted Diseases

Disease	Cause	Symptoms	Treatment
Chlamydia (klă-mĭd´ ē-ă)	*Chlamydia trachomatis* (bacterium)	Can be asymptomatic or exhibit the following: **MALE:** Mucopurulent discharge from penis; burning, itching in genital area; dysuria; swollen testes; can cause nongonococcal urethritis (NGU) and sterility **FEMALE:** Mucopurulent discharge from vagina, cystitis, pelvic pain, cervicitis; can lead to pelvic inflammatory disease (PID) and sterility **NEWBORN:** Eye infection, pneumonia; can cause death	Antibiotics—Zithromax (azithromycin) and Doxycycline (tetracycline) or erythromycin
Genital warts (jĕn´ ĭ-tăl)	Human papilloma-virus (HPV)	**MALE:** Cauliflowerlike growths on the penis and perianal area **FEMALE:** Cauliflowerlike growths around vagina and perianal area	Laser surgery, chemotherapy, cryosurgery, cauterization **Note:** GARDASIL is the only HPV vaccine that helps protect against four types of HPV. In girls and young women ages 9–26, it helps protect against two types of HPV that cause about 75% of cervical cancer cases, and two more types that cause 90% of genital warts cases. In boys and young men ages 9–26, GARDASIL helps protect against 90% of genital warts cases. GARDASIL also helps protect girls and young women ages 9–26 against 70% of vaginal cancer cases and up to 50% of vulvar cancer cases.
Gonorrhea (gŏn˝ ŏ-rē´ā)	*Neisseria gonorrhoeae* (bacterium)	**MALE:** Purulent urethral discharge, dysuria, urinary frequency **FEMALE:** Purulent vaginal discharge, dysuria, urinary frequency, abnormal menstrual bleeding, abdominal tenderness; can lead to PID and sterility **NEWBORN:** Gonorrheal ophthalmia neonatorum, purulent eye discharge; can cause blindness	Antibiotics—ceftriaxone, cefixime, ciprofloxacin, or ofloxacin

TABLE 18.2 Sexually Transmitted Diseases *(continued)*

Disease	Cause	Symptoms	Treatment
Herpes genitalis (hĕr´ pēz jĕn-ĭ-tāl´ ĭs)	Herpes simplex virus–2 (HSV-2)	**ACTIVE PHASE** **MALE:** Fluid-filled vesicles (blisters) on penis; caused by acute pain and itching **FEMALE:** Blisters in and around vagina **NEWBORN:** Can be infected during vaginal delivery; severe infection, physical and mental damage **GENERALIZED:** Flulike symptoms, fever, headache, malaise, anorexia, muscle pain	No cure; antiviral drugs acyclovir (Zovirax), famciclovir (Famvir), or valacyclovir hydrochloride (Valtrex) can be used to relieve symptoms during acute phase
Syphilis (sĭf´ ĭ-lĭs)	*Treponema pallidum* (bacterium)	**PRIMARY STAGE:** Chancre at point of infection; see Figure 18.15 ■	Antibotics—penicillin, tetracycline, or erythromycin

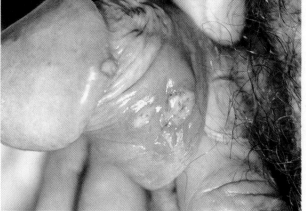

■ **Figure 18.15** Chancre.

(Courtesy of Jason L. Smith, MD)

MALE: penis, anus, rectum

FEMALE: vagina, cervix

BOTH: lips, tongue, fingers, nipples

TABLE 18.2 Sexually Transmitted Diseases *(continued)*

Disease	Cause	Symptoms	Treatment
		SECONDARY STAGE: Flulike symptoms with a skin rash over moist, fatty areas of the body; see Figure 18.16 ■	

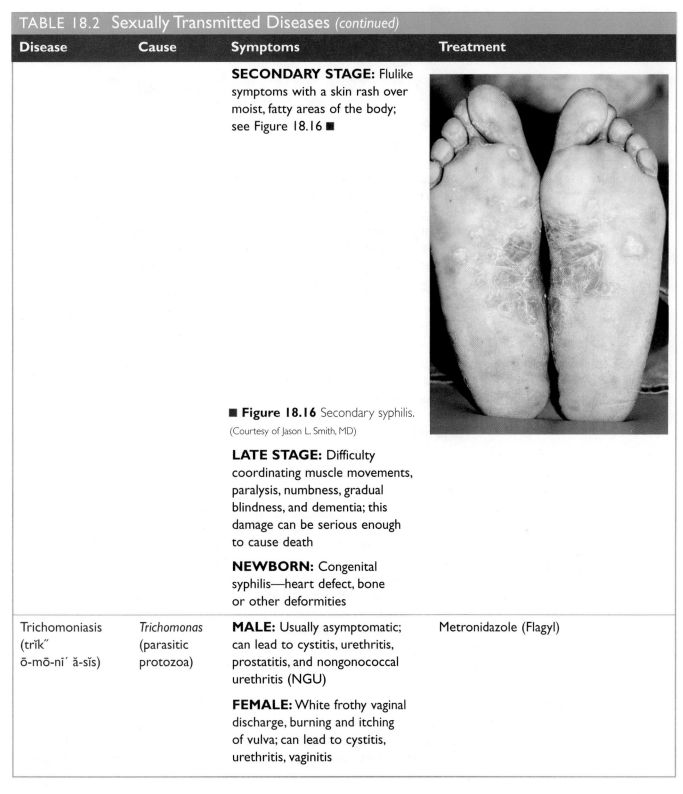

■ **Figure 18.16** Secondary syphilis.
(Courtesy of Jason L. Smith, MD)

Disease	Cause	Symptoms	Treatment
		LATE STAGE: Difficulty coordinating muscle movements, paralysis, numbness, gradual blindness, and dementia; this damage can be serious enough to cause death	
		NEWBORN: Congenital syphilis—heart defect, bone or other deformities	
Trichomoniasis (trĭk″ ō-mō-nī′ ă-sĭs)	*Trichomonas* (parasitic protozoa)	**MALE:** Usually asymptomatic; can lead to cystitis, urethritis, prostatitis, and nongonococcal urethritis (NGU)	Metronidazole (Flagyl)
		FEMALE: White frothy vaginal discharge, burning and itching of vulva; can lead to cystitis, urethritis, vaginitis	

• Drug Highlights •

TYPE OF DRUG	DESCRIPTION AND EXAMPLES
testosterone (male hormone)	Responsible for growth, development, and maintenance of the male reproductive system and secondary sex characteristics.
therapeutic use	As replacement therapy in primary hypogonadism and to stimulate puberty in carefully selected males. It can be used to relieve symptoms of the male climacteric due to androgen deficiency and to help stimulate sperm production in oligospermia and impotence due to androgen deficiency. It can also be used with advanced inoperable metastatic breast cancer in women who are 1–5 years postmenopausal. EXAMPLES: AndroGel (testosterone), DepoTestosterone (testosterone cypionate in oil), Delatestryl (testosterone enanthate in oil), and Androderm (testosterone transdermal systems)
patient teaching	Educate the patient to be aware of possible adverse reactions and report any of the following to the physician. *All patients:* nausea, vomiting, jaundice, edema. *Males:* frequent or persistent erection of the penis. *Females:* hoarseness, acne, changes in menstrual periods, growth of hair on face and/or body.
special considerations	Testosterone can decrease blood glucose and insulin requirements in diabetic patients. Testosterone can decrease the anticoagulant requirements of patients receiving oral anticoagulants. These patients require close monitoring when testosterone therapy is begun and then when it is stopped. Individuals who seek to increase muscle mass, strength, and overall athletic ability can abuse anabolic steroids (testosterone). This form is illegal; signs of abuse include flulike symptoms; headaches; muscle aches; dizziness; bruises; needle marks; increased bleeding (nosebleeds, petechiae, gums, conjunctiva); enlarged spleen, liver, and/or prostate; edema; and in the female increased facial hair, menstrual irregularities, and enlarged clitoris.
drugs used to treat benign prostatic hyperplasia (BPH)	5α-reductase inhibitor that lowers the levels of DHT, the major factor in enlargement of the prostate. Shrinkage of the enlarged prostate usually occurs in 6–12 months with medication therapy. Note: Proscar (5 mg) is one brand of finasteride that is prescribed for BPH, while Propecia (1 mg) is another brand of finasteride that is prescribed for male pattern baldness. EXAMPLES: Other medications used in the treatment of BPH include terazosin (Hytrin), doxazosin (Cardura), and tamsulosin (Flomax) Note: All three drugs act by relaxing the smooth muscle of the prostate and bladder neck to improve urine flow and to reduce bladder outlet obstruction.

TYPE OF DRUG	DESCRIPTION AND EXAMPLES
drugs used to treat erectile dysfunction (ED)	These drugs increase the body's ability to achieve and maintain an erection during sexual stimulation. They do not protect one from getting sexually transmitted diseases, including HIV. They are contraindicated in patients who use nitrates and they should not be used in men for whom sexual activity is inadvisable because of their underlying cardiovascular status. EXAMPLES: Viagra (sildenafil), Levitra (vardenafil), and Cialis (tadalafil)

• Diagnostic and Lab Tests •

TEST	DESCRIPTION
fluorescent treponemal antibody absorption (FTA-ABS) (floo-ō-rĕs´ ĕnt trĕp″ ō-nē măl ăn´ tĭ-bŏd″ ē ab-sorp´ shŭn)	Test performed on blood serum to determine the presence of *Treponema pallidum* to detect syphilis.
paternity (pă-tĕr´ nĭ-tē)	Test to determine whether a certain man is the father of a specific child. The most common and accurate test used is the DNA test, which compares a child's DNA pattern with that of the alleged father to check for evidence of inheritance. Result is either an exclusion (not the father) or inclusion (is the father). The mother's participation helps exclude half of the child's DNA, leaving the other half for comparison with the alleged father's DNA. A buccal (cheek) sample is taken from each participating person. Most states have laws that require an unmarried couple to fill out an Acknowledgment of Paternity (AOP) form to legally establish the identity of the father of a child.
prostate-specific antigen (PSA) immunoassay (prŏs´ tāt-spĕ-sĭf´ ĭk ăn´ tĭ-jĕn ĭm″ ū-nō-ăs´ sā)	Blood test that measures concentrations of a special type of protein known as *prostate-specific antigen*. An increased level indicates prostate disease or possibly prostate cancer.
semen (sē´ mĕn)	Test performed on semen that looks at the volume, pH, sperm count, sperm motility, and morphology to evaluate infertility in men.
testosterone toxicology (tĕs-tŏs´ tĕr-ōn tŏks″ ĭ-kŏl´ ō-jē)	Test performed on blood serum to identify the level of testosterone; increased level can indicate benign prostatic hyperplasia; decreased level can indicate hypogonadism, testicular hypofunction, hypopituitarism, and/or orchidectomy.
venereal disease research laboratory (VDRL) (vĕ-nē´ rē-ăl)	Test performed on blood serum to determine the presence of *Treponema pallidum* to detect syphilis.

• Abbreviations •

ABBREVIATION	MEANING
AIH	artificial insemination homologous
AOP	acknowledgment of paternity
BPH	benign prostatic hyperplasia (also denotes benign prostatic hypertrophy)
CAM	complementary and alternative medicines
DHT	dihydrotestosterone
DRE	digital rectal exam
ED	erectile dysfunction
FDA	Food and Drug Administration
FTA-ABS	fluorescent treponemal antibody absorption
GC	gonorrhea
HPV	human papillomavirus

ABBREVIATION	MEANING
HSV-2	herpes simplex virus–2
NGU	nongonococcal urethritis
PID	pelvic inflammatory disease
PSA	prostate-specific antigen
STDs	sexually transmitted diseases
TUIP	transurethral incision of the prostate
TUMT	transurethral microwave thermotherapy
TUNA	transurethral needle ablation
TUR	transurethral resection
TURP	transurethral resection of the prostate
VCD	vacuum constriction device
VD	venereal disease
VDRL	venereal disease research laboratory

y and Review • Study and Review • Study and Review
Review • Study and Review • Study and Review • St
ew • Study and Review • Study and Review • Study

Study and Review

Anatomy and Physiology

Write your answers to the following questions.

1. List the primary and accessory glands of the male reproductive system.

a. _____   b. _____

c. _____   d. _____

e. _____   f. _____

2. Name the supporting structure and accessory sex organs of the male reproductive system.

a. _____   b. _____

3. State the vital function of the male reproductive system. _____

4. The _____ _____ is the cone-shaped head of the penis.

5. Define *prepuce*. _____

6. Define *smegma*. _____

7. State two functions of the penis.

a. _____   b. _____

8. _____ _____ is the site of the development of spermatozoa.

9. List five effects of testosterone regarding male development.

a. _____   b. _____

c. _____   d. _____

e. _____

10. State two functions of the epididymis.

a. _____   b. _____

11. The excretory duct of the testes is known by two names, _____

_____ or _____ _____ .

12. State the function of the seminal vesicles. _____

13. Describe the prostate gland. _____

_____

14. Define the condition known as *benign prostatic hyperplasia.* _____

_____

15. The two small pea-sized glands located below the prostate and on either side of the urethra are known as the

_____ glands or as _____ glands.

16. Name the three sections of the male urethra.

a. _____   **b.** _____

c. _____

17. State a function of the male urethra. _____

18. The male urethra is approximately _____ cm long.

Word Parts

PREFIXES

Give the definitions of the following prefixes.

1. a-	_____	**2.** an-	_____
3. circum-	_____	**4.** epi-	_____
5. hydro-	_____	**6.** hypo-	_____
7. oligo-	_____	**8.** par-	_____
9. in-	_____	**10.** eu-	_____
11. heter-	_____	**12.** homo-	_____

ROOTS AND COMBINING FORMS

Give the definitions of the following roots and combining forms.

1. balan	_____	**2.** cis	_____
3. crypt	_____	**4.** artific/i	_____
5. didym	_____	**6.** enchyma	_____
7. orch	_____	**8.** orchid	_____
9. orchid/o	_____	**10.** phim	_____
11. prostat	_____	**12.** castr	_____

13. spadias _____   14. sperm _____

15. seminat _____   16. spermat/o _____

17. sperm/i _____   18. testicul _____

19. varic/o _____   20. vas _____

21. vesicul _____   22. zo/o _____

23. zoon _____   24. ejaculat _____

25. gon/o _____   26. gynec/o _____

27. mast _____   28. sexu _____

29. mit _____

SUFFIXES

Give the definitions of the following suffixes.

1. -al _____   2. -ar _____

3. -blast _____   4. -cele _____

5. -cide _____   6. -ectomy _____

7. -genesis _____   8. -ia _____

9. -ion _____   10. -ism _____

11. -it is _____   12. -ate _____

13. -osis _____   14. -genic(s) _____

15. -rrhea _____   16. -tomy _____

Identifying Medical Terms

In the spaces provided, write the medical terms for the following meanings.

1. _____ Inflammation of the glans penis

2. _____ Surgical excision of the epididymis

3. _____ Surgical excision of a testicle

4. _____ Foreskin over the glans penis

5. _____ Accumulation of fluid in a saclike cavity

6. _____ Wartlike growth on the skin

7. _____ Sperm germ cell

8. _____ Male sex cell

9. _____ Agent that kills sperm

10. _____ Pertaining to a testicle

Spelling

Circle the correct spelling of each medical term.

1. crptorchism / cryptorchidism

2. hypospadias / hyospadias

3. orchidotomy / orchdotomy

4. ugenics / eugenics

5. vasectomy / vasetomy

6. clamydia / chlamydia

7. gonorrhea / gonorhea

8. syphillis / syphilis

9. trichmoniasis / trichomoniasis

10. papillomavirus / papilomavirus

Matching

Select the appropriate lettered meaning for each of the following words.

_____ 1. circumcision

_____ 2. coitus

_____ 3. condom

_____ 4. gamete

_____ 5. genital warts

_____ 6. gonorrhea

_____ 7. infertility

_____ 8. prepuce

_____ 9. syphilis

_____ 10. trichomoniasis

a. Caused by the bacterium *Treponema pallidum*

b. Mature reproductive cell of the male or female

c. Sexual intercourse between a man and a woman

d. Caused by a parasitic protozoa

e. Surgical procedure of removing the foreskin of the penis

f. Thin, flexible protective sheath worn over the penis during copulation to help prevent impregnation or venereal disease

g. Disease caused by the human papillomavirus

h. Inability to produce a viable offspring

i. Causes purulent urethral discharge in the male and purulent vaginal discharge in the female

j. Caused by the bacterium *Chlamydia trachomatis*

k. The foreskin over the glans penis in the male

Abbreviations

Place the correct word, phrase, or abbreviation in the space provided.

1. benign prostatic hyperplasia _____

2. GC _____

3. human papillomavirus _____

4. HSV-2 _____

5. STDs _____

6. erectile dysfunction _____

7. TURP _____

8. NGU _____

9. venereal disease _____

10. prostate-specific antigen _____

Diagnostic and Laboratory Tests

Select the best answer to each multiple-choice question. Circle the letter of your choice.

1. Test performed on blood serum to detect syphilis.
   a. paternity   **c.** FTA-ABS
   b. semen   **d.** HSV-2

2. Test to determine whether a certain man is the father of a specific child.
   a. paternity   **c.** FTA-ABS
   b. semen   **d.** HSV-2

3. Increased level indicates prostate disease or possibly prostate cancer.
   a. fluorescent treponemal antibody   **c.** semen
   b. prostate-specific antigen   **d.** testosterone toxicology

4. Used to determine infertility in men.
   a. paternity   **c.** semen
   b. prostate-specific antigen   **d.** testosterone toxicology

5. Increased level can indicate benign prostatic hyperplasia.
   a. fluorescent treponemal antibody   **c.** testosterone toxicology
   b. prostate-specific antigen   **d.** venereal disease research laboratory

Read the adapted CDC Study and then answer the questions that follow.

CDC STUDY FINDS U.S. HERPES RATES REMAIN HIGH

1 in 6 Americans Infected; Highest Prevalence among Women and African Americans
About 1 in 6 Americans (16.2%) between the ages of 14 and 49 is infected with herpes simplex virus type 2 (HSV-2), according to a national health survey released today (March 9, 2010) by the Centers for Disease Control and Prevention. HSV-2 is a lifelong and incurable infection that can cause recurrent and painful genital sores.

The findings, presented at the 2010 National STD Prevention Conference, indicate that herpes remains one of the most common sexually transmitted diseases (STDs) in the United States. Research shows that people with herpes are two to three times more likely to acquire HIV, and that herpes can also make HIV-infected individuals more likely to transmit HIV to others. CDC estimates that over 80% of those with HSV-2 are unaware of their infection. Symptoms may be absent, mild, or mistaken for another condition. And people with HSV-2 can transmit the virus even when they have no visible sores or other symptoms.

"Many individuals are transmitting herpes to others without even knowing it," said John M. Douglas, Jr., M.D., director of CDC's Division of STD Prevention. "We can't afford to be complacent about this disease. It is important that persons with symptoms suggestive of herpes—especially recurrent sores in the genital area—seek clinical care to determine if these symptoms may be due to herpes and might benefit from treatment."

Combination of Prevention Approaches Needed to Reduce National Herpes Rates

Although HSV-2 infection is not curable, there are effective medications available to treat symptoms and prevent outbreaks. Those with known herpes infection should avoid sex when herpes symptoms or sores are present and understand that HSV-2 can still be transmitted when sores are not present. Effective strategies to reduce the risk of HSV-2 infection include abstaining from sexual contact, using condoms consistently and correctly, and limiting the number of sex partners.

CDC Study Questions

Place the correct answer in the space provided.

1. _____ remains one of the most common sexually transmitted diseases (STDs) in the United States.

2. About one in six Americans (16.2%) between the ages of _____ and _____ is infected with herpes simplex virus type 2 (HSV-2).

3. Is herpes a lifelong and incurable infection that can cause recurrent and painful genital sores? _____

4. The CDC estimates that over _____ percent of those with HSV-2 are unaware of their infection.

5. People with HSV-2 can transmit the virus even when they have no _____ sores or other symptoms.

PEARSON
mymedicalterminologylab

MyMedicalTerminologyLab is a premium online homework management system that includes a host of features to help you study. Registered users will find:

• Fun games and activities built within a virtual hospital

• Powerful tools that track and analyze your results—allowing you to create a personalized learning experience

• Videos, flashcards, and audio pronunciations to help enrich your progress

• Streaming lesson presentations and self-paced learning modules

• A space where you and your instructors can view and manage your assignments

ymphatic System • Respiratory System • Urinary System
ndocrine System • Nervous System • Special Senses: The
ar • Special Senses: The Eye • Female Reproductive Syst
n with an Overview of Obstetrics • Male Reproductive
em • **Oncology** • Radiology and Nuclear Medicine • N

19

LEARNING OUTCOMES

On completion of this chapter, you will be able to:

1. Define cancer.

2. Describe cell differentiation.

3. Identify the staging system that evaluates the spread of a tumor.

4. Contrast the characteristics of benign and malignant neoplasms.

5. List the seven warning signals of cancer.

6. Describe the methods that can be used in diagnosing cancer.

7. List the various forms of treatment for cancer.

8. Define radiation therapy.

9. Describe important factors that must be considered when determining the use of radiotherapy for the cancer patient.

10. Describe each of the types of cancer presented in Spotlight on Selected Cancers.

11. Analyze, build, spell, and pronounce medical words.

12. Identify and define selected abbreviations.

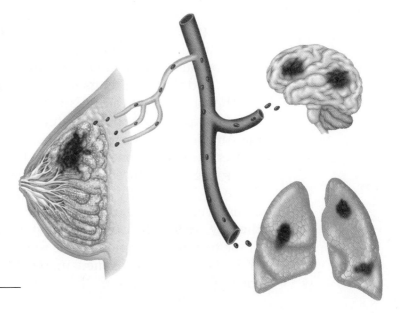

675

COMBINING FORMS OF ONCOLOGY

aden/o	gland	**mucos/o**	mucus
angi/o	vessel	**mutat/o**	to change
cancer/o	crab, cancer	**my/o**	muscle
capsul/o	a little box	**myc/o**	fungus
carcin/o	cancer	**myel/o**	bone marrow
chondr/o	cartilage	**nephr/o**	kidney
chori/o	chorion	**neur/o**	nerve
cyt/o	cell	**onc/o**	tumor
dendr/o	tree	**oste/o**	bone
duct/o	to lead	**palliat/o**	cloaked
fibr/o	fiber	**remiss/o**	remit
filtrat/o	to strain through	**reticul/o**	net
gli/o	glue	**retin/o**	retina
hem/o	blood	**rhabd/o**	rod
immun/o	safe, immunity	**sarc/o**	flesh
lei/o	smooth	**semin/i**	seed
leuk/o	white	**stom/o**	mouth
lip/o	fat	**suppress/o**	suppress
lymph/o	lymph	**terat/o**	monster
malign/o	bad kind	**thym/o**	thymus
medull/o	marrow	**tox/o**	poison
melan/o	black	**vir/o**	virus (poison)
mening/i	meninges, membrane	**xer/o**	dry

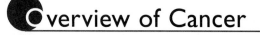verview of Cancer

Cancer (CA), a Latin word meaning **crab**, was first identified around 400 B.C. during the time of Hippocrates. Early reports on cancer compared the disease to a crab because of its tendency to stretch out and spread like the crab's four pairs of legs. Today, cancer refers to any malignant tumor (neoplasm, oncoma).

The incidence of cancer is now five times higher than it was 100 years ago. Cancer will strike one of every three Americans, according to recent statistics from the American Cancer Society (ACS). However, there is hope for those afflicted. Cancer has become one of the more treatable of the major diseases in the United States. Highly advanced **surgical techniques** are being used to remove cancerous tissue, and it is usually possible to excise all the cancer cells when the malignancy is discovered in its earliest stages (St). **Chemotherapy (chemo)** and **radiation therapy** are the other two principal means of treatment for patients with cancer. These treatments employ agents to kill cancerous cells that remain after surgery or in malignancies deemed inoperable. **Immunotherapy** and **photodynamic therapy** are two newer methods employed in the treatment of cancer.

Although the exact cause or causes remain unknown, research has shown that some cancers can be prevented, especially those associated with environmental factors. Oncologists searching for the causes of cancer have identified numerous factors that play a role in the development of cancer. See Figure 19.1 ■ These

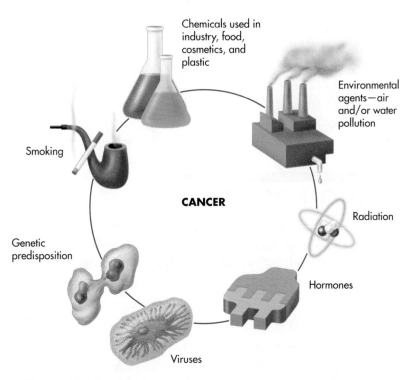

Chemicals used in industry, food, cosmetics, and plastic

Environmental agents—air and/or water pollution

Smoking

CANCER

Radiation

Genetic predisposition

Hormones

Viruses

■ **Figure 19.1** Possible causes of cancer.

factors are generally grouped under three main classifications: environmental, hereditary, and biological.

The American Cancer Society recommends various safeguards against cancer, which encourage individuals to take specific steps to safeguard their health and aid in the early detection of cancer. Some of these recommendations, according to site and action, are listed in Table 19.1 ■ For additional information, go to www.cancer.org.

TABLE 19.1 Early Detection of Cancer

Site	Action
Breast	Routine monthly breast self-examination; professional exam every 3 years from age 20 to 39 and yearly thereafter; screening mammography every year from age 40
Uterus	Yearly pelvic exam and Pap smear test for sexually active females over age 18; less often for women with three consecutive negative results
Lung	Regular chest x-ray for smokers
Skin	Regular skin check for those who are frequently exposed to the sun
Colon-rectum	Proctoscopy annually, especially after age 40; colonoscopy after age 50
Mouth	Exams regularly
Whole body	Annual health checkup including chest x-ray and various laboratory tests
Prostate	Annual digital rectal exam; PSA test yearly beginning at age 50 (men at higher risk should begin at age 40)
Testicles	Monthly testicular self-examination

CLASSIFICATION OF CANCER

Classification of cancer helps determine appropriate treatment and prognosis. Tumors are classified according to their anatomical site of origin, grading, and staging. Cell differentiation and the invasive process are also elements of the classification process.

Anatomical Site

The anatomical site indicates where the cancer originated in the body. **Carcinomas** make up the great majority of all cancers and are malignant tumors of epithelial tissues. Epithelial tissue lines body surfaces including those of glands and organs; therefore, carcinomas make up the majority of the glandular cancers and are generally found in the breast, stomach, uterus, tongue, and skin. They are named according to the type of epithelial cell in which the malignancy occurs or the primary site of the tumor. For instance, a cancer of squamous epithelium is called a **squamous carcinoma** (see Figure 19.2 ■ and Figure 5.41 on page 110), and a type of skin cancer is called a **basal cell carcinoma** (see Figure 19.8 on page 697 and Figure 5.9 on page 96). Likewise, a cancer originating in the bronchus of the respiratory tract is a **bronchogenic carcinoma.**

    Sarcomas originate in connective or supportive tissues of the body such as the muscles, tendons, fat, joints, and bone. They are named by adding the suffix *-oma* (tumor) with the root *sarc* (flesh) to the word part that identifies the tissue of origin. A cancer of the bone, for example, is an **osteosarcoma:** *osteo* (CF), bone; *sarc* (R), flesh; and *-oma* (S), tumor.

    Leukemias are cancers of the blood–forming tissues. **Lymphomas** are cancerous tumors of the lymph nodes, and **myelomas** are cancerous tumors arising in the hemopoietic portion of the bone marrow.

Cell Differentiation and Grading

Normal cells reproduce themselves through **mitosis**, an orderly process that ensures growth, tissue repair, and cell reproduction. Normal cells have a distinct appearance and a specialized function. In normal cell development, immature cells undergo normal changes as they mature and assume their specialized functions. This process

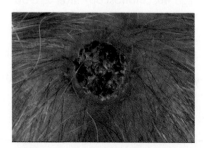

■ **Figure 19.2** Squamous cell carcinoma.

(Courtesy of Jason L. Smith, MD)

is called **differentiation.** Knowledge of cell differentiation allows a pathologist or histologist to identify the body area from which the tissue was removed by looking at a sample of tissue through a microscope. In cancer, an abnormal process in which a cell or group of cells undergoes changes and no longer carries on normal cell functions occurs. This failure of immature cells to develop specialized functions is called **dedifferentiation.** It is believed that this process involves a disturbance in the DNA of the affected cells. **Malignant cells** usually multiply rapidly, forming a mass of abnormal cells that enlarges, ulcerates, and sheds malignant cells that invade surrounding tissues. This process destroys the normal cells, and malignant cells take their places. Microscopic analysis of a malignant cell reveals a loss of differentiation, anaplasia, nuclei of various sizes that are hyperchromatic, and cells in the process of rapid and disorderly division.

Based on microscopic analysis, malignant tumors are further classified as grades I, II, III, or IV. The following describes each of the four grades of tumors in this system:

Grade I. The most differentiated and the least malignant tumors. Only a few cells are undergoing mitosis; however, some abnormality does exist.

Grade II. Moderately undifferentiated. More cells are undergoing mitosis, and the pattern is fairly irregular.

Grade III. Many undifferentiated cells. Tissue origin can be difficult to recognize. Many cells are undergoing mitosis.

Grade IV. The least differentiated and high degree of malignancy.

This system of grading tumors is used to report the prognosis of the disease and to determine whether the tumor is likely to respond to radiation therapy or chemotherapy, as well as the prognosis for surgery.

Invasive Process

Two ways in which malignant cells spread to body parts are by invasive growth and metastasis.

Invasive Growth

Invasive growth is the spreading process of a malignant tumor into adjacent normal tissue (see Figure 19.3 ■). Young malignant cells divide at the periphery of the tumor and spread by active migration or direct extension. In **active migration**, the malignant cells break away from the neoplasm (new growth), invade surrounding tissue, divide, form secondary neoplasms, and then reunite with the primary tumor as growth continues. In **direct extension**, multiplication of malignant cells is rapid, and subsequently spread into surrounding tissues via the interstitial (situated between the cells of a structure) spaces accompanied by engulfment and destruction of normal cells. As a tumor's mass enlarges, its weight is supported by connective fibers that attach to surrounding structures. These fibers invade adjacent veins and lymph vessels and become pathways for the spread of malignant cells to distant locations, such as breast cancer can spread to the bone, lung, or liver.

Metastasis

Metastasis is the process whereby cancer cells are spread from a primary site to distant secondary sites elsewhere in the body. This process usually occurs when malignant cells invade the bloodstream or lymph system and are transported to a secondary site where they become lodged and form a neoplasm (see Figure 19.5 on

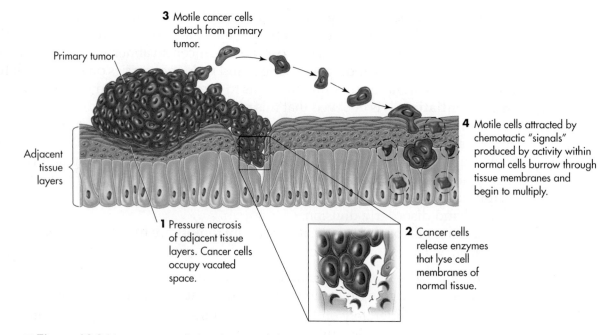

3 Motile cancer cells detach from primary tumor.

Primary tumor

4 Motile cells attracted by chemotactic "signals" produced by activity within normal cells burrow through tissue membranes and begin to multiply.

Adjacent tissue layers

1 Pressure necrosis of adjacent tissue layers. Cancer cells occupy vacated space.

2 Cancer cells release enzymes that lyse cell membranes of normal tissue.

■ **Figure 19.3** How cancer cells invade normal tissue.

page 688). Malignant cells carried in the bloodstream can lodge in highly vascular organs such as the lungs or liver, and the development of a secondary neoplasm depends on the viability and the receptivity of the organ.

Staging

Further reporting of the development and spread of cancer cells may be made through the use of a system that evaluates the spread of the tumor. The staging system uses the letters **T** (tumor), **N** (node), and **M** (metastasis) to indicate spread and uses numerical subscripts to indicate degree of tumor involvement. For example, $T_2N_1M_0$ indicates a primary tumor at stage II, abnormality of regional lymph nodes at stage I, and no evidence of distant metastasis.

A numerical system is also used to classify the staging of cancer. This system describes the various stages according to the extent of the spreading process.

Stage 0 Cancer in situ (limited to inner lining surface of the organ and not invading the organ)

Stage I Cancer limited to the tissue of origin and has not spread past the tissue or organ where it started

Stage II Limited local spread of cancerous cells, sometimes to lymph nodes

Stage III Extensive local and regional spread of cancer, usually to draining lymph nodes

Stage IV Distant metastasis, has spread beyond the regional lymph nodes to distant parts of the body

CHARACTERISTICS OF NEOPLASMS

Neoplasms or *tumors,* as they are commonly called, may be **benign** or **malignant.** See Table 19.2 ■ for characteristics that distinguish the differences between benign and malignant neoplasms.

TABLE 19.2 Characteristics of Benign and Malignant Tumors

Benign Tumors	Malignant Tumors
Grow slowly	Grow rapidly
Are encapsulated	Are not encapsulated
Have cells that resemble the normal cells from which they arose	Have cells that undergo permanent change, abnormal rapid proliferation
Grow by expansion and cause pressure on surrounding tissue	Have invasive growth and metastasis
Remain localized	Spread via the bloodstream
Do not recur when surgically removed	Can recur when surgically removed if invasive growth has occurred
Have minimal tissue destruction	Have extensive tissue destruction if invasive growth has occurred
Have no cachexia	Have cachexia (extreme weakness, fatigue, wasting, and malnutrition)
Are usually not a threat to life	Are threats to life unless detected early and properly treated

As malignant cells proliferate and begin the invasive process, the patient is unaware of the development of the cancer. In its early stages, cancer is said to be silent; however, cytological (at the cellular level) changes are occurring that could be detected if a tissue sample were taken and analyzed by a pathologist. With the proliferation of malignant cells and the continuation of the invasive process, tissues, organs, and surrounding structures become compressed, and ischemia can occur, causing necrosis, inflammation, ulceration, and bleeding. This bleeding is usually **occult** (*hidden*). Because of the silent development of cancer, the patient does not usually become aware of its symptoms until its systemic effects are evident. These systemic effects depend on the site and type of cancer but usually result in an imbalance in the patient's physiology, leading to subtle but noticeable changes that can warn of the disease.

The American Cancer Society lists seven warning signals of cancer. The first letters of each warning signal combine to spell the word **CAUTION**, and persons who develop any of the following symptoms should bring it to the attention of a physician immediately:

- **C**hange in bowel or bladder habits.
- **A** sore that does not heal.
- **U**nusual bleeding or discharge.
- **T**hickening or lump in breast or elsewhere.
- **I**ndigestion or difficulty in swallowing.
- **O**bvious change in a wart or mole.
- **N**agging cough or hoarseness.

DIAGNOSIS

A variety of *diagnostic tools* and *procedures* is used to detect the possible presence of cancer. Principal among these are examination, visualization by endoscopy, laboratory analysis, biopsy (Bx), and diagnostic radiology.

Examination

An *annual physical examination* could be the best means to protect a person's state of health. The American Cancer Society publishes a cancer detection examination that recommends certain tests be included in an annual physical examination in addition to the medical history and usual tests. For more specific information, visit the American Cancer Society's website at www.cancer.org.

Visualization by Endoscopy

Endoscopy provides the physician a direct view of certain portions of the body. The following is a list of endoscopic procedures used to assess specific locations within the body:

Sigmoidoscopy. Use of a sigmoidoscope to examine the lower 10 inches of the large intestines

Laryngoscopy. Use of a laryngoscope to examine the interior of the larynx.

Bronchoscopy. Use of a bronchoscope to examine the bronchi

Gastroscopy. Use of a gastroscope to examine the interior of the stomach

Cystoscopy. Use of a cystoscope to examine the bladder

Colposcopy. Use of a colposcope to examine the cervix and vagina

Proctoscopy. Use of a proctoscope to examine the anus and rectum

Colonoscopy. Use of a colonoscope to examine the colon

Laparoscopy. Use of a laparoscope to examine the abdomen

Laboratory Analysis

Laboratory analysis plays a key role in detecting specific types of cancer. The following are some of the laboratory tests that may be used to diagnose cancer:

Pap smear/test. Cytological screening test developed by Dr. George Papanicolaou and used to detect the presence of abnormal or cancerous cells from the cervix and vagina.

Fecal occult blood test. Test to detect occult (hidden) blood in the stool (feces); if present, further testing would be needed to check for possible cancer of the colon.

Sputum cytology test. Microscopic examination of sputum to detect abnormal or cancerous cells of the bronchi and lungs.

Blood serum test. Analysis of blood serum to obtain useful information about certain proteins synthesized by cancer; two such tests are the AFP and HCG.

Alpha-fetoprotein (AFP) test. Test to diagnose or monitor fetal distress or fetal abnormalities, diagnose some liver disorders, and screen for and monitor some cancers; higher than normal levels can indicate cancer in testes, ovaries, biliary tract, stomach, or pancreas.

Human chorionic gonadotropin (HCG) test. Test in which abnormal results can indicate ectopic pregnancy, miscarriage, **testicular cancer**, or trophoblastic tumor. It is used to monitor treatment in certain patients with cancer. During therapy, a falling HCG level indicates that the cancer is responding to treatment; rising levels can indicate that the cancer is not responding to therapy. Increased levels after treatment can indicate a recurrence of disease.

Bone marrow study. A test to detect abnormal bone marrow cells, which can indicate leukemia.

Urine assay test. Test providing useful information about catecholamines, which can indicate pheochromocytoma of the adrenal medulla.

Cancer antigen 125 (CA-125). Test that measures the amount of this protein in the blood. CA-125 is found on the surface of many ovarian cancer cells. It also can be found in other cancers and in small amounts in normal tissue.

Carcinoembryonic antigen (CEA). Test that measures the amount of a protein that can appear in the blood of some people who have certain kinds of cancers, especially large intestine (colon and rectal) cancer; also can be present in people with cancer of the pancreas, breast, ovary, or lung.

Human epidermal growth factor receptor–2 (HER-2/neu). Tests can be performed on breast cancer cells to determine the presence of HER-2/neu protein, a genetic protein that is in part responsible for how certain cancer cells grow, divide, and repair themselves. This information is useful when making treatment decisions.

Prostate-specific antigen (PSA). Blood test that measures the amount of PSA, a substance produced by the prostate gland; should be offered every year to men 50 years of age or older. The American Cancer Society recommends that screening tests start at age 40 for African American men or men with a family history of prostate cancer.

Biopsy

The surgical removal of a small piece of tissue for microscopic examination is known as biopsy (Bx). It is the method of providing the proof of cancer in the diagnosis of the disease. The following different types of biopsy can be used for tissue removal:

Excisional biopsy. Surgical removal of a piece of tissue from the suspected body site.

Incisional biopsy. Surgical incision to remove a section or wedge of tissue from the suspected body site.

Needle biopsy. Puncture of a tumor for the removal of a core of tissue through the lumen of a needle.

Fine needle aspiration (FNA). Form of breast biopsy in which a small needle is used to withdraw a sample of cells from the breast lump. If the lump is a cyst, removal of the fluid will cause the cyst to collapse. If the lump is solid, cells can be smeared onto slides for examination.

Stereotactic biopsy. Alternative to traditional surgical biopsy; the procedure, which uses a mammogram-guided needle, is performed by a radiologist and assisted by mammography technologists. It is most helpful when mammography shows a mass, a cluster of microcalcifications (tiny calcium deposits that are closely grouped together), or an area of abnormal tissue change but no lump can be felt on careful breast examination.

Core biopsy. Large-bore needle removal of a generous sample of breast tissue and a vacuum-assisted needle biopsy device (VAD), which uses vacuum suction to obtain a tissue sample.

Cone biopsy. Removal of a cone of tissue from the uterine cervix.

Sternal biopsy. Removal of a piece of bone marrow from the sternum.

Endoscopic biopsy. Removal of a piece of tissue through an endoscope.

Punch biopsy. Removal of a plug of tissue (epidermis, dermis, and subcutaneous tissue) from the skin.

Sentinel node biopsy. Process by which a physician pinpoints the first lymph node into which a tumor drains (the sentinel node) and removes only the nodes most likely to contain cancer cells. To locate the sentinel node, the physician injects a radioactive tracer in the area around the tumor. The tracer travels the same path to the lymph nodes that cancer cells would take, making it possible for the surgeon to determine the one or two nodes most likely to test positive. The surgeon then removes the nodes most likely to be cancerous for evaluation and staging.

Diagnostic Radiology

Encompassing a wide range of tests and procedures, **diagnostic radiology** can reveal tumors that were not detected by other diagnostic procedures. See Chapter 20, "Radiology and Nuclear Medicine," beginning on page 713 for a discussion of diagnostic radiology.

TREATMENT

The treatment of cancer can employ any one or a combination of the following methods: surgery, chemotherapy, radiation therapy, immunotherapy, or photodynamic therapy (PDT). The treatment of choice depends on the type of cancer, its location, its invasive process, and the patient's state of health. The ultimate goal of treatment is to kill every cancer cell. Therefore, the need to treat tumors at an early stage is critical. For example, a 1-cm breast tumor can contain 1 billion cancer cells before it is detected. A drug killing 99% of these cells would be considered an excellent drug, but 10 million cancer cells would still remain in the body. The relationship between cell kill and chemotherapy is shown in Figure 19.4 ■

Surgery

Surgery can be the treatment of choice when the tumor is small and localized and the surrounding tissue is accessible for removal. The aim of surgery is to remove all cancerous tissue plus some of the surrounding normal tissue. Surgery is also used to alleviate some of the complications of cancer, such as the obstruction of an area caused by the enlargement of a tumor.

A new type of microscopically controlled surgery, Mohs, created by a general surgeon, Dr. Frederic E. Mohs, can be used to remove the two most common forms of skin cancer, basal cell carcinoma and squamous cell carcinoma. The Mohs procedure is essentially a pathology sectioning method that allows for the complete examination of the surgical margin, while the patient is still present in the office. It is different from the standard technique of sectioning in which random samples of the surgical margin are examined, sent to a laboratory for analysis, and then the patient is notified of the results and, if indicated, must schedule another visit for further treatment. The Mohs surgery is performed in four steps during one visit:

1. Surgical removal of tissue
2. Mapping the piece of tissue, freezing and cutting the tissue between 5 and 10 micrometers using a cryostat (device for maintaining very low (cold) temperatures), and staining with hematoxylin and eosin (H&E), a popular stain used in medical diagnosis

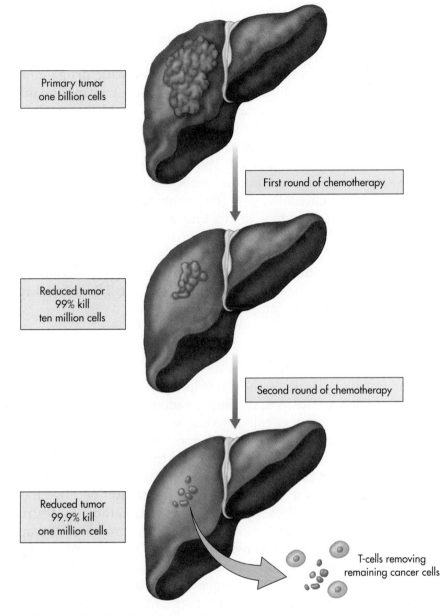

Primary tumor
one billion cells

First round of chemotherapy

Reduced tumor
99% kill
ten million cells

Second round of chemotherapy

Reduced tumor
99.9% kill
one million cells

T-cells removing
remaining cancer cells

■ **Figure 19.4** Cell kill and chemotherapy.

3. Interpretation of microscope slides for the presence of cancerous cells

4. Reconstruction of the surgical site as needed

The procedure is usually performed in a physician's office using a local anesthetic. A small scalpel is utilized to cut around the visible tumor. A very small surgical margin is utilized, usually with 1 to 1.5 mm of "free margin" or uninvolved skin. The amount of free margin removed is much less than the usual 4 to 6 mm required for the standard excision of skin cancers. After each surgical removal of tissue, the specimen is processed, cut on the cryostat and placed on slides, stained with H&E and then read by the Mohs surgeon/pathologist who examines the sections for cancerous cells. If cancer is found, its location is marked on the map (drawing of the tissue) and the surgeon removes the indicated cancerous tissue from the patient. This procedure is repeated until no further cancer is found.

Chemotherapy

Chemotherapy (chemo) can be the treatment of choice when the cancer is disseminated (widespread) and cannot be surgically removed. It is also used when a tumor fails to respond to radiation therapy. Antineoplastic drugs injure individual cells, interfere with their vital functions, and kill or destroy malignant cells. In rendering cancerous cells harmless, certain normal cells could also be destroyed. The normal cells with the greatest sensitivity to destruction are the hematopoietic cells, epithelial cells, and the hair follicles. The plan of treatment for patients undergoing chemotherapy is individualized. The aim of chemotherapy is to put the patient in remission so that life can continue without **exacerbation** of symptoms.

Combination chemotherapy (the combination of certain antineoplastic agents) has proven to be effective in treating acute leukemia; Hodgkin's disease; non-Hodgkin's lymphoma; carcinoma of the breast, testis, and ovary; childhood neuroblastoma; Wilms' tumor; and osteogenic sarcoma. The physician who prescribes combination chemotherapy weighs the anticipated benefits against the possible additive toxic effects of the drugs. Examples include TPE—Taxol (paclitaxel), Platinol (cisplatin), and VePesid (etoposide).

Radiation Therapy

The treatment of disease by the use of ionizing radiation is called **radiotherapy, x-ray therapy, cobalt treatment**, or simply **radiation therapy.** In all cases, this treatment seeks to deliver a precise, calculated dose of radiation to a tumor, while causing the least possible damage to surrounding normal tissue. **Radiation** therapy can be defined as the process whereby energy is beamed from its source to a selected target tissue. See Figure 19.10 on page 700. Substances that emit radiation are said to be *radioactive.*

Malignant cells are more sensitive to radiation because these cells divide frequently, making the DNA replication more vulnerable to destruction. Radiation is frequently used as either a *curative* or a *palliative* mode of therapy. Certain types of cancer cells can be destroyed by radiation therapy, thus preventing the unrestrained growth of such tumors. In other cancers, radiation has only a palliative effect, preventing cell growth, reducing pain, pressure, and bleeding but not providing complete tumor destruction. Important factors that must be considered when determining the use of radiotherapy for the cancer patient include the following:

* The tumor must be surrounded by normal tissue that can tolerate the radiation and then repair itself.
* The tumor must not be widespread. If the tumor has metastasized, radiation can be used as a palliative form of treatment.
* The tumor must be moderately sensitive to radiation (a radiosensitive tumor).

Radiotherapy is often the treatment of choice for cancers of the skin, uterus, cervix, or larynx or those located within the oral cavity. With other types of cancer, radiotherapy is frequently used in combination with other forms of treatment, including surgery and chemotherapy.

Techniques of Radiation Therapy

The two methods for the administration of radiation are **external radiation therapy (ERT)** and **internal radiation therapy (IRT).** The following is an overview of these two methods.

External Radiation Therapy. With the ERT method, the patient receives calculated doses of radiation from a machine located at some distance from the site of the tumor. The patient is carefully prepared for treatment by a radiation therapist, sometimes assisted by the **dosimetrist** or a radiation physicist. The precise size and location of the tumor are determined, and the **port**, or point of entry for the radiation, is marked using a dye or tattoo. In formulating the treatment plan, a computer is used to calculate the radiation dosage needed to effect maximal destruction of malignant cells and minimal damage to surrounding normal tissue. Special lead blockers or shields can be constructed by a radiation physicist to protect surrounding normal tissue from the harmful effects of radiation.

Internal Radiation Therapy. The IRT method of treatment can have two forms of administration, known as **sealed** and **unsealed radiation therapy.** Sealed radiation therapy involves the implantation of sealed containers of radioactive material near the tumor site within the body. Unsealed radiation therapy involves the introduction of a liquid containing a radioactive substance into the patient through the mouth, via the bloodstream, or by instillation into a body cavity.

- *Sealed Radiation Therapy.* Radioactive material such as *radium, cesium-137, cobalt-60,* and *iridium-192* is sealed in small gold containers called *seeds* or within molds, plaques, needles, or other devices designed to hold the radioactive substance near the malignancy. In some cases, the radiation source is implanted within the cancerous tissue. In other cases, special devices or applicators have been designed to hold the implant in position for the desired period of treatment.

- *Unsealed Radiation Therapy.* Radioactive *iodine-131, radioactive phosphorus-32,* and *radioactive gold-198* are some of the substances used in the unsealed form of internal radiation therapy. *Phosphorus-32* may be intravenously administered for use in the treatment of leukemia or lymphoma. *Gold-198* and/or *phosphorus-32* is placed in colloidal suspension and instilled in a body cavity for the palliative treatment of certain malignancies. *Iodine-131* can be orally administered, usually in conjunction with a thyroidectomy.

Side Effects of Radiation

Because radiotherapy unavoidably affects normal tissue while destroying malignant cells, patients usually experience some unpleasant **side effects**. The degree of severity associated with the side effects depends on the individual, the cancer, its location, and the amount of radiation. The following are some side effects that can occur as a result of radiation therapy: anorexia, nausea, vomiting, diarrhea, malaise, mild erythema, edema, ulcers, alopecia, taste blindness, stomatitis, mucositis, and xerostomia.

Immunotherapy

Immunotherapy is the treatment of disease by stimulation of the body's immune system. It may be used as an adjuvant to other types of treatment. There are three types of immunotherapy: **active specific** (the use of various agents to produce a specific host–immune response), **passive** (the use of serum or other products from an immunocompetent individual that are given to an immunodeficient individual to produce an immune response), and **adoptive** (the process of transferring a form of specific immune response from a donor to a recipient).

Photodynamic Therapy

Photodynamic therapy (PDT), a type of laser therapy, involves the use of a special chemical that is injected into the bloodstream and absorbed by cells all over the body. The chemical rapidly leaves normal cells but remains in cancer cells for a longer time. A *laser* light aimed at the cancer activates the chemical, which then kills the cancer cells that have absorbed it. Photodynamic therapy can be used to reduce symptoms of **lung cancer**, for example, to control bleeding or to relieve breathing problems due to blocked airways when the cancer cannot be removed through surgery. Photodynamic therapy can also be used to treat very small tumors in patients for whom the usual treatments for lung cancer are not appropriate.

SPOTLIGHT ON SELECTED TYPES OF CANCER

Breast Cancer

In 2009, approximately 192,370 new cases of invasive breast cancer were diagnosed in women. Of those, about 62,280 were cases of carcinoma in situ (CIS) (noninvasive and the earliest form of breast cancer). Approximately 40,170 women died from breast cancer.

Early detection of breast cancer is extremely important. The 5-year survival rate for women with *localized* and properly treated breast cancer is about 97%. For all stages of breast cancer, it is about 87%. If cancer is not detected and treated early, it will continue to grow, invade, and destroy adjacent tissue, and spread into surrounding lymph nodes. See Figure 19.5 ■ It can be carried by the lymph and/or blood to other areas of the body and once this process, known as metastasis, has occurred, the cancer is usually advanced and/or disseminated and the 5-year survival rate is low.

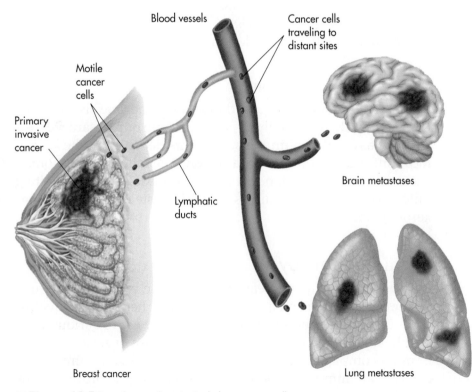

■ **Figure 19.5** Invasion and metastasis by cancer cells.

Approximately 50% of malignant tumors of the breast appear in the upper, outer quadrant and extend into the armpit. Eighteen percent of breast cancers occur in the nipple area, 11 percent in the lower outer quadrant, and 6 percent in the inner quadrant.

Signs and symptoms of breast cancer are generally insidious and may include:

- Unusual secretions from the nipple
- Changes in the nipple's appearance
- Nontender, movable lump
- Well-localized discomfort that may be described as burning, stinging, or aching sensation
- Dimpling or *peau d'orange* (orange-peel appearance) may be present over the area of cancer of the breast
- Asymmetry and an elevation of the affected breast
- Nipple retraction
- Pain in the later stages

Stages of breast cancer, according to the American Cancer Society, indicate the size of a tumor and how far the cancer has spread within the breast, to nearby tissues, and to other organs. Specific treatment is most often determined by the following stages of the disease:

Carcinoma in situ (CIS). Cancer is confined to the lobules (milk-producing glands) or ducts (passages connecting milk-producing glands to the nipple) and has not invaded nearby breast tissue. Also referred to as *ductal carcinoma in situ (DCIS)*.

Stage I. Tumor is smaller than or equal to 2 centimeters in diameter and axillary (underarm) lymph nodes test negative for cancer.

Stage II. Tumor is between 2 and 5 centimeters in diameter with or without positive lymph nodes, or tumor is greater than 5 centimeters without positive lymph nodes.

Stage III. This stage is divided into substages known as IIIA and IIIB:

- **IIIA.** Tumor is larger than 5 centimeters with positive movable lymph nodes, or tumor is any size with lymph nodes that adhere to one another or surrounding tissue.
- **IIIB.** Tumor of any size has spread to the skin, chest wall, or internal mammary lymph nodes (located beneath the breast and inside the chest).

Stage IV. Tumor, regardless of size, has metastasized (spread) to distant sites such as bones, lungs, or lymph nodes not near the breast.

Recurrent breast cancer. The disease has returned in spite of initial treatment.

Two genes have been identified as breast cancer genes. BRCA-1 and BRCA-2 are genes that, when changed, place a woman at greater risk of developing breast cancer compared to women who do not have either mutation. One single genetic mishap is not enough for a cell to become cancerous. It takes several changes. Women who have inherited mutations within the BRCA-1 and BRCA-2 genes are at higher risk for breast cancer than those who don't have the mutations. However, it still takes further events for cancer to occur in these women. There are internal factors, such as the hormone estrogen, and external factors that can contribute to this chain of events.

More than 90% of all breast lumps are discovered by women themselves. The majority of these lumps are benign (noncancerous), but for those that are not, early detection and treatment are essential. A woman should examine her breasts every month (Breast Self-Examination [BSE]—see Figure 19.6 ■).

WHY DO THE BREAST SELF-EXAM?

There are many good reasons for doing a breast self-exam each month. One reason is that it is easy to do and the more you do it, the better you will get at it. When you get to know how your breasts normally feel, you will quickly be able to feel any change, and early detection is the key to successful treatment and cure.

REMEMBER: A breast self-exam could save your breast – and save your life. Most breast lumps are found by women themselves, but in fact, most lumps in the breast are not cancer. Be safe, be sure.

WHEN TO DO BREAST SELF-EXAM

The best time to do breast self-exam is right after your period, when breasts are not tender or swollen. If you do not have regular periods or sometimes skip a month, do it on the same day every month.

NOW, HOW TO DO BREAST SELF-EXAM

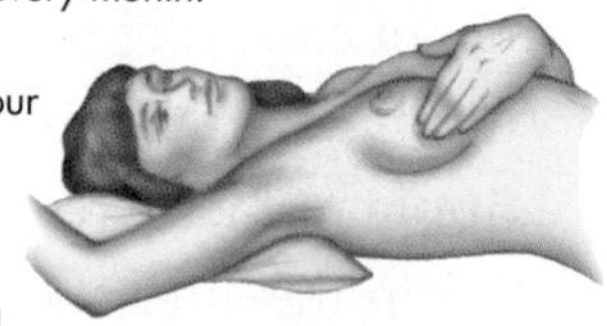

1. Lie down and put a pillow under your right shoulder. Place your right arm behind your head.

2. Use the finger pads of your three middle fingers on your left hand to feel for lumps or thickening. Your finger pads are the top third of each finger.

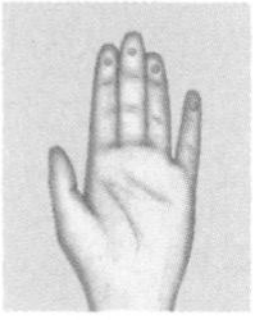

3. Press firmly enough to know how your breast feels. If you're not sure how hard to press, ask your health care provider. Or try to copy the way your health care provider uses the finger pads during a breast exam. Learn what your breast feels like most of the time. A firm ridge in the lower curve of each breast is normal.

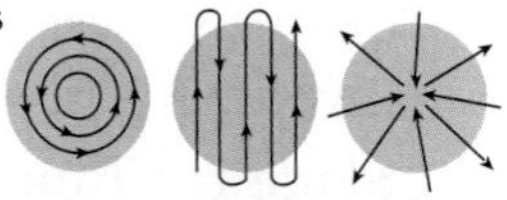

4. Move around the breast in a set way. You can choose either the circle (A), the up and down line (B), or the wedge (C). Do it the same way every time. It will help you to make sure that you've gone over the entire breast area, and to remember how your breast feels.

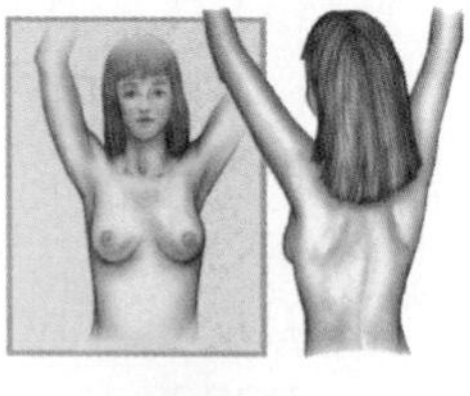

5. Now examine your left breast using your right hand finger pads.

6. If you find any changes, see your doctor right away.

FOR ADDED SAFETY:

You should also check your breasts while standing in front of a mirror right after you do your breast self-exam each month. See if there are any changes in the way your breasts look: dimpling of the skin, changes in the nipple, or redness or swelling.

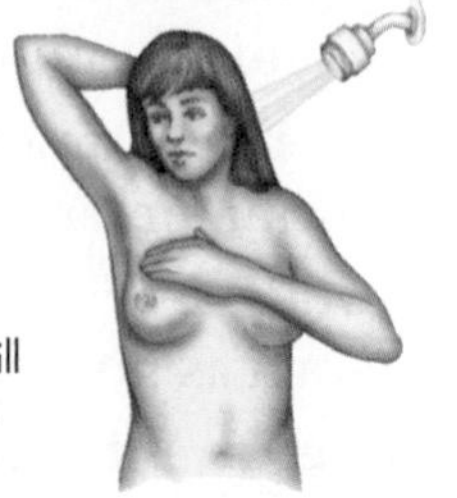

You might also want to do a breast self-exam while you're in the shower. Your soapy hands will glide over the wet skin, making it easy to check how your breasts feel.

■ **Figure 19.6** Breast self-examination.

Check for appearance, size, shape, symmetry, tenderness, thickening, and texture changes.

After increasing for more than 2 decades, female breast cancer incidence rates decreased by about 2% per year from 1999 to 2006. This decrease may be due at least in part to less use of hormone therapy (HT) after the results of the Women's Health Initiative were published in 2002. This study linked HT use to an increased risk of breast cancer and heart diseases.

Death rates from breast cancer have been declining since about 1990, with larger decreases in women younger than age 50. These decreases are believed to be the result of earlier detection through screening and increased awareness, as well as improved treatment.

Hodgkin's Disease

Hodgkin's disease (HD), sometimes called *Hodgkin's lymphoma,* is a cancer that starts in lymphatic tissue. There are two kinds of lymphomas: *Hodgkin's disease* (named after Dr. Thomas Hodgkin, who first recognized it in 1832) and *non-Hodgkin's lymphoma.*

Because lymphatic tissue is present in many parts of the body, Hodgkin's disease can start almost anywhere, but most often starts in lymph nodes in the upper part of the body. The most common sites are in the chest, neck, or under the arms. Hodgkin's disease enlarges the lymphatic tissue, which can then cause pressure on important structures. It can spread through the lymphatic vessels to other lymph nodes. Most Hodgkin's disease spreads to nearby lymph node sites in the body, not distant ones. It rarely gets into the blood vessels, but when it does, it can spread to almost any other site in the body, including the liver and lungs.

The cancer cells in Hodgkin's disease are called *Reed–Sternberg cells,* after the two doctors who first described them in detail. Under a microscope they look different from cells of non-Hodgkin's lymphomas and other cancers. Most scientists now believe that Reed–Sternberg cells are a type of malignant *B lymphocyte.* Normal B lymphocytes are the cells that make antibodies that help fight infections.

Before 1970 few people with diagnosed Hodgkin's disease recovered. Today, more than 80% of people who receive initial treatment experience a complete remission. Advances in diagnosis, staging, and treatment of Hodgkin's disease have helped to make this once uniformly fatal disease highly treatable with potential for full recovery.

Non-Hodgkin's lymphoma (NHL) is cancer that begins in the lymphatic system, usually in a B cell in a lymph node. The abnormal cell divides and makes copies of itself. The new cells divide again and again, making more and more abnormal (cancer) cells. The cancer cells can spread to nearly any other part of the body.

Symptoms of non-Hodgkin's lymphoma include swollen, painless lymph nodes in the neck, armpits, or groin; unexplained weight loss; fever; soaking night sweats; coughing, trouble breathing, or chest pain; weakness and tiredness that doesn't go away; and pain, swelling, or a feeling of fullness in the abdomen. Diagnosis is confirmed by either an *excisional biopsy* (entire lymph node is removed) or *incisional biopsy* (only part of a lymph node is removed). When lymphoma is found, the pathologist will report the type. The most common types are *diffuse large B-cell lymphoma* and *follicular lymphoma.* Lymphomas may also be grouped by how quickly they are likely to grow: indolent (low-grade) lymphomas grow slowly and aggressive (intermediate-grade and high-grade) lymphomas grow and spread more quickly.

Non-Hodgkin's lymphoma is more common than Hodgkin's disease. Survival rates are good with early diagnosis.

Leukemia

Leukemia is cancer that usually affects the white blood cells. White blood cells develop from stem cells in the bone marrow. Leukemia results when something goes wrong with the process of maturation from stem cell to white blood cell and a cancerous change occurs. The change often involves a rearrangement of pieces of chromosomes. Because the chromosomal rearrangements disturb the normal control of cell division, the affected cells multiply without restraint, becoming cancerous. They ultimately occupy the bone marrow, replacing the cells that produce normal blood cells. These leukemic (cancer) cells may also invade other organs, including the liver, spleen, lymph nodes, kidneys, and brain.

There are four major types of leukemia, named for how quickly they progress and which kind of white blood cell they affect. Acute leukemias progress rapidly; chronic leukemias progress slowly. Lymphocytic leukemias affect lymphocytes; myeloid (myelocytic) leukemias affect myelocytes.

- **Acute lymphocytic leukemia (ALL)** is a life-threatening disease in which the cells that normally develop into lymphocytes become cancerous and rapidly replace normal cells in the bone marrow. About 3,970 new cases of acute lymphocytic leukemia (ALL) are diagnosed each year in the United States. It is the most common type of leukemia in children and young people under the age of 19. Children are most likely to develop the disease, but it can occur at any age. Acute lymphocytic leukemia may be called by several names, including *acute lymphoid leukemia* and *acute lymphoblastic leukemia.*

- **Acute myeloid leukemia (AML)** is a life-threatening disease in which myelocytes become cancerous and rapidly replace normal cells in the bone marrow. This type of leukemia affects people of all ages, but mostly adults. Exposure to large doses of radiation and use of some cancer chemotherapy drugs increase the likelihood of developing acute myeloid leukemia. Acute myeloid leukemia may also be called by several names, including myelocytic, myelogenous, myeloblastic, and myelomonocytic leukemia.

- **Chronic lymphocytic leukemia (CLL)**, also referred to as *chronic lymphoid leukemia,* strikes nearly 9,730 people in the United States yearly. Chronic lymphocytic leukemia is characterized by a large number of cancerous mature lymphocytes (a type of white blood cell) and enlarged lymph nodes. More than three-fourths of the people who have this type of leukemia are over age 60; it affects men two to three times more often than women.

- **Chronic myelocytic leukemia (CML)** is a disease in which a cell in the bone marrow becomes cancerous and produces a large number of abnormal granulocytes. This disease may affect people of any age and of either sex but is uncommon in children under 10 years old. Chronic myelocytic leukemia may also be referred to as *myeloid, myelogenous,* and *granulocytic leukemia.*

Lung Cancer

Cancers that begin in the lungs are divided into two major types, **non–small cell lung cancer** and **small cell lung cancer**, depending on how the cells look under a microscope. Each type of lung cancer grows and spreads in different ways and is treated differently. There are three main types of non–small cell lung cancer. They are named for the type of cells in which the cancer develops: squamous cell carcinoma (also called *epidermoid carcinoma*), adenocarcinoma, and large cell carcinoma. Small cell lung cancer, sometimes called *oat cell cancer,* is less common than non–small cell lung cancer. This type of lung cancer grows more quickly and is more likely to spread to other organs in the body.

> **fyi** Common signs and symptoms of lung cancer include:
>
> - A cough that doesn't go away and gets worse over time
> - Constant chest pain
> - Coughing up blood
> - Shortness of breath, wheezing, or hoarseness
> - Repeated problems with pneumonia or bronchitis
> - Swelling of the neck and face
> - Loss of appetite or weight loss
> - Fatigue
>
> *Note:* These symptoms may be caused by lung cancer or by other conditions. It is important to see a physician if any of these symptoms persist.

To diagnose lung cancer, the doctor evaluates a person's medical history, smoking history, exposure to environmental and occupational substances, and family history of cancer. The doctor also performs a physical exam and may order a chest x-ray and other tests. If lung cancer is suspected, sputum cytology (the microscopic examination of cells obtained from a deep-cough sample of mucus in the lungs) is a simple test that may be useful in detecting lung cancer. To confirm the presence of lung cancer, the doctor must perform a biopsy and examine tissue from the lung.

Treatment depends on a number of factors, including the type of lung cancer (non-small or small cell lung cancer); the size, location, and extent of the tumor; and the general health of the patient. Many different treatments and combinations of treatments may be used for lung cancer, such as surgery, chemotherapy, radiation therapy, or photodynamic therapy (PDT).

> **fyi** The best way to prevent lung cancer is to quit (or never start) smoking. Researchers have discovered several causes of lung cancer—most are related to the use of tobacco, such as smoking cigarettes, cigars, pipes, and exposure to environmental tobacco smoke (ETS) or second-hand smoke. Other causes include exposure to radon, asbestos, and pollution.

Testicular Cancer

Testicular cancer (TC) is a disease in which malignant cells form in the tissues of one or both testicles. It is the most common cancer in men age 20 to 35. In a given year about 7,500 American men are diagnosed with this type of cancer.

> **fyi** For unknown reasons, the disease is about four times more common in white men than in black men. Some risk factors associated with testicular cancer include having had an undescended testicle, having had abnormal development of the testicles, and a personal or family history of testicular cancer.

Most testicular tumors are discovered by patients themselves, either by accident or while performing a testicular self-examination (TSE). It is most important that testicular cancer be diagnosed early, so young men should be taught how to examine their testicles. See Figure 19.7 ■

The most common presenting sign of testicular cancer is of an enlarged, painless lump or swelling in either testicle. The lump typically is pea-sized, but sometimes it might be as big as a marble or even an egg. Occasionally there may be pain. Besides lumps, if a man notices any other abnormality—an enlarged testicle, a feeling of heaviness or sudden collection of fluid in the scrotum, or a dull ache in the lower abdomen or groin—he should seek medical attention immediately. The origin and nature of scrotal masses must be determined as soon as possible because most testicular masses

Testicular Self-Examination

- Examine testicles while taking a warm shower or bath, or just after if using a mirror to compare size.

- The scrotum, testicles, and hands should be soapy to allow easy manipulation of the tissue.

- Gently roll each testicle between the thumb and fingers of each hand. If one testicle is substantially larger than the other, or if any hard lumps are detected, consult a physician immediately.

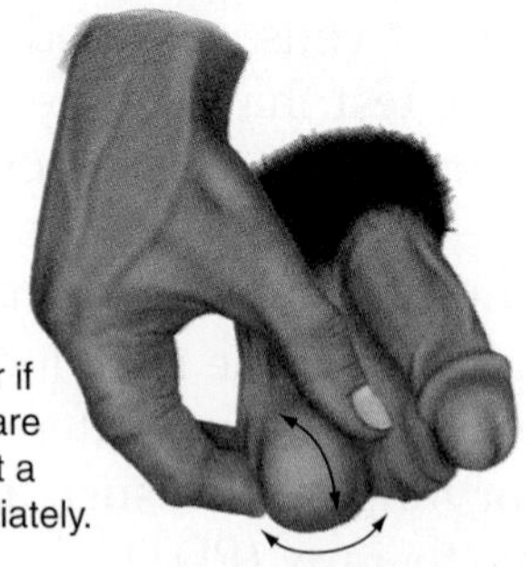

- Normal scrotal contents may be confusing. Just above and behind the testicle is the epididymis. It feels soft and tender overall, although parts of it may be rather firm. This is normal. The spermatic cord, a small, round, moveable tube, extends up from the epididymis. It feels firm and smooth. Of greatest concern is any hard lump felt directly on the testicle, even if it is painless.

- Choose a day out of each month on which to examine yourself. Most men choose an easy day to remember, such as the first or last day of the month.

■ **Figure 19.7** Procedure for testicular self-examination.

are malignant. Prognosis depends on the histology and extent of the tumor. With early detection, the survival rates for testicular cancer are approximately 95% at 5 years for seminomas and nonseminomas localized to the testis.

Nearly all testicular tumors stem from germ cells, the special sperm-forming cells within the testicles. These tumors fall into one of two types, seminomas or nonseminomas. Other forms of testicular cancer, such as sarcomas or lymphomas, are extremely rare.

Testicular cancer is diagnosed by a medical history and physical examination, ultrasound, serum tumor marker test, and a radical inguinal orchidectomy including a tissue biopsy. Imaging tests such as chest x-ray, computed tomography, magnetic resonance imaging, lymphangiogram, and positron emission tomography are often utilized to assess the spread of the disease and the staging of the cancer. Staging allows the doctor to plan the most appropriate treatment for each patient. Stages of testicular cancer are as follows:

Stage 1. Cancer confined to the testicle.

Stage 2. Disease spread to retroperitoneal lymph nodes, located in the rear of the body below the diaphragm.

Stage 3. Cancer spread beyond the lymph nodes to remote sites in the body, such as the lungs and/or liver.

Recurrent. Recurrent disease means that the cancer has come back after it has been treated. It may come back in the same place or in another part of the body.

No one treatment works for all testicular cancers. Seminomas and nonseminomas differ in their tendency to spread, their patterns of spread, and response to radiation therapy. Thus, they often require different treatment strategies, which doctors choose based on the type of tumor and the stage of the disease.

Because they are slow growing and tend to stay localized, seminomas generally are diagnosed in stage 1 or 2. Treatment might be a combination of testicle removal, radiation, or chemotherapy. Stage 3 seminomas are usually treated with a combination of chemotherapy drugs. Because certain treatments can cause infertility, the patient who wishes to have children should consider sperm banking before beginning treatment.

fyi For more information on testicular cancer, visit the Lance Armstrong Foundation website at www.livestrong.org.

• Building Your Medical Vocabulary •

This section provides the foundation for learning medical terminology. Review the following alphabetized word list. Note how common prefixes and suffixes are repeatedly applied to word roots and combining forms to create different meanings. The word parts are color-coded: prefixes are green, suffixes are blue, **roots/combining forms are red**.

You will find that some terms have not been divided into word parts. These are common words or specialized terms that are included to enhance your medical vocabulary. See Chapter 1, page 7, to review pronunciation guidelines.

MEDICAL WORD	WORD PARTS		DEFINITION
	Part	**Meaning**	
adenocarcinoma (Adeno-CA) (ăd″ ĕ-nō-kăr″ sĭn-ō′ mă)	aden/o carcin -oma	gland cancer tumor	Malignant tumor arising in a glandular organ
adjuvant therapy (ăd′ jū-vănt)			In breast cancer, adjuvant therapy includes chemotherapy, radiation therapy, or hormone therapy.
anaplasia (ăn″ ă-plā′ zĭ-ă)	ana- -plasia	up, apart, backward formation	Characteristic of most cancerous cells in which there is a loss of differentiation and an irreversible alteration in adult cells toward more embryonic cell types
astrocytoma (ăs″ trō-sĭ-tō′ mă)	astro- cyt -oma	star-shaped cell tumor	Tumor composed of star-shaped neuroglial cells
betatron (bā′ tă-trŏn)			Megavoltage machine used in administering external radiation therapy
brachytherapy (brăk″ ĭthĕr′ ă-pē)	brachy- -therapy	short treatment	Radiation therapy in which the radioactive substance is inserted into a body cavity or organ. The source of radiation is located a short distance from the body area being treated.
Burkitt's lymphoma (bŭrk′ ĭtz lĭm-fō′ mă)			Malignant tumor, most commonly found in Africa, that affects children; the characteristic symptom is a massive, swollen jaw
carcinogen (kăr″ sĭn′ ō-jĕn)	carcin/o -gen	cancer formation, produce	Agent or substance that incites or produces cancer

MEDICAL WORD	WORD PARTS		DEFINITION
	Part	**Meaning**	
carcinoid (kăr´ sĭ-nōīd)	carcin -oid	cancer resemble	Tumor derived from the argentaffin cells in the intestinal tract, bile duct, pancreas, bronchus, or ovary
carcinoma (kăr˝ sĭ-nō´ mă)	carcin -oma	cancer tumor	Malignant tumor arising in epithelial tissue. See Figure 19.8 ■

■ **Figure 19.8** Basal cell carcinoma.
(Courtesy of Jason L. Smith, MD)

MEDICAL WORD	WORD PARTS		DEFINITION
chondrosarcoma (kŏn˝ drō-săr-kō´ mă)	chondr/o sarc -oma	cartilage flesh tumor	Cancerous tumor derived from cartilage cells
choriocarcinoma (kō´ rĭ-ō-kăr˝ sĭ-nō´ mă)	chori/o carcin -oma	chorion cancer tumor	Cancerous tumor of the uterus or at the site of an ectopic pregnancy
cyclotron (sī´ klō-trŏn)			Megavoltage machine used in administering external radiation therapy
dedifferentiation (dē-dĭf˝ ĕr-ĕn´ shē-ā´ shŭn)			Process by which normal cells lose their specialization (*differentiation*) and become malignant
deoxyribonucleic acid (DNA) (dē-ŏk˝ sĭ-ri˝ bō- nū-klē´ ĭk)			Complex protein of high molecular weight found in the nucleus of every cell; controls all of the cell's activities and the genetic material necessary for the organism's heredity
differentiation (dĭf˝ ĕr-ĕn˝ shē-ā˝ shŭn)			Process by which normal cells have a distinct appearance and specialized function

MEDICAL WORD	WORD PARTS		DEFINITION
	Part	**Meaning**	
ductal carcinoma in situ (DCIS) (dŭk-tăl kăr′ sĭ-nō′ mă ĭn sī′ too)	duct -al carcin -oma in- situ	to lead pertaining to cancer tumor in place	Abnormal cells that involve only the lining of a duct and have not spread outside the duct to other tissues in the breast; also called *intraductal carcinoma*
encapsulated (ĕn-kăp″ sū-lā′ tĕd)	en- capsul -ate(d)	in a little box use, action	Enclosed within a site, sheath, or capsule
Ewing's sarcoma (ū′ ingz săr-kō′ mă)			Primary bone cancer occurring in the pelvic area or in one of the long bones; occurs mostly in children and adolescents
exacerbation (ĕks-ăs″ ĕr-bā′ shŭn)			Process of increasing the severity of symptoms; a time when the symptoms of a disease are most prevalent
external radiation (ĕk-stur′ năl rā-dĭ-ā′ shŭn)			Process of administering radiation to the patient via a radiation machine located outside the body
fibrosarcoma (fī″ brō-săr-kō′ mă)	fibr/o sarc -oma	fiber flesh tumor	Cancerous tumor arising in collagen-producing fibroblasts
fungating (fŭn′ gāt-ĭng)			Process of growing rapidly, like a fungus
glioblastoma (glī′ ō-blăs-tō′ mă)	gli/o -blast -oma	glue immature cell tumor	A rapidly growing cancerous tumor of the brain
glioma (glī-ō′ mă)	gli -oma	glue tumor	Cancerous tumor of the brain
hemangiosarcoma hē-măn″ jĭ-ō-săr-kō′ mă)	hem angi/o sarc -oma	blood vessel flesh tumor	Cancerous tumor originating in blood vessels

MEDICAL WORD	WORD PARTS		DEFINITION
	Part	**Meaning**	
Hodgkin's disease (HD) (hŏj´kĭns)			Form of lymphoma that occurs in children and young adults. The two kinds of lymphoma are *Hodgkin's disease* (named after Dr. Thomas Hodgkin, who first recognized it in 1832) and *non-Hodgkin's lymphoma.* See Figure 19.9 ■

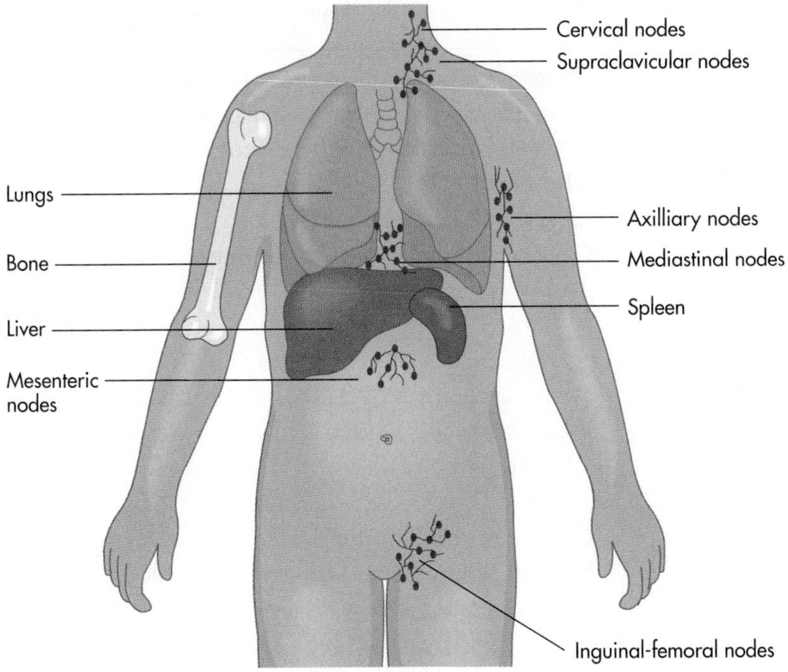

■ **Figure 19.9** Lymph nodes and organs affected in Hodgkin's disease in children.

MEDICAL WORD	WORD PARTS		DEFINITION
	Part	**Meaning**	
human T-cell leukemia-lymphoma virus (HTLV) (lū-kē´mĭ-ă-lĭm-fō´mă)			First virus known to cause cancer in humans
hyperplasia (hī˝pĕr-plā´zĭ-ă)	hyper- -plasia	excessive formation	Excessive formation and growth of normal cells
immunosuppression (ĭm˝ū-nō-sŭ-prĕsh´ŭn)	immun/o suppress -ion	safe, immunity suppress process	Process of preventing formation of the immune response
immunotherapy (ĭm˝mū-nō-thĕr´ă pē)	immun/o -therapy	safe, immunity treatment	Treatment of disease by active, passive, or adoptive immunity
infiltrative (ĭn´fĭl-trā˝tĭve)	in- filtrat -ive	into to strain through nature of	Pertaining to the process of extending or growing into normal tissue; invasive

MEDICAL WORD	WORD PARTS		DEFINITION
	Part	**Meaning**	
in situ (ĭn sī′ too)			Enclosed within a site; refers to tumor cells that remain at a site and have not invaded adjacent tissue
invasive			Pertaining to the spreading process of a malignant tumor into normal tissue
Kaposi's sarcoma (KS) (kăp′ ō-sēz săr-kō′ mă)			Malignant neoplasm that causes violaceous (purplish discoloration) vascular lesions and general lymphadenopathy; often seen in patients who have AIDS
leiomyosarcoma (lī″ ō-mī″ ō-săr-kō′ mă)	lei/o my/o sarc -oma	smooth muscle flesh tumor	Cancerous tumor of smooth muscle tissue
lesion (lē′ zhŭn)			Wound; an injury, altered tissue, or a single infected patch of skin
leukemia (lū-kē′ mĭ-ă)	leuk -emia	white blood condition	Cancer of the blood characterized by overproduction of leukocytes; cancer of the blood-forming tissues
leukoplakia (lū″ kō-plā′ kĭ-ă)	leuk/o -plakia	white plate	White, thickened patches formed on the mucous membranes of the inner cheeks, gums, or tongue that tend to become cancerous
linear accelerator (lĭn′ ē-ar ăk-sĕl′ ĕr-ā″ tŏr)			Megavoltage machine used in administering external radiation therapy. See Figure 19.10 ■

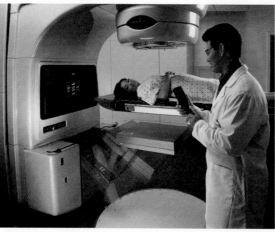

■ **Figure 19.10** Clinac® 23 EX linear accelerator. Used for the delivery of computer-driven intensity-modulated radiation therapy (IMRT), as well as conventional therapy in the treatment of cancer. (Courtesy of Varian Medical Systems of Palo Alto, CA. © 1999, Varian Medical Systems. All rights reserved.)

MEDICAL WORD	WORD PARTS		DEFINITION
	Part	Meaning	
liposarcoma (lĭp″ ō-săr-kō´ mă)	lip/o sarc -oma	fat flesh tumor	Cancerous tumor of fat cells
lobular carcinoma in situ (LCIS) (lŏb´ ū-lăr kăr´ sĭ-nō´ mă)	lobul -ar carcin -oma in- situ	small lobe pertaining to cancer tumor in place	Abnormal cells found in the lobules of the breast. This condition seldom becomes invasive cancer. However, having lobular carcinoma in situ increases the risk of developing cancer in either breast
lymphangiosarcoma (lĭm-făn″ jē-ō-săr-kō´ mă)	lymph angi/o sarc -oma	lymph vessel flesh tumor	Cancerous tumor of lymphatic vessels
lymphoma (lĭm-fō´ mă)	lymph -oma	lymph tumor	Cancerous tumor of lymphoid tissue
lymphosarcoma (lĭm″ fō-săr-kō´ mă)	lymph/o sarc -oma	lymph flesh tumor	Cancerous disease of lymphatic tissue; also called *lymphoblastoma*
malignant (mă-lĭg´ nănt)	malign -ant	bad kind forming	Pertaining to a bad wandering; refers to the spreading process of cancer from one area of the body to another
medulloblastoma (mě-dŭl″ ō-blăs-tō´ mă)	medull/o -blast -oma	marrow immature cell tumor	Cancerous tumor of the brain, the fourth ventricle, and the cerebellum
melanoma (měl″ ă-nō´ mă)	melan -oma	black tumor	Literally means *a cancerous black mole or tumor.* See Figure 19.11 ■

■ **Figure 19.11** Melanoma.

(Courtesy of Jason L. Smith, MD)

MEDICAL WORD	WORD PARTS		DEFINITION
	Part	**Meaning**	
meningioma (měn-ĭn″ jĭ-ō′ mă)	mening/i -oma	meninges, membrane tumor	Cancerous tumor originating in the arachnoidal (meninges) membrane of the brain
metastasis (mě-tăs′ tă-sis)	meta- -stasis	beyond control	Spreading process of cancer from a primary site to a secondary site. See Figure 19.5 on page 688. Similarly, *invasive growth* is the spreading process of a malignant tumor into adjacent normal tissue. See Figure 19.3 on page 680.
mucositis (mū″ kō-sī′ tĭs)	mucos -itis	mucus inflammation	Inflammation of the oral mucosa caused by exposure to high-energy beams delivered by radiation therapy
mutagen (mū′ tă-jěn)	muta -gen	to change formation, produce	Agent that causes a change in the DNA (genetic structure) of an organism
mutation (mū-tā′ shŭn)	mutat -ion	to change process	Process by which the DNA (genetic structure) is changed
mycotoxin (mī″ kō-tŏk′ sĭn)	myc/o tox -in	fungus poison substance	Substance produced by fungus growing in food or animal feed that, if ingested, can cause cancer
myeloma (mī″ ě-lō′ mă)	myel -oma	bone marrow tumor	Tumor arising in the hemopoietic portion of the bone marrow
myosarcoma (mī″ ō-săr-kō′ mă)	my/o sarc -oma	muscle flesh tumor	Cancerous tumor of muscle tissue
neoplasm (nē′ ō-plăzm)	neo- -plasm	new a thing formed	New tissue formed, such as an abnormal growth or tumor
nephroblastoma (něf″ rō-blăs-tō′ mă)	nephr/o -blast -oma	kidney immature cell tumor	Cancerous tumor of the kidney; also called *Wilms' tumor;* most often found in children 2–3 years of age
neuroblastoma (nū″ rō-blăs-tō′ mă)	neur/o -blast -oma	nerve immature cell tumor	Cancerous tumor composed chiefly of neuroblasts; can appear anywhere but usually in the abdomen as a swelling; most often diagnosed during the first year of life
oligodendroglioma (ŏl″ ĭ-gō-děn″ drō-glĭ-ō′ mă)	oligo- dendr/o gli -oma	little tree glue tumor	Cancerous tumor composed chiefly of neuroglial cells and located in the cerebrum

MEDICAL WORD	WORD PARTS		DEFINITION
	Part	Meaning	
oncogenes (ŏng″ kō-jēn z′)	onc/o -genes	tumor formation, produce	Cancer-causing genes; genes in a virus that can induce tumor formation
oncogenic (ŏng″ kō-jēn′ ĭk)	onc/o -genic	tumor formation, produce	Pertaining to the potential formation of tumors, especially cancerous ones
osteogenic sarcoma (ŏs″ tē-ō-jĕn′ ĭk săr-kō′ mă)	oste/o -genic sarc -oma	bone formation, produce flesh tumor	Cancerous tumor composed of osseous (bone) tissue
Paget's disease of the breast (păj′ ĕts)			Paget's disease of the breast (also called *mammary Paget's disease [MPD]*) is a rare form of breast cancer. The condition was originally reported in 1874 by Sir James Paget, an English surgeon, who also described an unrelated skeletal condition known as Paget's disease of the bone. These disorders are distinct disease entities that are medically unrelated. Paget's disease of the breast is characterized by inflammatory, "eczema-like" changes of the nipple that may extend to involve the areola. Initial findings often include itching, scaling, and crusting of and/or discharge from the nipple. In those with Paget's disease of the breast, distinctive tumor cells (known as Paget cells) are present within the outermost layer of skin of the nipple. In addition, the condition is often associated with an underlying malignancy of the milk ducts (ductal carcinoma). See Figure 19.12 ■

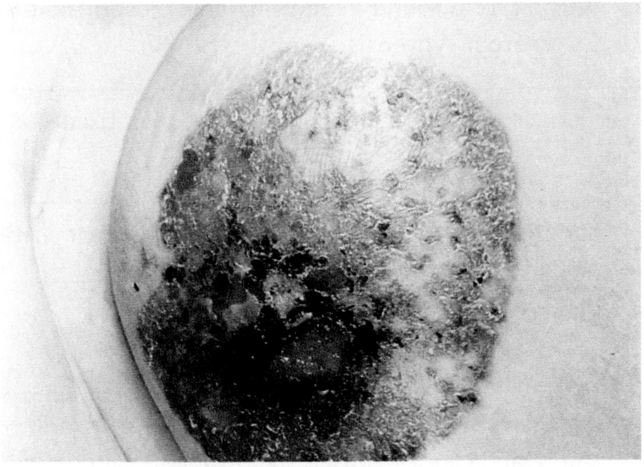

■ **Figure 19.12** Paget's disease of the breast.
(Courtesy of Jason L. Smith, MD)

MEDICAL WORD	WORD PARTS		DEFINITION
palliative (păl′ ĭ-ā-tĭv)	palliat -ive	cloaked nature of	Pertaining to a form of treatment to relieve or alleviate symptoms without curing
port			In radiation therapy, refers to the skin area of entry for the radiation
precancerous (prē-kăn′ sĕr-ŭs)	pre- cancer -ous	before crab, cancer pertaining to	Pertaining to changes or conditions before the onset of cancer
primary site			Original, initial, or principal site

MEDICAL WORD	WORD PARTS		DEFINITION
	Part	**Meaning**	
proliferation (prō-lĭf″ ĕr-ā′ shŭn)			Process of rapid production; growth by multiplying
remission (rē- mĭsh′ ŭn)	remiss -ion	remit process	Process of lessening the severity of symptoms; time when symptoms of a disease are controlled
reticulosarcoma (rĕ-tĭk″ ū-lō-săr-kō′ mă)	reticul/o sarc -oma	net flesh tumor	Cancerous tumor of the lymphatic system
retinoblastoma (rĕt″ ĭ-nō-blăs-tō′ mă)	retin/o -blast -oma	retina immature cell tumor	Cancerous tumor of the retina. Although relatively rare, it accounts for 5% of childhood blindness.
rhabdomyosarcoma (răb″ dō-mĭ″ ō-săr-kō′ mă)	rhabd/o my/o sarc -oma	rod muscle flesh tumor	Cancerous tumor originating from the same embryonic cells that develop into striated muscles. It is the most common soft tissue sarcoma in children.
ribonucleic acid (RNA) (rī″ bō-nū′ klē′ ĭk)			Nucleic acid found in all living cells; responsible for protein synthesis
sarcoma (săr-kō′ mă)	sarc -oma	flesh tumor	Cancerous tumor arising in connective tissue
secondary site			Second site usually derived from the primary site
seminoma (sĕm″ ĭ-nō′ mă)	semin -oma	seed tumor	Cancerous tumor of the testis
tamponade (cardiac) (tam′ pŏn-ād [kăr′ dē-ăk])			Excessive fluid in the pericardial sac surrounding the heart; can be caused by advanced cancer of the lung or a tumor that has metastasized to the pericardium
teletherapy (tĕl″ ĕ-thĕr′ ă-pē)			Radiation therapy in which the radioactive substance is at a distance from the body area being treated
teratoma (tĕr″ ă-tō′ mă)	terat -oma	monster tumor	Cancerous tumor of the ovary or testis; can contain embryonic tissues of hair, teeth, bone, or muscle
thymoma (thĭ-mō′ mă)	thym -oma	thymus tumor	Tumor of the thymus gland
trismus (trĭz′ mŭs)	trism -us	grating pertaining to	Pertaining to the inability to open the mouth fully; occurs in patients with oral cancer who undergo a combination of surgery and radiation therapy

MEDICAL WORD	WORD PARTS		DEFINITION
	Part	Meaning	
tumor (tū′ mor)			Abnormal growth, swelling, or enlargement
viral (vī′ răl)	vir -al	virus (poison) pertaining to	Pertaining to a virus, which means *poison* in Latin
Wilms′ tumor (vĭlmz tū′ mor)			Cancerous tumor of the kidney occurring mainly in children
xerostomia (zē″ rō-stō′ mē-ă)	xer/o stom -ia	dry mouth condition	Condition of dryness of the mouth; oral change caused by radiation therapy or chemotherapy

• Abbreviations •

ABBREVIATION	MEANING	ABBREVIATION	MEANING
ACS	American Cancer Society	**HD**	Hodgkin's disease
Adeno-CA	adenocarcinoma	**H & E**	hematoxylin and eosin
AFP	alpha-fetoprotein	**HER-2/neu**	human epidermal growth
AIDS	acquired immunodeficiency syndrome		factor receptor–2
ALL	acute lymphocytic leukemia	**HTLV**	human T-cell leukemia-lymphoma virus
AML	acute myeloid leukemia	**IRT**	internal radiation therapy
BRCA	breast cancer gene	**KS**	Kaposi's sarcoma
BSE	breast self-examination	**LCIS**	lobular carcinoma in situ
Bx	biopsy	**mL**	milliliter
CA	cancer	**mm**	millimeter
CA-125	cancer antigen 125	**MPD**	mammary Paget's disease
CEA	carcinoembryonic antigen	**NCI**	National Cancer Institute
chemo	chemotherapy	**NHL**	non-Hodgkin's lymphoma
CIS	carcinoma in situ	**PDT**	photodynamic therapy
CLL	chronic lymphocytic leukemia	**PSA**	prostate-specific antigen
cm	centimeter	**RNA**	ribonucleic acid
CML	chronic myelocytic leukemia	**St**	stage (of disease)
CT	computed tomography	**TC**	testicular cancer
DCIS	ductal carcinoma in situ	**TNM**	tumor, node, metastasis
DNA	deoxyribonucleic acid	**TPE**	Taxol, Platinol, and VePesid
ERT	external radiation therapy	**TSE**	testicular self-examination
ETS	environmental tobacco smoke	**VAD**	vacuum-assisted needle biopsy device
FNA	fine needle aspiration	**WHO**	World Health Organization
HCC	hepatocellular carcinoma		

• Study and Review • Study and Review • Study and Review
Review • Study and Review • Study and Review • Stu
w • Study and Review • Study and Review • Study a

Overview of Oncology

Write your answers to the following questions.

1. Name the three main classifications of cancer.

a. _____   b. _____

c. _____

2. Define *cell differentiation*. _____

_____

3. Define *dedifferentiation*. _____

_____

4. Name three ways that malignant cells spread to body parts.

a. _____   b. _____

c. _____

5. List the seven warning signals for cancer.

a. _____   b. _____

c. _____   d. _____

e. _____   f. _____

g. _____

6. Name four methods used in the treatment of cancer.

a. _____   b. _____

c. _____   d. _____

Word Parts

PREFIXES

Give the definitions of the following prefixes.

1. ana- _____
2. astro- _____
3. hyper- _____
4. neo- _____
5. oligo- _____
6. pre- _____
7. en- _____
8. in- _____
9. meta- _____
10. brachy- _____

ROOTS AND COMBINING FORMS

Give the definitions of the following roots and combining forms.

1. aden/o _____
2. angi/o _____
3. cancer _____
4. carcin _____
5. carcin/o _____
6. chondr/o _____
7. chori/o _____
8. cyt _____
9. dendr/o _____
10. fibr/o _____
11. gli _____
12. gli/o _____
13. hem _____
14. immun/o _____
15. lei/o _____
16. leuk _____
17. leuk/o _____
18. lip/o _____
19. lymph _____
20. lymph/o _____
21. medull/o _____
22. melan _____
23. mening/i _____
24. mucos _____
25. myc/o _____
26. myel _____
27. my/o _____
28. capsul _____
29. nephr/o _____
30. neur/o _____
31. onc/o _____
32. oste/o _____
33. reticul/o _____
34. retin/o _____
35. rhabd/o _____
36. sarc _____

37. duct _____

38. semin _____

39. stom _____

40. terat _____

41. thym _____

42. tox _____

43. trism _____

SUFFIXES

Give the definitions of the following suffixes.

1. -blast _____

2. -emia _____

3. -gen _____

4. -genes _____

5. -genic _____

6. -ia _____

7. -in _____

8. -itis _____

9. -oma _____

10. -ous _____

11. -plakia _____

12. -plasia _____

13. -plasm _____

14. -ate (d) _____

15. -therapy _____

16. -us _____

17. -al _____

18. -ar _____

19. -ion _____

20. -ive _____

21. -ant _____

22. -stasis _____

23. -oid _____

Identifying Medical Terms

In the spaces provided, write the medical terms for the following meanings.

1. _____ Agent or substance that incites or produces cancer

2. _____ Cancerous tumor derived from cartilage cells

3. _____ Cancerous tumor of the brain

4. _____ Cancerous tumor of smooth muscle tissue

5. _____ Cancer of the blood characterized by overproduction of leukocytes

6. _____ Cancerous tumor of lymphoid tissue

7. _____ Literally means a cancerous black mole or tumor

8. _____ Cancerous tumor of muscle tissue

9. _____ Cancerous tumor of the kidney occurring mainly in children

10. _____ Cancerous tumor arising in connective tissue

Spelling

Circle the correct spelling of each medical term.

1. anplasia / anaplasia

2. fibrsarcoma / fibrosarcoma

3. lymphosarcoma / lymphsarcoma

4. myeloma / myloma

5. oncgenic / oncogenic

6. seminoma / semioma

7. teletherapy / telethrapy

8. tertoma / teratoma

9. trismus / trimus

10. xerstomia / xerostomia

Matching

Select the appropriate lettered meaning for each of the following words.

_____ 1. Hodgkin's disease

_____ 2. exacerbation

_____ 3. differentiation

_____ 4. in situ

_____ 5. encapsulated

_____ 6. photodynamic therapy

_____ 7. fungating

_____ 8. hyperplasia

_____ 9. Kaposi's sarcoma

_____ 10. metastasis

a. Spreading process of cancer from a primary site to a secondary site

b. Excessive formation and growth of normal cells

c. Enclosed within a sheath

d. Process by which normal cells have a distinct appearance and specialized function

e. Form of lymphoma that occurs in young adults

f. Type of laser therapy that involves the use of a special chemical that is injected into the bloodstream and absorbed by cells all over the body

g. Enclosed within a site, sheath, or capsule

h. Malignant neoplasm that causes violaceous (purplish discoloration) vascular lesions and general lymphadenopathy

i. Process of increasing the severity of symptoms

j. Process of growing rapidly

k. Agent that causes a change in the genetic structure of an organism

Abbreviations

Place the correct word, phrase, or abbreviation in the space provided.

1. adenocarcinoma _____

2. biopsy _____

3. CA _____

4. chemo _____

5. deoxyribonucleic acid _____

6. IRT _____

7. acute lymphocytic leukemia _____

8. ductal carcinoma in situ _____

9. BRCA _____

10. tumor, node, metastases _____

PRACTICAL APPLICATION

MEDICAL RECORD ANALYSIS

This exercise contains information, abbreviations, and medical terminology from an actual medical record or case study that has been adapted for this text. The names and any personal information have been created by the author. Read and study each form or case study and then answer the questions that follow. You may refer to Appendix III, Abbreviations and Symbols, on page A41.

RIVER CITY PATHOLOGY
Paul Nelson, MD, Lab Director
1048 Peachtree Drive, Suite A 1040
Atlanta, GA 30328
(123)456-7890

PATHOLOGY REPORT

Path#: OB07-0000786	Patient: Betsy Parker	8234
Biopsy: 1/18/xx	DOB: 2/24/39 Sex: Female	SSN: xxx-xx-xxxx.....
Received: 1/18/xx	Physician: Jackson Lewis, MD	
Reported: 1/19/xx		

Diagnosis: Right Shoulder
Basal Cell Carcinoma, Nodular & Infiltrative Type, Margins Free, see description

---

Clinical data: Clinical BCC Check Margins, Suture Marks Superior Margin at
12 O'CLOCK

Specimen site: Right Shoulder-excision

Gross Description:

The specimen is a portion of skin measuring (cm) 2.4 x 1.3 x 0.3

Microscopic Description:

Present within the dermis are aggregates of basaloid cells with hyperchromatic nuclei, scant cytoplasm, and palisading of the peripheral nuclei. This neoplasm has an infiltrative pattern of growth in the submitted specimen. Sections have been taken to show the base and margins and reveal that the neoplastic process appears to be totally excised in these sections.

Paul Nelson, MD

Medical Record Questions

Place the correct answer in the space provided.

1. What is a neoplasm? _____

2. What is the meaning of BCC? _____

3. Why is it important to indicate "margins free" in the diagnosis? _____

4. What was the location of this specimen? _____

5. What is the meaning of cm? _____

PEARSON
mymedicalterminologylab

MyMedicalTerminologyLab is a premium online homework management system that includes a host of features to help you study. Registered users will find:

- Fun games and activities built within a virtual hospital

- Powerful tools that track and analyze your results—allowing you to create a personalized learning experience

- Videos, flashcards, and audio pronunciations to help enrich your progress

- Streaming lesson presentations and self-paced learning modules

- A space where you and your instructors can view and manage your assignments

m • Respiratory System • Urinary System • Endocrine
tem • Nervous System • Special Senses: The Ear • Spe
Senses: The Eye • Female Reproductive System with an
rview of Obstetrics • Male Reproductive System • Onc

20

gy • **Radiology and Nuclear Medicine** • Mental He

LEARNING OUTCOMES

On completion of this chapter, you will be able to:

1. Define radiology.

2. Explain the dangers and safety precautions associated with x-rays.

3. Identify the positions used in radiography.

4. Discuss diagnostic imaging as used by the radiologist and the computed-assisted x-ray machines that are described in this chapter.

5. Describe nuclear medicine and some of the general uses of this specialty.

6. Define interventional radiology and state some interventional procedures described in this chapter.

7. Analyze, build, spell, and pronounce medical words.

8. Identify and define selected abbreviations.

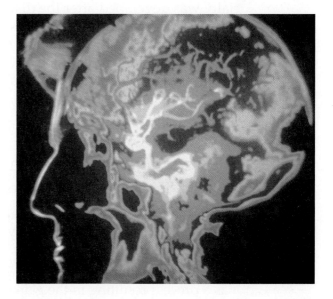

COMBINING FORMS OF RADIOLOGY AND NUCLEAR MEDICINE

act/o	acting		iont/o	ion
angi/o	vessel		lymph/o	lymph
arteri/o	artery		mamm/o	breast
arthr/o	joint		myel/o	spinal cord
bronch/o	bronchi		oscill/o	to swing
chol/e	gall, bile		phot/o	light
cinemat/o	motion		physic/o	nature
cyst/o	bladder		pyel/o	renal pelvis
dermat/o	skin		radi/o	ray, x-ray
digit/o	finger or toe		salping/o	fallopian tube
ech/o	echo		sial/o	salivary
encephal/o	brain		son/o	sound
fluor/o	fluorescence, luminous		therm/o	hot, heat
gen/o	kind		tom/o	to cut
hyster/o	womb, uterus		tract/o	to draw
ion/o	ion		ven/o	vein

Radiology and Nuclear Medicine

RADIOLOGY

Radiology is the scientific discipline of medical imaging using radionuclides, ionizing radiation, nuclear magnetic resonance, and ultrasound. This medical specialty was developed after the discovery of an unknown ray in 1895 by Wilhelm Konrad Roentgen, a German physicist, who called his discovery *x-ray.* An **x-ray** is produced by the collision of a stream of electrons against a target (usually an anode of one of the heavy metals) contained within a vacuum tube. This collision produces electromagnetic rays of short wavelengths and high energy. The physician who specializes in radiology, roentgen diagnosis, and roentgen therapy is called a **radiologist**.

Characteristics of X-Rays

The following are the characteristics of x-rays applicable to its medical use.

1. X-rays are an invisible form of radiant energy with short wavelengths traveling at 186,000 miles per second. They are able to penetrate different substances to varying degrees.

2. X-rays cause **ionization** of the substances through which they pass. Ionization is a process resulting in the gain or loss of one or more electrons in neutral atoms. The gain of an electron creates a negative electrical charge, whereas the loss of an electron results in a positively charged particle. These negatively or positively charged particles are called *ions.*

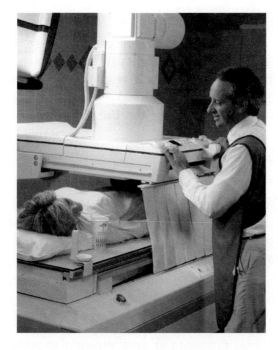

■ **Figure 20.1** Advantx™ radiography/fluoroscopy system. (Courtesy of GE Medical Systems)

3. X-rays cause fluorescence of certain substances, thus allowing for the process known as **fluoroscopy** (see Figure 20.1 ■), the examination of the tissues and deep structures of the body by x-ray, using the **fluoroscope**, a device that projects x-ray images in a movielike sequence onto a screen monitor. This process allows the physician to visualize internal structures that are in motion and to make permanent records of the examination for future study.

4. X-rays allow the x-ray beam to be directed at a specific site during radiotherapy or to produce high-quality shadow images on **film** (radiographs).

5. X-rays are able to penetrate substances of different densities. In the body, x-rays pass through air in the lungs, fluids such as blood and lymph, and fat around muscles. Such substances are said to be **radiolucent**. Substances that obstruct the passage of radiant energy, in other words absorb radiant energy, such as calcium in bones, lead, or barium (Ba), are called **radiopaque**. Control of the voltage and amperage applied to the x-ray tube plus the duration of the exposure allows images of body structures of varying densities. A contrast medium can be introduced into the body to enhance certain x-ray images. This characteristic allows x-rays to be used as a diagnostic tool.

6. X-rays can destroy body cells. Radiation can be used to destroy malignant tumors. In these cases, the x-ray voltage is administered by a radiotherapist using radiotherapy machines such as a linear accelerator or betatron. Care must be exercised in administering radiotherapy because x-rays can destroy healthy as well as abnormal tissue.

Dangers and Safety Precautions

Because x-rays are invisible and produce no sound or smell, those working around and with them need to take certain precautions to avoid unnecessary exposure. Following are some of the dangers known to be associated with x-rays and the safety precautions designed to prevent unnecessary exposure.

Prolonged Exposure

Prolonged and continued exposure to x-rays can cause damage to the gonads (testes or ovaries) and/or depress the hematopoietic system, which can cause leukopenia and/or leukemia. Personnel involved with radiation therapy should spend the minimal amount of time necessary when caring for patients receiving internal radiation therapy. The farther away an individual is from the source of radiation, the less the degree of exposure.

Secondary Radiation

X-rays can scatter or be diverted from their normal straight paths when they strike radiopaque objects. This scatter or secondary radiation tends to add unwanted density to the image; therefore, a device known as a **grid** is positioned between the x-ray machine and the patient to absorb scatter before it reaches the x-ray film.

Safety Precautions

Not all scatter or secondary radiation is absorbed by a grid; therefore, those working in areas adjacent to x-ray equipment risk unintentional exposure from this source unless proper safety precautions are observed. Generally, these safety precautions include the five described below.

1. *Film Badge.* A **film badge**, usually pinned to a medical worker's clothing, is a device that is sensitive to ionizing radiation and monitors exposure to beta and gamma rays. A periodic analysis of the film badge reveals the amount of radiation the individual has received. See Figure 20.2 ∎

2. *Lead Barrier.* Persons who operate x-ray machines do so from behind barriers equipped with a lead-treated window for viewing the patient.

3. *Lead-Lined Room.* X-ray equipment should be housed in an area featuring lead-lined walls, floors, and doors to prevent the escape of radiation from the room.

4. *Protective Clothing.* People who hold or position patients for x-ray examination should wear lead-lined gloves and aprons, especially if they hold a patient, such as a child, while an x-ray is being taken.

5. *Gonad Shield.* The reproductive organs are radiosensitive and must be protected by a lead shield while x-rays are being taken. X-rays can cause damage to the genetic material within the reproductive organs, which could lead to birth defects or cancer.

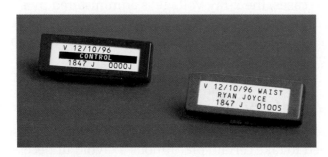

■ **Figure 20.2** Types of radiation badges to be worn by all staff around x-ray equipment.

Positions Used in Radiography

- **Anteroposterior Position (AP).** The patient is placed with the anterior (front) part of the body facing the x-ray tube and the posterior (back) of the body facing the film. X-rays pass through the body from the front to the back in reaching the film.

- **Posteroanterior Position (PA).** The patient is placed with the posterior (back) portion of the body facing the x-ray tube and the anterior (front) of the body facing the film. The x-rays pass through the body from the back to the front to reach the film.

- **Lateral Position (lat).** The x-ray beam passes from one side of the patient's body to the opposite side to reach the film. Placing the patient's right side next to the film and passing x-rays through the body from left to right is known as the *right lateral position*. Placing the patient's left side next to the film and passing x-rays through the body from right to left is known as the *left lateral position.*

- **Supine Position.** The patient rests on the back, face upward, allowing the x-rays to pass through the body from the front to the back.

- **Prone Position.** The patient is placed lying face down with the head turned to one side. The x-rays pass from the back to the front side of the body.

- **Oblique Position.** The patient is placed so that the body or body part to be imaged is at an angle to the x-ray beam.

Diagnostic Imaging

Diagnostic imaging involves the use of x-rays, ultrasound, radiopharmaceuticals, radiopaque media, and computers to provide the radiologist images of internal body organs and processes. These images are used to identify and locate tumors, fractures, hematomas, disease processes, and other abnormalities within the body. In recent years, advances in the field of electronics have produced a variety of computer-assisted x-ray machines to enhance the images obtained by the radiologist. These sophisticated machines now make possible noninvasive procedures for the visualization of organs and processes that were previously not accessible or that required exploratory surgical procedures for examination.

Pregnant health care practitioners are permitted to work in and around certain diagnostic imaging machines. Acceptable activities include, but are not limited to, positioning patients, scanning, archiving, injecting contrast, and entering the scan room in response to an emergency. Pregnant practitioners are requested not to remain in the room during the actual data acquisition or scanning. Pregnant patients may undergo certain scanning if, in the determination of a designated attending radiologist, the risk–benefit ratio for the patient warrants that the study be performed. The radiologist should confer with the referring physician and document that the data is needed and the physician does not believe that it is prudent to wait until the patient is no longer pregnant.

Computed Tomography

Computed tomography (CT) is sometimes referred to as a **CAT scan** (computerized axial tomography). It combines an advanced x-ray scanning system with a powerful minicomputer and has vastly improved imaging quality while making it possible to view parts of the body and abnormalities not previously open to

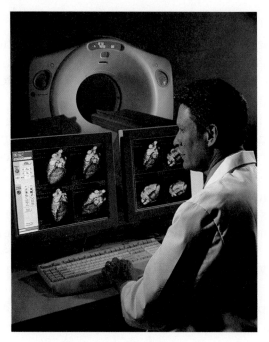

■ **Figure 20.3** LightSpeed[16]™ computed tomography system. (Courtesy of GE Medical Systems)

radiography. The CT scanner combines tomography, the process of imaging structures by focusing on a specific body plane and blurring all details from other planes, with a microprocessor that provides high-speed analysis of the tissue variances scanned (Figure 20.3 ■).

CT scans reveal both bone and soft tissues, including organs, muscles, and tumors (Figure 20.4 ■). Image tones can be adjusted to highlight tissues of similar density,

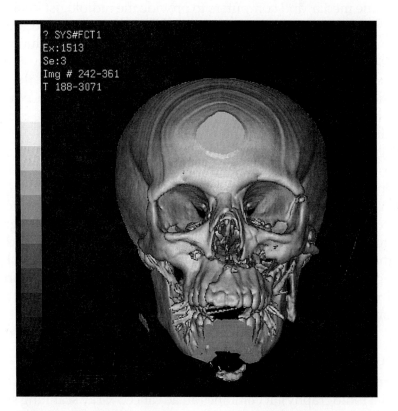

■ **Figure 20.4** 3D CT scan showing multiple facial fractures.

(Courtesy of Teresa Resch)

and, through graphics software, the data from multiple cross-sections can be assembled into three-dimensional images. CT aids diagnosis, surgery, and treatment, including radiation therapy, in which effective dosage depends highly on the precise density, size, and location of a tumor.

A person having a CT scan is asked to refrain from eating or drinking for 4 hours before the scan. All jewelry and metal objects that could interfere with the exam need to be removed beforehand. Women are asked if they are pregnant. A person having a CT scan needs to undress and put on an exam gown.

Next, the person lies on a narrow table that slides through the opening in a machine that is shaped like a doughnut with a hole in its center. The opening is called the *gantry*. While in the gantry, an x-ray tube travels around the individual, creating computer-generated x-ray images. Some types of exams require the patient to receive an intravenous injection of iodinated contrast, which is a dye that makes some tissues show up better. Scans of the intestines sometimes call for the person to drink diluted iodinated contrast solution prior to the exam. After the exam, the technologist views the pictures. If they are adequate, the person is free to leave.

Magnetic Resonance Imaging

Magnetic resonance imaging (MRI) is a noninvasive imaging technique. The MRI machine is used to view organs, bone, and other internal body structures. The imaged body part is exposed to radio waves while in a magnetic field. The picture is produced by energy emitted from hydrogen atoms in the human body. The patient is not exposed to radiation during this test.

MRI can be used for a variety of purposes. A physician can order an MRI of the brain, known as a *cranial MRI,* to evaluate a person's tumor, seizure disorder, or headache symptoms. See Figure 20.5 ■ An MRI of the spine examines a disk problem in a person's spine. If an individual has sustained injury to the shoulder or knee, an MRI is frequently used to study these large joints. Diseases of the heart, chest, abdomen, and pelvis are also commonly evaluated with MRI.

Before the test, the physician assesses the patient for any drug or food allergies (especially shellfish or foods with added iodine such as table salt) and whether the person has experienced claustrophobia or anxiety in enclosed spaces. If this is a problem, mild sedating medication may be given. A woman is asked if she is pregnant.

The person is asked to remove all metal objects such as belts, jewelry, and any pieces of removable dental work. Internal metal objects that cannot be removed can distort the final images so the person should inform the MRI technologist about any previous surgery that required placement of metal in the body, such as a hip pinning. Because the magnetic field can damage watches and credit cards, these objects are not taken into the MRI scanner.

Typically, the person having the test does not need to restrict food or fluids before an MRI scan. Certain tests, such as an MRI-guided biopsy, do require certain food and fluid restrictions. The person should consult the health care provider for instructions prior to the MRI.

As the test begins, the person lying on his or her back slides into the **bore** (horizontal tube running through the magnet from front to back) on a special table. To prevent image distortion on the final images, the person must lie very still for the duration of the test. Commonly, a special substance called a *contrast agent* is administered prior to or during the test. The contrast agent is used to enhance internal

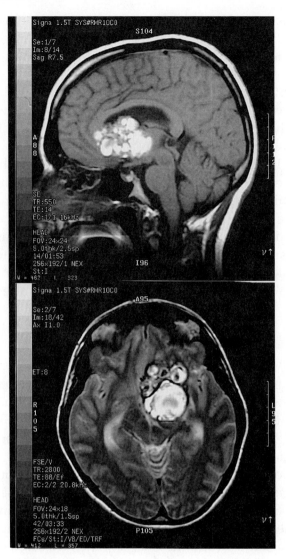

■ **Figure 20.5** MRI of the head showing large hemorrhagic lesion. (Courtesy of Teresa Resch)

structures and improve image quality. Typically, this material is injected into a vein in the arm.

The scanning process is painless. However, the part of the body being imaged can feel a bit warm. This sensation is harmless and normal. The person hears loud banging and knocking noises during many stages of the exam. Earplugs are provided for people who find the noises disturbing.

A radiologist analyzes the MRI images. Frequently, the MRI helps to better evaluate a disease or disorder affecting organs and blood vessels. MRI is particularly useful in evaluating the size and location of tumors as well as bleeding at various clotting stages. The health care provider and the radiologist use this information to help guide the next course of action for the individual's condition.

Ultrasound

Ultrasound literally means *beyond sound*. It is sound whose frequency is beyond the range of human hearing. Ultrasound is widely used in diagnostic imaging to evaluate a patient's internal organs. Its energy is transmitted into the patient and, because various internal organs and structures reflect and scatter sound differently, returning echoes can be used to form an image of a particular structure. These ultrasonic echoes are then recorded as a composite picture of the internal organ and/or structure. See Figure 20.13 on page 733 and Figure 20.14 on page 734.

Ultrasonography is the process of using ultrasound to produce a record of ultrasonic echoes as they strike tissues of different densities. The record produced by this process is called a **sonogram** or **echogram.** An adaptation of ultrasound technology is **Doppler echocardiography.** It is a noninvasive technique for determining the blood flow velocity in different locations in the heart. This same technique can be used to determine the uterine artery blood flow velocity during pregnancy as well as the fetal heart rate.

The test is done in the ultrasound or radiology department. The patient lies down for the procedure. A clear, water-based conducting gel is applied to the skin over the area being examined to help with the transmission of the sound waves. A handheld probe called a *transducer* is then moved over the area being examined. The patient can be asked to change position so that other areas can be examined.

Preparation for the procedure depends on the body region being examined. Ultrasound procedures generally cause little discomfort, although the conducting gel can feel slightly cold and wet.

Results are considered normal if the organs and structures in the area being examined are normal in appearance. The significance of abnormal results depends on the body region being examined and the nature of the symptom.

Other Imaging Techniques

Other diagnostic imaging techniques being used include **thermography,** in which detailed images of body parts are developed from data showing the degree of heat and cold present in areas being studied, and **scintigraphy,** which involves the production of two-dimensional images of tissue areas from the scintillations emitted by an internally administered radiopharmaceutical device that concentrates on a targeted site.

NUCLEAR MEDICINE

Nuclear medicine is a subspecialty within the field of radiology that uses radioactive substances to produce images of body anatomy and function. The images are developed based on the detection of energy emitted from the radioactive substance given to the patient either intravenously (IV) or by mouth (PO). These images are used to diagnose disease processes and evaluate organ functioning. Some of the general uses of nuclear medicine follow:

- Image blood flow and heart function.
- Scan lungs.
- Evaluate kidney function.
- Identify blockage of the gallbladder.
- Evaluate bones for fracture, infection, arthritis, tumors.

- Identify bleeding into the colon.
- Locate an infection site.
- Measure thyroid function for hyperactivity or hypoactivity.

Certain imaging procedures, including PET scanning, employ radionuclides to provide real-time visuals of biochemical processes. One device, a nuclear imaging machine, employs a scintillation camera that can rotate around the body to pick up radiation emitted by an injected substance, such as radioactive iodine, which localizes in the thyroid, or radioactive thallium, which localizes in the heart. Through computerization, a digitized image of a particular organ is produced.

Positron Emission Tomography

Positron emission tomography (PET), commonly called a **PET scan**, is a nuclear medicine imaging technique that helps physicians see how the organs and tissues inside the body are actually functioning. The test involves injecting a very small dose of a radioactive chemical, called a radiotracer, into the vein of the patient's arm. The tracer travels through the body and is absorbed by the organs and tissues being studied. The PET scan detects and records the energy given off by the tracer substance and, with the use of a computer this energy is converted into three-dimensional pictures. A physician can then look at cross-sectional images of the body organ from any angle in order to detect functional problems.

A PET scan can measure such vital functions as blood flow, oxygen use, and glucose metabolism, which helps doctors identify abnormal from normal functioning organs and tissues. The scan can also be used to evaluate the effectiveness of a patient's treatment plan, allowing the course of care to be adjusted if necessary.

PET scans are most commonly used to detect cancer, heart problems (such as coronary artery disease and damage to the heart following a heart attack), brain disorders (including brain tumors, memory disorders, seizures) and other central nervous system disorders.

INTERVENTIONAL RADIOLOGY

Interventional radiology (IR) is a branch of medicine in which certain diseases are treated nonoperatively. An **interventional radiologist** is a physician who has had special training in imaging and who specializes in treating diseases percutaneously. An interventional radiologist uses radiological imaging to guide catheters, balloons, stents, filters, and other tiny instruments through the body's vascular system and/or other systems.

The procedures and/or surgeries are performed in an interventional suite, generally on an outpatient basis. General anesthesia is usually unnecessary, and conscious sedation and/or local anesthesia is more commonly used. These procedures are cost effective and are increasingly replacing traditional surgery for certain conditions and procedures as described in Table 20.1 ■

TABLE 20.1 Selected Interventional Procedures

Balloon angioplasty	Opens blocked or narrowed blood vessels
Chemoembolization	Delivers cancer-fighting agents directly to the tumor site
Embolization	Delivers clotting agents directly to an area that is bleeding or to block blood flow to a problem area, such as a fibroid tumor
Fallopian tube catheterization	Opens blocked fallopian tubes, a cause of infertility in women
Needle biopsy	Diagnostic test for breast or other cancers; an alternative to surgical biopsy
Stent-graft placement	Reinforces a ruptured or ballooning section of an artery with a fabric-wrapped stent, a small cagelike tube that serves to patch the vessel
Thrombolysis	Dissolves blood clots
Transjugular intrahepatic portosystemic shunt (TIPS)	Improves blood flow for patients with severe liver dysfunction
Varicocele occlusion	Treats varicose veins in the testicles, a cause of infertility in men
Vena cava filters	Prevents blood clots from reaching the heart

Radiation Therapy

The treatment of disease by ionizing radiation is called **radiotherapy**, **x-ray therapy**, **cobalt treatment**, or simply **radiation therapy.** In all cases, this treatment seeks to deliver a precise, calculated dose of radiation to diseased tissue, such as a tumor, while causing the least possible damage to surrounding normal tissue. See pages 686–687 in Chapter 19, "Oncology," for more information about radiation therapy.

• Building Your Medical Vocabulary •

This section provides the foundation for learning medical terminology. Review the following alphabetized word list. Note how common prefixes and suffixes are repeatedly applied to word roots and combining forms to create different meanings. The word parts are color-coded: prefixes are green, suffixes are blue, roots/combining forms are red.

You will find that some terms have not been divided into word parts. These are common words or specialized terms that are included to enhance your medical vocabulary. See Chapter 1, page 7, to review pronunciation guidelines.

MEDICAL WORD	WORD PARTS		DEFINITION
	Part	Meaning	
angiocardiogram (ăn″ jĭ-ō-kăr′ dĭ-ō-grăm)	angi/o cardi/o -gram	vessel heart record	X-ray record of the heart and great vessels made visible through the use of a radiopaque contrast medium
angiogram (ăn′ jĭ-ō-grăm)	angi/o -gram	vessel record	X-ray record of the blood vessels made visible through the use of an injected radiopaque contrast medium
angiography (ăn″ jĭ- ŏg′ ră-fē)	angi/o -graphy	vessel recording	A medical imaging technique used to visualize the inside, or lumen, of blood vessels and organs of the body, with particular interest in the arteries, veins, and the heart chambers. This is traditionally done by injecting a radio-opaque contrast agent into the blood vessel and imaging using x-ray-based techniques such as fluoroscopy.
arteriography (ăr″ tē-rĭ-ŏg′ ră-fē)	arteri/o -graphy	artery recording	Process of making an x-ray record of the arteries
arthrography (ăr-thrŏg′ ră-fē)	arthr/o -graphy	joint recording	Process of making an x-ray record of a joint
barium (Ba) sulfate (bā′ rĭ-ŭm sŭl′ fāt)			Radiopaque barium compound used as a contrast medium in x-ray examination of the digestive tract; may be administered orally or via a barium enema (BE)
beam			Ray of light; in radiology and nuclear medicine, radiant energy emitted by a group of atomic particles traveling a parallel course
bronchogram (brŏng′ kō-grăm)	bronch/o -gram	bronchi record	X-ray record of the bronchial tree made visible through the use of a radiopaque contrast medium

MEDICAL WORD	WORD PARTS		DEFINITION
	Part	Meaning	
cassette			Light-proof case or holder for x-ray film
cathode (kăth´ ōd)			Negative pole of an electrical current
cholangiogram (kō-lăn´ jĭ-ō-grăm)	chol angi/o -gram	gall, bile vessel record	X-ray record of the bile ducts made visible through the use of a radiopaque contrast medium
cholecystogram (kō˝ lē-sĭs´ tō-grăm)	chole cyst/o -gram	gall bladder record	X-ray record of the gallbladder made visible through the use of a radiopaque contrast medium
cinematoradiography (sĭn˝ ĭ-măt˝ ō-rā˝ dĭ-ŏg´ ră-fē)	cinemat/o radi/o -graphy	motion x-ray recording	Process of making an x-ray record of an organ in motion
cineradiography (sĭn˝ ē-rā˝ dē-ŏg´ ră-fē)	cine radi/o -graphy	motion x-ray recording	Process of making a motion picture record of successive x-ray images appearing on a fluoroscopic screen
cobalt-60 (kō´ balt)			Radionuclide that serves as the radioactive substance in teletherapy machines; also used for implantation (interstitial) in the treatment of some malignancies
contrast medium			Radiopaque substance used in certain x-ray procedures to permit visualization of organs or structures
curie (Ci) (kūr´ e)			Unit of radioactivity
digital subtraction angiography (dĭj´ ĭ-tăl sŭb-trăk´ shŭn ăn˝ jĭ-ŏg´ ră-fē)	digit -al sub- tract -ion angi/o -graphy	finger or toe pertaining to below to draw process vessel recording	Method by which a computer performs instantaneous subtraction of x-ray images, giving high-quality x-ray images of blood vessels with less x-ray dye. *Note:* In this instance, digital refers to an Arabic number from 0 to 9, so named from counting on the fingers.
dose			Amount of medication or radiation to be administered

MEDICAL WORD	WORD PARTS		DEFINITION
	Part	Meaning	
echoencephalography (ĕk″ ō-ĕn-sĕf″ ă-lŏg′ ră-fē)	ech/o encephal/o -graphy	echo brain recording	Process of using ultrasound to study intracranial structures of the brain. Useful for diagnosing conditions that cause a shift in the midline structures of the brain.
echography (ĕk-ŏg′ ră-fē)	ech/o -graphy	echo recording	Process of using ultrasound as a diagnostic tool by making a record of the echo produced when sound waves are reflected back through tissues of different density
film			Thin, cellulose-coated, light-sensitive sheet or slip of material used in taking pictures
fluorescence (floo″ ō-rĕs′ ĕnts)			Property of certain substances to emit light as a result of exposure to and absorption of radiant energy
fluoroscopy (floo-räs′ kə-pē)	fluor/o -scopy	fluorescence, luminous visual examination, to view, examine	Process of examining internal structures by viewing the shadows cast on a fluorescent screen after the x-ray has passed through the body
hysterosalpingogram (hĭs″ tĕr-ō-săl-pĭn′ gō- grăm)	hyster/o salping/o -gram	uterus fallopian tube record	X-ray record of the uterus and fallopian tubes that is made visible through the use of a radiopaque contrast medium
intravenous pyelogram (ĭn″ tră-vē′ nŭs pī′ ĕ-lō-grăm)	intra- ven -ous pyel/o -gram	within vein pertaining to renal pelvis record	X-ray record of the kidney and renal pelvis made visible through the use of an injected radiopaque contrast medium
ion (ī-ŏn)			Atomic particle consisting of an atom or a group of atoms that carry an electrical charge, either negative or positive
ionization (ī″ ŏn-ĭ-zā′ shŭn)			Process of breaking up molecules into their component parts
ionizing radiation (ī′ ŏn-ĭ-zĭng rā″ dĭ-ā′ shŭn)			Powerful invisible energy capable of producing ions

MEDICAL WORD	WORD PARTS		DEFINITION
	Part	Meaning	
ionometer (ĭŏn´ ō-mē-tĕr)	ion/o -meter	ion instrument to measure	Instrument used to measure the amount of radiation used by x-rays or radioactive substances
ionotherapy (ī´´ ŏn-ō-thĕr´ ă-pē)	ion/o -therapy	ion treatment	Treatment by introducing ions into the body
iontoradiometer (ĭ-ŏn´´ tō-rā´´ dĭ-ŏm ĭ-tĕr)	iont/o radi/o -meter	ion x-ray instrument to measure	Instrument used to measure the amount and intensity of x-rays
irradiation (ĭ-rā´´ dē-ā´ shŭn)	ir (in)- radiat -ion	into radiant process	Process of using x-rays, radium rays, ultraviolet rays, gamma rays, or infrared rays in the diagnosis or therapeutic treatment of a patient
isotope (ī´ sō-tōp)			One of a series of nuclides that are chemically identical yet differ in atomic weight and electrical charge. Radioactive isotopes are composed of unstable atoms, and most are artificially produced. For example, cobalt-60 is a radioactive isotope artificially produced from naturally occurring cobalt-59.
lead (Pb) (lĕd)			Metallic chemical element; soft, heavy, inelastic, malleable, ductile, bluish-gray metallic element used in its metallic form as a protective shielding against x-rays. See Figure 20.6 ■

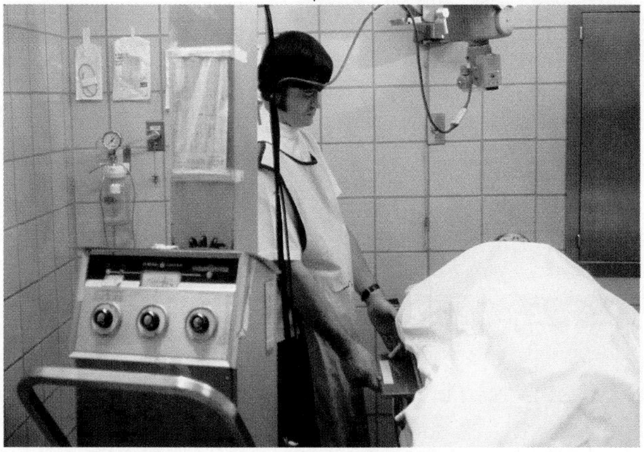

■ **Figure 20.6** X-ray technician in a lead apron positions a photographic plate beneath a patient undergoing an x-ray procedure. This apron is a protective shield of lead and rubber worn by a patient or those taking x-rays to protect the genitals and other vital organs from excessive exposure to x-rays.

MEDICAL WORD	WORD PARTS		DEFINITION
lymphangiogram (lĭm-fãn´´ jē-ō-grăm)	lymph angi/o -gram	lymph vessel record	X-ray record of the lymph vessels made visible with radiopaque contrast medium
lymphangiography (lĭm-fãn´´ jē-ŏg´ ră-fē)	lymph angi/o -graphy	lymph vessel recording	Process of making an x-ray record of the lymph vessels

MEDICAL WORD	WORD PARTS		DEFINITION
	Part	**Meaning**	
mammography (măm-ŏg´ ră-fē)	mamm/o -graphy	breast recording	Process of obtaining x-ray pictures of the breast using a low-dose x-ray system. The *mammogram* is the actual x-ray record (picture) of the breast. See Figures 20.7 ■ and 20.8 ■ The two types of mammograms are *screening*, which is generally used to detect breast cancer or other changes in the breast tissue in women who do not have symptoms, and *diagnostic*, which can be ordered when a screening mammogram shows something abnormal in the breast. A diagnostic mammogram can also be ordered if the woman has symptoms that suggest breast cancer.

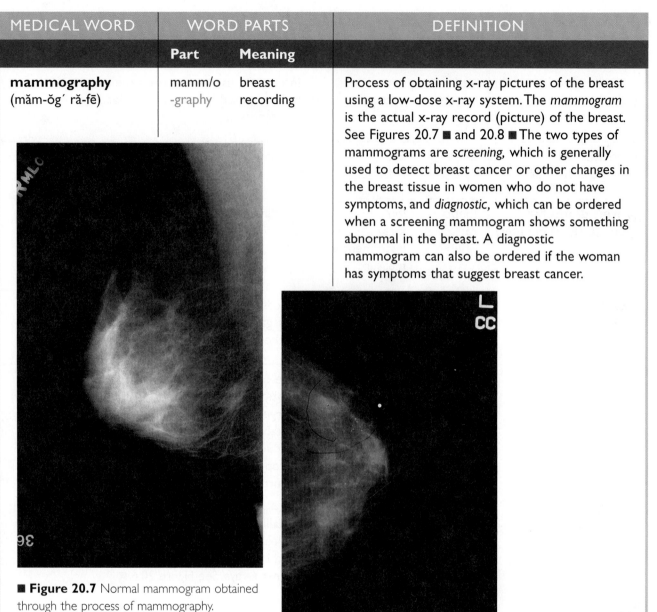

■ **Figure 20.7** Normal mammogram obtained through the process of mammography.
(Courtesy of Teresa Resch)

■ **Figure 20.8** Mammogram showing cancer with microcalcifications. (Courtesy of Teresa Resch)

LIFE SPAN CONSIDERATIONS

Breast cancer screening with mammograms has reduced deaths from breast cancer in women 40–69 years of age. A mammogram can detect changes in the breast, such as cancer, often before a lump can be felt. It can also show calcifications, or mineral deposits, cysts or fluid-filled masses, leaking breast implants, and noncancerous tumors or growths.

fyi Approximately 1,300 men a year are diagnosed with breast cancer. A male who is scheduled for a mammogram may be embarrassed because he believes that breast cancer is strictly a female disease. The male breast generally does not contain as much adipose tissue as the female breast, so it can be difficult to place the man's breast onto the film holder and obtain the proper amount of compression.

MEDICAL WORD	WORD PARTS		DEFINITION
	Part	**Meaning**	
millicurie (mCi) (mĭl˝ ĭ-kū´ rē)	milli- curie	one-thousandth curie	0.001 Ci
myelogram (mī´ ĕ-lō-grăm)	myel/o -gram	spinal cord record	X-ray record of the spinal cord made visible with a radiopaque contrast medium
oscilloscope (ŏ-sĭl´ ō-skōp)	oscill/o -scope	to swing instrument for examining	Instrument used to record an electrical wave visually on a fluorescent screen of a cathode-ray tube
photofluorogram (fō˝ tō-floo´ ĕr-ō-grăm)	phot/o fluor/o -gram	light fluorescence record	X-ray record of images seen during fluoroscopic examination
physicist (fĭz´ ĭ-sĭst)	physic -ist	nature one who specializes	Literally means *one who specializes in nature;* person who studies the energy, mass, and laws of nature
rad (răd)			Amount of radiation absorbed; the letters stand for **r**adiation **a**bsorbed **d**ose
radiation (rā-dĭ-ā´ shŭn)	radiat -ion	radiant process	Process by which radiant energy is propagated through space or matter
radioactive (rā˝ dĭ-ō-ăk´ tĭv)	radi/o act -ive	ray, x-ray acting nature of	Characterized by emitting radiant energy
radiodermatitis (rā˝ dĭ-ō-dur´ mă-tī´ tĭs)	radi/o dermat -itis	ray, x-ray skin inflammation	Inflammation of the skin caused by exposure to x-rays or radioactive substances
radiograph (rā´ dĭ-ō-grăf)	radi/o -graph	ray, x-ray instrument for recording	Picture produced on a sensitized film or plate by rays; an *x-ray record*
radiographer (rā˝ dĭ-ŏg´ ră-fĕr)	radi/o -graph -er	ray, x-ray instrument for recording one who	Person skilled in making x-ray records
radiography (rā˝ dĭ-ŏg´ ră-fē)	radi/o -graphy	ray, x-ray recording	Process of making an x-ray record

MEDICAL WORD	WORD PARTS		DEFINITION
	Part	**Meaning**	
radiologist (rā″ dĭ-ŏl′ ō-jĭst)	radi/o log -ist	ray, x-ray study of one who specializes	Literally means *one who specializes in radiology;* a physician who specializes in the production and interpretation of medical images See Figure 20.9 ■

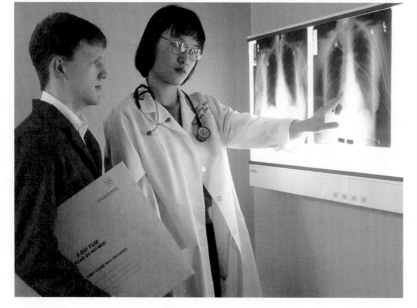

■ **Figure 20.9** Radiologist examines an x-ray of the chest.

MEDICAL WORD	WORD PARTS		DEFINITION
radiology (rā″ dĭ-ŏl′ ō-jē)	radi/o -logy	ray, x-ray study of	Scientific discipline of medical imaging using radionuclides, ionizing radiation, nuclear magnetic resonance, and ultrasound
radiolucent (rā″ dĭ-ō-lū′ sĕnt)	radi/o lucent	ray, x-ray to shine	Pertaining to property of permitting the passage of radiant energy
radionuclide (rā″ dĭ-ō-nū′ klĭd)	radi/o nucl -ide	ray, x-ray nucleus having a particular quality	Radioactive species of an atomic nucleus identified by its atomic number, mass, and energy state
radiopaque (rā″ dĭ-ō-pāk′)	radi/o paque	ray, x-ray dark	Pertaining to property of obstructing the passage of radiant energy
radioscopy (rā″ dĭ-ŏs′ kō-pē)	radi/o -scopy	ray, x-ray visual examination, to view, examine	Process of viewing and examining the inner structures of the body through the process of x-rays
radiotherapy (rā″ dĭ-ō-thĕr′ ă-pē)	radi/o -therapy	ray, x-ray treatment	Treatment of disease by the use of x-rays, radium, and other radioactive substances

MEDICAL WORD	WORD PARTS		DEFINITION
	Part	Meaning	
radium (Ra) (rā´ dǐ-ŭm)			Radioactive isotope used to treat certain malignant diseases
roentgen (R) (rĕnt´ gĕn)			International unit for describing exposure dose of x-ray or γ-radiation
roentgenology (rĕnt˝ gĕn-ŏl´ ō-jē)	roent gen/o -logy	roentgen kind study of	Study of roentgen rays for diagnostic and therapeutic purposes
scan			Process of using a moving device or a sweeping beam of radiation to produce images of organs or structures of the body. Figure 20.10 ■ shows a PET scan; Figure 20.11 ■ shows a CAT scan; and Figure 20.12 ■ shows a bone scan. A **bone scan** is a test used to find cancer, infection, fractures, or other injuries in the bone and to check a person's response to treatment for certain bone conditions, such as Paget's disease. A radioactive substance is injected into a vein in the arm of the person having the scan. The test usually begins after a wait of 2–3 hours.

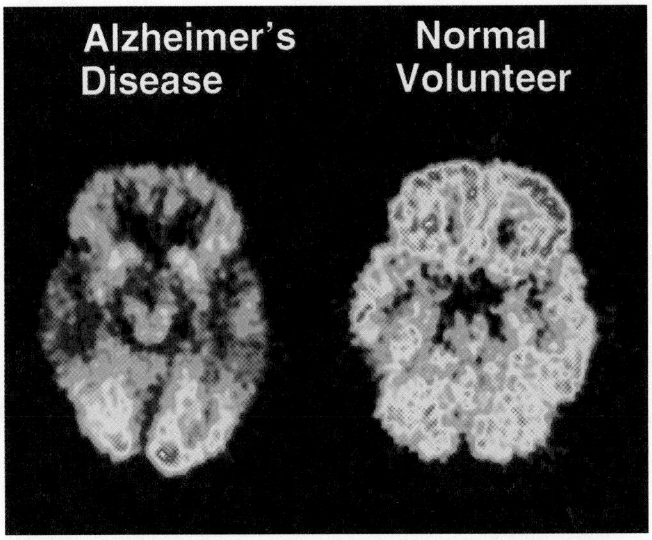

Alzheimer's Disease — **Normal Volunteer**

■ **Figure 20.10** PET scan comparing the metabolic activity levels of a normal brain and the brain of an Alzheimer's sufferer. Red and yellow colors indicate high activity levels; blue colors represent low activity levels.

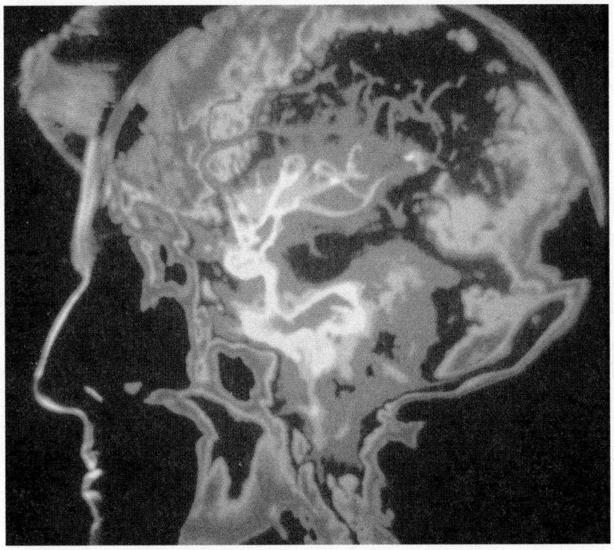

■ **Figure 20.11** CAT scan of a human head in profile.

MEDICAL WORD	WORD PARTS		DEFINITION
	Part	**Meaning**	

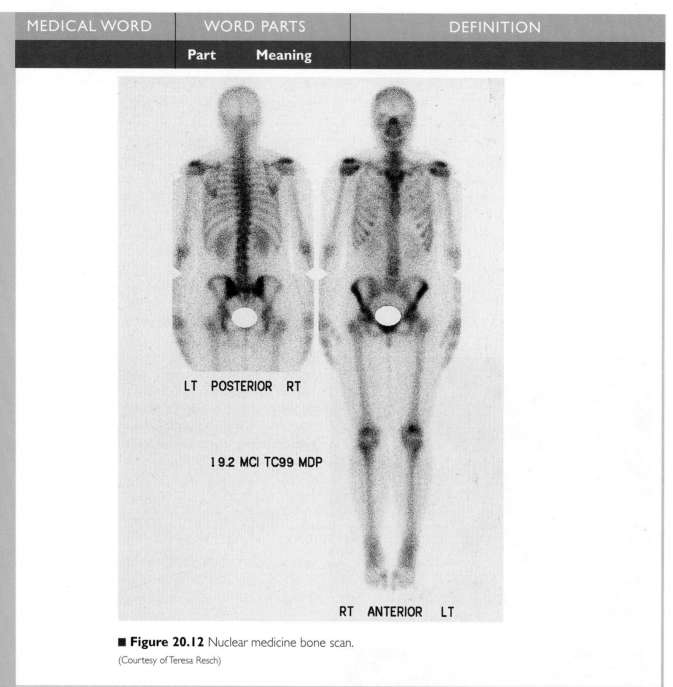

LT POSTERIOR RT

19.2 MCI TC99 MDP

RT ANTERIOR LT

■ **Figure 20.12** Nuclear medicine bone scan.

(Courtesy of Teresa Resch)

fyi A bone scan can:

- Show specific areas of irregular bone metabolism, which can suggest certain diseases based on the pattern of abnormality.
- Detect abnormal blood flow to a particular bony region.
- Help evaluate metabolic diseases that affect bones, such as certain thyroid conditions.
- Detect the spread of cancer to the bones and help the physician evaluate results of cancer treatment.
- Provide information for the physician to diagnose bone changes from a condition called *reflex sympathetic dystrophy*, a disorder of nerves that causes pain, usually in the hands or feet.

| **shield** | | | Protective structure used to prevent or reduce the passage of particles or radiation |

MEDICAL WORD	WORD PARTS		DEFINITION
	Part	**Meaning**	
sialography (sī″ ă-lŏg′ ră-fē)	sial/o -graphy	salivary recording	Process of making an x-ray record of the salivary ducts and glands
sonogram (sōn′ ō-grăm)	son/o -gram	sound record	Record produced by ultrasonography. See Figure 20.13 ■

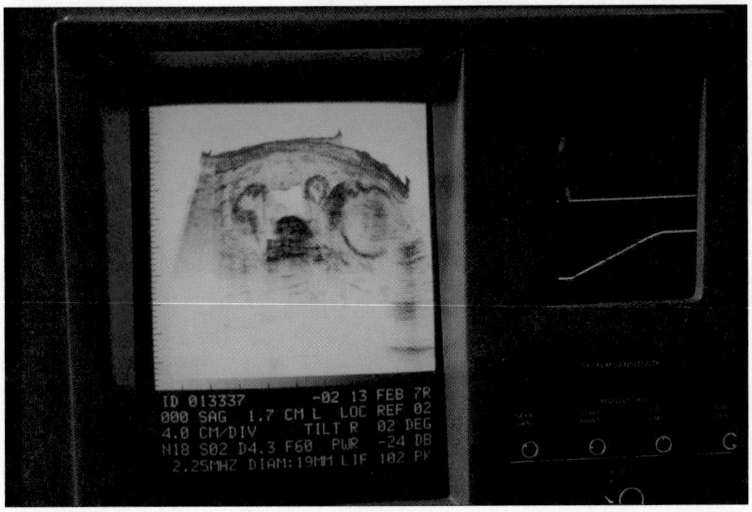

■ **Figure 20.13** Human fetus image called a sonogram is displayed on an ultrasound monitor.

MEDICAL WORD	WORD PARTS		DEFINITION
tagging			Process of tracing a radioactive isotope that has become involved in metabolic or chemical actions
thermography (thĕr-mŏg′ ră-fē)	therm/o -graphy	hot, heat recording	Process of recording heat patterns of the body's surface; useful in the detection of breast cancer
tomography (tō-mŏg′ ră-fē)	tom/o -graphy	to cut recording	Process of cutting across and producing images of single tissue planes that help place into focus a very particular object within a larger field
ultrasonic (ŭl″ tră-sŏn′ ĭk)	ultra- son -ic	beyond sound pertaining to	Pertaining to sounds beyond 20,000 cycles/sec

MEDICAL WORD	WORD PARTS		DEFINITION
	Part	**Meaning**	
ultrasonography (ŭl″ tră-sŏn-ŏg′ ră-fē)	ultra- son/o -graphy	beyond sound recording	Process of using ultrasound to produce a record of ultrasonic echoes as they strike tissues of different densities. See Figure 20.14 ■

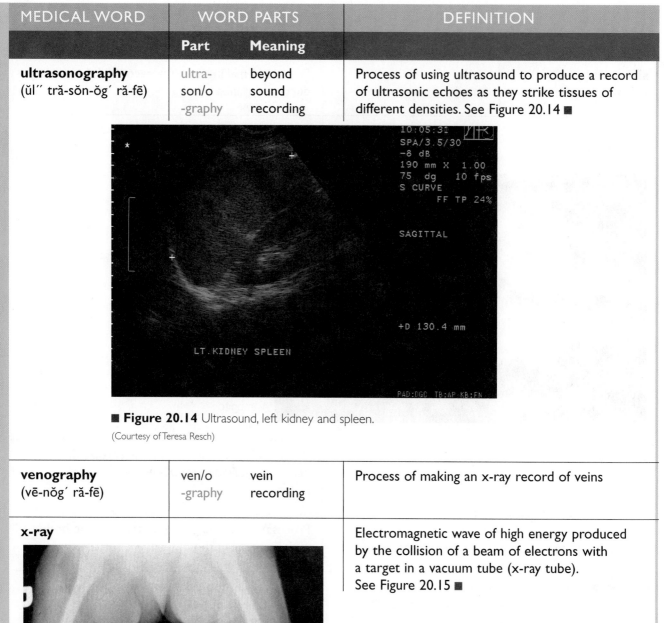

■ **Figure 20.14** Ultrasound, left kidney and spleen.
(Courtesy of Teresa Resch)

| **venography**
(vē-nŏg′ ră-fē) | ven/o
-graphy | vein
recording | Process of making an x-ray record of veins |
| **x-ray** | | | Electromagnetic wave of high energy produced by the collision of a beam of electrons with a target in a vacuum tube (x-ray tube). See Figure 20.15 ■ |

■ **Figure 20.15** X-ray of a child's lower legs showing fractures in the right tibia and left tibia.

• Abbreviations •

ABBREVIATION	MEANING	ABBREVIATION	MEANING
AP	anteroposterior	MRI	magnetic resonance imaging
Ba	barium	PA	posteroanterior
BE	barium enema	Pb	lead
BSE	breast self-examination	PET	positron emission tomography
CAT	computerized axial tomography	PO	orally; by mouth
Ci	curie	R	roentgen
CT	computed tomography	Ra	radium
IR	interventional radiology	rad	radiation absorbed dose
IV	intravenous	TIPS	transjugular intrahepatic portosystemic shunt
lat	lateral		
mCi	millicurie		

• Study and Review • Study and Review • Study and Review
Review • Study and Review • Study and Review • Stu
• Study and Review • Study and Review • Study

• Study and Review •

Overview of Radiology and Nuclear Medicine

Write your answers to the following questions.

1. Define radiology. _____

2. Name three characteristics of x-rays.

   a. _____   b. _____

   c. _____

3. Name two dangers of x-rays.

   a. _____   b. _____

4. List five safety precautions designed to prevent unnecessary exposure to x-rays.

   a. _____   b. _____

   c. _____   d. _____

   e. _____

5. Name five techniques used in diagnostic imaging.

   a. _____   b. _____

   c. _____   d. _____

   e. _____

Word Parts

PREFIXES

Give the definitions of the following prefixes.

1. sub- _____   2. intra- _____

3. milli- _____   4. ultra- _____

5. ir- (in-) _____

ROOTS AND COMBINING FORMS

Give the definitions of the following roots and combining forms.

1. act _____

2. angi/o _____

3. digit _____

4. arteri/o _____

5. arthr/o _____

6. bronch/o _____

7. cardi/o _____

8. chol _____

9. chole _____

10. cine _____

11. cinemat/o _____

12. tract _____

13. curie _____

14. cyst/o _____

15. dermat _____

16. ech/o _____

17. encephal/o _____

18. fluor/o _____

19. gen/o _____

20. hyster/o _____

21. ion/o _____

22. iont/o _____

23. nucl _____

24. log _____

25. lucent _____

26. lymph _____

27. mamm/o _____

28. myel/o _____

29. oscill/o _____

30. paque _____

31. phot/o _____

32. physic _____

33. pyel/o _____

34. radiat _____

35. radi/o _____

36. roent _____

37. salping/o _____

38. sial/o _____

39. son _____

40. son/o _____

41. therm/o _____

42. tom/o _____

43. ven _____

44. ven/o _____

SUFFIXES

Give the definitions of the following suffixes.

1. -er _____

2. -genic _____

3. -al _____

4. -gram _____

5. -graph _____

6. -graphy _____

7. -ic _____

8. -ion _____

9. -ist _____

10. -itis _____

11. -ive _____

12. -logy _____

13. -meter _____

14. -ous _____

15. -scope _____

16. -scopy _____

17. -therapy _____

18. -ide _____

Identifying Medical Terms

In the spaces provided, write the medical terms for the following meanings.

1. _____ A medical imaging technique used to visualize the inside, or lumen, of blood vessels and organs of the body

2. _____ Process of making an x-ray record of a joint

3. _____ X-ray record of the gallbladder made visible through the use of a radiopaque contrast medium

4. _____ Treatment by introducing ions into the body

5. _____ Process of obtaining x-ray pictures of the breast

6. _____ 0.001 Ci

7. _____ Literally means one who specializes in nature

8. _____ Process whereby radiant energy is propagated through space or matter

9. _____ Characterized by emitting radiant energy

10. _____ Person skilled in making x-ray records

11. _____ Pertaining to property of permitting the passage of radiant energy

12. _____ Pertaining to property of obstructing the passage of radiant energy

13. _____ Record produced by ultrasonography

Spelling

Circle the correct spelling of each medical term.

1. hystersalpingram / hysterosalpingogram

2. echography / echgraphy

3. lymphangiography / lymphangography

4. myleogram / myelogram

5. casette / cassette

6. radioactive / radiactive

7. radigraphy / radiography

8. silography / sialography

9. tomography / tomgraphy

10. venograpohy / venography

Matching

Select the appropriate lettered meaning for each of the following words.

_____ 1. PET scan

_____ 2. cathode

_____ 3. beam

_____ 4. cassette

_____ 5. rad

_____ 6. lead

_____ 7. radium

_____ 8. scan

_____ 9. shield

_____ 10. tagging

a. Protective structure used to prevent or reduce the passage of particles or radiation

b. Radioactive isotope used to treat certain malignant diseases

c. Ray of light

d. Nuclear medicine imaging technique that helps physicians see how the organs and tissues inside the body are actually functioning

e. Negative pole of an electrical current

f. Loss of energy

g. Light-proof case or holder for x-ray film

h. Process of tracing a radioactive isotope that has become involved in metabolic or chemical reactions

i. Process of using a moving device or sweeping beam of radiation to produce images of organs or structures of the body

j. Amount of radiation absorbed

k. Metallic chemical element

Abbreviations

Place the correct word, phrase, or abbreviation in the space provided.

1. anteroposterior _____

2. barium _____

3. computed tomography _____

4. IR _____

5. lat _____

6. Ra _____ _____

7. magnetic resonance imaging _____

8. PA _____

9. curie _____

10. PET _____

PRACTICAL APPLICATION

MEDICAL RECORD ANALYSIS

This exercise contains information, abbreviations, and medical terminology from an actual medical record or case study that has been adapted for this text. The names and any personal information have been created by the author. Read and study each form or case study and then answer the questions that follow. You may refer to Appendix III, Abbreviations and Symbols, on page A41.

LA VISTA WOMEN'S CENTER
7785 West Walnut Drive
Clifton Park, NY 12065-2919
(123) 456-7890

Sarah Jane Justice
2345 Maple Avenue
Clifton Park, NY 12065-2919
Date of Mammogram <u>7-6-xx</u>

We wish to report the following on your mammography examination. A report will be sent to your referring physician or other health care provider.

☐ Normal/Negative. No evidence of cancer.

☐ No abnormality seen but comparison with previous mammograms will be performed when and if they can be obtained.

☐ Probably benign (not cancer). Recommended repeat mammogram in 6 months. Please call your physician for an order, then call for appointment at (518) 789-1234.

☐ Additional imaging studies are needed to complete evaluation, such as ultrasound or additional mammographic views. Please call your physician for an order, then call for appointment.

☐ Previous films needed. There is a finding on your mammogram that needs to be compared to previous mammograms.

■ Abnormal. There is a finding on your mammogram that requires further tests for a more thorough evaluation. You should contact your physician or other health care provider as soon as possible.

Interpreting Radiologists: Steven Presley Woods, MD

Should you develop a lump or any changes in your breast before your next screening mammogram, contact your physician or other health care provider for an exam without delay.

Medical Record Questions

Place the correct answer in the space provided.

1. Define mammography. _____

2. Why is there a box for previous films needed? _____

3. This patient had an abnormal mammogram. What does this indicate? _____

4. What does a normal/negative mammogram indicate? _____

5. Who else is sent a copy of the report? _____

PEARSON
mymedicalterminologylab

MyMedicalTerminologyLab is a premium online homework management system that includes a host of features to help you study. Registered users will find:

- Fun games and activities built within a virtual hospital

- Powerful tools that track and analyze your results—allowing you to create a personalized learning experience

- Videos, flashcards, and audio pronunciations to help enrich your progress

- Streaming lesson presentations and self-paced learning modules

- A space where you and your instructors can view and manage your assignments

Urinary System • Endocrine System • Nervous System
pecial Senses: The Ear • Special Senses: The Eye • Femal
eproductive System with an Overview of Obstetric •
Reproductive System • Oncology • Radiology and Nu
Medicine • **Mental Health** • Introduction to Medical

21

LEARNING OUTCOMES

On completion of this chapter, you will be able to:

1. Define mental health.

2. Describe mental illness and six posssible contributing factors.

3. Identify general symptoms (according to age group) that can suggest a mental disorder.

4. Explain how the diagnosis of mental illness may be obtained.

5. Describe three basic forms of treatment that can be employed.

6. Analyze, build, spell, and pronounce medical words.

7. Comprehend the drugs highlighted in this chapter.

8. Identify and define selected abbreviations.

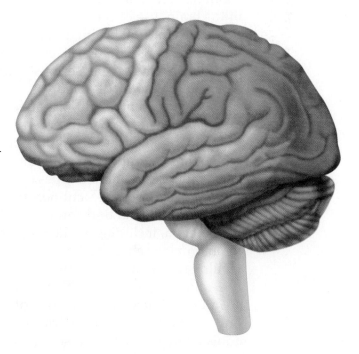

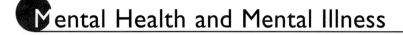

COMBINING FORMS OF MENTAL HEALTH			
agor/a	marketplace	**phren/o**	mind
centr/o	center	**psych/o**	mind
cycl/o	circle, cycle	**schiz/o**	to divide
delus/o	to cheat	**somat/o**	body
neur/o	nerve	**thym/o**	mind, emotion
path/o	disease		

Mental Health and Mental Illness

Please note that much of the information on mental disorders has been adapted from the National Institute of Mental Health (NIMH), which is a component of the National Institutes of Health (NIH), a part of the U.S. Department of Health and Human Services (HHS).

The World Health Organization (WHO) defines **health** as a state of complete physical, mental, and social well-being, not merely the absence of disease or infirmity. It defines **mental health** as a state of well-being in which an individual realizes his or her own abilities, can cope with the normal stresses of life, can work productively and fruitfully, and is able to make a contribution to his or her community.

Mental illness is an abnormal condition of the brain or mind. It affects the way a person thinks, feels, behaves, and relates to others and to his or her surroundings. In most cases, the exact cause of mental illness is not known. Possible contributing factors include genetics, the environment, chemical changes occurring in the brain, use of certain drugs, and psychological, social, and cultural conditions. Most mental health disorders are caused by a combination of factors, such as biological, psychological, environmental, and social. See Figure 21.1 ■ These disorders can be severe, seriously interfere with a person's life, and even cause a person to become disabled.

Many different conditions are classified as mental illnesses. The more common types include mood disorders (depression and bipolar disorder), anxiety disorders, attention-deficit hyperactivity disorder (ADHD), eating disorders, schizophrenia, impulse control and addiction disorders, and personality disorders. Other, less common types of mental illnesses include adjustment disorder, dissociative disorders, factitious disorders, sexual and gender disorders, somatoform disorders, and tic disorders. Various sleep-related problems and some forms of dementia, including Alzheimer's disease (see Chapter 14, pages 494 and 498, for information about Alzheimer's disease and dementia), can be classified as mental illnesses because they involve the brain.

According to the U.S. Surgeon General, during a given year, an estimated 44 million adults and about 20% of American children suffer from a mental disorder. About 5 million American adults and more than 5 million children and adolescents suffer from a serious mental condition. Major depression, bipolar disorder, and schizophrenia are among the top 10 leading causes of disability in the United States.

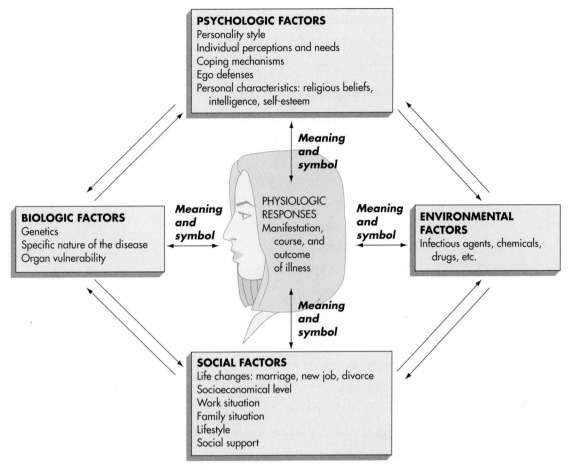

■ **Figure 21.1** Multicausational concept of the illness process. The phrase *meaning and symbol* refers to the fact that a patient interprets all experiences in a highly individual manner according to his or her specific meaning and the broader meaning in the patient's culture.

SYMPTOMS OF A MENTAL DISORDER

Symptoms of a mental disorder vary according to the type and severity of the condition and the age of the individual. The following are some general symptoms (according to age group) that can suggest a mental disorder

In an adult:

- Confused thinking
- Long-lasting sadness or irritability
- Extreme highs and lows in mood
- Excessive fear, worry, or anxiety
- Social withdrawal
- Dramatic changes in eating or sleeping patterns
- Strong feelings of anger
- Delusion or hallucinations
- Increasing inability to cope with daily problems and activities
- Thoughts of suicide
- Denial of obvious problems

- Many unexplained physical problems
- Abuse of drugs and/or alcohol

In an adolescent:

- Abuse of drugs and/or alcohol
- Inability to cope with daily problems and activities
- Changes in eating or sleeping patterns
- Excessive complaints of physical problems
- Defying authority, skipping school, stealing, or damaging property
- Intense fear of gaining weight
- Long-lasting negative mood
- Thoughts of death
- Frequent outbursts of anger

In younger children:

- Changes in school performance
- Poor grades despite strong efforts
- Excessive worry or anxiety
- Hyperactivity
- Persistent nightmares
- Continual disobedience and/or aggressive behavior
- Frequent temper tantrums

DIAGNOSIS OF MENTAL ILLNESS

The standard manual used by experts for the diagnosis of recognized mental illness in the United States is the *Diagnostic and Statistical Manual of Mental Disorders*, Fourth Edition, Text Revision (DSM-IV-TR). This official manual of mental health disorders is compiled by the American Psychiatric Association (APA) and identifies categories of adult mental illness. Psychiatrists, psychologists, social workers, and other health care providers use it to understand and diagnose mental health disorders. Insurance companies and health care providers also use it to classify and code mental health disorders for reimbursment of services rendered.

Psychiatry is the branch of medicine that deals with the study, diagnosis, and treatment of mental illness. A person who specializes in this field of medicine is a **psychiatrist** who is a medical doctor (MD) with specialized training in **psychotherapy** and drug therapy. The psychiatrist can further specialize in the treatment of children (child psychiatry) or in the legal aspects of psychiatry, such as the determination of mental competence in criminal cases (forensic psychiatry). **Psychoanalysts** are psychiatrists with specialized training in **psychoanalysis**, a method of obtaining a detailed account of past and present mental and emotional experiences and repressions.

Psychology is the study of the mind. A **psychologist** is a person who is not a medical doctor but has a master's degree or doctor of philosophy (PhD) degree in a specific field of psychology, such as clinical, experimental, or social.

Clinical psychologists are patient-oriented and can use various methods of psychotherapy to treat patients but cannot prescribe medications or electroconvulsive therapy (ECT). They are trained in the use of tests to evaluate various aspects of a patient's mental health and intelligence. Examples are **intelligence quotient (IQ)** tests such as the **Stanford–Binet Intelligence Scale** and the **Wechsler Adult Intelligence Scale (WAIS).** Other tests used are the **Rorschach Inkblot Test** and the **Thematic Apperception Test (TAT)**, in which pictures are used as stimuli for the patient to create stories. The **Minnesota Multiphasic Personality Inventory (MMPI)** consists of true–false questions that can reveal aspects of personality, such as dominance, sense of duty or responsibility, and ability to relate to others; it is used as an objective measure of psychological disorders in adolescents and adults. A patient's responses to the questions can be compared with responses made by individuals with diagnoses of schizophrenia, depression, and many other mental disorders.

Psychiatrists and psychologists also use specially designed interview and assessment tools to evaluate a person for a mental illness. The therapist bases the diagnosis on the person's report of symptoms, including any social or functional problems caused by the symptoms. The therapist then determines whether the person's symptoms and degree of disability indicate a diagnosis of a specific disorder.

TREATMENTS FOR MENTAL ILLNESS

The three basic forms of treatment for mental illness are **drug therapy**, **psychotherapy**, and **electroconvulsive therapy.**

Drug Therapy

Drugs that are generally used to treat mental disorders include antianxiety agents, antidepressant agents, antimanic agents, and antipsychotic agents. Drugs used for attention-deficit hyperactivity disorder (ADHD) include stimulants. See Drug Highlights on page 762 for more information on drug therapy for mental disorders.

Psychotherapy

Psychotherapy is a method of treating mental disorders using psychological techniques instead of physical methods. It involves talking, interpreting, listening, rewarding, and role-playing. Psychotherapy should be performed by a trained mental health professional, such as a psychiatrist, psychologist, social worker, or counselor.

Types of psychotherapy include cognitive-behavioral therapy, family therapy, group therapy, play therapy, art therapy, hypnosis, and psychoanalysis.

- **Cognitive-behavioral therapy (CBT)** has two components. The cognitive component helps people change thinking patterns that keep them from overcoming their fears. The behavioral component seeks to change people's reactions to anxiety-provoking situations. A key element of this component is exposure, in which people confront the things they fear. Research has shown that CBT is an effective form of psychotherapy for several anxiety disorders, particularly panic disorder and social phobia.
- **Family therapy** involves an entire family. The focus is on resolving and understanding conflicts and problems as a *family* situation, not just as an individual member's problem.
- **Group therapy** involves small groups of people with similar problems attending meetings together. There are discussions and interactions between group participants; a therapist helps to focus and guide the therapy sessions.

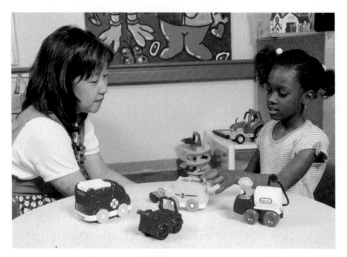

■ **Figure 21.2** Psychologist using play therapy to help Cassandra reenact her car crash. This helps her gain control over the event so that it is not so frightening.

- **Play therapy** involves a child using toys, such as dolls and puppets, to express thoughts, feelings, fantasies, and conflicts. Because most emotionally disturbed children will not talk about their problems, play therapy provides an alternative method to encourage children to open up about what is troubling them. Children reveal themselves when they play with toys provided by the therapist and often act out their problems (see Figure 21.2 ■).

- **Art therapy** can be used to encourage a child to portray his or her feelings in drawings. When asked to draw the family or a picture of him- or herself, information about the child, the family, and their interactions can be revealed.

- **Hypnosis** is a state of altered consciousness, usually artificially induced, used in treating mental illness by lessening the mind's unconscious defenses and allowing some patients to be able to recall and even re-experience important childhood events that have long been forgotten or repressed. Historically, Dr. Sigmund Freud, a noted Austrian neurologist and psychoanalyst, developed the theory of the unconscious as a result of his experiments with a hypnotized patient.

- **Psychoanalysis** is a method of obtaining a detailed account of past and present mental and emotional experiences and repressions. It also was developed by Dr. Freud. Psychoanalysis attempts, through free association and dream interpretation, to reveal and resolve the unconscious conflicts that are considered to be at the root of some mental illnesses. It is believed that these conflicts have been repressed since childhood and after being brought to the conscious level can be resolved.

Electroconvulsive Therapy

Electroconvulsive therapy (ECT) is the use of an electric shock to produce convulsions. It is useful for individuals whose depression is severe or life threatening, particularly for those who cannot take antidepressant medication. In recent years, ECT has been much improved. A muscle relaxant is given to the patient before treatment, which is performed under brief anesthesia. Electrodes are placed at precise locations on the head to deliver electrical impulses. The stimulation causes a brief (about 30-second) seizure within the brain. The person receiving ECT does not consciously experience the electrical stimulus. For full therapeutic benefit, at least several sessions of ECT, typically given at the rate of three per week, are required.

• Building Your Medical Vocabulary •

This section provides the foundation for learning medical terminology. Review the following alphabetized word list. Note how common prefixes and suffixes are repeatedly applied to word roots and combining forms to create different meanings. The word parts are color-coded: prefixes are green, suffixes are blue, roots/combining forms are red.

You will find that some terms have not been divided into word parts. These are common words or specialized terms that are included to enhance your medical vocabulary. See Chapter 1, page 7, to review pronunciation guidelines.

MEDICAL WORD	WORD PARTS		DEFINITION
	Part	Meaning	
affect (ăf´ fĕkt)			In psychology, observable evidence of an individual's emotional reaction associated with an experience
affective disorder (ă f-fĕk´ tĭv)			Characterized by a disturbance of mood accompanied by a manic or depressive syndrome; this syndrome is not caused by any other physical or mental disorder
agoraphobia (ăg″ ō-ră-fō´ bĭă)	agor/a -phobia	marketplace fear	Abnormal fear of being in public places; fear of leaving the safety of home; an anxiety syndrome and panic disorder
anorexia nervosa (ăn″ ō -rĕk-sē-ă nĕr-vō-să)	an- -orexia	lack of, without appetite	Complex psychological disorder in which the individual refuses to eat or has an abnormally limited eating pattern. People with eating disorders may engage in self-induced vomiting and abuse of laxatives, diuretics, or prolonged exercise to control their weight. The condition could lead them to become excessively thin or even emaciated. In severe cases, this condition can be life threatening. See Figure 21.3 ■

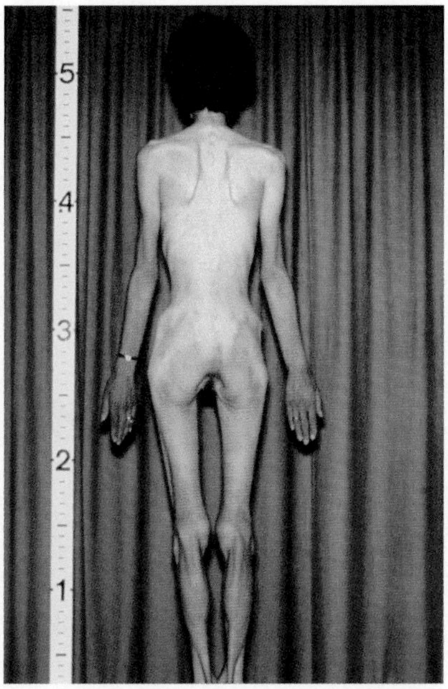

■ **Figure 21.3** Emaciated young woman with anorexia nervosa. (Source: Custom Medical Stock Photo, Inc.)

MEDICAL WORD	WORD PARTS		DEFINITION
	Part	**Meaning**	
anxiety (ăng-zī′ ě -tē)			Feeling of uneasiness, apprehension, worry, or dread; involuntary or reflex reaction of the body to stress
anxiety disorders			Serious mental illnesses that affect approximately 19 million American adults. Anxiety disorders share the common theme of excessive, irrational fear and dread and are chronic, growing progressively worse if not treated. See Figure 21.4 ■ for physiological responses in anxiety disorders.

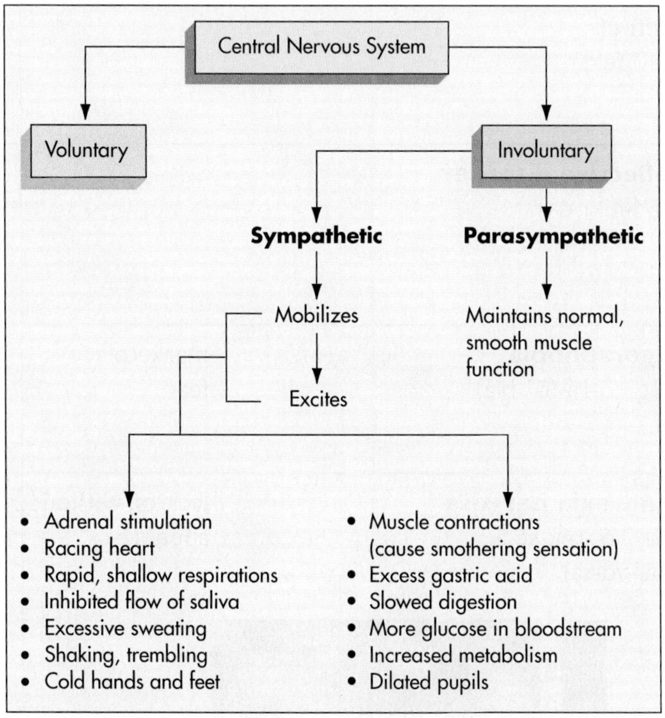

■ **Figure 21.4** Physiological responses in anxiety disorders.

A form of anxiety disorder, **panic disorder** (often called *panic attacks*) causes feelings of terror that strike suddenly and repeatedly with no warning. People with this disorder cannot predict when an attack will occur, and many develop intense anxiety between episodes, worrying about when and where the next one will strike.

When having a panic attack, a person feels sweaty, flushed or chilled, weak, faint, or dizzy. The hands can tingle or feel numb. There can be nausea, chest pain or a smothering sensation, a sense of unreality, or fear of impending doom or loss of control. The individual can genuinely believe that he or she is having a heart attack, losing his or her mind, or on the verge of death.

MEDICAL WORD	WORD PARTS		DEFINITION
	Part	Meaning	
apathy (ăp´ ă-thē)			Condition in which a person lacks feelings and emotions and is indifferent
apperception (ăp˝ ĕ r-sĕp´ shŭn)			Comprehension or assimilation of the meaning and significance of a particular sensory stimulus as modified by an individual's own experiences, knowledge, thoughts, and emotions
attention-deficit hyperactivity disorder (ADHD)			One of the most commonly diagnosed behavioral disorders among children and adolescents, it often continues into adulthood. Children with ADHD have impaired functioning in multiple settings, including home, school, and in relationships with peers. If untreated, the disorder can have long-term adverse effects. Symptoms of ADHD will appear over the course of many months, and include: *Impulsiveness:* a child who acts quickly without thinking first. *Hyperactivity:* a child who can't sit still, walks, runs, or climbs when others are seated; talks when others are talking. *Inattention:* a child who daydreams or seems to be in another world; is sidetracked by what is going on around him or her.
autism (ŏ´ tĭ zm)	aut -ism	self condition	Mental disorder in which the individual may be self-absorbed, inaccessible, unable to relate to others, and has language disturbances. It is a syndrome usually beginning in infancy and becoming apparent in the first or second year of life. See Figure 21.5 ■

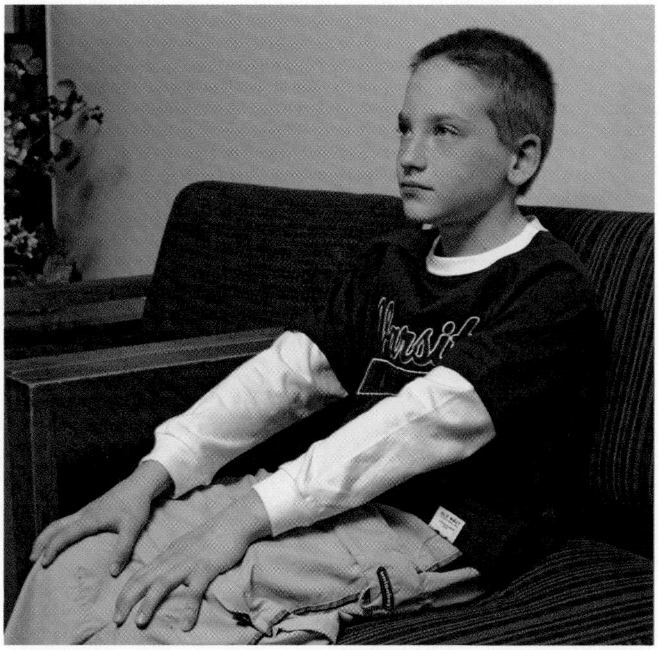

■ **Figure 21.5** This child with autism sits stiffly in the chair. He has a disengaged look and does not readily interact with other children or adults who are in his environment.

MEDICAL WORD	WORD PARTS		DEFINITION
	Part	Meaning	

> **fyi** According to the National Institute of Neurological Disorders and Stroke (NINDS), autism spectrum disorder (ASD) is a range of complex neurodevelopment disorders, characterized by social impairments, communication difficulties, and restricted, repetitive, and stereotyped patterns of behavior. Autistic disorder, sometimes called autism or classic ASD, is the most severe form of ASD, while other conditions along the spectrum include a milder form known as Asperger syndrome, a rare condition called Rett syndrome, and childhood disintegrative disorder and pervasive developmental disorder not otherwise specified (usually referred to as PDD-NOS). Although ASD varies significantly in character and severity, it occurs in all ethnic and socioeconomic groups and affects every age group. Experts estimate that three to six children out of every 1,000 will have ASD. Males are four times more likely to have ASD than females. The hallmark feature of ASD is impaired social interaction.

MEDICAL WORD	WORD PARTS		DEFINITION
	Part	Meaning	
bipolar disorder (bĭ-pōl´ ăr)			Brain disorder also known as *manic-depressive illness* that causes unusual shifts in a person's mood, energy, and ability to function. Bipolar disorder is characterized by cycling mood changes: severe highs (*mania*) and lows (*depression*). Sometimes, severe episodes of mania or depression include symptoms of *psychosis* (psychotic symptoms) such as *hallucinations* and *delusions*.
compulsion (kŏm-pŭl´ ŭn)			Uncontrollable, recurrent, and distressing urge to perform an act in order to relieve fear connected with obsession. Common compulsions involve excessive handwashing, touching objects, and continual counting and checking.
cyclothymic disorder (sĭ″klŏ-thī´mĭ k)	cycl/o thym -ic	circle, cycle mind, emotion pertaining to	Mood disorder characterized by alternating moods of elation and depression, similar to bipolar disorder but of milder intensity
delirium (dē-lĭr´ ĭ-ŭm)			State of mental confusion marked by illusions, hallucinations, excitement, restlessness, delusions, and speech incoherence
delusion (dē-loo´ zhŭn)	delus -ion	to cheat process	Characterized by bizarre thoughts that have no basis in reality; a fixed, false belief or abnormal perception held by a person despite evidence to the contrary

MEDICAL WORD	WORD PARTS		DEFINITION
	Part	Meaning	
dementia (dē-měn´ shē-ă)			Problem in the brain that makes it difficult for a person to remember, learn, and communicate and eventually to take care of him- or herself; can also affect a person's mood and personality. Dementia of the Alzheimer's type is the most common form. See Chapter 14, "Nervous System," for more information about this condition.
depression (dē-prěsh´ ŭn)			Mental disorder marked by altered mood and loss of interest in things that are usually pleasurable such as food, sex, work, friends, hobbies, or entertainment. See Figure 21.6 ■ A less severe type of depression, *dysthymia*, involves long-term, chronic symptoms that do not disable but keep an individual from functioning well or feeling good. Many people with dysthymia also experience major depressive episodes at some time in their lives.

Mood depressed; Memory problems
Anxious; Apathetic; Appetite changes
"**J**ust no fun"
Occupational impairment
Restlessness; Ruminative

Doubts self; Difficulty making decisions
Empty feeling
Pessimistic; Persistent sadness; Psychomotor retardation
Report vague pains
Energy gone
Suicidal thoughts and impulses
Sleep disturbances
Irritability; Inability to concentrate
Oppressive guilt
"**N**othing can help" (Hopelessness)

■ **Figure 21.6** Characteristics of major depression.

MEDICAL WORD	WORD PARTS		DEFINITION
	Part	**Meaning**	

LIFE SPAN CONSIDERATIONS

The depressed child can pretend to be sick, refuse to go to school, cling to a parent, or worry that the parent could die. Older children sulk; get into trouble at school; and are negative, grouchy, and feel misunderstood. Because normal behaviors vary from one childhood stage to another, it can be difficult to tell whether a child is just going through a temporary phase or suffering from depression. Symptoms of depression in the child:

Toddlers. Sadness, inactivity, complaints of stomachaches, and, in rare cases, self-destructive behavior.

Elementary school–age children. Unhappiness, poor school performance, irritability, refusal to take part in activities he or she used to enjoy, and occasional thoughts of suicide.

Adolescents. Sadness, withdrawal, feelings of hopelessness or guilt, changes in sleeping or eating habits, and frequent thoughts of suicide.

A child does not understand feelings of stress, anxiety, or depression and does not know how to ask for help, so when a child exhibits dramatic mood or behavior shifts, a physician should be consulted immediately. The physician could recommend psychotherapy or prescribe an antidepressant for children who are at least 5 years of age or older.

MEDICAL WORD	WORD PARTS		DEFINITION
	Part	**Meaning**	
dissociation (dĭs-sō″ sē-ā′ shun)			Defense mechanism in which a group of mental processes become separated from normal consciousness and, thus separated, function as a unitary whole. In *dissociative disorder* there is a severe disturbance or trauma that causes changes in memory, consciousness, identity, and general awareness of oneself and one's environment. There are four primary types of dissociative disorders: *psychogenic amnesia, psychogenic fugue, multiple personality disorder,* and *depersonalization disorder.*
eating disorder			Health condition characterized by a preoccupation with weight that results in severe disturbances in eating behavior; *anorexia nervosa* and *bulimia* are the most common types. According to the APA, between 0.5% and 3.7% of females experience anorexia nervosa, and between 1.1% and 4.2% of females experience bulimia in their lifetime.
egocentric (ē″ gō-sĕn′ trĭk)	ego centr -ic	I, self center pertaining to	Pertaining to being self-centered

MEDICAL WORD	WORD PARTS		DEFINITION
	Part	**Meaning**	
factitious disorder (făk-tĭsh´ ŭs)			Disorder that is not real, genuine, or natural. The physical and psychological symptoms are produced by the person to place him- or herself or another in the role of a patient or someone in need of help. These patients have a severe personality disturbance. *Munchausen's syndrome* is a chronic factitious disorder in which a healthy person habitually seeks medical treatment; in the rare *Munchausen by proxy syndrome (MBPS),* a parent (usually the mother) or other caregiver is the deliberate cause of a child's illness (by poisoning, for instance) to gain sympathy or attention.
fugue (fūg)			Dissociative disorder in which amnesia is accompanied by physical flight from customary surroundings. In psychogenic fugue, there is sudden, unexpected travel away from an individual's home or place of work with inability to recall the past. The individual can assume a partial or completely new identity. This condition is usually of short duration but can last for months. Following recovery, the person does not recall anything that happened during the fugue.
generalized anxiety disorder (GAD)			Characterized by much higher levels of anxiety than people normally experience day to day. It is chronic and fills a person's day with exaggerated worry and tension. Having this disorder means always anticipating disaster, often worrying excessively about health, money, family, or work.
hallucination (hă-loo-sĭ-nā´ shŭ n)	hallucinat -ion	to wander in mind process	Process of experiencing sensations that have no source. Some examples of hallucinations include hearing nonexistent voices, seeing nonexistent things, and experiencing burning or pain sensations with no physical cause.
hypomania (hī˝ pō-mā´ nē -ă)	hypo- -mania	deficient, below madness	Abnormal mood of mild mania characterized by hyperactivity, inflated self-esteem, talkativeness, heightened sexual interest, quickness to anger, irritability, and a decreased need for sleep

MEDICAL WORD	WORD PARTS		DEFINITION
	Part	**Meaning**	
impulse control disorder			Mental condition in which the person is unable to resist urges or impulses to perform acts that could be harmful to him- or herself or others. *Pyromania* (starting fires), *kleptomania* (stealing), and compulsive gambling are examples of impulse control disorders.
mania (mă´ nĕ -ă)			Mental disorder characterized by excessive excitement; literally means *madness*
mood			Pervasive and sustained emotion that plays a key role in an individual's perception of the world. Examples include depression, joy, elation, anger, and anxiety.
neurotic (nŭ-rōt´ ĭk)	neur/o -tic	nerve pertaining to	Pertaining to one who has an abnormal emotional or mental disorder
norepinephrine (nor-ĕpĭ-nĕf´ rĭn)			Hormone produced by the adrenal medulla that acts as a neurotransmitter. It is believed that disturbances in its metabolism at important brain sites can be implicated in affective disorders.
obsession			Neurotic state in which an individual has a recurrent, persistent thought, image, or impulse that is unwanted and distressing and comes involuntarily to mind despite attempts to resist

fyi **Obsessive–compulsive disorder (OCD)** involves persistent, unwelcome thoughts or images or the urgent need to engage in certain rituals that the person cannot control. For example, individuals can exhibit the following:

- Obsession with germs or dirt, thus they repeatedly wash their hands
- Doubt and the need to check things repeatedly
- Frequent thoughts of violence and the fear that they will harm someone close to them
- Long periods of touching or counting things or being preoccupied with order or symmetry
- Persistent thoughts of performing repulsive sexual acts
- Thoughts against their religious beliefs

The disturbing thoughts or images are called *obsessions,* and the rituals performed to try to prevent or get rid of them are called *compulsions.* The person experiences only temporary relief not pleasure in carrying out the rituals, caused by the anxiety that increases when they are not performed.

MEDICAL WORD	WORD PARTS		DEFINITION
	Part	**Meaning**	
paranoia (păr″ ă-noy′ ă)	para- -noia	beside, abnormal mind	Mental disorder characterized by highly exaggerated or unwarranted mistrust or suspiciousness; generally classified into three categories: *paranoid personality disorder, delusional (paranoid) disorder,* and *paranoid schizophrenia.* Delusional (paranoid) disorder is characterized by persistent delusions of persecution or grandeur, or a combination of the two.
personality disorder			Mental disorder characterized by inflexible and maladaptive personality traits that are distressing to the person and/or cause problems in work, school, or social relationships. In addition, the person's pattern of thinking and behavior significantly differ from the expectations of society and are so rigid that he or she does not function well.
phobia (fō′ bē-ă)			Morbid and persistent fear of a specific object, activity, or situation that results in a compelling desire to avoid the feared stimulus. Examples include *claustrophobia* (fear of enclosed places), *acrophobia* (fear of heights), *photophobia* (fear of light), *arachnophobia* (fear of spiders), *nyctophobia* (fear of darkness/night), and *hematophobia* or *hemophobia* (fear of blood/bleeding).
post-traumatic stress disorder (PTSD)			Debilitating anxiety disorder that can develop following a terrifying event. It was brought to public attention by war veterans, but it can result from any number of traumatic incidents, such as a mugging, rape, or torture; being kidnapped or held captive; child abuse; serious accidents; and nautral disasters. Some people with PTSD repeatedly relive the trauma in the form of nightmares and disturbing recollections during the day.
psychiatrist (sī-kī′ ă-trĭst)	psych iatr -ist	mind treatment one who specializes	Physician who specializes in the study and treatment of mental disorders

MEDICAL WORD	WORD PARTS		DEFINITION
	Part	**Meaning**	
psychoanalysis (sī″ kō-ă-năl′ ĭ-sĭs)			Method of investigating the mental processes of an individual using the techniques of free association, interpretation, and dream analysis
psychologist (sī-kŏl′ ō-jĭst)	psych/o log -ist	mind study of one who specializes	Person who specializes in the study of the mind and behavior
psychology (sī-kŏl′ ō-jē)	psych/o -logy	mind study of	Study of the mind and behavior, both normal and pathological
psychopath (sī′ kō-păth)	psych/o path	mind disease	Mentally ill individual with an antisocial personality disorder; also called *sociopath*
psychosis (sī-kō′ sĭs)	psych -osis	mind condition	Serious, abnormal mental condition in which the individual's mental capacity to recognize reality and communicate with and relate to others is impaired; the person can experience delusions and hallucinations
psychosomatic (sī″ kō-sō-măt′ ĭk)	psych/o somat -ic	mind body pertaining to	Pertaining to the interrelationship of the mind and the body; a manifestation of physical disease that has a mental origin
psychotherapy (sī′ kō-thĕr′ ă-pē)	psych/o -therapy	mind treatment	Method of treating mental disorders by using psychological techniques instead of physical methods; may involve talking, interpreting, listening, rewarding, and role-playing
psychotropic (sī′ kō -trŏ″ ĭk)			Drug that affects psychic function, behavior, or experience
pyromania (pī″ rō-mā′ (nĭ-ă)	pyro- -mania	fire madness	Impulsive disorder consisting of a compulsion to set fires or to watch fires; literally means *a madness for fire*; person suffering from this disorder (pyromaniac) receives pleasure and emotional relief from these activities

MEDICAL WORD	WORD PARTS		DEFINITION
	Part	**Meaning**	
schizophrenia (skĭz″ō-frĕn′ē-ă)	schiz/o phren -ia	to divide mind condition	Mental disorder characterized by *positive* and *negative* symptoms. Positive (psychotic) symptoms include delusions, hallucinations, and disordered thinking (apparent from a person's fragmented, disconnected, and sometimes nonsensical speech). Negative symptoms include social withdrawal, extreme apathy, diminished motivation, and blunted emotional expression.
seasonal affective disorder (SAD)			Form of depression that appears related to fluctuations in a person's exposure to natural light; usually strikes during autumn and often continues through the winter when natural light is reduced. Researchers have found that people who have SAD can be helped if they spend blocks of time bathed in light from a special full-spectrum light source called a *light box*.
serotonin (sēr″ō-tōn′ĭn)			Chemical present in gastrointestinal mucosa, platelets, mast cells, and carcinoid tumors; a vasoconstrictor and a neurotransmitter in the central nervous system (CNS); affects sleep and sensory perception
sexual disorders			Disorders that affect sexual desire, performance, and behavior. *Sexual dysfunction, gender identity disorder* (characterized by a persistent discomfort concerning one's anatomical sexual makeup and the desire to live as a member of the opposite sex), and *paraphilias* are examples. In paraphilia, sexual arousal requires unusual or bizarre fantasies or acts involving nonhuman objects, sexual activity with humans in which real or simulated suffering or humiliation occurs, or sexual activity with nonconsenting partners. Included in this disorder are *bestiality, fetishism, transvestism, zoophilia, pedophilia, exhibitionism, voyeurism, sexual masochism,* and *sexual sadism.*

MEDICAL WORD	WORD PARTS		DEFINITION
	Part	**Meaning**	
somatoform disorder (sŏ-măt´ ō-fŏrm)	somat/o -form	body shape	Mental disorder, previously known as *psychosomatic disorder,* in which the person experiences physical symptoms of an illness that are not explained by medical condition or medication. Included in this disorder are *body dysmorphic disorder (BDD),* which involves a disturbed body image; *hypochondriasis,* which is a preoccupation with fears of having or the belief that one has a serious disease based on misinterpretation of bodily symptoms; *somatization disorder,* a chronic condition in which there are numerous physical complaints; *conversion disorder,* in which emotional distress or unconscious conflicts are expressed through physical symptoms; and *somatoform pain disorder,* in which persistent and chronic pain is experienced by a person in the absence of physiological causes.
substance abuse			Misuse of medications, alcohol, or illegal substances
suicide			Willfully ending one's own life. In the United States, suicide is the seventh leading cause of death for males, the 16th for females, and the third for young people 15–24 years of age. Suicide attempts are among the leading causes of hospital admissions in persons under age 35. Of persons who commit or attempt suicide, 90% have depression or another diagnosable mental or substance abuse disorder.

LIFE SPAN CONSIDERATIONS

According to the National Institute of Mental Health (NIMH), older Americans are disproportionately likely to die by suicide. Of every 100,000 people ages 65 and older, 14.2 died by suicide in 2006. This figure is higher than the national average of 10.9 suicides per 100,000 people in the general population. Non-Hispanic white men age 85 or older had an even higher rate, with 48 suicide deaths per 100,000.

Depression, which can lead to suicide, is a serious problem in the older adult. Depressive symptoms are *not* a normal part of aging. Persistent sadness or grief or loss of interest in food, sex, work, family, friends, and hobbies should be noted in an older person.

Depression often co-occurs with other serious illnesses such as heart disease, stroke, diabetes, cancer, and Parkinson's disease. Because many older adults face these illnesses as well as various social and economic difficulties, health care professionals often mistakenly conclude that depression is a normal consequence of these problems—an attitude often shared by patients themselves. These factors together contribute to the underdiagnosis and undertreatment of depressive disorders in older people. See Figure 21.7 ∎

MEDICAL WORD	WORD PARTS		DEFINITION
	Part	Meaning	

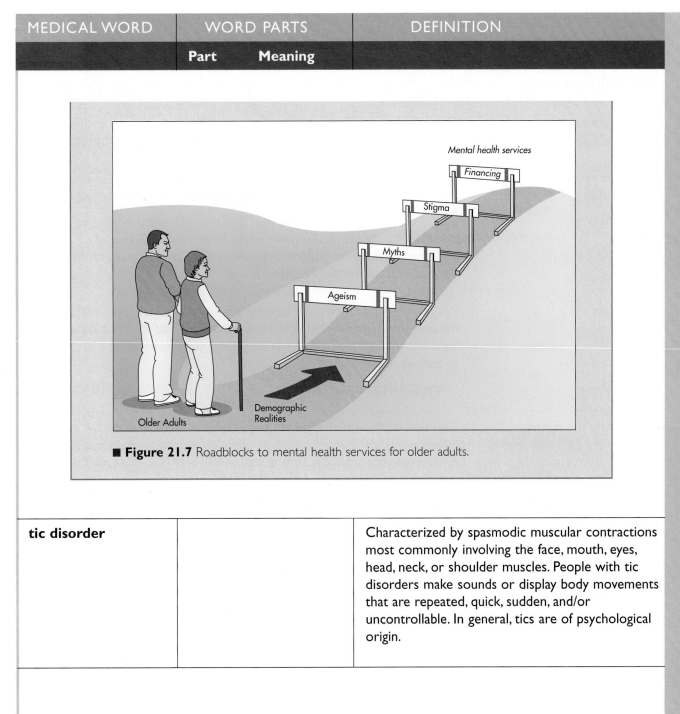

■ **Figure 21.7** Roadblocks to mental health services for older adults.

tic disorder			Characterized by spasmodic muscular contractions most commonly involving the face, mouth, eyes, head, neck, or shoulder muscles. People with tic disorders make sounds or display body movements that are repeated, quick, sudden, and/or uncontrollable. In general, tics are of psychological origin.

• Drug Highlights •

TYPE OF DRUG	DESCRIPTION AND EXAMPLES
antianxiety agents	Chemical substances that relieve anxiety and muscle tension are indicated when anxiety interferes with a person's ability to function properly.
benzodiazepines	The *benzodiazepines* are a group of drugs with similar chemical structures and pharmaceutical activities. They are the most widely prescribed drugs for the treatment of anxiety. EXAMPLES: Xanax (alprazolam), Klonopin (clonazepam), Tranxene (clorazepate), Librium (chlordiazepoxide HCl), Valium (diazepam), Ativan (lorazepam), and Serax (oxazepam)
azipirones	Antianxiety medication used to treat generalized anxiety disorder (GAD). Possible side effects include dizziness, headaches, and nausea. Unlike the benzodiazepines, buspirone must be taken consistently for at least 2 weeks to achieve an antianxiety effect. EXAMPLE: BuSpar (buspirone)
antidepressant agents	Chemical substances that relieve the symptoms of depression are indicated when depression interferes with a person's ability to function properly. Antidepressant agents can be grouped as SSRIs, SNRIs, TCAs, or MAOIs.
selective serotonin reuptake inhibitors (SSRIs)	Drugs in this group specifically block reabsorption of serotonin. EXAMPLES: Prozac (fluoxetine), Zoloft (sertraline), Paxil (paroxetine), and Luvox (fluvoxamine)
serotonin-norepinephrine reuptake inhibitors (SNRIs)	Drugs in this group block the reabsorption of serotonin and norepinephrine. EXAMPLE: Effexor (venlafaxine)
tricyclic antidepressants (TCAs)	Drugs in this group raise the level of norepinephrine and serotonin in the brain by slowing the rate at which they are reabsorbed by nerve cells. EXAMPLES: Tofranil (imipramine), Pamelor (nortriptyline), and amoxapine
monoamine oxidase inhibitors (MAOIs)	Drugs in this group work by blocking the breakdown of two potent neurotransmitters—norepinephrine and serotonin—and by allowing them to bathe the nerve endings for an extended length of time. EXAMPLES: Nardil (phenelzine) and Parnate (tranylcypromine)

TYPE OF DRUG	DESCRIPTION AND EXAMPLES
lithium carbonate	Although not a group of drugs, various lithium medications control mood disorders by directly affecting internal nerve cell processes in all of the neurotransmitter systems. Lithium is best known as an antimanic drug used in the treatment of bipolar disorder. EXAMPLE: Eskalith (lithium carbonate)
miscellaneous drugs	Many newly created drugs treat depression. Some of these drugs are used for other illnesses and are being tested for treating depression; others do not fit into any of the described groups. EXAMPLES: Mirapex (pramipexole), nefazodone, Wellbutrin (bupropion), and Remeron (mirtazapine)
antipsychotic agents	Called *neuroleptics,* these agents modify psychotic behavior. Many antipsychotic agents are derivatives of phenothiazine (an organic compound used in the manufacture of certain of these drugs). These agents are used in the treatment of acute and chronic schizophrenia, organic psychoses, the manic phase of bipolar disorder, and psychotic disorders. EXAMPLE: chlorpromazine HCl Some antipsychotic agents are not actually phenothiazines but resemble them in action. Others resemble tricyclic antidepressants, while some are miscellaneous compounds. EXAMPLES: Clozaril (clozapine), Zyprexa (olanzapine), Loxitane (loxapine), and Orap (pimozide)
atypical antipsychotics	Drugs in this group affect serotonin and dopamine. EXAMPLES: Risperdal (risperidone), Clozaril (clozapine), and Syprexa (olanzapine)
stimulants	These drugs stimulate the central nervous system (CNS) and are generally prescribed for attention-deficit hyperactivity disorder. Patients using these drugs must take care to avoid abuse and excessive CNS stimulation by overdose. Many of these drugs are Schedule II agents with a very high potential for abuse. EXAMPLES: Dexedrine (dextroamphetamine sulfate), Ritalin (methylphenidate HCl), and Adderall, which is a combination of amphetamine salts

• Abbreviations •

ABBREVIATION	MEANING	ABBREVIATION	MEANING
ADHD	attention-deficit hyperactivity disorder	NIMH	National Institute of Mental Health
APA	American Psychiatric Association	NINDS	National Institute of Neurological Disorders and Stroke
ASD	autism spectrum disorder		
BDD	body dysmorphic disorder	OCD	obsessive–compulsive disorder
CBT	cognitive-behavioral therapy	PhD	doctor of philosophy (also doctor of pharmacy)
CNS	central nervous system		
DSM-IV-TR	*Diagnostic and Statistical Manual of Mental Disorders,* Fourth Edition, Text Revision	PDD-NOS	pervasive developmental disorder not otherwise specified
ECT	electroconvulsive therapy	PTSD	post-traumatic stress disorder
GAD	generalized anxiety disorder	SAD	seasonal affective disorder
HHS	Department of Health and Human Services	SNRI	serotonin-norepinephrine reuptake inhibitor
IQ	intelligence quotient	SSRIs	selective serotonin reuptake inhibitors
MAOIs	monoamine oxidase inhibitors		
MBPS	Munchausen by proxy syndrome	TAT	Thematic Apperception Test
MD	medical doctor	TCAs	tricyclic antidepressants
MMPI	Minnesota Multiphasic Personality Inventory	WAIS	Wechster Adult Intelligence Scale
NIH	National Institutes of Health	WHO	World Health Organization

Overview: Mental Health and Mental Illness

Write your answers to the following questions.

1. _____ is an abnormal condition of the brain or mind.

2. List the three mental disorders that are listed among the top 10 causes of disability in the United States.

   a. _____   b. _____

   c. _____

3. _____ is the branch of medicine that deals with the study, diagnosis, and treatment of mental illness.

4. Give the three basic forms of treatment for mental illness.

   a. _____   b. _____

   c. _____

5. _____ is a method of obtaining a detailed account of past and present mental and emotional experiences and repressions.

Word Parts

PREFIXES

Give the definitions of the following prefixes.

1. an-   _____   2. hypo- _____

3. para- _____   4. pyro- _____

ROOTS AND COMBINING FORMS

Give the definitions of the following roots and combining forms.

1. agor/a _____   2. aut   _____

3. centr   _____   4. cycl/o _____

5. delus   _____   6. ego   _____

7. hallucinat _____   8. iatr   _____

9. log _____ 10. neur/o _____

11. path _____ 12. phren _____

13. psych _____ 14. psych/o _____

15. schiz/o _____ 16. somat _____

17. somat/o _____ 18. thym _____

SUFFIXES

Give the definitions of the following suffixes.

1. -form _____ 2. -ia _____

3. -ic _____ 4. -ion _____

5. -ism _____ 6. -ist _____

7. -logy _____ 8. -mania _____

9. -noia _____ 10. -orexia _____

11. -osis _____ 12. -phobia _____

13. -therapy _____ 14. -tic _____

Identifying Medical Terms

In the spaces provided, write the medical terms for the following meanings.

1. _____ Abnormal fear of being in public places

2. _____ Condition in which a person lacks feelings and emotions

3. _____ Fixed, false belief or abnormal perception

4. _____ Mental disorder marked by altered mood and loss of interest in things that are usually pleasurable

5. _____ Pertaining to being self-centered

6. _____ Mental disorder characterized by excessive excitement; literally means *madness*

7. _____ Morbid and persistent fear of a specific object, activity, or situation that results in a compelling desire to avoid the feared stimulus

8. _____ Physician who specializes in the study and treatment of mental disorders

9. _____ Method of treating mental disorders by using psychological techniques instead of physical methods

10. _____ Literally means a madness for fire

Spelling

Circle the correct spelling of each medical term.

1. anxeity / anxiety

2. autism / autesm

3. bulimia / bulemia

4. dementia / dementea

5. factious / factitious

6. hallucination / halluciation

7. parnoia / paranoia

8. psychosomatic / psychomatic

9. schizphrenia / schizophrenia

10. somatoform / somatform

Matching

Select the appropriate lettered meaning for each of the following words.

_____ 1. dysthymia

_____ 2. seasonal affective disorder

_____ 3. bipolar disorder

_____ 4. schizophrenia

_____ 5. delusion

_____ 6. hallucination

_____ 7. obsessive–compulsive disorder

_____ 8. post-traumatic stress disorder

_____ 9. generalized anxiety disorder

_____ 10. attention-deficit hyperactivity disorder

a. Mental disorder characterized by positive, negative, and cognitive symptoms

b. Process of experiencing sensations that have no source

c. Brain disorder also known as *manic-depressive illness* that causes unusual shifts in a person's mood, energy, and ability to function

d. Less severe type of depression involving long-term, chronic symptoms that do not disable but keep the person from functioning well or from feeling good

e. Debilitating condition that can develop following a terrifying event

f. Characterized by bizarre thoughts that have no basis in reality

g. Form of depression that appears related to fluctuations in a person's exposure to natural light

h. Chronic condition that fills the person's day with exaggerated worry and tension

i. Characterized by anxious thoughts or rituals that the person feels compelled to perform and cannot control

j. One of the most commonly diagnosed behavioral disorders among children and adolescents and often continues into adulthood

k. Anxiety syndrome and panic disorder

Abbreviations

Place the correct word, phrase, or abbreviation in the space provided.

1. cognitive-behavioral therapy _____

2. *Diagnostic and Statistical Manual of Mental Disorders,* Fourth Edition,

   Text Revision _____

3. ECT _____

4. MMPI _____

5. National Institute of Mental Health _____

6. OCD _____

7. post-traumatic stress disorder _____

8. SAD _____

9. TAT _____

10. World Health Organization _____

PRACTICAL APPLICATION

MEDICAL RECORD ANALYSIS

This exercise contains information, abbreviations, and medical terminology from an actual medical record or case study that has been adapted for this text. The names and any personal information have been created by the author. Read and study each form or case study and then answer the questions that follow. You may refer to Appendix III, Abbreviations and Symbols, on page A41.

June 20, 20xx

DEPARTMENT OF SOCIAL SERVICES
Disability Evaluation Division
1888 Golden Gate Blvd., Suite 10
San Francisco, CA 94132
Re: Rotha, Maly # 123-45-6789

Dear Staff:

Thank you for referring to me the case of Ms. Rotha for psychiatric evaluation. She was examined in psychiatric consultation on June 17, 20xx. No physical exam was performed. No psychological testing was given. Medical records provided were reviewed. The patient was a clean, neatly dressed, well-groomed Asian female. She understood English and responded to questions. There was no evidence of any ambulation difficulties or speech impediments. Energy level was described as poor, with description of fatigue with minimal exertion.

History of Present Illness

Ms. Rotha is a 42-year-old Cambodian female. She lives in an apartment with her husband and three children. She describes feeling sick all the time and too weak and tired, dizzy and depressed to do anything except "rest." Currently, she is taking a combination of five different medications under the care of two different physicians. She takes Proventil inhaler for relief of asthmatic symptoms, analgesics, decongestants, and two different forms of tricyclic antidepressants. She feels that the medications are helping her. She is not receiving any formal psychiatric treatment with or without medication.

Mental Examination

There is no evidence or history of alcoholism or illicit drug use. She is oriented to time, place, persons, and events. There is no evidence of delusion or hallucinations at the present time and no history of such in the past. There is no evidence of paranoia such as feelings of being persecuted or plotted against. Thought content is generally well organized, coherent, and relevant without flight of ideas or loose associations.

Depression is manifested by occasional crying, usually occurring every other day. There is fitful sleep. There are occasional nightmares. There is no suicidal ideation or history of any suicide attempts.

Memory for recent and remote events, she feels, is impaired. She cannot recall her Social Security number. She can recall her address and phone number. She can do simple arithmetic.

Medical Opinion

It is my medical opinion that at Ms. Rotha's current level of daily functioning, she has minimal difficulty in relating to others. In appearance she seems to have the ability to care for her personal needs. How much her interest, habits, and daily activities are constricted as a result of mental impairments is difficult to assess because it is my medical opinion that this represents a factitious disorder, although post-traumatic stress disorder should be ruled out.

Very truly yours,

Hana Eun Kim, MD

Medical Record Questions

Place the correct answer in the space provided.

1. State the symptoms Ms. Rotha described. _____

2. What medications did this patient take? _____

3. What is a delusion? _____

4. Define hallucination. _____

5. Define factitious disorder. _____

Answer Key

APPENDIX I

• CHAPTER I
WORD PARTS
Prefixes
1. without
2. away from
3. against
4. self
5. bad
6. one hundred, one hundredth
7. through
8. different
9. bad
10. small
11. one thousandth
12. many, much
13. new
14. beside
15. before
16. together
17. apart
18. upon
19. out
20. in, into

Roots and Combining Forms
1. stuck to
2. armpit
3. center
4. chemical
5. a shaping
6. formation, produce
7. a thousand
8. large
9. death
10. law
11. rule
12. tumor
13. organ
14. fever
15. heat, fire
16. ray, x-ray

17. to examine
18. putrefaction
19. hot, heat
20. place
21. cough
22. to infect
23. people
24. cause
25. to cut
26. bad kind
27. greatest
28. least
29. palm
30. guarding

Suffixes
1. pertaining to
2. pertaining to
3. surgical puncture
4. that which runs together
5. shape
6. to flee
7. formation, produce
8. knowledge
9. a step
10. a weight
11. recording
12. condition
13. pertaining to
14. process
15. condition
16. nature of, quality of
17. liter
18. study of
19. instrument to measure
20. condition
21. pertaining to
22. disease
23. to carry
24. instrument for examining
25. decay
26. treatment
27. pertaining to
28. condition

IDENTIFYING MEDICAL TERMS
1. adhesion
2. asepsis
3. axillary
4. chemotherapy
5. heterogeneous
6. malformation
7. microscope
8. multiform
9. neopathy
10. oncology

SPELLING
1. antiseptic
2. autonomy
3. centimeter
4. diaphoresis
5. milligram
6. necrosis
7. paracentesis
8. radiology

MATCHING
1. f	2. d
3. j	4. g
5. a	6. k
7. b	8. i
9. c	10. e

ABBREVIATIONS
1. abnormal
2. axillary
3. Bx
4. cardiovascular
5. neurology
6. ENT
7. FP
8. g
9. gynecology
10. pediatrics

PRACTICAL APPLICATION

1. written transcript of information about a patient and his or her health care
2. Health Insurance Portability and Accountability Act of 1996
3. **a.** patient information form
   b. medical history
   c. physical examination
   d. consent form
   e. informed consent form
   f. physician's orders
   g. nurse's notes
   h. physician's progress notes
   i. consultation report
   j. ancillary/miscellaneous reports
   k. diagnostic tests/laboratory reports
   l. operative report
   m. anesthesiology report
   n. pathology report
   o. discharge summary
4. **a.** subjective
   b. objective
   c. assessment
   d. plan
5. diagnosis
6. plan

• CHAPER 2

IDENTIFYING SUFFIXES

1. card**iac**
2. cephal**ad**
3. enur**esis**
4. obstet**rician**
5. bronch**iole**
6. pust**ule**
7. dent**algia**
8. dia**betes**
9. hyper**emesis**
10. hemo**ptysis**

DEFINING SUFFIXES

1. weakness
2. process
3. inflammation
4. softening
5. enlargement, large
6. disease
7. deficiency
8. to digest
9. fear
10. rupture
11. pertaining to
12. pertaining to
13. use, action
14. condition
15. to make
16. resemble
17. one who
18. pertaining to
19. pertaining to
20. nourishment
21. tissue, structure

SPELLING

1. auricle
2. bronchiole
3. cardiologist
4. cephalad
5. cyanotic
6. embolism
7. podiatry
8. pustule

USING SUFFIXES TO BUILD MEDICAL WORDS

1. hyperhidrosis
2. muscular
3. macula
4. alopecia
5. ventricle
6. decubitus
7. integumentary
8. penile
9. congenital
10. anterior

IDENTIFYING MEDICAL TERMS

1. abrasion
2. anesthetize
3. arousal
4. asymmetry
5. asystole
6. comatose
7. dysarthria
8. grandiose
9. gynecoid
10. palpate

• CHAPTER 3

IDENTIFYING PREFIXES

1. apnea
2. bradypnea
3. dyspnea
4. eupnea
5. hyperpnea
6. hypopnea
7. tachypnea
8. binary
9. concentration
10. extraocular

DEFINING PREFIXES

1. against
2. short
3. through
4. different
5. similar, same
6. water
7. micro, small
8. scanty, little
9. all
10. false
11. without
12. without
13. two
14. twice
15. with, together
16. down, away from
17. outside
18. excessive
19. under
20. not
21. between
22. many
23. beside
24. around
25. many
26. before
27. again, backward
28. below
29. upper, above
30. not

SPELLING

1. binary
2. concentration
3. occlusion
4. parasternal
5. pericardial
6. latent
7. patent
8. unconscious

USING PREFIXES TO BUILD MEDICAL WORDS

1. anicteric
2. hyperactive
3. multifocal
4. decompensation
5. intermediary
6. bifurcate
7. polydactyly
8. hypoplasia
9. subacute
10. unconscious

IDENTIFYING MEDICAL TERMS

1. afebrile
2. extraocular
3. insomnia
4. arrest
5. enucleate
6. lumen
7. patent
8. react
9. sign
10. symptom

• CHAPTER 4

ANATOMY AND PHYSIOLOGY LABELING

1. posterior
2. anterior
3. cranial cavity
4. spinal cavity
5. thoracic cavity
6. diaphragm
7. abdominal cavity
8. pelvic cavity
9. pericardial membranes
10. heart

ANATOMY AND PHYSIOLOGY

1. body … cells … sustain
2. cell membrane
3. cell membrane … cytoplasm … nucleus
4. metabolism … growth … reproduction
5. embryonic cell
6. **a.** protection
   b. absorption
   c. secretion
   d. excretion
   e. sensation
   f. diffusion
7. Connective
8. **a.** striated (voluntary)
   b. cardiac
   c. smooth (involuntary)
9. excitability … conductivity
10. tissue serving a common purpose
11. group of organs functioning together for a common purpose
12. **a.** integumentary
    b. skeletal
    c. muscular
    d. digestive
    e. cardiovascular
    f. blood and lymphatic
    g. respiratory
    h. urinary
    i. endocrine
    j. nervous
    k. reproductive
13. **a.** above, in an upward direction
    b. in front of, before
    c. toward the back
    d. pertaining to the head
    e. nearest the midline or middle
    f. to the side, away from the middle
    g. nearest the point of attachment
    h. away from the point of attachment
14. midsagittal plane
15. transverse or horizontal
16. coronal or frontal
17. **a.** thoracic
    b. abdominal
    c. pelvic
18. **a.** cranial
    b. spinal

WORD PARTS

Prefixes

1. both
2. up, apart
3. two
4. color
5. down, away from
6. apart
7. outside
8. within
9. similar, same
10. middle
11. through
12. first
13. one
14. upper, above

Roots and Combining Forms

1. fat
2. man
3. life
4. tail
5. cell
6. cell
7. to pour
8. tissue
9. water
10. cell's nucleus
11. side
12. disease
13. nature
14. to drink
15. body
16. place
17. a turning
18. body organs
19. toward the front
20. cranium
21. away from the point of origin
22. back
23. to strain through
24. horizon

25. below
26. groin
27. within
28. side
29. toward the middle
30. organ
31. to show
32. behind, toward the back
33. near the point of origin
34. a composite whole
35. near the belly side

Suffixes
1. pertaining to
2. use, action
3. formation, produce
4. pertaining to
5. process
6. study of
7. form, shape
8. resemble
9. pertaining to
10. a thing formed, plasma
11. body
12. control, stop, stand still
13. incision
14. pertaining to
15. type

IDENTIFYING MEDICAL TERMS
1. android
2. bilateral
3. cytology
4. ectomorph
5. karyogenesis
6. somatotrophic
7. unilateral

SPELLING
1. adipose
2. caudal
3. cytology
4. diffusion
5. histology
6. mesomorph
7. perfusion
8. proximal
9. somatotrophic
10. unilateral

MATCHING
1. c	2. d
3. e	4. f
5. a	6. i
7. g	8. h
9. j	10. b

ABBREVIATIONS
1. abdomen
2. anatomy and physiology
3. deoxyribonucleic acid
4. ENT
5. GI
6. water
7. left lower quadrant
8. O_2
9. OTC
10. right upper quadrant

• CHAPTER 5
ANATOMY AND PHYSIOLOGY LABELING
1. epidermis
2. dermis
3. subcutaneous layer
4. sweat gland
5. sebaceous gland
6. hair
7. nerve
8. artery
9. vein

ANATOMY AND PHYSIOLOGY
1. skin
2. **a.** hair
   b. nails
   c. sebaceous glands
   d. sweat glands
3. **a.** protection
   b. regulation
   c. sensory reception
   d. secretion
4. epidermis ... dermis
5. **a.** stratum germinativum
   b. stratum spinosum
   c. stratum granulosum
   d. stratum lucidum
   e. stratum corneum
6. Keratin
7. Melanin
8. dermis
9. **a.** papillary layer
   b. reticular layer
10. lunula

WORD PARTS
Prefixes
1. without, lack of
2. self
3. out
4. down
5. out
6. excessive
7. under
8. within
9. around
10. below

Roots and Combining Forms
1. extremity
2. ray
3. gland
4. white
5. cancer
6. heat
7. juice
8. corium
9. skin
10. skin
11. skin
12. skin
13. skin
14. skin
15. fox mange
16. red
17. sweat
18. jaundice
19. tumor
20. horn
21. white
22. study of
23. black
24. black
25. fungus
26. nail
27. little cell
28. nail
29. thick
30. a louse

31. cord
32. wrinkle
33. hard, hardening
34. oil
35. old
36. hot, heat
37. to pull
38. hair
39. nail
40. yellow
41. dry
42. to lie
43. little bag
44. a covering
45. yellow
46. plate
47. millet (tiny)
48. itching
49. end, distant
50. vessel

Suffixes
1. pertaining to
2. pain
3. pertaining to
4. pertaining to
5. skin
6. pertaining to
7. sensation
8. pencil, grafting knife
9. condition
10. pertaining to
11. process
12. condition
13. one who specializes
14. inflammation
15. study of
16. dilatation
17. resemble
18. tumor
19. condition
20. pertaining to
21. surgical repair
22. flow, discharge
23. instrument to cut

IDENTIFYING MEDICAL TERMS

1. actinic dermatitis
2. cutaneous
3. dermatitis

4. dermatology
5. pruritus
6. hyperhidrosis
7. hypodermic
8. icteric
9. onychitis
10. pachyderma
11. thermanesthesia
12. xanthoderma

SPELLING

1. causalgia
2. dermomycosis
3. ecchymosis
4. excoriation
5. hyperhidrosis
6. melanoma
7. onychomycosis
8. rhytidoplasty
9. scleroderma
10. seborrhea

MATCHING

1. d	2. f
3. e	4. h
5. j	6. i
7. b	8. g
9. a	10. c

ABBREVIATIONS

1. BCC
2. biopsy
3. decubitus
4. intradermal
5. I&D
6. purified protein derivative
7. SG
8. staphylococcus
9. streptococcus
10. TIMs

DIAGNOSTIC AND LABORATORY TESTS

1. c	2. d
3. a	4. b
5. a	

PRACTICAL APPLICATION

1. Dx
2. basal cell carcinoma

3. a solid, circumscribed, elevated area of the skin
4. telangiectasia
5. solar elastosis

• CHAPTER 6

ANATOMY AND PHYSIOLOGY LABELING

1. cranium
2. mandible
3. clavicle
4. scapula
5. sternum
6. humerus
7. ulna
8. radius
9. femur
10. tibia

ANATOMY AND PHYSIOLOGY

1. 206
2. **a.** axial
   b. appendicular
3. **a.** flat . . . ribs, scapula, parts of the pelvic girdle, bones of the skull
   b. long . . . tibia, femur, humerus, radius
   c. short . . . carpal, tarsal
   d. irregular . . . vertebrae, ossicles of the ear
   e. sesamoid . . . patella

*Optional answer to question 3:

   f. sutural or wormian . . . between the flat bones of the skull
4. **a.** Provide shape, support, and the framework of the body
   b. Provide protection for internal organs
   c. Serve as a storage place for mineral salts, calcium, and phosphorus
   d. Play an important role in the formation of blood cells (hematopoiesis)

e. Provide areas for the attachment of skeletal muscles

f. Help make movement possible through articulation

5. **a.** ends of a developing bone

b. shaft of a long bone

c. membrane that forms the covering of bones except at their articular surfaces

d. dense, hard layer of bone tissue

e. narrow space or cavity throughout the length of the diaphysis

f. tough connective tissue membrane lining the medullary canal and containing the bone marrow

g. reticular tissue that makes up most of the volume of bone

6. Matching

1. f	**2.** k
3. d	**4.** m
5. h	**6.** j
7. i	**8.** n
9. a	**10.** l
11. b	**12.** c
13. g	**14.** e

7. **a.** synarthrosis

b. amphiarthrosis

c. diarthrosis

8. Abduction

9. moving a body part toward the midline

10. Circumduction

11. bending a body part backward

12. Eversion

13. straightening a flexed limb

14. Flexion

15. turning inward

16. Pronation

17. moving a body part forward

18. Retraction

19. moving a body part around a central axis

20. Supination

WORD PARTS

Prefixes

1. without
2. apart
3. water
4. between
5. beyond
6. around
7. many, much
8. under, beneath
9. together
10. back

Roots and Combining Forms

1. acetabulum, hip socket
2. gristle
3. extremity, point
4. extremity
5. stiffening, crooked
6. joint
7. joint
8. a pouch
9. heel bone
10. to place
11. cancer
12. wrist
13. wrist
14. cartilage
15. cartilage
16. clavicle, collarbone
17. fastened
18. coccyx, tail bone
19. coccyx, tail bone
20. glue
21. to lead
22. to bind together
23. rib
24. rib
25. crescent
26. light
27. skull
28. skull
29. finger or toe
30. finger or toe
31. femur
32. carrying
33. fibula
34. x-ray
35. humerus
36. ilium
37. ilium
38. ischium
39. a hump
40. lamina (thin plate)
41. bending, curve, swayback
42. loin, lower back
43. loin
44. lower jawbone
45. jawbone
46. jaw
47. bone marrow
48. bone marrow
49. discharge
50. elbow
51. bone
52. kneecap
53. to draw
54. foot
55. phalanges (finger/toe bones)
56. a passage
57. spine
58. radius
59. sacrum
60. flesh
61. shoulder blade
62. curvature
63. curvature
64. spine
65. vertebra
66. sternum, breastbone
67. sternum, breastbone
68. tendon
69. tibia
70. ulna, elbow
71. ulna, elbow
72. vertebra
73. vertebra
74. sword

Suffixes

1. pertaining to
2. pertaining to
3. pain
4. pertaining to
5. pertaining to
6. immature cell, germ cell
7. surgical puncture
8. related to
9. process
10. pain
11. excision
12. swelling

13. formation, produce
14. formation, produce
15. mark, record
16. instrument for recording
17. pertaining to
18. inflammation
19. nature of
20. instrument for examining
21. softening
22. structure
23. resemble
24. tumor
25. shoulder
26. condition
27. deficiency
28. growth
29. formation, produce
30. surgical repair
31. formation
32. instrument to cut
33. incision
34. structure, tissue

IDENTIFYING MEDICAL TERMS

1. acroarthritis
2. ankylosis
3. arthritis
4. calcaneal
5. chondral
6. coccygodynia
7. costal
8. craniectomy
9. dactylic
10. osteotome
11. intercostal
12. ischialgia
13. lumbar
14. myeloma
15. osteoarthritis
16. osteomyelitis or myelitis
17. osteopenia
18. pedal
19. xiphoid

SPELLING

1. acromion
2. arthroscope
3. bursitis
4. chondrocostal
5. connective

6. craniotomy
7. dislocation
8. ischial
9. myelitis
10. osteoporosis
11. phosphorus
12. patellar
13. phalangeal
14. rachigraph
15. scoliosis
16. spondylitis
17. symphysis
18. tendonitis
19. ulnocarpal
20. vertebral

MATCHING

1. i	2. j
3. e	4. c
5. b	6. h
7. g	8. a
9. d	10. f

ABBREVIATIONS

1. CDH
2. DJD
3. long leg cast
4. osteoarthritis
5. PEMFs
6. rheumatoid arthritis
7. SPECT
8. thoracic vertebra, first
9. temporomandibular joint
10. Tx

DIAGNOSTIC AND LABORATORY TESTS

1. c	2. d
3. c	4. b
5. b	

PRACTICAL APPLICATION

1. dual-energy X-ray absorptiometry scan
2. bone mineral density (test)
3. lumbar vertebra, first
4. osteopenia
5. XRDXA/76075

• CHAPTER 7

ANATOMY AND PHYSIOLOGY LABELING

Anterior View:
1. trapezius
2. deltoid
3. rectus femoris
4. sternocleidomastoid
5. pectoralis major
6. biceps brachii

Posterior View:
7. gluteus maximus
8. biceps femoris
9. gastrocnemius
10. latissimus dorsi
11. triceps
12. Achilles tendon

ANATOMY AND PHYSIOLOGY

1. **a.** skeletal
   b. smooth
   c. cardiac
2. 42
3. **a.** nutrition
   b. oxygen
4. **a.** origin
   b. insertion
5. voluntary or striated
6. aponeurosis
7. **a.** body
   b. origin
   c. insertion
8. **a.** muscle that counteracts the action of another muscle; when one contracts the other relaxes
   b. muscle that is primary in a given movement produced by its contraction
   c. muscle that acts with another muscle to produce movement
9. involuntary, visceral, or unstriated
10. **a.** digestive tract
    b. respiratory tract
    c. urinary tract

d. eye
e. skin
11. Cardiac
12. a. movement
    b. maintain posture
    c. produce heat

WORD PARTS
Prefixes
1. lack of
2. away from
3. toward
4. against
5. two
6. slow
7. with
8. through
9. difficult
10. into
11. within
12. water
13. four
14. with, together
15. three

Roots and Combining Forms
1. agony
2. arm
3. clavicle
4. to cut through
5. neck
6. finger or toe
7. to lead
8. work
9. a band
10. skin
11. discharge
12. fiber
13. fiber
14. equal
15. a rind
16. lifter
17. an addition
18. breast
19. hot, heat
20. to measure
21. muscle
22. muscle
23. muscle
24. muscle
25. nerve

26. disease
27. to loosen
28. rod
29. to turn
30. a turning
31. flesh
32. hardening
33. to gain
34. convulsive
35. sternum
36. tendon
37. tone, tension
38. twisted
39. to draw
40. will
41. synovial membrane
42. twisted

Suffixes
1. pain
2. pertaining to
3. pertaining to
4. weakness
5. immature cell, germ cell
6. head
7. binding
8. pain
9. chemical
10. treatment
11. instrument for recording
12. condition
13. pertaining to
14. process
15. agent
16. inflammation
17. condition
18. motion
19. motion
20. study of
21. process
22. softening
23. resemble
24. tumor
25. a doer
26. condition
27. weakness
28. disease
29. a fence
30. surgical repair
31. stroke, paralysis
32. suture

33. pertaining to
34. tension, spasm
35. order
36. instrument to cut
37. incision
38. nourishment, development
39. condition
40. condition

IDENTIFYING MEDICAL TERMS
1. atonic
2. bradykinesia
3. dactylospasm
4. dystrophy
5. intramuscular
6. levator
7. myasthenia gravis
8. myology
9. myoparesis
10. myoplasty
11. myosarcoma
12. myotomy
13. polyplegia
14. tenodesis
15. synergetic
16. triceps

SPELLING
1. fascia
2. myokinesis
3. dermatomyositis
4. rhabdomyoma
5. sarcolemma
6. sternocleidomastoid
7. dystrophin
8. torticollis

MATCHING
1. d   2. i
3. g   4. e
5. j   6. a
7. h   8. c
9. b   10. f

ABBREVIATIONS
1. above elbow
2. aspartate aminotransferase
3. Ca

4. EMG
5. full range of motion
6. musculoskeletal
7. ROM
8. sh
9. total body weight
10. triceps jerk

DIAGNOSTIC AND LABORATORY TESTS

1. b
2. d
3. b
4. c
5. a

PRACTICAL APPLICATION

1. waddling
2. electromyography
3. **a.** minimize deformities
   b. preserve mobility
4. Test to measure electrical activity across muscle membranes by means of electrodes attached to a needle that is inserted into the muscle.
5. Surgical removal of a small piece of muscle tissue for examination.

• CHAPTER 8

ANATOMY AND PHYSIOLOGY LABELING

1. right lobe of liver
2. gallbladder
3. appendix
4. parotid gland
5. pharynx
6. esophagus
7. spleen
8. body of stomach
9. pancreas
10. small intestine

ANATOMY AND PHYSIOLOGY

1. **a.** mouth
   b. pharynx
   c. esophagus
   d. stomach
   e. small intestine
   f. large intestine
2. **a.** salivary glands
   b. liver
   c. gallbladder
   d. pancreas
3. **a.** digestion
   b. absorption
   c. elimination
4. soft mass of chewed food ready to be swallowed
5. series of wavelike muscular contractions that are involuntary
6. hydrochloric acid and gastric juices
7. duodenum
8. chyme
9. circulatory system
10. cecum, colon, rectum, and anal canal
11. liver
12. stores and concentrates bile
13. produces digestive enzymes
14. **a.** plays an important role in metabolism
    b. manufactures bile
    c. stores iron and vitamins B_{12}, A, D, E, and K
15. small intestine
16. parotid, sublingual, submandibular
17. **a.** insulin
    b. glucagon

WORD PARTS

Prefixes

1. lack of
2. difficult
3. above
4. excessive, above
5. deficient, below
6. bad
7. around
8. after
9. through
10. below

Roots and Combining Forms

1. to suck in
2. gland
3. starch
4. a building up
5. a casting down
6. orange-yellow
7. appendix
8. appendix
9. gall, bile
10. cheek
11. abdomen, belly
12. lip
13. gall, bile
14. common bile duct
15. colon
16. colon
17. colon
18. colon
19. bladder
20. tooth
21. to press together
22. diverticula
23. duodenum
24. small intestine
25. to remove dregs
26. esophagus
27. stomach
28. stomach
29. gums
30. tongue
31. sweet, sugar
32. blood
33. liver
34. liver
35. hernia
36. ileum
37. ileum
38. lip
39. abdomen
40. to loosen
41. tongue
42. fat
43. study of
44. middle
45. pancreas
46. to digest
47. pharynx
48. meal
49. to vomit
50. anus and rectum
51. pylorus, gatekeeper
52. rectum
53. saliva, salivary

54. sigmoid
55. spleen
56. mouth
57. poison
58. a breaking out
59. worm
60. breath
61. vein liable to bleed
62. nourishment
63. to chew
64. to disable; paralysis
65. hair
66. nest
67. to roll
68. tooth

Suffixes
1. pertaining to
2. pertaining to
3. pain, ache
4. pertaining to
5. enzyme
6. hernia
7. resemble
8. condition
9. surgical excision
10. vomiting
11. shape
12. formation, produce
13. pertaining to
14. pertaining to
15. process
16. condition
17. one who specializes
18. inflammation
19. nature of, quality of
20. study of
21. destruction, to separate
22. enlargement, large
23. tumor
24. appetite
25. condition
26. flow
27. to digest
28. pertaining to
29. to eat, to swallow
30. instrument for examining
31. visual examination, to view, examine
32. contraction
33. new opening

34. incision
35. pertaining to
36. suture

IDENTIFYING MEDICAL TERMS
1. amylase
2. anabolism
3. anorexia
4. appendectomy
5. appendicitis
6. biliary
7. celiac
8. dysphagia
9. hepatitis
10. herniorrhaphy
11. postprandial
12. splenomegaly
13. sigmoidoscope

SPELLING
1. biliary
2. colonoscopy
3. deglutition
4. gastroenterology
5. halitosis
6. laxative
7. peristalsis
8. sialadenitis
9. periodontal
10. vermiform

MATCHING
1. e   2. f
3. d   4. b
5. i   6. h
7. j   8. a
9. g   10. c

ABBREVIATIONS
1. ac
2. bowel movement
3. bowel sounds
4. cholesterol
5. GB
6. HAV
7. nasogastric
8. nothing by mouth
9. pc
10. TPN

DIAGNOSTIC AND LABORATORY TESTS
1. a   2. c
3. d   4. c
5. c

PRACTICAL APPLICATION
1. Appointment Date: October 17, 2011 Time: 8:45 A.M.
2. Referred to: Seymour Butts, MD Endoscopy Center 14 Maddox Drive Rome, GA 30165
3. For: _____X___ Diagnostic Procedure Screening Colonoscopy _____ Consultation _____ Evaluate and treat, initiating appropriate diagnostic and/or therapeutic services _____ Report test results to: Angel De'Crohn, MD Fax (706) 235-6676
4. Patient Instructions: Bring a driver, all current medications, driver's license, and proof of insurance
5. Referring Physician's Name: Angel De'Crohn, MD Date: 09/28/11 Phone #: (706) 235-7765 Fax #: (706) 235-6676

• CHAPTER 9
ANATOMY AND PHYSIOLOGY LABELING
1. superior vena cava
2. aorta
3. right atrium
4. tricuspid valve
5. right ventricle
6. inferior vena cava
7. mitral valve

8. endocardium
9. myocardium
10. pericardium

ANATOMY AND PHYSIOLOGY

1. **a.** heart
   b. arteries
   c. veins
   d. capillaries
2. **a.** endocardium
   b. myocardium
   c. pericardium
3. 300
4. atria … interatrial
5. ventricles …
   interventricular
6. electrocardiogram
7. autonomic nervous system
8. sinoatrial node
9. Purkinje network
10. **a.** radial … on the radial
    side of the wrist
    b. brachial … in the
    antecubital space of the
    elbow
    c. carotid … in the neck
11. **a.** pressure exerted by the
    blood on the walls of the
    vessels
    b. difference between the
    systolic and diastolic
    readings
12. person's fist … 60–90 and
    80–89
13. 120 and 139
14. transport blood from the
    right and left ventricles of
    the heart to all body parts;
    transports blood away
    from the heart
15. transport blood from
    peripheral tissues back to
    the heart

WORD PARTS
Prefixes
1. lack of
2. two
3. slow

4. together
5. within
6. within
7. outside
8. excessive, above
9. deficient, below
10. around
11. difficult, abnormal
12. half
13. rapid
14. three

Roots and Combining Forms
1. vessel
2. to choke
3. vessel
4. opening
5. aorta
6. artery
7. artery
8. artery
9. fatty substance, porridge
10. fatty substance, porridge
11. atrium
12. atrium
13. heart
14. heart
15. heart
16. dark blue
17. listen to
18. to widen
19. electricity
20. a throwing in
21. sweet, sugar
22. blood
23. to hold back
24. bile
25. study of
26. moon
27. thin
28. mitral valve
29. muscle
30. circular
31. sour, sharp, acid
32. vein
33. vein
34. sound
35. lung
36. rhythm
37. hardening
38. a curve

39. pulse
40. narrowing
41. chest
42. to draw, to bind
43. to limp
44. pressure
45. clot of blood
46. small vessel
47. vessel
48. reflected sound
49. vein
50. body
51. ventricle
52. fibrils (small fibers)
53. blood
54. power
55. infarct (necrosis of an area)
56. to close up
57. oxygen
58. throbbing
59. a partition
60. end
61. clot of blood
62. solid (fat)
63. chest
64. fat

Suffixes
1. pertaining to
2. pertaining to
3. pertaining to
4. record
5. surgical puncture
6. point
7. measurement
8. dilatation
9. surgical excision
10. blood condition
11. relating to
12. formation, produce
13. instrument for recording
14. recording
15. condition
16. pertaining to
17. having a particular quality
18. process
19. condition
20. one who specializes
21. inflammation
22. nature of, quality of
23. study of

24. softening
25. enlargement, large
26. instrument to measure
27. tumor
28. one who
29. condition
30. disease
31. surgical repair
32. to pierce
33. instrument for examining
34. contraction, spasm
35. incision
36. tissue
37. pertaining to

IDENTIFYING MEDICAL TERMS

1. angioma
2. angiocardiography
3. angioplasty
4. angiostenosis
5. arrhythmia
6. arteritis
7. bicuspid
8. cardiologist
9. cardiomegaly
10. cardiopulmonary
11. constriction
12. embolism
13. phlebitis
14. tachycardia
15. vasodilator

SPELLING

1. anastomosis
2. atherosclerosis
3. atrioventricular
4. endocarditis
5. extracorporeal
6. ischemia
7. myocardial
8. oxygen
9. phlebitis
10. palpitation

MATCHING

1. d   2. e
3. f   4. g
5. b   6. c
7. a   8. i
9. j   10. h

ABBREVIATIONS

1. AMI
2. A-V, AV
3. blood pressure
4. coronary artery disease
5. CC
6. electrocardiogram
7. high-density lipoprotein
8. H & L
9. myocardial infarction
10. tissue plasminogen activator

DIAGNOSTIC AND LABORATORY TESTS

1. c   2. a
3. b   4. c
5. b

PRACTICAL APPLICATION

1. dyspnea
2. blood enzyme
3. oxygenated
4. electrocardiogram
5. coronary vasodilator

• CHAPTER 10

ANATOMY AND PHYSIOLOGY LABELING

1. cervical nodes
2. thoracic duct
3. axillary nodes
4. pectoral nodes
5. cisterna chyli
6. abdominal nodes
7. pelvic and inguinal nodes
8. popliteal nodes

ANATOMY AND PHYSIOLOGY

1. **a.** erythrocytes
   b. thrombocytes
   c. leukocytes
2. transport oxygen and carbon dioxide
3. 5
4. 80–120 days
5. body's main defense against the invasion of pathogens

6. 8,000
7. **a.** neutrophils
   b. eosinophils
   c. basophils
   d. lymphocytes
   e. monocytes
8. play an important role in the clotting process
9. 200,000–500,000
10. **a.** A
    b. B
    c. AB
    d. O
11. **a.** transports proteins and fluids
    b. protects the body against pathogens
    c. serves as a pathway for the absorption of fats
12. **a.** spleen
    b. tonsils
    c. thymus

WORD PARTS

Prefixes
1. lack of
2. against
3. self
4. up
5. beyond
6. excessive
7. deficient
8. one
9. all
10. many
11. before
12. across
13. deficient

Roots and Combining Forms
1. gland
2. gland
3. clumping
4. other
5. vessel
6. unequal
7. base
8. lime, calcium
9. color
10. to pour

11. clots, to clot
12. flesh, creatine
13. cell
14. blood
15. cell
16. rose-colored
17. red
18. globe
19. little grain, granular
20. blood
21. blood
22. blood
23. white
24. white
25. fat
26. study of
27. lymph
28. lymph
29. large
30. neither
31. kernel, nucleus
32. eat, engulf
33. a thing formed, plasma
34. net
35. putrefying
36. whey, serum
37. iron
38. fiber
39. spleen
40. sea
41. clot
42. clot
43. thymus
44. fiber
45. tonsil
46. formation
47. immunity
48. vessel
49. whey
50. a developing
51. vessel
52. small vessel

Suffixes
1. capable
2. forming
3. immature cell, germ cell
4. body
5. swelling
6. to separate
7. cultivation

8. cell
9. surgical excision
10. blood condition
11. work
12. formation, produce
13. protection
14. protein
15. tissue
16. pertaining to
17. chemical
18. process
19. one who specializes
20. inflammation
21. study of
22. destruction
23. enlargement
24. tumor
25. condition
26. lack of
27. removal
28. attraction
29. attraction
30. formation
31. bursting forth
32. control, stop, stand still
33. incision
34. condition
35. oxygen

IDENTIFYING MEDICAL TERMS
1. agglutination
2. allergy
3. antibody
4. anticoagulant
5. antigen
6. basophil
7. coagulable
8. creatinemia
9. eosinophil
10. granulocyte
11. hematologist
12. hemoglobin
13. hyperglycemia
14. hyperlipidemia
15. leukocyte
16. lymphostasis
17. mononucleosis
18. prothrombin
19. splenomegaly
20. thrombocyte

SPELLING
1. allergy
2. creatinemia
3. extravasation
4. erythrocytosis
5. thromboplastin
6. hematocrit
7. hemorrhage
8. leukemia
9. lymphadenotomy
10. anaphylaxis

MATCHING
1. h 2. d
3. e 4. g
5. f 6. c
7. b 8. a
9. j 10. i

ABBREVIATIONS
1. AIDS
2. BSI
3. chronic myelogenous leukemia
4. Hb, Hgb
5. hematocrit
6. HIV
7. *Pneumocystis carinii* pneumonia
8. prothrombin time
9. red blood cell (count)
10. RIA

DIAGNOSTIC AND LABORATORY TESTS
1. d 2. c
3. c 4. b
5. a

PRACTICAL APPLICATION
1. complete blood count
2. differential count
3. MCH (mean corpuscular hemoglobin)
4. WBC: 4.0–10.0 (4,000–10,000)
5. RBC: 3.80–5.80 (3.8 million–5.8 million)

• CHAPTER II

ANATOMY AND PHYSIOLOGY LABELING

1. nasopharynx
2. hard palate
3. soft palate
4. oropharynx
5. larygopharynx
6. epiglottis
7. larynx
8. trachea
9. cricoid cartilage
10. thyroid cartilage

ANATOMY AND PHYSIOLOGY

1. a. nose
   b. pharynx
   c. larynx
   d. trachea
   e. bronchi
   f. lungs
2. to furnish oxygen for use by individual cells and to take away their gaseous waste product, carbon dioxide
3. process in which the lungs are ventilated and oxygen and carbon dioxide are exchanged between the air in the lungs and the blood within capillaries of the alveoli
4. process in which oxygen and carbon dioxide are exchanged between the bloodstream and the cells of the body
5. a. serves as an air passageway
   b. warms and moistens inhaled air
   c. its cilia and mucous membrane trap dust, pollen, bacteria, and foreign matter
   d. contains special smell receptor cells (nerve cells), which assist in distinguishing various smells
   e. contributes to phonation and the quality of voice
6. a. serves as a passageway for air
   b. serves as a passageway for food
   c. contributes to phonation as a chamber where the sound is able to resonate
7. acts as a lid to prevent aspiration of food into the trachea
8. narrow slit at the opening between the true vocal folds
9. production of vocal sounds
10. serves as a passageway for air
11. provide a passageway for air to and from the lungs
12. conical-shaped, spongy organs of respiration lying on both sides of the heart
13. serous membrane composed of several layers
14. diaphragm
15. mediastinum
16. 3 … 2
17. alveoli
18. to bring air into intimate contact with blood so that oxygen and carbon dioxide can be exchanged in the alveoli
19. temperature, pulse, respiration, and blood pressure
20. a. amount of air in a single inspiration and expiration
    b. amount of air remaining in the lungs after maximal expiration
    c. volume of air that can be exhaled after maximal inspiration
21. medulla oblongata … pons
22. 30–80
23. 12–20

WORD PARTS

Prefixes
1. lack of
2. upon
3. difficult
4. within
5. good
6. out
7. below, deficient
8. excessive
9. in
10. rapid

Roots and Combining Forms
1. to draw in
2. small, hollow air sac
3. coal
4. imperfect
5. bronchi
6. bronchi
7. bronchiole
8. bronchi
9. dust
10. dark blue
11. breathe
12. blood
13. larynx, voice box
14. larynx, voice box
15. larynx, voice box
16. lobe
17. sac
18. fiber
19. nose
20. straight
21. middle
22. a little swelling
23. palate
24. breast, chest
25. pharynx, throat
26. pharynx, throat
27. nipple
28. partition
29. pleura
30. pleura
31. pleura
32. lung, air
33. lung, air
34. lung
35. lung
36. pus
37. nose

38. a curve, hollow
39. breath
40. breathing
41. chest
42. to air
43. almond, tonsil
44. trachea, windpipe
45. trachea, windpipe
46. snore
47. flesh
48. diaphragm, partition

Suffixes
1. pertaining to
2. pain
3. hernia, tumor, swelling
4. surgical puncture
5. pain
6. dilation
7. surgical excision
8. pertaining to
9. condition
10. process
11. inflammation
12. instrument to measure
13. condition
14. tumor
15. dripping
16. surgical repair
17. a doer
18. breathing
19. to spit
20. flow, discharge
21. instrument for examining
22. new opening
23. incision
24. pertaining to

IDENTIFYING MEDICAL TERMS
1. alveolus
2. bronchiectasis
3. bronchitis
4. dysphonia
5. eupnea
6. hemoptysis
7. inhalation
8. laryngitis
9. pneumothorax
10. rhinoplasty
11. rhinorrhea
12. sinusitis

SPELLING
1. bronchoscope
2. diaphragmatocele
3. expectoration
4. laryngeal
5. orthopnea
6. pleuritis
7. pulmonectomy
8. rhonchus
9. tachypnea
10. tracheal

MATCHING
1. h   2. i
3. k   4. f
5. c   6. b
7. d   8. a
9. e   10. G

ABBREVIATIONS
1. AFB
2. cystic fibrosis
3. CXR
4. COPD
5. endotracheal
6. postnasal drip, paroxysmal nocturnal dyspnea
7. R
8. sudden infant death syndrome
9. SOB
10. tuberculosis

DIAGNOSTIC AND LABORATORY TESTS
1. b   2. c
3. c   4. d
5. a

PRACTICAL APPLICATION
1. abnormal sound heard on auscultation of the chest; a crackling, rattling, or bubbling sound
2. directly observed therapy
3. pertaining to without fever
4. no
5. occasional cough, nonproductive

• CHAPTER 12

ANATOMY AND PHYSIOLOGY LABELING
1. kidney
2. ureter
3. bladder
4. urethra

ANATOMY AND PHYSIOLOGY
1. **a.** kidneys
   b. ureters
   c. bladder
   d. urethra
2. extraction of certain wastes from the bloodstream, conversion of these materials to urine, and transport of the urine from the kidney, via the ureters, to the bladder for elimination
3. a notch
4. saclike collecting portion of the kidney
5. inner
6. structural and functional unit of the kidney
7. renal corpuscle … tubule
8. glomerulus … Bowman's capsule
9. filtration … reabsorption
10. 1,000–1,500
11. narrow, muscular tubes that transport urine from the kidneys to the bladder
12. muscular, membranous sac that serves as a reservoir for urine
13. urinary meatus
14. laboratory test that evaluates the physical, chemical, and microscopic properties of urine

15. **a.** yellow to amber
    b. clear
    c. 4.6–8.0
    d. 1.003–1.030
    e. aromatic
    f. 1000–1500 mL/day
16. diabetes mellitus
17. renal disease, acute glomerulonephritis, pyelonephritis

WORD PARTS

Prefixes
1. without
2. against
3. complete, through
4. complete, through
5. difficult, painful
6. within
7. water
8. outside, beyond
9. not
10. scanty
11. through
12. beyond
13. excessive

Roots and Combining Forms
1. sifted out
2. protein
3. bacteria
4. bile
5. calcium
6. colon
7. to hold
8. bladder
9. body
10. bladder
11. skin
12. glomerulus, little ball
13. glomerulus, little ball
14. glucose, sugar
15. blood
16. ketone
17. stone
18. study of
19. blood
20. passage
21. to urinate
22. kidney
23. kidney
24. night
25. peritoneum
26. perineum
27. sound
28. to tighten, contraction
29. pus
30. renal pelvis
31. kidney
32. hardening
33. trigone
34. urine
35. urine
36. ureter
37. urethra
38. urethra
39. urine
40. urine
41. urine
42. urination

Suffixes
1. pertaining to
2. pain
3. pertaining to
4. hernia
5. pain
6. pertaining to
7. pertaining to
8. surgical excision
9. blood condition
10. a mark, record
11. pertaining to
12. chemical
13. process
14. one who specializes
15. inflammation
16. stone
17. study of
18. separation, loosening, dissolution
19. crushing
20. process
21. instrument to measure
22. tumor
23. condition
24. disease
25. surgical repair
26. instrument for examining
27. condition
28. new opening
29. incision
30. urine

IDENTIFYING MEDICAL TERMS
1. antidiuretic
2. cystectomy
3. cystitis
4. dysuria
5. glomerulitis
6. hypercalciuria
7. micturition
8. nephrolith
9. periurethral
10. pyuria
11. ureteropathy
12. urethralgia
13. urologist

SPELLING
1. excretory
2. enuresis
3. glycosuria
4. hematuria
5. incontinence
6. nephrocystitis
7. nocturia
8. ureteroplasty
9. urinalysis
10. urobilin

MATCHING
1. d   2. e
3. b   4. f
5. a   6. g
7. j   8. c
9. h   10. i

ABBREVIATIONS
1. ARF
2. blood urea nitrogen
3. CRF
4. cystoscopy
5. genitourinary
6. hemodialysis
7. IVP
8. peritoneal dialysis
9. hydrogen ion concentration
10. UA

DIAGNOSTIC AND LABORATORY TESTS

1. c   2. c
3. b   4. c
5. b

PRACTICAL APPLICATION

1. yellow to amber
2. weight of a substance compared with an equal amount of water; urine has a specific gravity of 1.003–1.030
3. higher
4. yes
5. early warning of hepatic or hemolytic disease

• CHAPTER 13

ANATOMY AND PHYSIOLOGY LABELING

1. hypohysis (pituitary) gland
2. thyroid and parathyroid gland
3. adrenal gland
4. testis (male)
5. ovary (female)
6. pancreas
7. thymus gland
8. pineal gland

ANATOMY AND PHYSIOLOGY

1. a. pituitary
   b. pineal
   c. thyroid
   d. parathyroid
   e. islets of Langerhans
   f. adrenals
   g. ovaries
   h. testes
2. involves the production and regulation of chemical substances (hormones) that play an essential role in maintaining homeostasis
3. chemical transmitter that is released in small amounts and transported via the bloodstream to a targeted organ or other cells
4. synthesizes and secretes releasing hormones, releasing factors, release-inhibiting hormones, and release-inhibiting factors
5. because of its regulatory effects on the other endocrine glands
6. a. growth hormone (GH)
   b. adrenocorticotropin (ACTH)
   c. thyroid-stimulating hormone (TSH)
   d. follicle-stimulating hormone (FSH)
   e. luteinizing hormone (LH)
   f. prolactin (PRL)
   g. melanocyte-stimulating hormone (MSH)
7. a. antidiuretic hormone (ADH)
   b. oxytocin
8. melatonin … serotonin
9. plays a vital role in metabolism and regulates the body's metabolic processes
10. a. thyroxine (T4)
    b. triiodothyronine (T3)
    c. calcitonin
11. serum calcium … phosphorus
12. blood sugar
13. glucocorticoids, mineralocorticoids, and the androgens
14. a. regulates carbohydrate, protein, and fat metabolism
    b. stimulates output of glucose from the liver (gluconeogenesis)
    c. increases the blood sugar level
    d. regulates other physiological body processes

*Optional answers to question 14:

   e. promotes the transport of amino acids into extracellular tissue

   f. influences the effectiveness of catecholamines such as dopamine, epinephrine, and norepinephrine
   g. has an anti-inflammatory effect
   h. helps the body cope during times of stress
15. a. use of carbohydrates
    b. absorption of glucose
    c. gluconeogenesis
    d. potassium and sodium metabolism
16. Aldosterone
17. substance or hormone that promotes the development of male characteristics
18. a. dopamine
    b. epinephrine
    c. norepinephrine
19. a. elevates the systolic blood pressure
    b. increases the heart rate and cardiac output
    c. Increases glycogenolysis, thereby hastening release of glucose from the liver. This action elevates the blood sugar level and provides the body with a spurt of energy.

*Optional answers to question 19:

   d. dilates the bronchial tubes
   e. dilates the pupils
20. estrogen … progesterone
21. testosterone
22. a. thymosin
    b. thymopoietin
23. a. gastrin
    b. secretin
    c. pancreozymincholecystokinin
    d. enterogastrone

WORD PARTS

Prefixes
1. through
2. within

3. good, normal
4. out, away from
5. out, away from
6. excessive
7. deficient, under
8. beside
9. before
10. upon
11. water

Roots and Combining Forms
1. acid
2. extremity, point
3. gland
4. gland
5. cortex
6. flesh
7. cretin
8. man
9. to secrete
10. to secrete
11. small
12. milk
13. old age
14. giant
15. little acorn
16. sweet, sugar
17. seed
18. hairy
19. insulin
20. cortex
21. insulin
22. potassium
23. drowsiness
24. study of
25. mucus
26. eye
27. pine cone
28. kidney
29. pituitary gland
30. kidney
31. kidney
32. mad desire
33. thymus
34. to bear
35. thyroid, shield
36. thyroid, shield
37. poison
38. nourishment
39. masculine
40. body

41. testicle
42. solid
43. thyroid, shield
44. vessel
45. to press
46. adrenal gland
47. adrenal gland
48. pancreas

Suffixes
1. pertaining to
2. formation, produce
3. pertaining to
4. to go
5. surgical excision
6. swelling
7. blood condition
8. formation, produce
9. condition
10. pertaining to
11. condition
12. one who specializes
13. inflammation
14. study of
15. hormone
16. enlargement, large
17. resemble
18. tumor
19. condition
20. disease
21. substance
22. growth
23. chemical
24. flow, discharge
25. pertaining to

IDENTIFYING MEDICAL TERMS
1. adenosis
2. cretinism
3. diabetes
4. endocrinology
5. euthyroid
6. exocrine
7. gigantism
8. glucocorticoid
9. hyperkalemia
10. hypogonadism
11. lethargic
12. thymitis

SPELLING
1. catecholamines
2. cretinism
3. exophthalmic
4. hypothyroidism
5. myxedema
6. pineal
7. pituitary
8. thyroid
9. oxytocin
10. virilism

MATCHING
1. e   2. f
3. b   4. g
5. h   6. i
7. c   8. j
9. d   10. a

ABBREVIATIONS
1. BMR
2. DM
3. fasting blood sugar
4. glucose tolerance tests
5. PBI
6. parathyroid hormone (parathormone)
7. radioimmunoassay
8. STH
9. thyroid function studies
10. vasopressin

DIAGNOSTIC AND LABORATORY TESTS
1. a   2. c
3. c   4. b
5. c

PRACTICAL APPLICATION
1. because his dad and grandfather both take insulin
2. Hb A1C and FBS
3. thirsty (polydipsia), hungry (polyphagia), and urinating (polyuria) a lot
4. fasting blood sugar
5. 25

• CHAPTER 14

ANATOMY AND PHYSIOLOGY LABELING

1. cerebrum
2. frontal lobe
3. parietal lobe
4. occipital lobe
5. cerebellum
6. spinal cord
7. medulla
8. pons
9. temporal lobe
10. lateral fissure

ANATOMY AND PHYSIOLOGY

1. **a.** central
   b. peripheral
2. Neurons
3. long process reaching from the cell body to the area to be activated
4. resembles the branches of a tree and has short, unsheathed processes that transmit impulses to the cell body
5. sensory nerves transmit impulses to the central nervous system
6. **a.** single elongated process
   b. bundle of nerve fibers
   c. groups of nerve fibers
7. brain … spinal cord
8. **a.** dura mater
   b. arachnoid
   c. pia mater
9. **a.** cerebrum
   b. diencephalon
   c. midbrain
   d. cerebellum
   e. pons
   f. medulla oblongata
   g. reticular formation
10. frontal lobe
11. somesthetic area
12. auditory … language
13. vision
14. **a.** relay center for all sensory impulses
    b. relays motor impulses from the cerebellum to the cortex
15. **a.** is a regulator
    b. produces neurosecretions
    c. produces hormones
16. sensory perception and motor output
17. **a.** regulates and controls breathing
    b. regulates and controls swallowing
    c. regulates and controls coughing
    d. regulates and controls sneezing
    e. regulates and controls vomiting
18. **a.** conducts sensory impulses
    b. conducts motor impulses
    c. is a reflex center
19. 120 … 150
20. **a.** controls sweating
    b. controls the secretions of glands
    c. controls arterial blood pressure
    d. controls smooth muscle tissue
21. **a.** sympathetic
    b. parasympathetic

WORD PARTS

Prefixes

1. lack of
2. lack of
3. star-shaped
4. slow
5. down
6. difficult
7. upon
8. half
9. water
10. excessive
11. within
12. small
13. little
14. beside
15. beside
16. many
17. four
18. below

Roots and Combining Forms

1. to walk
2. dura, hard
3. head
4. side
5. little brain
6. cerebrum
7. color
8. shaken violently
9. skull
10. skull
11. cell
12. tree
13. a disk
14. dura, hard
15. electricity
16. brain
17. brain
18. feeling
19. numbness, sleep, stupor
20. knot
21. glue
22. sleep
23. globus pallidus
24. thin plate
25. lobe
26. study of
27. membrane, meninges
28. membrane, meninges
29. membrane, meninges
30. mind
31. memory
32. bone marrow, spinal cord
33. bone marrow, spinal cord
34. muscle
35. nerve
36. nerve
37. nerve
38. papilla
39. dusky
40. gray
41. hardening
42. a thorn
43. vertebra
44. sleep

45. sympathy
46. vagus, wandering
47. ventricle

Suffixes
1. pertaining to
2. condition of pain
3. pain
4. pertaining to
5. weakness
6. germ cell
7. hernia
8. cell
9. binding
10. surgical excision
11. swelling
12. feeling
13. glue
14. mark, record
15. instrument for recording
16. recording
17. condition
18. pertaining to
19. process
20. condition
21. one who specializes
22. inflammation
23. motion, movement
24. motion
25. seizure
26. a sheath, husk
27. diction, word, phrase
28. study of
29. nourishment, development
30. measurement
31. visual examination, to view, examine
32. tumor
33. condition
34. weakness
35. disease
36. to eat, swallow
37. speak, speech
38. action
39. nourishment
40. order, coordination
41. incision
42. pertaining to
43. condition

IDENTIFYING MEDICAL TERMS
1. amnesia
2. analgesia
3. aphagia
4. ataxia
5. cephalalgia
6. cerebellar
7. craniectomy
8. dyslexia
9. encephalitis
10. epidural
11. hemiparesis
12. meningitis
13. neuralgia
14. neuritis
15. neurocyte
16. neurology
17. neuroma
18. palsy
19. polyneuritis
20. somnambulism
21. vagotomy
22. ventriculometry

SPELLING
1. anesthesia
2. bradykinesia
3. cerebrospinal
4. craniotomy
5. epilepsy
6. meningioma
7. meningomyelocele
8. neuropathy
9. poliomyelitis
10. ventriculometry

MATCHING
1. g	2. d
3. c	4. b
5. e	6. h
7. j	8. f
9. a	10. i

ABBREVIATIONS
1. AD
2. ALS
3. central nervous system
4. cerebral palsy
5. CT
6. HDS
7. intracranial pressure
8. lumbar puncture
9. multiple sclerosis
10. PET

DIAGNOSTIC AND LABORATORY TESTS
1. a	2. b
3. c	4. d
5. c	

PRACTICAL APPLICATION
1. cognition
2. tremor
3. difficult articulation of speech
4. antiparkinsonism
5. used for palliative relief from such major symptoms of Parkinson's disease as bradykinesia, rigidity, tremor, and disorder of equilibrium and posture

• CHAPTER 15
ANATOMY AND PHYSIOLOGY LABELING
1. external auditory canal
2. auricle
3. malleus
4. incus
5. stapes
6. cochlea
7. eustachian tube
8. round window
9. tympanic membrane

ANATOMY AND PHYSIOLOGY
1. hearing … balance
2. external … middle … inner
3. auricle or pinna and the external acoustic meatus
4. auricle
5. **a.** to lubricate the ear
   b. to protect the ear

6. **a.** malleus (hammer)
   b. incus (anvil)
   c. stapes (stirrup)
7. mechanically transmit sound vibrations from the tympanic membrane to the oval window
8. **a.** transmits sound vibrations from the tympanic membrane to the cochlea
   b. equalizes external/internal air pressure on the tympanic membrane
9. cochlea, vestibule, and the semicircular canals
10. **a.** cochlear duct
    b. semicircular ducts
    c. utricle and saccule
11. organ of Corti
12. vestibule
13. acoustic or eighth cranial nerve
14. motion sickness
15. **a.** endolymph
    b. perilymph

WORD PARTS

Prefixes
1. within
2. within
3. around
4. twice
5. one

Roots and Combining Forms
1. hearing
2. to hear
3. to hear
4. hearing
5. the ear
6. gall, bile
7. land snail
8. electricity
9. maze, inner ear
10. maze, inner ear
11. larynx, voice box
12. study of
13. mastoid process, breast-shaped
14. fungus
15. eardrum, tympanic membrane
16. eardrum, tympanic membrane
17. nerve
18. ear
19. ear
20. pharynx
21. voice
22. old
23. pus
24. nose
25. hardening
26. stapes, stirrup
27. fat
28. drum
29. ear
30. window
31. middle
32. eardrum, tympanic membrane

Suffixes
1. pertaining to
2. pain
3. hearing
4. pain
5. surgical excision
6. a mark, record
7. recording
8. pertaining to
9. one who specializes
10. inflammation
11. stone
12. study of
13. serum, clear fluid
14. instrument to measure
15. measurement
16. resemble
17. tumor
18. condition
19. surgical repair
20. flow
21. instrument for examining
22. instrument to cut
23. incision
24. pertaining to
25. small
26. process
27. condition

IDENTIFYING MEDICAL TERMS
1. audiologist
2. audiometry
3. auditory
4. endaural
5. labyrinthitis
6. myringoplasty
7. myringotome
8. otodynia
9. otolaryngology
10. otopharyngeal
11. otoscope
12. perilymph
13. stapedectomy
14. tympanectomy
15. tinnitus

SPELLING
1. acoustic
2. audiology
3. cholesteatoma
4. electrocochleography
5. labyrinthitis
6. myringoplasty
7. otomycosis
8. otosclerosis
9. tympanic
10. tympanitis

MATCHING
1. h	2. e
3. i	4. a
5. g	6. b
7. j	8. c
9. d	10. f

ABBREVIATIONS
1. AC
2. BC
3. decibel
4. ENG
5. ear, nose, throat
6. HD
7. OM

DIAGNOSTIC AND LABORATORY TESTS
1. a   2. b
3. d   4. b
5. a

PRACTICAL APPLICATION
1. 102.2° F; pulling
2. otoscopy
3. analgesic/antipyretic; pain; fever
4. antibiotic; infection
5. acid; antibiotic

• CHAPTER 16
ANATOMY AND PHYSIOLOGY LABELING
1. cornea
2. pupil
3. iris
4. lens
5. vitreous humor
6. uvea
7. optic nerve
8. retina
9. choroid
10. sclera

ANATOMY AND PHYSIOLOGY
1. orbit, muscles, eyelids, conjunctiva, and the lacrimal apparatus
2. fatty tissue
3. optic nerve … ophthalmic artery
4. **a.** support
   b. rotary movement
5. intense light, foreign particles … impact
6. mucous membrane that acts as a protective covering for the exposed surface of the eyeball
7. structures that produce, store, and remove the tears that cleanse and lubricate the eye
8. eyeball, its structures, and the nerve fibers

9. vision
10. optic disk
11. process of sharpening the focus of light on the retina
12. Matching answers:
    1. c   **2.** e
    3. b   **4.** a
    5. f   **6.** d
    7. h   **8.** i
    9. j   **10.** g

WORD PARTS
Prefixes
1. lack of, without
2. two
3. in
4. in
5. inward
6. beyond
7. within
8. three
9. out
10. half
11. lack of
12. behind

Roots and Combining Forms
1. dull
2. to join together, conjunctiva
3. unequal
4. eyelid
5. eyelid
6. choroid
7. cold
8. pupil
9. cornea
10. ciliary body
11. ciliary body
12. to remove the kernel of
13. tear, lacrimal duct, tear duct
14. less, smaller
15. electricity
16. focus
17. angle
18. iris
19. iris
20. cornea
21. cornea
22. tear
23. study of

24. measure
25. to shut
26. muscle
27. night
28. eye
29. eye
30. eye
31. eye
32. eye
33. lens
34. lentil, lens
35. light
36. old
37. pupil
38. retina
39. retina
40. sclera, hardening
41. point
42. tone, tension
43. turn
44. uvea
45. foreign material
46. dry
47. dilation, widen
48. straight
49. disintegrate
50. to clot
51. radiating out from a center
52. lens
53. fiber
54. a squinting
55. hair

Suffixes
1. pertaining to
2. pertaining to
3. pertaining to
4. germ cell
5. condition
6. surgical excision
7. mark, record
8. recording
9. condition
10. pertaining to
11. specialist
12. process
13. condition
14. one who specializes
15. inflammation
16. study of
17. destruction, to separate

18. formation
19. instrument to measure
20. tumor
21. sight, vision
22. condition
23. disease
24. fear
25. surgical repair
26. stroke, paralysis
27. prolapse, drooping
28. instrument for examining
29. pertaining to
30. incision
31. structure

IDENTIFYING MEDICAL TERMS

1. amblyopia
2. bifocal
3. blepharoptosis
4. corneal
5. dacryoma
6. diplopia
7. emmetropia
8. intraocular
9. keratitis
10. keratoplasty
11. lacrimal
12. ocular
13. photophobia

SPELLING

1. astigmatism
2. cycloplegia
3. iridectomy
4. ophthalmologist
5. phacosclerosis
6. pupillary
7. retinoblastoma
8. scleritis
9. tonometer
10. uveal

MATCHING

1. e 2. f
3. j 4. h
5. c 6. d
7. g 8. b
9. a 10. i

ABBREVIATIONS

1. Acc
2. emmetropia
3. hypermetropia (hyperopia)
4. IOL
5. ST
6. myopia
7. visual acuity
8. intraocular pressure
9. VF
10. exotropia

DIAGNOSTIC AND LABORATORY TESTS

1. c 2. b
3. c 4. d
5. d

PRACTICAL APPLICATION

1. antibiotic to prevent/treat bacterial infection
2. antibiotic to prevent/treat bacterial infection
3. yes
4. anytime before the day of surgery
5. Tylenol

• CHAPTER 17

ANATOMY AND PHYSIOLOGY LABELING

1. fundus of uterus
2. bladder
3. clitoris
4. labia minora
5. vagina
6. labia majora
7. Bartholin's gland
8. rectum
9. cervix
10. sacrum

ANATOMY AND PHYSIOLOGY

1. a. ovaries
   b. fallopian tubes
   c. uterus
   d. vagina
   e. vulva
   f. breasts
2. anteflexion
3. rounded portion of the uterine body superior to the attachment of the fallopian tube
4. a. perimetrium
   b. myometrium
   c. endometrium
5. a. provides a place for the nourishment and development of the fetus during pregnancy
   b. contracts rhythmically and powerfully to help push out the fetus during the process of birthing
6. a. bent backward at an angle with the cervix usually unchanged from its normal position
   b. fundus forward toward the pubis with the cervix tilted up toward the sacrum
   c. bent backward with the cervix pointing forward toward the symphysis pubis
7. uterine tubes or oviducts
8. fertilization
9. a. production of ova
   b. production of hormones
10. a. female organ of copulation
    b. passageway for discharge of menstruation
    c. passageway for birth of the fetus
11. mammary glands
12. areola … nipple
13. thin yellowish secretion containing mainly serum and white blood cells; the "first milk"
14. a. follicular phase
    b. ovulation
    c. luteal phase

OVERVIEW OF OBSTETRICS

1. Obstetrics
2. Fertilization
3. zygote
4. yolk sac and amniotic cavity
5. **a.** time period from conception to onset of labor
   b. last phase of pregnancy to the time of delivery
   c. act of giving birth, also known as *childbirth* or *delivery*
   d. the 6 weeks following childbirth and expulsion of the placenta
6. **a.** begins from the onset of true labor and lasts until the cervix is fully dilated to 10 cm
   b. continues after the cervix is dilated to 10 cm until the delivery of the baby
   c. delivery of the placenta

WORD PARTS

Prefixes
1. lack of
2. against
3. difficult, painful
4. out
5. within
6. within
7. scanty
8. around
9. after
10. backward
11. before

Roots and Combining Forms
1. to miscarry
2. Bartholin's glands
3. receive
4. cervix, neck
5. a coming together
6. vagina
7. cul-de-sac
8. bladder
9. fibrous tissue
10. belonging to birth
11. female
12. hymen
13. womb, uterus
14. womb, uterus
15. to shine
16. study of
17. breast
18. breast
19. month, menses, menstruation
20. month, menses, menstruation
21. womb, uterus
22. womb, uterus
23. muscle
24. ovum, egg
25. ovary
26. ovary
27. to bear
28. cessation
29. rectum
30. fallopian tube
31. fallopian tube
32. uterus
33. vagina
34. sexual intercourse
35. turning
36. lump
37. lying beside, sexual intercourse

Suffixes
1. pertaining to
2. beginning
3. hernia
4. surgical puncture
5. surgical excision
6. formation, produce
7. condition
8. pertaining to
9. process
10. one who specializes
11. inflammation
12. tumor
13. condition
14. surgical repair
15. to burst forth
16. flow
17. instrument for examining
18. resemble

IDENTIFYING MEDICAL TERMS
1. cervicitis
2. dysmenorrhea
3. fibroma
4. gynecology
5. hymenectomy
6. mammoplasty
7. menorrhea
8. oogenesis
9. dyspareunia
10. genitalia

SPELLING
1. bartholinitis
2. hysterotomy
3. menorrhagia
4. oophorectomy
5. salpingitis
6. vaginitis
7. venereal
8. menarche
9. oligomenorrhea
10. postcoital

MATCHING
1. e.   2. b.
3. a   4. c.
5. d   6. h
7. j   8. g
9. i   10. f

ABBREVIATIONS
1. abdominal hysterectomy
2. diethylstilbestrol
3. BCP
4. IUD
5. PID
6. CIN
7. dysfunctional uterine bleeding
8. premenstrual syndrome
9. D&C
10. TSS

DIAGNOSTIC AND LABORATORY TESTS
1. a   2. c
3. d   4. b
5. d

PRACTICAL APPLICATION

1. GYN
2. hot flashes
3. dyspareunia
4. two pregnancies
5. rule out uterine fibroid tumor

• CHAPTER 18

ANATOMY AND PHYSIOLOGY LABELING

1. bladder
2. vas deferens
3. seminal vesicles
4. prostate
5. urethra
6. epididymis

ANATOMY AND PHYSIOLOGY

1. **a.** testes
   b. various ducts
   c. urethra
   d. bulbourethral gland
   e. prostate gland
   f. seminal vesicles
2. **a.** scrotum
   b. penis
3. provide the sperm cells necessary to fertilize the ovum, thereby perpetuating the species
4. glans penis
5. loose skin folds that cover the penis
6. lubricating fluid
7. **a.** male organ of copulation
   b. site of the orifice for the elimination of urine and semen from the body
8. seminiferous tubules
9. **a.** responsible for the development of secondary male characteristics during puberty
   b. essential for normal growth and development of the male accessory sex organs

c. plays a vital role in the erection process of the penis
   d. affects the growth of hair on the face
   e. affects muscular development and vocal timbre
10. **a.** storage site for sperm
    b. duct for the passage of sperm
11. vas deferens or ductus deferens
12. production of a slightly alkaline fluid
13. about 4 cm wide and weighs about 20 g; composed of glandular, connective, and muscular tissues and lies behind the urinary bladder
14. enlargement of the prostate that can occur in older men
15. bulbourethral … Cowper's
16. **a.** prostatic
    b. membranous
    c. penile
17. transmits urine and semen out of the body
18. 20

WORD PARTS

Prefixes

1. lack of
2. lack of
3. around
4. upon
5. water
6. under
7. scanty
8. beside
9. into
10. good
11. different
12. similar, same
13. three

Roots and Combining Forms

1. glans penis
2. to cut
3. hidden

4. not natural
5. testis
6. to pour
7. testicle
8. testicle
9. testicle
10. a muzzle
11. prostate
12. to prune
13. a rent (opening)
14. seed
15. seed, semen
16. seed, sperm
17. seed, sperm
18. testicle
19. twisted vein
20. vessel
21. vesicle
22. animal
23. life
24. to throw out
25. genitals
26. female
27. breast
28. sex
29. thread
30. body

Suffixes

1. pertaining to
2. pertaining to
3. immature cell, germ cell
4. hernia, swelling, tumor
5. to kill
6. surgical excision
7. formation, produce
8. condition
9. process
10. condition
11. inflammation
12. use
13. condition
14. formation, produce
15. flow
16. incision
17. pertaining to

IDENTIFYING MEDICAL TERMS

1. balanitis
2. epididymectomy

3. orchidectomy
4. prepuce
5. hydrocele
6. condyloma
7. spermatoblast
8. spermatozoon
9. spermicide
10. testicular

SPELLING

1. cryptorchidism
2. hypospadias
3. orchidotomy
4. eugenics
5. vasectomy
6. chlamydia
7. gonorrhea
8. syphilis
9. trichomoniasis
10. papillomavirus

MATCHING

1. e	2. c
3. f	4. b
5. g	6. i
7. h	8. k
9. a	10. d

ABBREVIATIONS

1. BPH
2. gonorrhea
3. HPV
4. herpes simplex virus–2
5. sexually transmitted diseases
6. ED
7. transurethral resection of the prostate
8. nongonococcal urethritis
9. VD
10. PSA

DIAGNOSTIC AND LABORATORY TESTS

1. c	2. a
3. b	4. c
5. c	

PRACTICAL APPLICATION

1. Herpes
2. 14 and 49

3. yes
4. 80
5. visible

• CHAPTER 19

AN OVERVIEW OF CANCER

1. **a.** carcinomas
   b. sarcomas
   c. mixed cancers
2. process in which normal cells have a distinct appearance and specialized function
3. process in which normal cells lose their specialization and become malignant
4. **a.** active migration
   b. direct extension
   c. metastasis
5. **a.** Change in bowel or bladder habits
   b. Sore that does not heal
   c. Unusual bleeding or discharge
   d. Thickening or lump in breast or elsewhere
   e. Indigestion or difficulty in swallowing
   f. Obvious change in a wart or mole
   g. Nagging cough or hoarseness
6. **a.** surgery
   b. chemotherapy
   c. radiation therapy
   d. immunotherapy

WORD PARTS

Prefixes

1. up, apart, backward
2. star-shaped
3. excessive
4. new
5. little
6. before
7. in
8. in
9. beyond
10. short

Roots and Combining Forms

1. gland
2. vessel
3. cancer, crab
4. cancer
5. cancer
6. cartilage
7. chorion
8. cell
9. tree
10. fiber
11. glue
12. glue
13. blood
14. safe
15. smooth
16. white
17. white
18. fat
19. lymph
20. lymph
21. marrow
22. black
23. meninges, membrane
24. mucus
25. fungus
26. bone marrow
27. muscle
28. a little box
29. kidney
30. nerve
31. tumor
32. bone
33. net
34. retina
35. rod
36. flesh
37. to lead
38. seed
39. mouth
40. monster
41. thymus
42. poison
43. grating

Suffixes

1. immature cell
2. blood condition
3. formation, produce
4. formation, produce
5. formation, produce

6. condition
7. substance
8. inflammation
9. tumor
10. pertaining to
11. plate
12. formation
13. a thing formed
14. use, action
15. treatment
16. pertaining to
17. pertaining to
18. pertaining to
19. process
20. nature of
21. forming
22. control
23. resemble

IDENTIFYING MEDICAL TERMS

1. carcinogen
2. chondrosarcoma
3. glioma
4. leiomyosarcoma
5. leukemia
6. lymphoma
7. melanoma
8. myosarcoma
9. Wilms' tumor
10. sarcoma

SPELLING

1. anaplasia
2. fibrosarcoma
3. lymphosarcoma
4. myeloma
5. oncogenic
6. seminoma
7. teletherapy
8. teratoma
9. trismus
10. xerostomia

MATCHING

1. e   2. i
3. d   4. g
5. c   6. f
7. j   8. b
9. h   10. a

ABBREVIATIONS

1. Adeno-CA
2. Bx
3. cancer
4. chemotherapy
5. DNA
6. internal radiation therapy
7. ALL
8. DCIS
9. breast cancer gene
10. TNM

PRACTICAL APPLICATION

1. new growth or tumor, may be benign or malignant
2. basal cell carcinoma
3. to reveal that the neoplastic process appears to be totally excised
4. right shoulder
5. centimeter

• CHAPTER 20

AN OVERVIEW OF RADIOLOGY AND NUCLEAR MEDICINE

1. scientific discipline of medical imaging using radionuclides, ionizing radiation, nuclear magnetic resonance, and ultrasound
2. **a.** invisible
   b. cause ionization
   c. cause fluorescence

*Alternate characteristics to those listed:

   d. allow the x-ray beam to be directed at a specific site or to produce high-quality shadow images on film
   e. able to penetrate substances
   f. destroy cells
3. **a.** can depress the hematopoietic system, cause leukopenia, leukemia

   b. can damage the gonads
4. **a.** wearing a film badge
   b. lead screens
   c. lead-lined room
   d. protective clothing
   e. gonad shield
5. **a.** computed tomography
   b. magnetic resonance imaging
   c. ultrasound
   d. thermography
   e. scintigraphy

WORD PARTS

Prefixes

1. below
2. within
3. one-thousandth
4. beyond
5. into

Roots and Combining Forms

1. acting
2. vessel
3. finger or toe
4. artery
5. joint
6. bronchi
7. heart
8. gall, bile
9. gall
10. motion
11. motion
12. to draw
13. curie
14. bladder
15. skin
16. echo
17. brain
18. fluorescence
19. kind
20. uterus
21. ion
22. ion
23. nucleus
24. study of
25. to shine
26. lymph
27. breast
28. spinal cord
29. to swing

30. dark
31. light
32. nature
33. renal pelvis
34. radiant
35. ray, x-ray
36. roentgen
37. fallopian tube
38. salivary
39. sound
40. sound
41. hot, heat
42. to cut
43. vein
44. vein

Suffixes
1. one who
2. formation, produce
3. pertaining to
4. record
5. instrument for recording
6. recording
7. pertaining to
8. process
9. one who specializes
10. inflammation
11. nature of
12. study of
13. instrument to measure
14. pertaining to
15. instrument for examining
16. visual examination, to view, examine
17. treatment
18. having a particular quality

IDENTIFYING MEDICAL TERMS
1. angiography
2. arthrography
3. cholecystogram
4. ionotherapy
5. mammography
6. millicurie
7. physicist
8. radiation
9. radioactive
10. radiographer
11. radiolucent

12. radiopaque
13. sonogram

SPELLING
1. hysterosalpingogram
2. echography
3. lymphangiography
4. myelogram
5. cassette
6. radioactive
7. radiography
8. sialography
9. tomography
10. venography

MATCHING
1.	d	2.	e
3.	c	4.	g
5.	j	6.	k
7.	b	8.	i
9.	a	10.	h

ABBREVIATIONS
1. AP
2. Ba
3. CT
4. interventional radiology
5. lateral
6. radium
7. MRI
8. posteroanterior
9. Ci
10. positron emission tomography

PRACTICAL APPLICATION
1. a specific type of imaging that uses a low-dose x-ray system for examination of the breasts
2. because if there is a finding on the mammogram it needs to be compared to previous mammograms
3. there is a finding on the mammogram that requires further tests for a more thorough evaluation
4. no evidence of cancer
5. the referring physician or other health care provider

• CHAPTER 21

AN OVERVIEW: MENTAL HEALTH AND MENTAL ILLNESS
1. Mental illness
2. **a.** major depression
   b. bipolar disorder
   c. schizophrenia
3. Psychiatry
4. **a.** drug therapy
   b. psychotherapy
   c. electroconvulsive therapy
5. Psychoanalysis

WORD PARTS
Prefixes
1. lack of, without
2. deficient, below
3. beside, abnormal
4. fire

Roots and Combining Forms
1. marketplace
2. self
3. center
4. circle, cycle
5. to cheat
6. I, self
7. to wander in mind
8. treatment
9. study of
10. nerve
11. disease
12. mind
13. mind
14. mind
15. to divide
16. body
17. body
18. mind, emotion

Suffixes
1. shape
2. condition
3. pertaining to
4. process
5. condition
6. one who specializes
7. study of

8. madness
9. mind
10. appetite
11. condition
12. fear
13. treatment
14. pertaining to

IDENTIFYING MEDICAL TERMS

1. agoraphobia
2. apathy
3. delusion
4. depression
5. egocentric
6. mania
7. phobia
8. psychiatrist
9. psychotherapy
10. pyromania

SPELLING

1. anxiety
2. autism
3. bulimia
4. dementia
5. factitious

6. hallucination
7. paranoia
8. psychosomatic
9. schizophrenia
10. somatoform

MATCHING

1. d   2. g
3. c   4. a
5. f   6. b
7. i   8. e
9. h   10. j

ABBREVIATIONS

1. CBT
2. DSM-IV-TR
3. electroconvulsive therapy
4. Minnesota Multiphasic Personality Inventory
5. NIMH
6. obsessive–compulsive disorder
7. PTSD
8. seasonal affective disorder
9. Thematic Apperception Test
10. WHO

PRACTICAL APPLICATION

1. feels sick all the time, too weak and tired, dizzy and depressed, to do anything except "rest"
2. proventil inhaler for relief of asthmatic symptoms, analgesics, decongestants, and two different forms of tricyclic antidepressants
3. a fixed, false belief or abnormal perception held by a person despite evidence to the contrary
4. process of experiencing sensations that have no source
5. disorder that is not real, genuine, or natural; the physical and psychological symptoms are produced by the person to place him- or herself or another in the role of a patient or someone in need of help

Glossary of Word Parts

APPENDIX II

PREFIXES

Prefix	Meaning
a-	no, not, without, lack of, apart
ab-	away from
ad-	toward, near
ambi-	both, both sides, around, about
an-	no, not, without, lack of
ana-	up, apart, backward, again, anew
ant-	against
ante-	before, forward
anti-	against
apo-	separation
astro-	star-shaped
auto-	self
bi-	two, double
bin-	twice, two
brachy-	short
brady-	slow
cac-	bad
centi-	one hundred, one hundredth
chromo-	color
circum-	around
con-	with, together
contra-	against, opposite
de-	down, away from
deca-	ten
di-	two, double
di(a)-	through, between, complete
dia-	through, between, complete
dif-	apart, free from, separate
di(s)-	two, apart
dis-	apart
dys-	bad, difficult, painful, abnormal
ec-	out, outside, outer
ecto-	out, outside, outer
em-	in
en-	in, within
end-	within, inner
endo-	within, inner
ep-	upon, over, above
epi-	upon, over, above
eso-	inward
eu-	good, normal
ex-	out, away from
exo-	out, away from
extra-	outside, beyond
hemi-	half
heter-	different
hetero-	different
homeo-	similar, same, likeness, constant
homo-	similar, same
hydr-	water
hydro-	water
hyp-	below, deficient
hyper-	above, beyond, excessive
hypo-	below, under, deficient
in-	in, into, not
infer-	below
inter-	between
intra-	within
ir-	not
mal-	bad
mega-	large, great
meso-	middle
meta-	beyond, over, between, change
micro-	small
milli-	one-thousandth
mon(o)-	one
mono-	one
multi-	many, much
neo-	new
nulli-	none
olig-	little, scanty
oligo-	little, scanty
pan-	all
par-	around, beside
para-	beside, along side, abnormal
per-	through
peri-	around
poly-	many, much, excessive
post-	after, behind
pre-	before, in front of
primi-	first
pro-	before, in front of
proto-	first
pseudo-	false
pyro-	fire
quadri-	four
re-	back, backward, again
retro-	backward

semi-	half	sym-	together, with	tri-	three
sub-	below, under, beneath	syn-	together, with	ultra-	beyond
supra-	above, beyond, superior	tachy-	rapid, fast	un-	back, reversal, not, annulment
super-	upper, above	trans-	across	uni-	one

WORD ROOTS/COMBINING FORMS

abdomin	abdomen	ambly, ambly/o	dull	arter, arter/i, arteri/o	artery
abort, abort/o	to miscarry	ambul	to walk	arthr, arthr/o	joint, to articulate
absorpt, absorpt/o	to suck in	amni/o	amniotic fluid	artific/i	not natural
acanth	thorn	ampere	ampere	aspirat, aspirat/o	to draw in
acetabul, acetabul/o	acetabulum, hip socket	amputat, amputat/o	to cut through	atel, atel/o	imperfect
acid, acid/o	acid	amyl, amyl/o	starch	ather, ather/o	fatty substance, porridge
acoust	hearing	anabol, anabol/o	building up		
acr, acr/o	extremity, point	anastom	opening	atri, atri/o	atrium
act, act/o	acting, act	andr, andr/o	man	aud/i, audi/o	to hear
actin	ray	ang, ang/i	vessel	auditor	hearing
acute	sharp	angin, angin/o	to choke	aur, aur/i	ear
aden, aden/o	gland	angi/o	vessel	auscultat, auscultat/o	listen to
adhes	stuck to	anis/o	unequal	aut	self
adip, adip/o	fat	ankyl, ankyl/o	stiffening, crooked	axill	armpit
adren, adren/o	adrenal gland	an/o	anus	bacter/i	bacteria
agglutinat	clumping	anter, anter/o	toward the front	balan, balan/o	glans penis
agglutin/o	clumping	anthrac, anthrac/o	coal	bartholin	Bartholin's glands
agon, agon/o	agony	aort, aort/o	aorta	bas/o	base
agor/a	marketplace	append, append/o	appendix	bil, bil/i	bile, gall
albin, albin/o	white	appendic, appendic/o	appendix	bi/o	life
albumin, albumin/o	protein	arachn	spider	blast/o	germ cell
aliment, aliment/o	nourishment	arche	beginning	blephar, blephar/o	eyelid
all, all/o	other	arous	alertness, to rise	brach/i	arm
alveol, alveol/o	small, hollow air sac			bronch, bronch/i, bronch/o	bronchi
				bronchiol, bronchiol/o	bronchiole

bucc,		choledoch/o	common	constipat	to press
bucc/o	cheek		bile duct		together
burs,		chondr,		continence	to hold
burs/o	pouch	chondr/o	cartilage	cor, cor/o	pupil
calc, calc/i,		chord	cord	cord/o	cord
calc/o	lime, calcium	chori/o	chorion	coriat	corium
calcan/e	heel bone	choroid,		corne,	
cancer,		choroid/o	choroid	corne/o	cornea
cancer/o	crab, cancer	chromat,		corpor,	
capn	smoke	chromat/o	color	corpor/e	body
capsul,		chrom/o	color	cortic,	
capsul/o	little box	chym	juice	cortic/o	cortex
carcin,		cine	motion	cortis	cortex
carcin/o	cancer	cinemat/o	motion	cost, cost/o	rib
card, card/i,		circulat,		cox	hip
cardi/o	heart	circulat/o	circular	crani,	
carp,		cirrh,		cran/i,	
carp/o	wrist	cirrh/o	orange-yellow	crani/o	skull
cartil	gristle	cis, cis/o	to cut	creat	flesh
cartilagin/o	cartilage	claudicat,		creatin	flesh, creatine
castr	to prune	claudicat/o	to limp	crine, crin/o	to secrete
catabol,	casting	clavicul,	clavicle,	crur	leg
catabol/o	down	clavicul/o	collar bone	cry/o	cold
caud,		cleid/o	clavicle	crypt,	
caud/o	tail	clon/o	turmoil	crypt/o	hidden
caus, caus/o	heat	coagul,		cubit	elbow, to lie
cavit	cavity	coagulat,		culd/o	cul-de-sac
celi,	abdomen,	coagul/o	to clot	curie	curie
celi/o	belly	coccyg/e,	coccyx,	cutane,	
cellul,		coccyg/o	tailbone	cutan/e,	
cellul/o	little cell	cochle/o	land snail	cutane/o	skin
centr,		coit, coit/o	coming	cyan, cyan/o	dark blue
centr/i,			together	cycl, cycl/o	ciliary body
centr/o	center	col, col/o	colon		of eye, circle,
centrat	center	coll/a	glue		cycle
cephal,		collis	neck	cyst, cyst/o	bladder, sac
cephal/o	head	colon,		cyt, cyt/o	cell
cept	receive	colon/o	colon	cyth	cell
cerebell,		colp/o	vagina	dacry,	tear, lacrimal
cerebell/o	little brain	comat	a deep sleep	dacry/o	duct, tear duct
cerebr/o	cerebrum	compensat	to make good	dactyl,	
cervic,		concuss	shaken	dactyl/o	finger or toe
cervic/o	cervix, neck		violently	defecat	to remove
cheil,		condyle	knuckle		dregs
cheil/o	lip	con/i	dust	delus,	
chem/o	chemical	conjunctiv,	conjunctiva,	delus/o	to cheat
chir/o	hand	conjunctiv/o	to join together	dem	people
chlor/o	green	connect	to bind	dendr/o	tree
chol, chole,			together	dent, dent/i,	
chol/e	gall, bile	consci	aware	dent/o	tooth

derm, derm/a, derm/o	skin
dermat, dermat/o	skin
dextr/o	to the right
diaphrag- mat/o	diaphragm, partition
didym, didym/o	testis
digit, digit/o	finger or toe
dilat, dilat/o	to widen
dipl/o	double
disk, disk/o	disk
dist, dist/o	away from the point of origin
diverticul, diverticul/o	diverticula
dors, dors/i, dors/o	backward
duct, duct/o	to lead
duoden, duoden/o	duodenum
dur, dur/o	dura, hard
dwarf	small
dynam, dynam/o	power
ech/o	echo, reflected sound
ectop	displaced
eg/o	I, self
ejaculat, ejaculat/o	to throw out
electr/o	electricity
embol, embol/o	to cast, to throw
eme	to vomit
emulsificat	disintegrate
encephal, encephal/o	brain
enchyma	to pour
enter/o	intestines (usually small intestine)
enucleat	to remove the kernel of

eosin/o	rose-colored
episi/o	vulva, pudenda
erget	work
erg/o	work
eructat	breaking out
erysi	red
erythr/o	red
esophag/e	esophagus
esophage/o	esophagus
esthesi/o	feeling, sensation
esthet	feeling, sensation
estr/o	mad desire
eti/o	cause
excret/o, excretor	sifted out
fasc	band (fascia)
fasci/o	band (fascia)
febr	fever
femor, femor/o	femur, thigh bone
fenestrat	window
fibr, fibr/o	fibrous tissue, fiber
fibrillat	fibrils (small fibers)
fibrin/o	fiber
fibul, fibul/o	fibula
filtrat, filtrat/o	to strain through
fixat, fixat/o	fastened
flex	to bend
fluor/o	fluorescence, luminous
foc, foc/o	focus
follicul, follicul/o	little bag
format	shaping
fungat	mushroom, fungus
furc	fork
fus, fus/o	to pour
galact/o	milk
ganglion	knot
gastr, gastr/o	stomach
gen, gene,	formation,

genet	produce
genital	belonging to birth
gen/o	kind
ger, ger/o	old age
gester	to bear
gigant, gigant/o	giant
gingiv, gingiv/o	gums
glandul	little acorn
gli, gli/o	glue
globin	globule
glob, globul, globul/o	globe
glomerul, glomerul/o	glomerulus, little ball
gloss/o	tongue
gluc/o	sweet, sugar
glyc, glyc/o, glycos, glycos/o	glucose, sweet, sugar
gnost	knowledge
gonad, gonad/o	seed
goni/o	angle
gon/o	genitals
grand/i	great
granul/o	little grain, granular
gravida, gravidar	pregnancy
gryp	curve
gurgitat	to flood
gynec/o	female
halat, halat/o	breathe
halit/o	breath
hallucinat	to wander in mind
hallux	great (big) toe
hem, hem/o, hemat, hemat/o	blood
hemorrh, hemorrh/o	vein liable to bleed
hepat, hepat/o	liver

Word part	Meaning
herni/o	hernia
hidr, hidr/o	sweat
hirsut, hirsut/o	hairy
hist/o	tissue
hol/o	whole
horizont	horizon
humer, humer/o	humerus
hydr, hydr/o	water
hymen	hymen
hypn, hypn/o	sleep
hyster, hyster/o	womb, uterus
iatr	treatment
icter, icter/o	jaundice
ile, ile/o	ileum
ili, ili/o	ilium
illus	foot
immun/o	safe, immunity
infarct, infarct/o	infarct (necrosis of an area)
infect	to infect
infer, infer/o	below
inguin, inguin/o	groin
insul, insul/o	insulin
insulin/o	insulin
integument, integument/o	covering
intern	within
ionizat	ion (going)
ion/o	ion
iont/o	ion
irid, irid/o	iris
isch, isch/o	to hold back
ischi	ischium
is/o	equal
jaund	yellow
kal, kal/i	potassium
kary/o	cell's nucleus
kel, kel/o	tumor
kerat, kerat/o	horn, cornea
keton, keton/o	ketone
kil/o	one thousand
kinet	motion
kyph, kyph/o	hump
labi, labi/o	lip
labyrinth, labyrinth/o	maze
lacrim, lacrim/o	tear, lacrimal duct, tear duct
lamin, lamin/o	lamina, thin plate
lamp(s)	to shine
lapar/o	abdomen
laryng, laryng/e, laryng/o	larynx, voice box
later, later/o	side
laxat	to loosen
lei/o	smooth
lemma	rind, sheath, husk
lent, lent/o	lens
lept	seizure
letharg	drowsiness
leuk, leuk/a, leuk/o	white
levat	lifter
lingu, lingu/o	tongue
lip, lip/o	fat
lipid, lipid/o	fat
lith, lith/o	stone
lob, lob/o	lobe
lobul	small lobe
locat	to place
log	study
log/o	word
lopec	fox mange
lord, lord/o	bending, curve, swayback
lucent	to shine
lumb, lumb/o	loin, lower back
lump	lump
lun, lun/o	moon
lymph, lymph/o	lymph, clear fluid
macr/o	large
malign, malign/o	bad kind
mamm/o	breast
mandibul, mandibul/o	lower jawbone
man/o	thin
mast, mast/o	mastoid process, breast-shaped, breast
masticat	to chew
mat	to ripen
maxill, maxill/o	jawbone
maxilla	jaw
maxim	greatest
meat, meat/o	passage
med	middle
medi, medi/o	toward the middle
medull, medull/o	marrow
melan, melan/o	black
men, men/o	month, menses, menstruation
mening, mening/i, mening/o	membrane, meninges
menisc, menisc/i, menisc/o	meniscus, crescent-shaped
men/o	month, menses, menstruation
menstru	to discharge the menses
ment, ment/o	mind
mes, mes/o	middle
mester	month

metr,		occlus,		papill,	
metr/i,	to measure,	occlus/o	to close up	papill/o	papilla
metr/o	womb,	ocul, ocul/o	eye	paque	dark
	uterus	odont,		para	to bear,
micturit,		odont/o	tooth		bring forth
micturit/o	to urinate	olecran,		paralyt	to disable,
miliar	millet (tiny)	olecran/o	elbow		paralysis
minim	least	olfact/o	smell	pareun,	
mi/o	less, smaller	omphal/o	navel,	pareun/o	lying beside,
mit, mit/o	thread		umbilicus		sexual
mitr, mitr/o	mitral valve	onc/o	tumor		intercourse
mnes	memory	onych,		partum	labor
mucos,		onych/o	nail	parturit	in labor
mucos/o,		o/o	ovum, egg	patell,	
mucus	mucus	oophor,		patell/o	kneecap,
muscul,		oophor/o	ovary		patella
muscul/o	muscle	ophthalm,		path, path/o	disease
muta,		ophthalm/o	eye	pause	cessation
mutat,		opt, opt/o	eye	pector,	
mutat/o	to change	or, or/o	mouth	pector/o	chest
my, my/o	muscle	orch, orch/o	testicle	pector(at)	breast, chest
myc, myc/o	fungus	orchid,		ped, ped/o,	
mydriat	dilation,	orchid/o	testicle	ped/i	foot, child
	widen	organ,		pedicul,	
myel,		organ/o	organ	pedicul/o	louse
myel/o	bone marrow,	orth, orth/o	straight	pelv/i	pelvis
	spinal cord	oscill,		penile	penis
my/o,		oscill/o	to swing	pept, pept/o	to digest
my/o(s)	muscle	oste,		perine,	
myring,		oste/o	bone	perine/o	perineum
myring/o	eardrum,	ot, ot/o	ear	periton/e	peritoneum
	tympanic	ovar	ovary	phac,	
	membrane	ovul, ovulat	ovary	phac/o	lens
myx, myx/o	mucus	ox, ox/i,		phag,	
narc/o	numbness,	ox/o	oxygen	phag/o	to eat,
	sleep, stupor	oxy	sour, sharp,		engulf
nas/o	nose		acid	phak,	
nat, nat/o	birth			phak/o	lentil, lens
necr, necr/o	death	pachy,		phalang/e	phalanges,
nephr,		pachy/o	thick		finger/toe
nephr/o	kidney	palat/o	palate		bones
neur, neur/i,		palliat,			
neur/o	nerve	palliat/o	cloaked	pharyng,	
neutr/o	neither	pallid/o	globus	pharyng/e,	pharynx,
nid	nest		pallidus	pharyng/o	throat
noct, noct/o	night	palm	palm	phas	speech
nom	law	palp	touch	phen/o	to show
norm	rule	palpitat,		phe/o	dusky
nucl	nucleus	palpit/o	throbbing	phim	muzzle
nucle	kernel, nucleus	pancreat,		phleb,	
nyctal	night	pancreat/o	pancreas	phleb/o	vein

phon,	
phone	voice
phon/o	sound
phor	carrying
phos	light
phot/o	light
phragm	partition
phras	speech
phren,	
phren/o	mind
physic,	
physic/o	nature
pil/o	hair
pine	pine cone
pineal	pineal body
pin/o	to drink
pituitar	pituitary
	gland
plak, plak/o	plate
plasma,	
plasm/o	plasma
plast	developing
pleur,	
pleura,	
pleur/o	pleura
plicat	to fold
pneum/o	lung, air
pneumon,	
pneumon/o	lung
pod/o	foot
poiet	formation
poli/o	gray
pollex	thumb
por	passage
porphyr	purple
poster,	behind,
poster/o	toward the
	back, back
prand/i	meal
presby,	
presby/o	old
press	to press
proct,	anus and
proct/o	rectum
prophylact	guarding
prostat,	
prostat/o	prostate
prosth/e	an addition
proxim,	near the point
proxim/o	of origin

prurit,	
prurit/o	itching
psych,	
psych/o	mind
pudend	external
	genitals
pulm/o	lung
pulmon,	
pulmon/o	lung
pulmonar,	
pulmonar/o	lung
pupill,	
pupill/o	pupil
purpur	purple
py, py/o	pus
pyel,	
pyel/o	renal pelvis
pylor,	
pylor/o	pylorus,
	gatekeeper
pyret	fever
pyr/o	heat, fire
rach, rach/i	spine
radi/o	ray, x-ray
radiat	radiant
radic/o	spinal nerve
	root
radicul	spinal nerve
	root
ras	to scrape off
rect/o	rectum
regul	rule
relaxat	to loosen
remiss,	
remiss/o	remit
ren, ren/o	kidney
respirat,	
respirat/o	breathing
reticul/o	net
retin, retin/o	retina
rhabd/o	rod
rheumat,	
rheumat/o	discharge
rhin/o	nose
rhonch,	
rhonch/o	snore
rhytid/o	wrinkle
roent	roentgen
rotat,	
rotat/o	to turn

rrhyth,	
rrhythm,	
rrhythm/o	rhythm
rube/o	red
sacr, sacr/o	sacrum
salping,	
salping/o,	tube, fallopian
salpinx	tube
sarc, sarc/o	flesh
scapul,	shoulder
scapul/o	blade
schiz/o	to divide
scler, scler/o	hard, harden-
	ing, sclera
scoli, scoli/o	curvature
scop	to examine
seb/o	oil
secund	second
semin,	
semin/i	seed, semen
seminat	seed, semen
senil, senile	old
sept	putrefaction
septic,	
septic/o	putrefying
sept/o	a partition
ser(a), ser/o	whey, serum
sert	to gain
sexu	sex
sial, sial/o	saliva,
	salivary
sider/o	iron
sigmoid,	
sigmoid/o	sigmoid
sin/o	curve
sinus	a hollow
	curve
situ	place
som, somat,	
somat/o	body
somn,	
somn/o	sleep
son, son/o	sound
spadias	rent, opening
spastic	convulsive
sperm,	
sperm/i,	
sperm/o	seed (sperm)
spermat,	
spermat/o	seed (sperm)

sphygm/o	pulse	testicul,		ungu	nail
spin, spin/o	spine, thorn	testicul/o	testicle	ur, ur/o	urinate,
spir/o	breath	test/o	testicle		urination
splen/o	spleen	thalass	sea	urea	urea
spondyl,		thel/i	nipple	uret	urine
spondyl/o	vertebra	therm,		ureter,	
staped,		therm/o	hot, heat	ureter/o	ureter
staped/o	stapes, stirrup	thorac,		urethr,	
steat,		thorac/o	chest	urethr/o	urethra
steat/o	fat	thorax	chest	urin,	
sten, sten/o	narrowing	thromb,		urin/o	urine
ster	solid	thromb/o	clot	urinat	urine
stern,	sternum,	thym,	thymus, mind,	uter, uter/o	uterus
stern/o	breast bone	thym/o	emotion	uve, uve/o	uvea
sterol	solid (fat)	thyr, thyr/o	thyroid,	vagin,	
steth,			shield	vagin/o	vagina
steth/o	chest	thyrox	thyroid, shield	vag/o	vagus,
stigmat,		tibi, tibi/o	tibia		wandering
stigmat/o	point	toc	birth	valvul/o	valve
stom,		tom/o	to cut	varic/o	twisted vein
stom/o	mouth	ton, ton/o	tone, tension	vas, vas/o	vessel
stomat,		tonsill,		vascul,	
stomat/o	mouth	tonsill/o	tonsil, almond	vascul/o	small vessel
strabism	squinting	topic, top/o	place	vector	carrier
strict	to tighten,	tors, tors/o	twisted	ven, ven/i,	
	contraction	tort/i	twisted	ven/o	vein
suppress,		tox, tox/o	poison	venere,	sexual
suppress/o	suppress	toxic,		venere/o	intercourse
surrog	substitute	toxic/o	poison	ventilat,	
symmetric	symmetry	trach/e,		ventilat/o	to air
sympath	sympathy	trache/o	trachea	ventr,	near or
synov,	synovial	tract,		ventr/o	on the
synov/o	membrane	tract/o	to draw		belly side of
system	composite	trephinat	bore		the body
	whole	trich,		ventricul,	ventricle,
systol	contraction	trich/o	hair	ventricul/o	little belly
systole	contraction	trigon	trigone	vermin,	
tars/o	ankle, tarsus	trism	grating	verm/i	worm
tel	end, distant	trop, trop/o	turning	vers,	
tele	distant	troph,		vers/o	turning
tempor	temples	troph/o	a turning	vertebr,	
tendin	tendon	tuber	bulge	vertebr/o	vertebra
tend/o	tendon	tubercul,		vesic	bladder
tendon,		tubercul/o	little swelling	vesicul,	seminal
tendon/o	tendon	turg	swelling	vesicul/o	vesicle
ten/o	tendon	tuss	cough	vir, vir/o	virus (poison)
tenos	tendon	tympan,	eardrum,	viril,	
tens	tension	tympan/o	drum	viril/o	masculine
tentori	tentorium, tent	uln, uln/o	ulna, elbow	viscer,	
terat, terat/o	monster	umbilic	navel	viscer/o	body organs

volt	volt
volunt,	
volunt/o	will
volvul	to roll
vuls, vuls/o	to pull

watt	watt
xanth/o	yellow
xen, xen/o	foreign
	material
xer, xer/o	dry

xiph,	
xiph/o	sword
zo/o	animal
zoon	life

Suffixes

-able	capable
-ac	pertaining to
-act	to act
-ad	pertaining to
-age	related to
-al	pertaining to
-algesia	condition of pain
-algia	pain, ache
-ant	forming
-ar	pertaining to
-arche	beginning
-ary	pertaining to
-ase	enzyme
-asthenia	weakness
-ate, -ate(d)	use, action, having the form of, possessing
-betes	to go
-blast	immature cell, germ cell, embryonic cell
-body	body
-cele	hernia, tumor, swelling
-centesis	surgical puncture
-ceps	head
-cide	to kill
-clasia	a breaking
-clasis	crushing, breaking up
-cle	small
-clysis	injection
-cope	strike
-crit	to separate
-culture	cultivation
-cusis	hearing

-cuspid	point
-cyesis	pregnancy
-cyst	bladder, sac
-cyte	cell
-derma	skin
-dermis	skin
-desis	binding
-dipsia	thirst
-drome	course
-dynia	pain, ache
-ectasia	dilatation
-ectasis	dilatation, dilation, stretching, expansion
-ectasy	dilation
-ectomy	surgical excision, surgical removal, resection
-edema	swelling
-emesis	vomiting
-emia	blood condition
-er	relating to, one who
-ergy	work
-esis	condition
-esthesia	feeling
-form	shape
-fuge	to flee
-gen	formation, produce
-genes	produce
-genesis	formation, produce
-genic	formation, produce

-glia	glue
-globin	protein
-gnosis	knowledge
-grade	step
-graft	pencil, grafting knife
-gram	weight, mark, record
-graph	to write, record, instrument for recording
-graphy	recording
-hexia	condition
-ia	condition
-iasis	condition
-iatrics	treatment
-iatry	treatment
-ic	pertaining to
-ician	specialist, physician
-ide	having a particular quality
-ile	pertaining to substance
-in	pertaining to
-ine	pertaining to, substance
-ing	quality of
-ion	process
-ior	pertaining to
-is	pertaining to
-ism	condition
-ist	one who specializes, agent
-itis	inflammation
-ity	condition

-ive	nature of, quality of	-ous	pertaining to	-rrhea	flow, discharge
-ize	to make, to treat or combine with	-oxia	oxygen	-rrhexis	rupture
		-paresis	weakness	-scope	instrument for examining
-kinesia	motion, movement	-pathy	disease, emotion	-scopy	to view, examine, visual examination
-kinesis	motion, movement	-penia	lack of, deficiency, abnormal reduction	-sepsis	decay
-lalia	to talk	-pepsia	to digest	-sis	state of, condition
-lemma	sheath, rind	-pexy	surgical fixation	-some	body
-lepsy	seizure			-sound	sound
-lexia	diction, word, phrase	-phagia	to eat, to swallow	-spasm	tension, spasm, contraction
-liter	liter	-phasia	to speak, speech		
-lith	stone	-pheresis	removal, remove	-stalsis	contraction
-logy	study of			-stasis	control, stop, stand still
-lymph	clear fluid, serum, pale fluid	-phil	attraction	-staxis	dripping, trickling
		-philia	attraction		
-lysis	destruction, separation, breakdown, loosening, dissolution	-phobia	fear	-sthenia	strength
		-phoresis	to carry	-stomy	new opening
		-phragm	fence	-systole	contraction
		-phraxis	to obstruct	-taxia	order, coordination
		-phylaxis	protection		
-malacia	softening	-physis	growth	-therapy	treatment
-mania	madness	-plakia	plate	-thermy	heat
-megaly	enlargement, large	-plasia	formation, produce	-tic	pertaining to
-meter	instrument to measure	-plasm	thing formed, plasma	-tome	instrument to cut
-metry	measurement	-plasty	surgical repair	-tomy	incision
-mnesia	memory			-tone	tension
-morph	form, shape	-plegia	stroke, paralysis, palsy	-tripsy	crushing
-noia	mind			-troph(y)	nourishment, development
-oid	resemble, like, similar	-pnea	breathing	-trophy	nourishment, development
-ole	opening, small	-poiesis	formation		
-oma	tumor, mass, fluid collection	-praxia	action	-type	type
		-ptosis	prolapse, drooping, sagging, falling down	-um	tissue, structure
-omion	shoulder			-ure	process
-on	pertaining to hormone			-uria	urination, condition of urine
-one		-ptysis	to spit, spitting		
-opia	sight, vision	-puncture	to pierce		
-opsia	sight, vision	-rrhage	to burst forth, bursting forth	-us	pertaining to, structure
-opsy	to view				
-or	one who, doer	-rrhagia	to burst forth, bursting forth	-y	condition, pertaining to, process
-orexia	appetite				
-ose	pertaining to				
-osis	condition	-rrhaphy	suture		

Abbreviations and Symbols

APPENDIX III

ABBREVIATIONS

A

17-KS	17-ketosteroids
17-OHCS	17-hydroxycorticosteroids
a	ampere; anode; anterior; aqua; area; artery
a̅a̅	of each
A/G	albumin/globulin ratio
A&P	auscultation and percussion; anatomy and physiology
AB	abortion; abnormal
Ab	antibody
ABC	aspiration biopsy cytology
Abd	abdomen
ABGs	arterial blood gases
ABLB	alternate binaural loudness balance
ABMS	American Board of Medical Specialties
ABO	blood group
ABR	auditory brainstem response
AC	air conduction; anticoagulant
ac	before meals (ante cibum); acute
Acc	accommodation
ACE	angiotensin converting enzyme (inhibitor)
ACG	angiocardiography
ACh	acetylcholine
ACL	anterior cruciate ligament
ACOG	American College of Obstetrics and Gynecology
ACR	American College of Rheumatology
ACS	American Cancer Society
ACTH	adrenocorticotropic hormone
AD	Alzheimer's disease; advance directive
ad lib	as desired; freely
ADA	American Diabetes Association
adeno-CA	adenocarcinoma
ADH	antidiuretic hormone (vasopressin)

ADHD	attention-deficit hyperactivity disorder
ADL	activities of daily living
adm	admission
ADP	adenosine diphosphate
AE	above elbow
AED	automated external defibrillator
AF	atrial fibrillation
AFB	acid-fast bacilli
AFP	alpha-fetoprotein
Ag	antigen
AGN	acute glomerulonephritis
AH	abdominal hysterectomy
AHD	arteriosclerotic heart disease
AHF	antihemophilic factor VIII
AHG	antihemophillic globulin factor VIII
AI	artificial insemination; aortic insufficiency
AIDS	acquired immunodeficiency syndrome
AIH	artificial insemination homologous
AJ	ankle jerk
AK	above knee
AKA	above-knee amputation
alk phos	alkaline phosphatase
ALD	aldolase
ALL	acute lymphocytic leukemia
ALS	amyotrophic lateral sclerosis
ALT	argon laser trabeculoplasty; alanine aminotransferase
alt dieb	every other day
alt hor	every other hour
alt noc	every other night
AM, am	before noon (ante meridiem); morning
AMA	against medical advice; American Medical Association
Amb	ambulate; ambulatory
AMD	age-related macular degeneration

AMI	acute myocardial infarction
AML	acute myeloid leukemia
ANA	antinuclear antibodies
ANS	autonomic nervous system
ant	anterior
AOM	acute otitis media
AOP	acknowledgment of paternity
AP	anteroposterior
A-P	anterior–posterior
APA	American Psychiatric Association
approx	approximately
APTT	activated partial thromboplastin time
AQ, aq	water
ARD	acute respiratory disease
ARDS	acute respiratory distress syndrome
ARF	acute renal failure
ARMD	age-related macular degeneration
AROM	artificial rupture of membranes
AS	aortic stenosis
As, Ast, astigm	astigmatism
ASAP	as soon as possible
Ascus	atypical squamous cells of undetermined significance
ASD	atrial septal defect
ASH	asymmetrical septal hypertrophy
ASHD	arteriosclerotic heart disease
ASO	antistreptolysin O
AST	aspartate aminotransferase
ATN	acute tubular necrosis
ATP	adenosine triphosphate
A-V, AV	atrioventricular; arteriovenous
AVMs	arteriovenous malformations
AVR	aortic valve replacement
ax	axillary
AZT	zidovudine

B

Ba	barium
BAC	blood alcohol concentration
BaE	barium enema
baso	basophil
BBB	bundle branch block
BBT	basal body temperature
BC	bone conduction
BCC	basal cell carcinoma
BCP	birth control pill
BDD	body dysmorphic disorder
BE	below elbow; barium enema

BG, bG	blood glucose
bid	twice a day
BIN, bin	twice a night
BK	below knee
BKA	below-knee amputation
BM	bowel movement
BMD	bone mineral density (test)
BMI	body mass index
BMR	basal metabolic rate
BNO	bladder neck obstruction
BP	blood pressure
BPH	benign prostatic hyperplasia (hypertrophy)
BRCA	breast cancer gene
BRP	bathroom privileges
BS	blood sugar; breath sounds; bowel sounds
BSE	breast self-examination
BSI	body systems isolation
BSP	bromsulphalein
BT	bleeding time
BUN	blood urea nitrogen
Bx	biopsy

C

c̄	with (cum)
C	centigrade, Celsius
C1, C2, etc.	first cervical vertebra; second cervical vertebra
C&S	culture and sensitivity
CA	cancer; carcinoembryonic antigen
CA-125	cancer antigen 125
Ca	calcium
CABG	coronary artery bypass graft
CAD	coronary artery disease
CAM	complementary and alternative medicines
cap	capsule
CAPD	continuous ambulatory peritoneal dialysis
CAT	computerized axial tomography
cath	catheterization; catheter
CBC	complete blood count
CBR	complete bed rest
CBS	chronic brain syndrome
CBT	cognitive-behavioral therapy
CC	cardiac catheterization; chief complaint; clean catch (urine)
CCU	coronary care unit
CDC	Centers for Disease Control and Prevention

CDH	congenital dislocation of hip
CEA	carcinoembryonic antigen
CF	cystic fibrosis
CGN	chronic glomerulonephritis
CHD	coronary heart disease
chemo	chemotherapy
CHF	congestive heart failure
CHO	carbohydrate
chol	cholesterol
CHT	congenital hypothyroidism
Ci	curie
Cib	food (cibus)
CIN	cervical intraepithelial neoplasia
CIS	carcinoma in situ
CK	creatine kinase
Cl	chlorine
CLI	critical limb ischemia
CLIA	clinical laboratory improvement amendments
CLL	chronic lymphocytic leukemia
cm	centimeter
CMG	cystometrogram
CML	chronic myelocystic leukemia
CMP	cardiomyopathy
CMV	cytomegalovirus
CNS	central nervous system
c/o	complains of
CO	cardiac output
CO_2	carbon dioxide
COLD	chronic obstructive lung disease
cont	continue
COPD	chronic obstructive pulmonary disease
CP	cerebral palsy
CPD	cephalopelvic disproportion
CPK	creatine phosphokinase
CPM	continuous passive motion
CPR	cardiopulmonary resuscitation
CPS	cycles per second
CR	computerized radiography
CRF	chronic renal failure; corticotropin-releasing factor
CS, C-section	cesarean section
CSF	cerebrospinal fluid
CT	computed tomography
CTA	clear to auscultation
CTS	carpal tunnel syndrome
CUC	chronic ulcerative colitis
CV	cardiovascular
CVA	cerebrovascular accident (stroke)
CVD	cardiovascular disease

CVP	central venous pressure
CVS	chorionic villus sampling
CWP	childbirth without pain
CXR	chest x-ray; chest radiograph
cysto	cystoscopic examination; cystoscopy

D

/d	per day
D	diopter (lens strength)
D&C	dilation (dilatation) and curettage
D&E	dilation and evacuation
db, Db	decibel
DBS	deep brain stimulation
DCIS	ductal carcinoma in situ
DDS	doctor of dental surgery; dorsal cord stimulation
decub	decubitus
Derm	dermatology
DES	diethylstilbestrol
DHT	dihydrotestosterone
DI	diabetes insipidus; diagnostic imaging
diff	differential count (white blood cells)
dil	dilute; diluted
DJD	degenerative joint disease
DM	diabetes mellitus
DMARDs	disease-modifying antirheumatic drugs
DMD	Duchenne muscular dystrophy
DNA	deoxyribonucleic acid; does not apply
DNR	do not resuscitate
DNS	did not show
DO	doctor of osteopathy
DOA	dead on arrival
DOB	date of birth
DOT	directly observed therapy
Dr.	doctor
DRE	digital rectal examination
DRGs	diagnostic related groups
DS	double strength
DSA	digital subtraction angiography
DSM-IV-TR	*Diagnostic and Statistical Manual of Mental Disorders*, Fourth Edition, Text Revision
DTaP	diphtheria, tetanus, and pertussis (vaccine)
DTRs	deep tendon reflexes
DUB	dysfunctional uterine bleeding

DVA	distance visual acuity
DVT	deep vein thrombosis
D/W	dextrose in water
Dx	diagnosis
DXA	dual-energy X-ray absorptiometry scan

E

EBV	Epstein–Barr virus
ECC	extracorporeal circulation
ECCE	extracapsular cataract extraction
ECF	extracellular fluid; extended care facility
ECG, EKG	electrocardiogram
ECHO	echocardiogram
E. coli	*Escherichia coli*
ECSL	extracorporeal shockwave lithotriptor
ECT	electroconvulsive therapy
ED	erectile dysfunction
EDB	estimated date of birth
EDC	estimated date of confinement (delivery)
EDD	estimated date of delivery
EEG	electroencephalogram; electroencephalograph
EENT	eye, ear, nose, and throat
EFM	electronic fetal monitor
EGD	esophagogastroduodenoscopy
EHR	electronic health record
ELISA	enzyme-linked immunosorbent assay
EM	emmetropia
EMG	electromyography
EMR	electronic medical record
ENG	electronystagmography
ENT	ear, nose, throat (otorhinolaryngology)
EOM	extraocular movement; extraocular muscles
eos, eosin	eosinophil
EPS	electrophysiology study (intracardiac)
ER	emergency room; endoplasmic reticulum
ERCP	endoscopic retrograde cholangiopancreatography
ERT	estrogen replacement therapy; external radiation therapy
ERV	expiratory reserve volume

ESL, ESWL	extracorporeal shock-wave lithotripsy
ESR	erythrocyte sedimentation rate
ESRD	end-stage renal disease
EST	electroshock therapy
ESWL	extracorporeal shockwave lithotripsy
ET	esotropia; endotracheal
Ex	examination

F

F	Fahrenheit; female
FACP	Fellow of the American College of Physicians
FACS	Fellow of the American College of Surgeons
FBG	fasting blood glucose
FBS	fasting blood sugar
FDA	Food and Drug Administration
FEF	forced expiratory flow
FEKG	fetal electrocardiogram
FEV	forced expiratory volume
FFA	free fatty acids
FH	family history
FHB	fetal heartbeat
FHR	fetal heart rate
FHS	fetal heart sound
FHT	fetal heart tone
FIV	forced inspiratory volume
FMS	fibromyalgia syndrome
FNA	fine needle aspiration
FP	family practice
FRC	forced residual capacity
FROM	full range of motion
FS	frozen section
FSH	follicle-stimulating hormone
FTA-ABS	fluorescent treponemal antibody absorption
FTND	full-term normal delivery
F-V loop	flow volume loop
FVC	forced vital capacity
Fx	fracture

G

g	gram
GAD	generalized anxiety disorder
GB	gallbladder
GBS	group B streptococcus
GC	gonorrhea

GCSF	granulocyte colony-stimulating factor
GERD	gastroesophageal reflux disease
GFR	glomerular filtration rate
GGT	gamma-glutamyl transferase
GH	growth hormone
GHRF	growth hormone–releasing factor
GI	gastrointestinal
GIFT	gamete intrafallopian transfer
GnRF	gonadotropin-releasing factor
GOT	glutamic oxaloacetic transaminase
Gpi	globus pallidus
GPT	glutamic pyruvic transaminase
grav I	pregnancy one
GTT	glucose tolerance test
GU	genitourinary
GYN	gynecology

H

H_2O	water
H, hr	hour
H	hydrogen
H&E	hematoxylin and eosin
H&L	heart & lungs
HAA	hepatitis-associated antigen
HAART	highly active antiretroviral therapy
HAV	hepatitis A virus
Hb, Hgb, HGB	hemoglobin
HBIG	hepatitis B immune globulin
HBOT	hyperbaric oxygen therapy
HBP	high blood pressure
HBV	hepatitis B virus
HCC	hepatocellular carcinoma
hCG, HCG	human chorionic gonadotropin
HCl	hydrochloric acid
HCO_3	bicarbonate
Hct, HCT	hematocrit
HD	hip disarticulation; hearing distance; Hodgkin's disease; hemodialysis
HDL	high-density lipoprotein
HDS	herniated disk syndrome
HEENT	head, eyes, ears, nose, throat
HER-2/neu	human epidermal growth factor receptor–2
HF	heart failure
Hg	mercury
HHS	Health and Human Services (Department of)

HIPAA	Health Insurance Portability and Accountability Act of 1996
HIV	human immunodeficiency virus
HLA	human leukocyte antigen
HMD	hyaline membrane disease
HNP	herniated nucleus pulposus (herniated disk)
Hpd	hematoporphyrin derivative
H. pylori	*Heliocobacter pylori*
HPV	human papillomavirus
HT	hormone therapy
HSG	hysterosalpingography
HSV	herpes simplex virus
HSV-2	herpes simplex virus–2
HT	hyperopia
Ht	height
HTLV	human T-cell leukemia-lymphoma virus
HTN	hypertension
Hx	history
hypo	hypodermic injection

I

I&D	incision and drainage
I&O	intake and output
IAS	interatrial septum
IBS	irritable bowel syndrome
IC	interstitial cystitis; inspiratory capacity
ICCE	intracapsular cataract cryoextraction
ICF	intracellular fluid
ICP	intracranial pressure
ICSH	interstitial cell-stimulating hormone
ICU	intensive care unit
ID	intradermal
IDDM	insulin-dependent diabetes mellitus
Ig	immunoglobulin
IH	infectious hepatitis
IHSS	idiopathic hypertropic subaortic stenosis
IL-2	interleukin-2
IM	intramuscular
inj	injection
IOL	intraocular lens
IOP	intraocular pressure
IPD	intermittent peritoneal dialysis
IPPB	intermittent positive-pressure breathing

IQ	intelligence quotient
IR	interventional radiology
IRDS	infant respiratory distress syndrome
IRT	internal radiation therapy
IRV	inspiratory reserve volume
IS	intercostal space
ITP	idiopathic thrombocytopenia purpura
IUD	intrauterine device
IUGR	intrauterine growth rate; intrauterine growth retardation
IV	intravenous
IVC	inferior vena cava; intravenous cholangiography; intraventricular catheter
IVF	in vitro fertilization
IVP	intravenous pyelogram
IVS	interventricular septum
IVU	intravenous urogram

J

J	joule
JNC	Joint National Committee
JRA	juvenile rheumatoid arthritis
jt	joint
JVD	jugular vein distention

K

K	potassium
KD	knee disarticulation
kg	kilogram
KJ	knee jerk
KS	Kaposi's sarcoma
KUB	kidney, ureter, and bladder
kV	kilovolt

L

L1, L2, etc.	first lumbar vertebra, second lumbar vertebra, etc.
L	liter
L&A	light and accommodation
L&W	living and well
LA	left atrium
lab	laboratory
LAC	long arm cast
LAK	lymphokine-activated killer (cells)
LAT, lat	lateral
LB	large bowel
lb	pound

LBBB	left bundle branch block
LCIS	lobular carcinoma in situ
LD, LDH	lactate dehydrogenase
LDL	low-density lipoprotein
LE	lupus erythematosus; lower extremity; left eye
LEDs	light-emitting diodes
LES	lower esophageal sphincter
LH	luteinizing hormone
LH-RH	luteinizing hormone–releasing hormone
lig	ligament
liq	liquid
LLC	long leg cast
LLCC	long leg cylinder cast
LLQ	left lower quadrant
LMP	last menstrual period
LOA	left occipitoanterior
LOC	level of consciousness
LOM	limitation or loss of motion
LP	lumbar puncture
LPI	laser peripheral iridotomy
LRQ	lower right quadrant
lt	left
LTH	lactogenic hormone
LUQ	left upper quadrant
LV	left ventricle
lymphs	lymphocytes

M

M	molar; thousand; muscle; male
m	male; meter; minim
mA	milliampere
mAs	milliampere second
MALT	mucosa-associated lymphoid tissue; mucosal-associated-lymphoid type (lymphoma)
MAOIs	monoamine oxidase inhibitors
MBC	maximal breathing capacity
MBPS	Munchausen by proxy syndrome
mcg	microgram
MCH	mean corpuscular hemoglobin
MCHC	mean corpuscular hemoglobin concentration
mCi	millicurie
MCV	mean corpuscular volume
MD	medical doctor; muscular dystrophy
MDR TB	multidrug-resistant tuberculosis
mEq	milliequivalent
mets	metastases

MG	myasthenia gravis
mg	milligram (0.001 gram)
MH	marital history
MHT	minor head trauma
MI	myocardial infarction; mitral insufficiency
MIF	melanocyte-stimulating hormone release-inhibiting factor
mix astig	mixed astigmatism
mL	milliliter (0.001 liter)
mm	millimeter (0.001 meter; 0.039 inch)
mMol	millimole
MMPI	Minnesota Multiphasic Personality Inventory
MMR	measles, mumps, and rubella (vaccine)
MMSE	Mini Mental State Examination
mol wt	molecular weight
mono	monocyte
MPD	mammary Paget's disease
MR	mental retardation
MRF	melanocyte-stimulating hormone–releasing factor
MRI	magnetic resonance imaging
MS	mitral stenosis; multiple sclerosis; musculoskeletal
MSH	melanocyte-stimulating hormone
MTBI	mild traumatic brain injury
MTD	right eardrum (membrana tympani dexter)
MTS	left eardrum (membrana tympani sinister)
MV	mitral valve; minute volume
mV	millivolt
MVP	mitral valve prolapse
MVV	maximal voluntary ventilation
MY	myopia

N

n	nerve
Na	sodium
NaCl	sodium chloride
N&V	nausea & vomiting
NANBH	non-A, non-B hepatitis virus
NB	newborn
NCI	National Cancer Institute
nCi	nanocurie
NCV	nerve conduction velocity
neg	negative
Neuro	neurology

NG	nasogastric (tube)
ng	nanogram
NGU	nongonococcal urethritis
NH$_3$	ammonia
NHLBI	National Heart, Lung and Blood Institute
NIDDM	noninsulin-dependent diabetes mellitus
NIH	National Institute of Health
NIMH	National Institute of Mental Health
NINDS	National Institute of Neurological Disorders and Stroke
NK	natural killer (cells)
NKDA	no known drug allergies
NMR	nuclear magnetic resonance
NPH	nonprotein nitrogen
NPO, npo	nothing by mouth
NPT	nocturnal penile tumescence
NREM	no rapid eye movement (sleep)
NS	normal saline
NSAIDs	nonsteroidal anti-inflammatory drugs
NSSC	normal size, shape, and consistency
NST	nonstress test
NVA	near visual acuity

O

O	pint
O, O$_2$	oxygen
O&P	ova and parasites
OA	osteoarthritis
OB	obstetrics
OB-GYN	obstetrics and gynecology
OC	oral contraceptive
OCD	obsessive–compulsive disorder
OCPs	oral contraceptive pills
OD	overdose
OHS	open heart surgery
OM	otitis media
OP	outpatient
OPCAB	off-pump coronary artery bypass surgery
OR	operating room
ORTH, ortho	orthopedics; orthopaedics
os	mouth opening; bone
OTC	over-the-counter
oto	otology
OV	office visit
oz	ounce

P

P	pulse; phosphorus
PA	posteroanterior; pernicious anemia
PAC	premature arterial contraction
PAD	peripheral artery disease
Pap	Papanicolaou (smear)
PAT	paroxysmal atrial tachycardia
Path	pathology
PBI	protein bound iodine
PC	professional corporation
pc	after meals (post cibum)
PCL	posterior cruciate ligament
PCP	*Pneumocystis carinii* pneumonia
PCV	packed cell volume
PD	peritoneal dialysis
PDD-NOS	pervasive developmental disorder not otherwise specified
PDR	*Physicians' Desk Reference*
PE	physical examination; pulmonary embolism
Peds	pediatrics
PEEP	positive end-expiratory pressure
PEG	percutaneous endoscopic gastrostomy
PEMFs	pulsing electromagnetic fields
PERRLA	pupils equal, round, react to light and accommodation
PET	positron emission tomography
PE tube	polyethylene tube
PFT	pulmonary function test
pH	hydrogen ion concentration; degree of acidity
PH	past history
Ph.D.	doctor of philosophy, doctor of pharmacy
phaco	phacoemulsification
PHI	protected health information
PI	present illness
PID	pelvic inflammatory disease
PIF	prolactin release-inhibiting factor
PIH	pregnancy-induced hypertension
PIP	proximal interphalangeal
PKU	phenylketonuria
PM	physical medicine
PM, pm	afternoon, evening
PMH	past medical history
PMI	point of maximal impulse
PMN	polymorphonuclear neutrophil
PMP	previous menstrual period
PMR	physical medicine and rehabilitation

PMS	premenstrual syndrome
PND	paroxysmal nocturnal dyspnea; postnasal drip
PNS	peripheral nervous system
PO	orally, by mouth
poly	polymorphonuclear
PP	postprandial (after meals)
PPD	purified protein derivative (TB test); pack(s) per day
PPI	proton pump inhibitor
pr	per rectum
PRF	prolactin-releasing factor
PRL	prolactin hormone
PRN, prn	as necessary; as required; when necessary; as needed
PSA	prostate-specific antigen
Psych	psychiatry, psychology
PT	physical therapy; prothrombin time
pt	patient; pint
PTC	percutaneous transhepatic cholangiography
PTCA	percutaneous transluminal coronary angioplasty
PTH	parathyroid hormone (parathormone)
PTS	permanent threshold shift
PTSD	post-traumatic stress disorder
PTT	partial thromboplastin time
PUBS	percutaneous umbilical blood sampling
PUD	peptic ulcer disease
PUL	percutaneous ultrasonic lithotropsy
PVC	premature ventricular contraction
PVD	peripheral vascular disease
PWB	partial weight bearing

Q

q	every (quaque)
q2h	every 2 hours
q4h	every 4 hours
qh	every hour
qid	four times a day
qm	every morning (quaque mane)
qns	quantity not sufficient
qs	quantity sufficient
qt	quart

R

R	respiration
R, rt	right

RA	right atrium; rheumatoid arthritis
Ra	radium
rad	radiation absorbed dose
RAI	radioactive iodine
RAIU	radioactive iodine uptake
RBC	red blood cell; red blood cell (count)
RD	respiratory disease
RDA	recommended dietary or daily allowance
rDNA	recombinant deoxyribonucleic acid
RDS	respiratory distress syndrome
RE	right eye
REM	rapid eye movement (sleep)
resp	respiratory
RF	rheumatoid factor
Rh	Rhesus blood factor (Rh+ or Rh–)
RIA	radioimmunoassay
RLF	retrolental fibroplasias
RLQ	right lower quadrant
RNA	ribonucleic acid
R/O	rule out
ROM	range of motion; read-only memory
RP	retrograde pyelography
RPE	retinal pigment epithelium
RPM	revolutions per minute
RQ	respiratory quotient
RRR	regular rate and rhythm
RSV	respiratory syncytial virus
RT	radiation therapy
RUQ	right upper quadrant
RV	right ventricle; residual volume
Rx	take thou; prescribe; treatment; therapy

S

s̄	without
SA, S-A	sinoatrial (node)
SAB	spontaneous abortion
SAC	short arm cast
SAD	seasonal affective disorder
SAH	subarachnoid hemorrhage
SALT	serum alanine aminotransferase
SARS	severe acute respiratory syndrome
SAST	serum aspartate aminotransferase
SBFT	small-bowel followthrough
SCA	sudden cardiac arrest
SCC	squamous cell carcinoma
SCD	sudden cardiac death

SD	shoulder disarticulation; standard deviation
seg, poly	polymorphonuclear neutrophil
segs	segmented (mature RBCs)
SG	skin graft
SGOT	serum glutamic oxaloacetic transaminase
SGPT	serum glutamic pyruvic transaminase
SH	serum hepatitis
sh	shoulder
SIDS	sudden infant death syndrome
SK	streptokinase
SLC	short leg cast
SLT	selective laser trabeculoplasty
SMBG	self-monitoring of blood glucose
SNRI	serotonin-norepinephrine reuptake inhibitor
SOAP	subjective, objective, assessment, plan
SOB	shortness of breath
SOM	serous otitis media
sono	sonogram, sonography
SOP	standard operating procedure
SOS	if necessary (si opus sit)
SPECT	single photon emission computed tomography
sp. gr, SG	specific gravity
SPP	suprapubic prostatectomy
SR, sed rate	sedimentation rate
SS	Social Security
ss	one half
SSN	Social Security number
SSRIs	selective serotonin reuptake inhibitors
ST	esotropia
St	stage (of disease)
staph	staphylococcus
stat	immediately
STDs	sexually transmitted diseases
STH	somatotropin hormone
strep	streptococcus
STS	serologic test for syphilis
STSS	streptococcal toxic shock syndrome
Sub-Q, subQ	subcutaneous
SVC	superior vena cava
SVD	spontaneous vaginal delivery
Sx	symptom
syr	syrup

T

T1, T2, etc.	thoracic vertebrae first, thoracic vertebrae second, etc.
T_3	triiodothyronine
T_3RU	triiodothyronine resin uptake
T_3U	triiodothyronine uptake
T_4	thyroxine
T, temp	temperature
T&A	tonsillectomy and adenoidectomy
Tab, tab	tablet
TAH	total abdominal hysterectomy
TAT	Thematic Apperception Test
TB	tuberculosis
TBW	total body weight
TC	testicular cancer
TCAs	tricyclic antidepressants
TENS	transcutaneous electrical nerve stimulation
TFS	thyroid function studies
TH	thyroid hormone
THA	total hip arthroplasty
THR	total hip replacement
TIAs	transient ischemic attacks
tid	three times a day
TIMs	topical immunomodulators
TIPS	transjugular intrahepatic portosystemic shunt
TJ	triceps jerk
TKA	total knee arthroplasty
TKR	total knee replacement
TLC	tender loving care; total lung capacity
TM	tympanic membrane
TMJ	temporomandibular joint
TNF	tumor necrosis factor
TNM	tumor, node, metastasis
TNS	transcutaneous nerve stimulation
TOF	tetralogy of Fallot
top	topically
TPA	*Treponema pallidum* agglutination (test)
TPA, tPA	tissue plasminogen activator
TPE	Taxol, Platinol, and VePesid
TPN	total parenteral nutrition
TPR	temperature, pulse, respiration
tr, tinct	tincture
trans	transverse
TRH	thyrotropin-releasing hormone
TSE	testicular self-exam
TSH	thyroid-stimulating hormone
TSS	toxic shock syndrome
TTH	thyrotropic hormone
TUIP	transurethral incision of the prostrate
TUMT	transurethral microwave thermotherapy
TUNA	transurethral needle ablation
TUR	transurethral resection
TURP	transurethral resection of the prostate
TV	tidal volume
Tx	traction; treatment; transplant

U

UA	urinalysis
U&L, U/L	upper and lower
UC	uterine contractions
UCHD	usual childhood diseases
UG	urogenital
UGI	upper gastrointestinal
ULQ	upper left quadrant
URI	upper respiratory infection
URQ	upper right quadrant
US	ultrasound
USP	United States Pharmacopeia
UTI	urinary tract infection

V

v	vein
VA	visual acuity
VAD	vacuum-assisted needle biopsy device
VC	vital capacity
VCD	vacuum constriction device
VCG	vectorcardiogram
VCU, VCUG	voiding cystourethrogram
VD	venereal disease
VDRL	Venereal Disease Research Laboratory (syphilis test)
VF	visual field
VHD	ventricular heart disease
VLDL	very low-density lipoprotein
vol	volume
vol %	volume percent
VMA	vanillylmandelic acid
VP	vasopressin
VS, V/S	vital signs
VSD	ventricular septal defect
VT	ventricular tachycardia

W

WAIS	Wechster Adult Intelligence Scale
WBC	white blood cell; white blood (cell) count
WDWN	well developed, well nourished
WF, BF	white female, black female
WHO	World Health Organization
WM, BM	white male, black male
WNL	within normal limits
Wt	weight
w/v	weight by volume

X

XM	cross match for blood (type and cross match)

XP

XP	xeroderma pigmentosum
XR	x-ray
XT	exotropia
XX	female sex chromosomes
XY	male sex chromosomes

Y

YAG	yttrium-aluminum-garnet (laser)
y/o	year(s) old
YOB	year of birth
yr	year

Z

z	atomic number

SYMBOLS

×	times, power
−	negative
+	positive
+/−	positive or negative
*	birth
†	death
%	percent
#	number; pound
=	equal
?	question
™	trademark
©	copyright
®	registered
¶	paragraph

Laboratory Reference Values

APPENDIX IV

ABBREVIATIONS USED IN REPORTING LABORATORY VALUES

cm^3	cubic centimeter
cu μ	cubic micron
dL	deciliter
fL	femtoliter
g	gram
g/dL	grams per deciliter
kg	kilogram
L	liter
mcg	microgram
μL	microliter
mEq	milliequivalent
mg	milligram
mg/dL	milligram per deciliter
mL	milliliter
mm	millimeter
mm^3	cubic millimeter
mm Hg	millimeter of mercury
mmol	millimole
mol (M)	mole
ng	nanogram
ng/dL	nanogram per deciliter
ng/mL	nanogram per milliliter
pg	picogram

HEMATOLOGY TESTS

	Normal Ranges
Differential	
Neutrophils	37–80%
Lymphocytes	10–50%
Monocytes	0.1–10%
Eosinophils	0.1–6%
Basophils	0.0–3%
Erythrocytes—red blood cells (RBC)	
Females	4.2–5.4 million/mm^3
Males	4.6–6.2 million/mm^3
Children	4.5–5.1 million/mm^3

Hemoglobin (HGB, Hgb)

Females	12.0–14.0 g/dL
Males	14.0–16.0 g/dL
Hematocrit (HCT)	37.0–54%
Females	37–47%
Males	40–54%
Leukocytes— white blood cells (WBC)	4000–10,000/mm^3
Thrombocytes— Platelets	115,000– 436,000/mm^3
Mean corpuscular hemoglobin (MCH)	27.0–32.0 pg
Mean corpuscular hemoglobin concentration (MCHC)	32.0–36.0 g/dL
Mean corpuscular volume (MCV)	80–100 fL

COAGULATION TESTS

Bleeding time	2.75–8.0 min
Coagulation time	5–15 min
Prothrombin time (PT)	12–14 sec

CHEMISTRIES

	Normal Ranges
Sodium (Na)	136–145 mEq/L
Potassium (K)	3.5–5.1 mEq/L
Calcium (Ca)	8.6–10.8 mg/dL
Chloride (Cl)	99–111 mmol/L
CO_2	22–29 mmol/L
Phosphate (PO_4)	3.0–4.5 mg/dL
Glucose (fasting)	70–99 mg/dL
Blood urea nitrogen (BUN)	7–18 mg/dL
Creatinine	0.6–1.1 mg/dL
Creatine phosphokinase (CPK)	
Females	30–135 U/L
Males	55–170 U/L

Anion gap	10–17 mEq/L
Alkaline phosphatase (ALP)	20–90 U/L
Alanine aminotransferase (ALT, SGPT)	5–30 U/L
Albumin	3.5–5.5 g/dL
Globulin	1.4–4.8 g/dL
A/G ratio	0.7–2.0 g/dL
Aspartate aminotransferase (AST, SGOT)	10–30 U/L
Bilirubin	0.0–1.2 mg/dL
Cholesterol	<200 mg/dL
High-density lipoprotein (HDL)	>60 mg/dL
Low-density lipoprotein (LDL)	<100 mg/dL
Triglycerides	<150 mg/dL
Uric acid	
Females	1.5–7.0 mg/dL
Males	2.5–8.0 mg/dL
Lactate dehydrogenase (LDH)	100–190 U/L
Thyroxine (T_4)	4.4–9.9 μg/dL
Free T_4	0.8–1.8 ng/dL
Thyroid stimulating hormone (TSH)	0.5–6.0 uIU/mL
Prostate specific antigen (PSA) Male	0.0–4.0 ng/mL
Testosterone	241–827 ng/dL

URINALYSIS

	Normal Ranges
Color	Yellow to amber
Turbidity (Appearance)	Clear
Specific gravity	1.003–1.030
Reaction (pH)	4.6–8.0
Odor	Faintly aromatic
Protein	Negative
Glucose	Negative
Ketones	Negative
Bilirubin	Negative
Blood	Negative
Urobilinogen	0.1–1.0
Nitrite	Negative
Leukocytes	Negative

Index